Bioceramics

Volume 8

Edited by

June Wilson
Larry L. Hench
University of Florida, USA

David Greenspan
U.S. Biomaterials Corp., Florida, USA

PERGAMON

Pergamon/Elsevier Titles of Related Interest

BOOKS

W. BONFIELD, G. W. HASTINGS and K. E. TANNER: Bioceramics 4
(ISBN 0 7506 0269 4)

P. DUCHEYNE and D. CHRISTIANSEN: Bioceramics 6
(ISBN 0 7506 1884 1)

Ö. H. ANDERSSON, R.-P. HAPPONEN and A. YLI-URPO: Bioceramics 7
(ISBN 0 7506 2175 3)

JOURNALS

Biomaterials

Full details of all Elsevier Science publications/free specimen copy of any Elsevier Science journal are available on request from your nearest Elsevier Science office.

Bioceramics

Volume 8

Proceedings of the 8th International Symposium on
Ceramics in Medicine

Ponte Vedra, Florida, USA, November 1995

Edited by
June Wilson
Larry L. Hench
David Greenspan

U.K. Elsevier Science Ltd, The Boulevard, Langford Lane, Kidlington, Oxford OX5 1GB, U.K.

U.S.A. Elsevier Science Inc., 660 White Plains Road, Tarrytown, New York 10591-5153, U.S.A.

JAPAN Elsevier Science Japan, Tsunashima Building Annex, 3-20-12 Yushima, Bunkyo-ku, Tokyo 113, Japan

---

First Edition 1995

Library of Congress Cataloging in Publication Data
A catalog record for this book is available from the Library of Congress

British Library Cataloguing in Publication Data
A catalogue record for this book is available from the British Library

ISBN 0 08 042677 8

Cover picture

Protected by ceramic tiles, the orbiter Atlantis is launched into space in November 1994. On board were astronauts from the United States and France. Photograph: N.A.S.A.

Printed in Great Britain by Alden Press, Oxford

Local Committee

Chairmen Larry L. Hench
June Wilson

Committee David Greenspan
Alice Greenspan
Jon West
A.E. (Buddy) Clark

Secretary Waverly Munn

International Advisory Board

Orjan Andersson
William Bonfield
Klaas de Groot
Ulrich Gross
Sam Hulbert
Tadeshi Kokubo
Hironubo Oonishi
Takao Yamamuro
Antti Yli-Urpu

In Memoriam

Toshiaki Kitsugi, M.D. 1952-1995
Assistant Professor, Department of Orthopaedic Surgery
Kyoto University

Preface

Bioceramics 8, the latest in the series of annual, international meetings was held in November 1995 in Florida, 26 years after the discovery of Bioglass® at the University of Florida.

This series, now in its eighth year, has established itself as the forum in which the most important work in the field of Bioceramics is regularly presented. The series of volumes, of which this is the eighth, have become valuable research tools, not least because of the timeliness of their publication.

The size of the meetings has remained relatively small, wherever possible the organizers have avoided parallel sessions so that all present can take part in discussions and be exposed to areas other than their own.

There is no question as to their international status, as can be seen from the list below, which is based on the country of origin of the center where the work was done, not on the nationality of attendees.

Year	Location	Countries represented
1988	Kyoto, Japan	6
1989	Heidelberg, Germany	9
1990	Terre Haute, Ind. USS	7
1991	London, England	11
1992	Kyoto, Japan	10
1993	Philadelphia, PA USA	13
1994	Turku, Finland	12
1995	Ponte Vedra, FL USA	14

The distribution of presentations between the various classes of materials demonstrates a certain consistency in the relative proportions of the different materials being studied, allowing that the "other" category includes invited and review papers.

These data must not, however, be taken too seriously. The interests of the host institution, location of the meeting site, and availability of travel funding all play a part in determining what is done, where it is done and how easy it is to attend a meeting to talk about it.

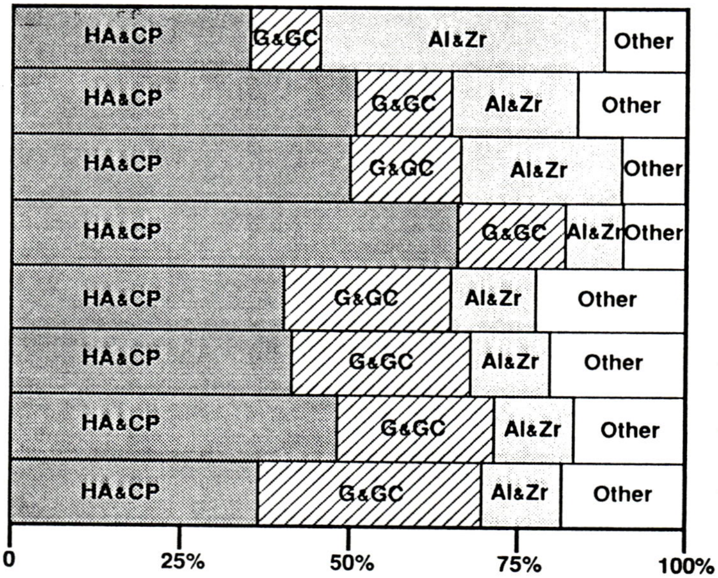

This volume would not have been possible without the contributions of both the International and Local Advisory Boards, who reviewed both abstracts and manuscripts in a timely fashion; without the financial support of U.S. Biomaterials Corporation or without the expert editorial assistance of Waverly Munn, Alice Holt, Holly Richardson and Minnie Stavely.

We hope that Bioceramics 8 will allow many of us to pick up our discussions where we left off in Turku and, for many others, introduce them to the valuable and friendly forum which is the Ceramics in Medicine series.

June Wilson | Larry L. Hench | David Greenspan

Ponte Vedra, Florida USA, November 1995

CONTENTS

BONE BIOLOGY

NEW DIRECTIONS

COMPOSITES

BIOACTIVE GLASSES

BONE BIOLOGY

BONE AND ITS REPAIR

Jeffrey Hollinger* and Bradley McAllister**

*Oregon Health Sciences University, Department of Surgery Divsion of Plastic and Reconstructive Surgery, L352-A, School of Medicine, 3181 SW Sam Jackson Park Road, Portland, OR 97201-3098 **Oregon Health Sciences University, Departments of Periodontics and Oral Molecular Biology, School of Dentistry, 3181 SW Sam Jackson Park Road, Portland, OR 97201-3097

ABSTRACT

Bones and teeth are the only structures within the body where calcium and phosphate participate as functional pillars. Despite their calcific nature, both organs are vital and dynamic. The maintenance and renewal of bone is a physiologic marvel of nature. Sadly, structural deficits to teeth only can be renewed by nonphysiologic means.

This review will focus on the biologic hierarchy of bone and its capacity for repair and regeneration. The macrostructural and microstructural components, including the organic, mineral, and cellular composition will be described. Dynamic aspects of bone will be defined according to prevailing concepts of modeling and remodeling.

Terminology associated with reparative processes of bone will be introduced. In addition, therapeutic modalities that promote formation will be highlighted. The goal of this review is to consolidate contemporary knowledge of bone physiology with exciting therapeutic prospects for its repair.

DEVELOPMENTAL HIERARCHY

Histogenesis of bone is either directly from *mesenchymal connective tissue* or from preexisting *cartilage.* Biochemically and morphologically, the end-products of both developmental pathways are indistinguishable.

Intramembranous bone

Mesenchymal cells within the connective tissue stroma give rise directly to *intramembranous bone* in the mandibulo-craniofacial complex, ilium, clavicle, and scapula. The *flat bones* of the bony vault of the cranium (extending from the supraorbital ridge posteriorly to the external occipital protuberance) include the paired parietal bones, squamous portion of the occipital and temporal bones, the squama frontalis, and part of the greater wing of the sphenoid bone. The mandible, except for the a section of the coronoid process and the midsymphyseal region, are derived from mesenchymal lineage cells that convert directly to *osteoblasts* [1].

Endochondral bone

Appendicular and axial bones (exclusive of the claniofacial complex) are derived from a *cartilaginous precursor* and are referred to as *endochondral bone.* Endochrondal bone formation begins when pluripotential mesenchymal stem cells *convert* to *chondroblasts* following interaction with a *morphogen (e.g.*, bone morphogenetic protein). Chondroblasts proliferate into *theques* (collections) of *chondrocytes* entrapped witbin an amorphous, acellular matrix: *the cartilage anlage* (i.e., bone precursor). Vascular ingress heralds cartilage calcification, its resorption, and replacement with bone.

MACROSTRUCTURAL HIERARCHY

Cortical bone

Tubular bone of the appendicular skeleton, axial bones, and the inner and outer tables of the flat bones of the craniofacial complex are composed of *cortical bone* (also known as the *compacta).* Cortical bone is engineered to protect vital organs and to endure and respond to biofunctional loading. Buttresses designed to meet biofunctional loading are *anistropical ly* patterned as *haversian systems* (or *osteons).* A haversian system consists of 4-20 circumferential layers of concentrically arranged *lamellae* encompassing a central canal *(haversian canal)* 22-110 μm in diameter, containing blood vessels and lymphatics. The average haversian system diameter in man is about 200 μm [2].

Cancellous bone

Interposed between bone cortices is the *cancellous (spongy) bone*. A three dimensional lattice work of *trabeculae* is the hallmark of this structure. In the skull, it is referred to as the *diploë.* Approximately 70-85% of the bony interface and other tissues occurs with cancellous bone; therefore, it is best suited for metabolic roles.

MICROSTRUCTURAL HIERARCHY

Cells: osteoblast

A nondifferentiated, pluripotential mesenchymal cell (e.g., *osteoprogenitor cell)* can develop into a bone-forming *osteoblast* [3-5]. Why osteoprogenitor *(stem)* cells convert to *osteoblasts is* a question that is being explored. Osteoblasts elaborate an organic matrix *(osteoid),* vectorially directed, that averages 8-10 μm in thickness [6]. Osteoid consists principally of *type I collagen* admixed with *ground substance.* After approximately 10-20 days, the osteoid will *calcify* at a rate of 0.75-1.0 μm/day [6]. The process of *calcification (mineralization)* requires cells (i.e., chondrocytes for cartilage, osteoblasts for bone) coupled with sulfated and/or phosphorylated proteins that both nucleate and regulate calcium-phosphate crystal growth. Alkaline phosphatase localized to the plasma membrane of osteoblasts increases concomitantly with bone formation. However, its role in mineralization is unclear. It may be involved with phosphate transport.

Type I bone collageo is a highly oriented *substratum* onto which bone mineral crystal may be deposited. Mineralization of collagen has been associated with *matrix vesicles:* outpockettings from osteoblasts and chondrocytes that contain calciumphosphate and assorted enzymes requisite for mineralization [7,8]. Collagen may act as a template for mineral deposition with the process modulated by collagen- associated phosphorylated sialoproteins: *osteopontin, bone sialoprotein, and bone acidic glycoprotein* [9]. *Osteopontin* functions as ao inhibitor of mineralization; *bone sialoprotein is* a nucleator; the role of *bone acidic glycoprotein* has yet to be determined. Mechanisms of actions and interactions between these noncollagenous proteins and collagen remained to be elucidated.

Osteocyte

An osteoblast entombed in its bony sarcophagus is an *osteocyte.* There is an extensive web of cytoplasmic, cell-cell communications among osteocytes residing within *haversian systems.* The cytoplasmic processes traverse *canaliculi,* interacting by *gap junctions* with neighboriog osteocytes, and ultimately connectiog to processes of surface osteoblasts. Direct passage of molecules between cells occurs at the gap junction *(nexus).* While the complete, complex regulatory influences of osteocytes have not yet been uncovered, these cells assist in calcium regulation and ensure viability of bone.

Osteoclast

Bone resorption is accomplished by a specialized type of multinucleated giant cell: the *osteoclast.* These leviathans originate from a granulocytic-macrophage precursor found in bone marrow that circulates as a monocytic cell, and through asynchronous fusion, derives an osteoclast[10-13]. Osteoblast migration (perhaps in response to parathyroid hormone, PTH) leaves an exposed osteoid-mineralized surface for osteoclast attachment. Attachment involves an interaction between osteoclast surface adhesion molecules *(integrins)* and proteins located on the bone surface [14]. *Osteopontin* a *sialophosphoprotein*), is believed to be the key receptor for this attachment, possessing an RGD (Arginine-Glycine-Aspartic acid) motif [15].

The attaching end of the osteoclast is recognized as a *ruffled border* and constitutes the resorptive territory where enzymatic breakdown of bone surface occurs. Enzymatic factors consist of *acid phosphatase, aryl-sulfatase, beta-glucuronidase,* and *beta--glycerophosphatase,* as well as the *metalloproteoases, collagenase and stromelsin* [14] . A *sealing zone* (or *zone of attachment)* between the ruffled border and bone surface isolates the microenvironment, and osteoclastic *carbonic anhydrase* lowers the pH, allowing solubilization of calcium-phosphate, and exposing organic components [16]. These are internalized, proteolysed tbxugh acidification, or exocytosed.

Following bone resorption to a certain depth and extent, which is determined by unknown mechanisms, the osteoclast detaches and may move along the surface to reattach and resorb another site or become inactivated. The resorptive sites (pits) are referred to as *Howship's lacunae.* Pits become sites for bone formation within a couple of days. The *coupling* of resorption with formation is part of the *remodeling* aspect of bone. It is hypothesized that coupling is mediated by a factor secreted by osteoblasts that stimulates osteoclasts [17].

COMPOSITIONAL HIERARCHY

Extracellular Matrix

The *organic extracellular matrix* of bone constitutes approximately 35% of its dry weight. It is comprised of principally type I collagen, an exploding universe of noncollagenous proteins, and ground substance. The crucial *regulatory and instructive* roles of *extracellular matrix (ECM)* in bone repair, renewal, and regeneration reside in several key features of this complex consorlium of molecules. Components of the ECM (e.g., collagens, proteoglycans) may bind growth factors (i.e., transforming growth factor beta, platelet derived growth factor) and differentiating factors (i.e., bone morphogenetic proteins), thus presenting them in the proper *configuration* to cell surface reseptors. Moreover, the binding can *protect and facilitate controlled release* of factors to promote, augment, and terminate the *bone formation cascade.*

Ground substance

Glycosaminoglycans constitute the lion's share of the ground substance and include: *chondroitin sulfate, keratan sulfate,* and *hyaluronic acid.* The extracellularmatrix assumes an important instructive role for the repair and regeneration of connective tissues by providing key attachment and regulatory ligands. For example, it has been shown that for the CD44 cell adhesion receptor, hyaluronan is one of its ligands [18].

Collagen

Type I collagen comprises about 90% of the organic extracellular matrix and serves as an anchorage platform for cell attachment and provides the infrastructure for mineral deposition. Collagen is expressed by osteoblasts as parallel, quarter-staggered arrays of *tropocollagen fibrils.* Fibrils become organized into *fibers.* Consecutive fibrils assume a head-to-tail relationship with *hole regions* interposed. Along sides of contiguous fibrils are *pores. Amorphous calcium phosphate is* preferentially deposited in *hole regions.*

Noncollagenous proteins

A considerable number of *noncollagenous proteins* function as regulatory molecules for mineralization, calcium modulation, cell regulation, and bone regeneration. *Osteonectin is* the most abundant noncollagenous protein and may direct calcium concentration, potentiate nucleation, or stabilize calcium-phosphate. *Osteocalcin is* another noncollagenous protein, but with an as yet unidentified role. *Bone sialoprotein* (e.g., *osteopontin)* may be involved with attachment of osteoblasts and osteoclasts to bone. Many types of cytokines, growth and differentiating factors have been isolated from bone [19,20]. Space limitations prohibit discussing these powerful regulatory molecules; however, several incisive reviews are offered in the bibliography [19-23]. We will discuss a few regulatory molecules later in the review.

Inorganic matrix

The *inorganic matrix* of bone accounts for 60-70% of the total dry weight of bone. The principal component in mature bone is hydroxyapatite (HA): $Ca_{10}(PO_4)_6(OH)_2$. During *osteogenesis* (bone formation), *amorphous* forms of calcium-phosphate are deposited first, maturing to crystalline HA. HA is a *plate-like crystal* measuring 20-80 nm by 2-5 nm.

The *inorganic matrix* fulfills significant functional and physiological roles. *Functionally,* it provides rigidity to bone, enabling us to escape the bond of gravity by allowing us to walk upright. Serving as origins and insertions for muscles, ingeniously engineered lever arms develop sufficient power for locomotion. *Physiologically,* the *inorganic matrix* provides life sustaining aliquots of minerals needed for *homeostasis.* For example, through *hormonal* (parathyroid hormone, vitanin D, calcitonin) and *cellular* (osteoclastic and osteoblastic) regulation, serum calcium is closely titrated, under homeostatic conditions varying only between 9.0-10.0 mg/dl.

BONE REPAIR

The *goals* in *bone repair* are to *regenerate form* thereby reestablishing *function* with *enduring bone.* Cellular and biochemical events ensuring for regeneration of bone recapitulate skeletal morphogenesis of embryological development [24]. Fracture repair often has been investigated to elucidate the morphological processes of bone repair. Healing time for a simple fracture is in excess of 4 weeks. Significant emphasis has been placed on modulating *molecular regulators* of the bone healing process, thereby compressing the duration of time for repair and ensuring for healing in compromised medical situations, for example, in diabetic and geriatric patients.

Initial event: Hematoma and blood clot

The initial events following fracture include *hematoma* formation and the resultant *blood clot.* An entourage of mediators are released or synthesized at this stage, such as growth and differentiation factors that promote biological responses through specific cell surface receptor binding. This results in activation of signal transduction pathways[25]. Molecular mediators released by platelet degranulation within the hematoma and blood clot are chemoattractants to recruit inflammatory cells and undifferentiated mesenchymal cells. *Platelet derived-growth factor* (PDGF) is a chemoattractant for mesenchymal cells and inflammatory cells [26]. *Transforming growth factor-beta* (TGF-beta) is a chemoattractant for monocytes [27] and fibroblasts [28].

The addition of molecular mediators to fractures profoundly influences its repair. For example, application of PDGF, FGF (fibroblast growth factor) and TGF-beta to fractures in rats, augments the osteogenic response [29-31]. Moreover, *osteogenic protein-l* Cnown as either OP-1 or bone morphogenetic protein 7, BMP-7) [32] and the tandem PDGF and *insulin-like growth factor-l* (IGF-1) [33], enhance early bone formation in defects around dental titanium implants.

Callus

The term *callus* has been applied imprecisely to describe granulation tissue, unmineralized osteoid, and the calcified hard tissue forming over a fracture site. Callus usually is associated with long bone fracture repair, and its formation is proportional to the amount of movement of the fracture fragments. Morphologically, the callus has been divided into *soft* and *hard* stages. These designators are arbitrary, in that different regions within a fracture progress at different rates of repair. Vascular invasion of the callus increases oxygen tension, heralding chondrocyte death. However, excessive mobility of a fracture site disrupts the angiogenic process and leads to non-union *(fibrous union, pseudoarthrosis).*

Vascularity

The role of *vascularly* in *osteogenesis* has been stressed, beginning with the preeminent study by Trueta [34]. Vascular dependency of bone is emphasized in its structural hierarchy, where concentric orbs of osteocytes are no more than 0.2 mm from the central haversian canal. Moreover, for *cancellous* and *compact* bone, in general, osteocytes are between 0.1-0.3 mm from a vascular conduit.

Blood vessels perpetuate bone viability and provide regulatory modulation for its repair and regeneration. *Endothelium* binds the *angiogenic factor* bFGF [35] in addition to BMP-3 *(osteogenin),* BMP4, and transforming growth factor-beta$_1$ (reviewed by

Ripamooti and Reddi) [36]. BMPs provide morphogenetic signals to lineage cells leading to conversion to osteoblasts; while bFGF provokes angiogenesis. Moreover, *pericytes* lining walls of capillary webs advancing into zones of bone repair, are speculated to be *osteoprogenitor cell candidates* [37]. Consequently, binding localization of growth and differentiating factors (such as the BMPs) and their presentation to pericytes, can lead to osteoblast expression, bone formation and its regeneration.

Remodeling

The term *remodeling* has been applied to the processes that sculpt the fracture callus, yielding a finished product reminiscent of the preinjured form. In simplistic terms, as a consequence of micro- and macrodamage, *remodeling* may be viewed as the process that repairs and shapes bone, ensuring for its renewal of form and function. *Modeling,* on the other hand, may be viewed as the processes associated with the development of bone form through embryogenesis to maturation. The remodeling of the callus involves the replacement of immature lamellar bone with mature lamellar bone. Lamellar bone orientation is consistent with the strains and loads of bone in function.

TERMINOLOGY AND CONCEPTS

Grafting techniques may involve the following materials: *autograft* (derived from the host), *allograft* (derived from the same species), *alloplast* (animal derivatives, synthetics, metals), or *recombinant molecular factors.*

Osteogenesis has been coined to describe the direct cell transfer in autografting. Osteoblasts and osteoprogenitor cells survive the grafting to promote bone regeneration.

Osteoconduction embraces the principle of providing a substratum for the cellular and biochemical events progressing to bone formation. Allografts and alloplasts may be osteoconductive.

The *principle of autoinduction* promulgated by Urist in 1965, described heterotopic ossicle formation induced by a diffusible glycoprotein delivered by a collagenous matrix [40]. Shortly thereafter, he introduced the term *bone morphogenetic protein* and the concept of *osteoinduction [41] . Osteoinduction* embodies dhe principle of converting pluripotential, mesenchymal-derived cells into a chondro osteoblast pathway with their subsequent expression of cartilage and bone.

Following Urist's seminal work, a legion of investigators explored BMPs, and in 1988, Wozney's group shared their work on recombinant human BMP [42]. The most exciting recombinant molecular factors for calcified tissues are *bone morphogenetic proteins* (BMPs *1-9) [38,39].* Their emergence as pivotal agents in *osteoinduction* has lead to a flurry of activity to develop a delivery system applicable to human therapeutic applications.

Despite the prevalence of recombinant human BMPs, the challenge to regenerate skeletal structures still remains: *a delivery system must be designed to present a therapeutic dose of BMP.*

SUMMARY

This review focused on the biologic hierarchy of bone and its capacity for repair and regeneration. The goal of this review was to introduce contemporary knowledge of bone physiology along with exciting therapeutic prospects for its regeneration.

REFERENCES

1. Paff, G.H. Anatomy of the Head and Neck. Philadelphia W.B. Saunders. 1973, 77.
2. Jowsey, J. *JAnat 1966,* 100: 857-864.
3. Owen, M. *Arthritis Rheum* 1980, 23: 1073-1080.
4. Owen, M. Lineage of osteogenic cells and their relationship to the stromal system. Elsevier Science Publishers. 1985, 1-25.
5. Owen, T.A., Aronow, M., Shalhoub, V., Barone, L M., Wuning, L., Tassinari, M.S., Kennedy, M.B., Pockwinse, S., Lian, J.B., and Stein, G.S. J *Cell. Physiol.* 1990,143: 420-430.
6. Parfitt, M.A. *Calcif. Tissue Int.* 1984, 36: 37-45.
7. Anderson, H.C. J. *CellBiology* 1969, 41: 59-72.
8. Anderson, H.C. *Bone Mineral Res.* 1985, 3: 109-149.
9. Boskey, A. In: BoneFormation and Repair, C.T. Brighton, G. Friedlacnder, and JM. Lane (Ed.), Rosemont American Academy of Orthopaedic Surgeons. 1994, 23-38.
10. Burger, E.H., Van der Meer, J., Van de Gevel, J.S., Gribnau, J.C., Thesingh, C.W., and Van Furth, R. In: Current Advances in Skeletonogenesis: Development, Bimineralization, Mediators, and Metabolic Bone Disease, M. Silbermann and H.C. Slavkin (Eds.), Amsterdam: Excerpta Medica, 1982.
11. Baron, R, Neff, L., Louvard, D., and Courtoy, P.J. *J.Cell Biol.* 1985, 101: 2210-2222.
12. Alvarez, J., Ross, P., Atbanasou, N., Blair, H., Greenfield, E., and Teitelbaum, S. *Calcif Tissue Int* 1992, 51: 48-53.
13. Rodan, G.A. *Bone* 1992, 13: S3-S6.
14. Baron, R. In: Bone Formation and Repair, C.T. Brighton, G. Friedlaender, and J M. Lane (Eds.), Rosemont American Academy of Orthopaedic Surgeons. 1994, 247-252.
15. Reinholt, F.P., Hultenby, K., Oldberg, A., and Heinegard, D. *Proc. Natl. Acad. Sci USA* 1990, 87: 4473-4475.
16. Kaplan, F.S., Hayes, W.C., Keavrny, TM., Boskey, A., Einhom, T.A., and Iannoni, J.P In: Orthopedic Basic Science, S.R. Simmon (Ed.), Chicago: Port City Press. 1994, 133.
17. Watrous, D.A. and Andrews, B. *SeminarsArthritisRheumatism* 1989, 19: 45-65.
18. Lesley, J., Hyman, R., and Kincade, P.W. *Advances Immunol.* 1993, 54: 271-335.
19. Goldring, M.B. and Goldring, S.R. *Clin Orthop Rel Res,* 1990, 258: 245.
20. Hauschka, P.V. In: The Osteoblast and Osteocycte, B.K. Hall (Ed), The Telfor Press, Inc. 1990, 103-170.
21. Bolander, ME. *Proc. Soc. Exp. Biol. Med.* 1992, 200: 165-170.
22. Pan, W.T. and Einhorn, T.A. *Current Orthop.* 1992, 6: 207-213.
23. Hollinger, J.O. *J. Craniofac. Surg.* 1993, 4: 115-121.
24. Erlbacher, A., Fllvaroff, E.H., Giteman, S.E., and Derynck, R. *Cell* 1995, 80: 371-378.
25. McAllister, B.S., Walters, J.D., and Olson, M.S. *Critical Reviews in Oral Biology and Medicine* 1994, 5: 291-310.
26. Graves, D. and Cochran, D. *Critical Reviews in Oral Biology and Medicine* 1990, 1: 17-36.
27. Wahl, S.M., Hunt, D.A., Wakefield, L.M., McCarlney-Francis, N., Wahl, L.M., Roberts, A.B., and Sporn, M.B. *Proc. Natl. Acad. Sci. U SA* 1987, 84: 57885792.

28. Postlethwaite, A.E., Keski-Oja, J., Moses, HL., and Kang, A.H. J. Sp. *Med.* 1987, 65: 251-256.
29. Joyce, M.E., Roberts, A.B., Sporn, M.B., and Bolander, ME. J. *Cell. Biol.* 1990, 110: 2195-2207.
30. Joyce, ME., Jingushi, S., and Bolander, ME. *Orthop. Clin. N. Am.* 1990, 21: 199-209.
31. Joyce, ME., Heydemann, A., and Bolander, ME. *Orthop. Trans.* 1990, 14: 363.
32. Rutherford, RB., Ryan, M.E., Kennedy, JE., Tucker, MM., and Charette, M.F. *J. Clin. Periodontol.* 1993, 20: 537544.
33. Becker, W., Lynch, S.E., Lekhohm, U., Becker, B.E., Caffesse, R., Donath, K., and Sanchez, R A *J. Periodontol.* 1992, 63: 929-940.
34. Trueta, J. *J. Bone Joint Surg.* 1963, 45B: 402-418.
35. Folknan, J., Klagsbrun, M., Sasse, J., Wadzinski, M., Ingber, D., and Vldavsky, I. *Am. J. Path.* 1988, 130: 393 400.
36. Ripamonti, U. and Reddi, A.H. *J. Periodont. Res* 1994, 29: 225-235.
37. Brighton, C.T., Lorich, D.G., Kupcha, R, Reilly, TM., Jones, A.R., and Woodbury, R.A. *Clin. Orthop. Rel. Res.* 1992, 275: 287-299.
38. Wozney, J.M. *Molecular Reproduct. Develop.* 1992, 32: 160-167.
39. Celeste, A.J., Song, J.J., Cox, K., Rosen, V., and Wozney, J.M. *J. Bone Us Res. 1994, 9: S137*
40. Urist, M.R *Science l965, 150 893-899.*
41. Urist, M.R and Strates, B.S. *J. Dent. Res.* 1971,50: 1392-1406.
42. Wozney, J.M., Rosen, V., Celeste, AJ., Mitsock, LM., Whittiers, M.J., Kriz, R.W., Hewick, R.M., and Wang, E.A. *Science* 1988,242: 1528-1534.

IMMUNOHISTOCHEMISTRY AND BONE: CHARACTERISATION OF THE TISSUE REACTIONS TO ORTHOPAEDIC IMPLANTS, INCLUDING THE CHANGES IN ASEPTIC LOOSENING AND THOSE RELATED TO BIOACTIVE MATERIALS

P.A. Revell

Osteoarticular Research Group and U.K. Interdisciplinary Research Centre in Biomaterials Department of Histopathology, Royal Free Hospital School of Medicine, Rowland Hill Street, London NW3 2PF

ABSTRACT

While a large number of orthopaedic joint replacment devices function satisfactorily for the remaining life-time of the often elderly patient, a proportion of cases develop loosening in the absence of infection or a mechanical problem in the process known as aseptic loosening. This account describes the results of studies performed to identify the inflammatory reactions occurring around such loosened implants and outlines the histological features present in relation to 'bioactive' materials. The latter are coating materials used to bring about bone growth in intimate contact with the implant.

THE INFLAMMATORY REACTION AND ASEPTIC LOOSENING OF ORTHOPAEDIC IMPLANTS

In the process of aseptic loosening, a fibrous tissue layer (or membrane) forms around the implant between the biomaterial and bone. Micromovement and the presence of wear debris are the two reasons for the development of the fibrous membrane and increasingly the cellular reaction to debris is considered to be of major importance. The features of the tissue usually found between the biomaterial and bone in aseptic loosening are illustrated in Fig. 1. Macrophages and fibroblasts are the cells found immediately next to the biomaterial, be it polymethyl methacrylate (bone cement), metal alloy (cobalt-chromium-molybdenum; titanium-aluminium-vanadium; stainless steel), plastic (ultrahigh molecular weight polyethylene) or ceramic (alumina, zirconia). These cells form a synovium-like structure next to the implant, as demonstrated by conventional histology [1] and by immuno-histochemistry with monoclonal antibody (MAB) markers [2,3]. There is some evidence that macrophages are also recruited to the surface of well-fixed components [4]. Recent studies have shown that a proportion of the macrophages in this layer are activated, since they express the CD11b and CD11c epitopes [3,5], HLA-DR [6] and show evidence of antigen-presentation in the form of MAB RFD1 positivity [7]. The region between this synovial layer and the surface of the bone is where particulate wear

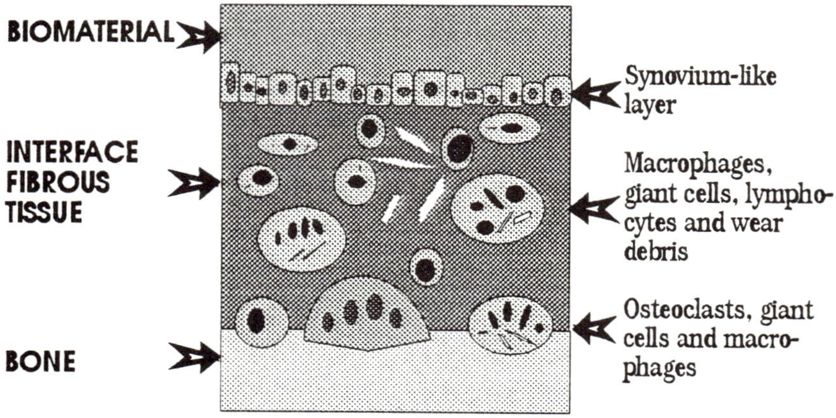

Figure 1. Diagram to show the cell populations in the interface tissues and adjacent to the biomaterial and bone

debris accumulates, and the principal inflammatory response occurs. Metal alloy and ceramic debris is found predominantly in macrophages, while UHMWPE and bone cement are accompanied by macrophages and macrophage polykaryons (foreign body giant cells). These cells show a variety of patterns of staining with MAB markers. The macrophages and their polykaryons are CD11b and CD68 positive, and the majority of the latter are also CD13 (aminopeptidase) and CD71 (transferrin receptor) positive [8]. Strong expression of HLA-DR and CD11b is found on debris-containing cells [9]. That there is heterogeneity among the cells recruited in response to wear debris is further evidenced by our studies. Thus 20-40% of the total macrophage (CD68 reactive) population is RFD1 positive (dendritic antigen-presenting cells), while the other debris-containing macrophages are RFD7 positive (mature macrophages) and RFD9 positivity is entirely confined to macrophage polykaryons [10]. The relationship between macrophages, their polykaryons and the bone-resorbing multinucleated osteoclasts at bone surfaces has been debated recently [11]. Markers previously thought specific for osteoclasts, like tartrate-resistant acid phosphatase [12] and MAB against vitronectin receptor (VNR) [13], have been shown to cross-react with macrophages and other cells of the monuclear phagocyte system, including macrophage polykaryons [8,14]. As well as there being heterogeneity in the macrophage population, it is beginning to appear that there is heterogeneity among foreign body giant cells, some of which are CD11b negative, VNR positive, while others are CD11b positive, VNR negative [8]. Controversy over whether macrophages and foreign body giant cells can resorb bone persists [15] though mounting evidence suggests this is a strong possibility [8,16,17].

These macrophages and their polykaryons can be shown by immunohistochemistry to contain a number of different inflammatory chemical mediators called cytokines. Interleukin 1β (IL1β) is found in the largest proportion of cells and in the greater percentage of interface fibrous membranes [18], though tumour necrosis factor α (TNFα) (which has similar actions) [19] and granulocyte-macrophage colony stimulating factor

(GM-CSF) [20] are also present. The message for interleukin 6 (IL6) (mRNA by in situ hybridisation) has been detected [21]. The effect of these pro-inflammatory cytokines is to stimulate the production of enzymes such as the metalloproteinases (MMPs) [22] and recruit and/or activate osteoclasts [23,24]. Osteoclastic and macrophage polykaryon acid phosphatase as well as MMP production have been demonstrated in relation to the cells resorbing bone adjacent to the inflammation at the implant interface [8,19]. The IL-1, TNFα and MMP-1 producing cells are of the RFD-7 mature macrophage phenotype [10]. IL1 and GM-CSF may have a synergistic role in the proliferation and activation of macrophages and GM-CSF affect polykaryon or osteoclast formation [20]. Considerable further work is required before the inflammatory mechanism which gives rise to aspetic loosening and removal of bone (osteolysis) is properly understood. Results so far point to the central role of wear particles. Two approaches may be made to decrease the effects of wear particles and so prolong the implant life-time: (a) improvement of wear conditions at the bearing surface; (b) integration of bone with implant at the prosthesis-tissue interface. It is this second area which will form the second part of this account.

THE TISSUE REACTION TO HYDROXYAPATITE AND BIOACTIVE GLASS

Because hydroxyapatite (HA) is brittle and relatively weak compared with the metal alloys and ceramics used in orthopaedic implants, its best use in load bearing implants is as a coating on the surface of one of these implant materials. Such an HA coating extends the functional life of the prosthesis because there is no longer a fibrous membrane in which debris can accumulate, bone growing instead in continuity with the coating. The coating must be of a type which will elicit the optimum tissue response by way of bone formation. The percentage crystallinity of the HA coating can affect its solubility and the surface of more amorphous coatings is subject to more prominent cell-mediated changes than highly crystalline ones in tissue culture [25]. Greater cell growth and attachment occurs in tissue culture with lower crystallinity HA [26]. Our own studies have shown that amorphous hydroxyapatite has better bone integration/bonding properties in rat bone than crystalline hydroxyapatite and that both of these are superior to β tricalcium phosphate [27]. Many studies have now examined the long-term effects of hydroxyapatite, fluorapatite and related materials in relation to bone bonding. Direct bone bonding with no fibrous tissue interposition is the norm. It is known that certain other biomaterials, notably titanium, can have direct contact with bone and this is thought to be through the initial formation of a calcium phosphate layer on the surface of the metal [28,29]. In a study of the early changes next to HA coated and uncoated titanium rods and perspex, new bone was found in relation to both forms of titanium implant by 6 days in the rabbit and by 17 days it had formed a circumferential cylinder with bone in contact. At 84 days, the number of bone contact points were the same for all three implants and there were no differences in the amount of bone apposition (surface area) between HA coated and uncoated titanium implants though this was less for perspex [30] (Fig. 2). The figures for percentage of bonding to the surface are similar to those reported recently in studies of the early bone response to HA [31]. It has been shown from tissue culture studies that fibronectin and vitronectin are needed for cell attachment to metal and ceramic surfaces [32,33], and that these two proteins together with laminin, type IV collagen and osteopontin are associated with HA-coated implants in vivo within 6 days [34]. Recent studies with bioactive glass (Bioglass® 45S5) show the absorption of albumin, fibronectin, vitronectin and immunoglobulins A and G as soon as 1 day after subcutaneous implantation, with a decrease in fibronectin by 3 days and of all these proteins by 14 days [35].

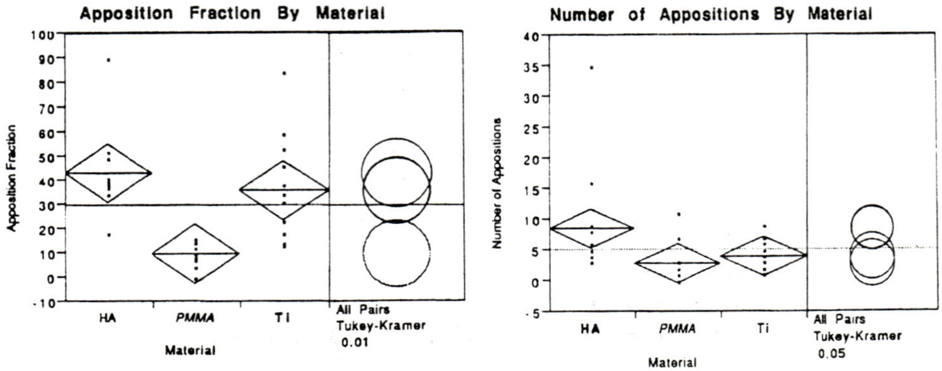

Figure 2. Appositional fraction and number of appositions for hydroxyapatite coated (HA) and uncoated (Ti) titanium, compared with perspex (PMMA). Showing means with confidence intervals (left) and Tukey-Kramer plot for p values of 0.01 (apposition fraction) and 0.05 (number of appositions)

Bonding of this material to bone is well documented, with firm union and bone ongrowth demonstrable from between 10 days and 2 years [36,37]. The formation of a silica gel layer and calcium phosphate deposition at the surface of this material occurs within one hour in vitro [38], and it is on this that subsequent hydroxyapatite formation, bone cell attachment and growth occur [29]. Our own recent studies have shown that silica gel and outer calcified layers are detectable after 1 day in vivo for 45S5 Bioglass and that this pattern of surface appearance remained over the next 3 weeks of the experiment [35]. By contrast, a related glass known not to bond to bone (60S), showed no surface silica gel or calcified zones and by 6 days showed an irregular crenated surface to which there was macrophage recruitment.

The above is part of an ever enlarging literature which is developing around the cellular and chemical reactions occurring in the presence of HA, bioactive glasses and similar materials. A wide variety of methods has been applied in vitro and in vivo and studies performed at light microscopical and ultrastructural level. While there is much commonality in the results, there remain many aspects yet to be investigated, particularly in relation to early chemical and cellular events occurring in vivo. Considerable scope exists for future work in this bone healing and formation field with the techniques of immunohistochemistry and the study of chemical mediators currently used for studies of inflammation and bone resorption as described in the first part of this article.

REFERENCES

1. Goldring, S.R., Schiller, A.L., Roelke, M., Rourke, C.M., O'Neill, D.A., Harris, W.H., *J. Bone Jt. Surg.* 1983, 65A, 575-584.
2. Revell, P.A., Lalor P.A., *Proc. Bone-Biomaterial Interface Workshop*, Toronto, 1990. ed. Davies.
3. Lalor, P.A., Revell, P.A., *Clin. Materials,* 1993, 14, 91-100.
4. Levade, B., Revell, P.A., Freeman, M.A.R., *Acta.Orthop.Scand.*, 1987, 58, 384-387.

5. Revell, P.A., AL-Saffar, N. In *Failure of Joint Replacement. A biolog*ical, mechanical or surgical problem?* Institute of Orthopaedics, London 1994, eds. Downes and Dabestani .
6. Lalor, P.A. *PhD Thesis,* University of London, 1991.
7. AL-Saffar, N., Mah, J.T.L., Revell, P.A. *J. Pathol.* 1993, 170 (Suppl.), 348A.
8. Kadoya, Y.,AL-Saffar, N.,Kobayashi, A., Revell, P.A. *Bone Miner.* 1994, 27, 85-96.
9. AL-Saffar, N., Mah, J.T.L., Revell, P.A. *J. Pathol.* 1994, 172 (Suppl.), 103A.
10. AL-Saffar, N., Revell, P.A. *Trans. Soc. Biomater.* 1994, 17, 233.
11. Revell, P.A. *Pathol. Society of Great Britain* meeting, Oxford, January 1995.
12. Minkin, C. *Calif. Tiss. Int.* 1982, 34, 285-290.
13. Horton, M.A., Lewis, D., McNulty, K., Pringle, J.A.S., Chambers, T.J. *Cancer Res.* 1985, 45, 5663-5669.
14. Athanasou, N.A., Quinn, J., Horton, M.A., McGee, J.O'D. *Bone Miner.* 1990, 8, 7-22.
15. Chambers, T.J., Horton, M.A. *Calif. Tiss. Int.* 1984, 36, 556-558.
16. Quinn, J., Joyner, C., Triffit, J.T., Athanasou, N.A. *J. Bone Jt. Surg.* 1992, 74B, 652-658.
17. Revell, P.A., Kadoya, Y., AL-Saffar, N., Kobayashi, A., Scott, G., Freeman, M. *Proc. Austral. Soc. Biomater.* 1995, Melbourne, Australia, 5, B3.
18. AL-Saffar, N., Kadoya, Y., Revell, P.A. *Brit. J. Rheumat.* 1994, 33, 309-316.
19. AL-Saffar, N., Kadoya, Y., Revell, P.A. *J. Pathol.* 1994, 172 (Suppl.), 103A.
20. AL-Saffar, N., Khwaja, H., Revell, P.A. *J. Pathol.* 1994, 173 (Suppl.), 154A.
21. Goodman, S.B., Sibley, R., Huie, P., Lee, K., Doshi, A., Roshdieh, B., Woolson, S.T., Maloney, W.J., Schuman, D.J. *Trans. Soc. Biomater.* 1994, 17, 55.
22. Krane, S.M., Amento, E.P., Goldring, M.B., Goldring, S.R. et al. In *Articular Biochemistry*, 1986, Raven Press, New York, eds. Kuettner, Schleyerback and Hascall, 413-422.
23. Gowen, M., Wood, D.D., Ihrie, E.J., McGuire, M.K.F., Russell, G.R. *Nature* 1983, 306, 378-380.
24. Bertolini, D.R., Nedwon, G.E., Brigman, T.S., Smith, D.D., Mundy, G.R. *Nature* 1986, 319, 516-518.
25. van Blitterswijk, C.A., van den Brink, J., Bovell, Y.P., Leenders, H., Flach, J., de Bruijn, J.D., Radder, A.M. *Trans. Soc. Biomater.* 1994, 17, 432.
26. Maxian, S.H., Melican, M.C., Gross, K.A., Berndt, C.C., Zawadsky, J.P. *Trans. Soc. Biomater.* 1995, 18, 200.
27. Revell, P.A., Chalkley, S., (unpublished findings).
28. Ducheyne, P., Bianco, P., Radin, S., Schepers, E. In *Bone Bonding*, 1992, Reed Healthcare Communications, eds. Ducheyne, Kokubo and van Blitterswijk. 1-12.
29. Kokubo, T. In *An Introduction to Bioceramics,* 1993, World Scientific, Singapore, eds. Hench and Wilson, 5, 75-103.
30. Fegan, A., Pirie, C., Revell, P.A. *J. Pathol.* 1992, 168 (Suppl.), 109A.
31. Spector, M., Prabhakor, R., Bignami, A., Lalor, P.A., Bearcroft, J., Beals, N., Nancollas, G.H. *Trans. Soc. Biomater.* 1995, 18, 122.
32. Howlett, C.R., Evans, M.D.M., Walsh, W.R., Johnson, G., Steele, J.G. *Biomaterials,* 1994, 15, 213-222.
33. Seitz, T.L., Noonon, K.D., Hench, L.L., Noonon, N.E. *J.Biomed. Mater. Res.* 1982, 16, 195-207.

34. Benezra, V., Hoang, L., Hobbs, L.W. *Trans. Soc. Biomater.* 1995, 18, 69.
35. Revell, P.A., Wilson, J., Osei, D., Smith, S. (Unpublished findings).
36. Hench, L.L., Splinter, R.J., Allen, W.C., Greenlee, T.K. *J. Biomed. Mater. Res.* 1971, 5, 117-141.
37. Hench, L.L., Paschall, H.A. *J. Biomed. Mater. Res.* 1973, 7, 25-42.
38. Hench, L.L., Andersson, Ő.H., La Torre, G.P. In *Bioceramics 4,* 1991, Butterworth, London, eds. Bonfield, W., Hastings, G., Tanner, K.E., 155-162.

BONE IN-FILL OF NON-HEALING CALVARIAL DEFECTS USING PARTICULATE BIOGLASS® AND AUTOGENOUS BONE

Stewart A. Bergman and Leonard J. Litkowski*

Department of Oral and Maxillofacial Surgery,*Department of Restorative Dentistry Dental School, University of Maryland at Baltimore, 666 West Baltimore Street, MD.

ABSTRACT
The purpose of this study was to evaluate the bone in-fill of surgically created non-healing calvarial defects in the rabbit model, when using particulate Bioglass® 90-710, μm, 110-310 μm, and spherical, alone and in combination with autogenous calvarial cortical bone dust. Results indicate that the combination of particulate Bioglass®, 90-710 μm and 50% autogenous calvarial cortical bone dust was the most efficacious combination in inducing bone in-fill of non-healing calvarial defects in the rabbit model. This was followed by particulate Bioglass® 90-710 μm alone. The particulate Bioglass® 110-310 μm showed little if any bone in-fill at all time intervals after placement as did the spherical Bioglass® particles.

INTRODUCTION
A significant problem for oral and maxillofacial and orthopedic reconstructive surgery, where large areas of bone may be removed as result of tumor resection, or cyst removal, is the identification of a material which will promote host bone replacement that rapidly fills-in and bridges the defect thereby restoring both form and function. The material of choice has been and remains autogenous bone. Autogenous bone is composed of organic and inorganic structures. The organic component is primarily collagen which provides resilience and toughness and the inorganic component is primarily hydroxyapatite which provides hardness and rigidity. The inorganic matrix also contains organic components of osteocytes, osteoblasts, and various amounts of mesenchymal cells. Because of the presence of this viable cellular component, autogenous bone is the only osteogenic material presently available. However, in order to obtain this bone it is frequently necessary to surgically harvest the bone from a second or donor site. This adds to the surgical morbidity that the patient must endure, increases anesthesia and surgical time, increases blood loss, and possible surgical complications. The iliac crest because of its relatively rich supply of cortical and cancellous bone is often used as the donor site. However, even here there is a limit to the supply of bone which can be harvested

necessitating the use of additional donor sites. Consequently, there may be inadequate bone to fill a large defect [1].

When autogenous bone was insufficient to completely fill a defect, freeze dried lyophilized or demineralized banked allogeneic bone has been used to augment the available bone. However, there is increasing reluctance to used banked bone if alternatives are available due to the added risk of infection (AIDS, hepatitis B & C, and sexually transmitted diseases) [2]. Alloplastic materials have been used as an alternative to allografts. Alloplastic materials for bone replacement are synthetic or deorganified biocompatible materials. They are primarily ceramics which are either inert or bioactive. Inert ceramics do not bond with the host tissues. Rather there is an intimate mechanical contact which permits force transfer. Such materials are rarely used as bone augmentation materials. Bioactive ceramics are frequently used as a bone substitute. They include calcium phosphate materials ie. hydroxyapatite (HA), or tricalcium phosphate (TCP). A chemical contact between the host bone and the grafted material may develop as well as possible stimulus of bone formation activity [3]. Bioglass® is a bioactive ceramic material. Previous work has shown that particulate Bioglass® allows bone reconstruction in the periodontium at a much faster rate than other calcium phosphate materials used for this purpose [4]. This is believed to be due to an osteoconductive effect upon the osteogenic cells in contact with the surface of the material. Pilot studies have shown that using a mixture of autogenous bone to provide osteogenic cells combined with particulate Bioglass® has produced bone augmentation in dog ribs, of up-to 12 times that of unaugmented bone at seven weeks and more that three times the augmentation produced by autogenous bone alone [5].

The purpose of this study was to develop bioactive Bioglass® materials in particulate form used alone or in combination with autogenous bone to fill osseous defects which result from disease, trauma or surgical resection of osseous tissue. A range of Bioglass® particles were used to determine the optimal size of the glass particle to be used alone or mixed with autogenous bone that would fill a non-healing bony defect. In a pilot study there was some evidence that significant augmentation occurred even when the particle size was small enough to be resorbable in areas of high blood flow. Comparison of the effect of sol-gel derived preparation and the standard preparation of the glass particles were also evaluated.

METHODS AND MATERIALS

Fifteen New Zealand white rabbits, 4.0 to 4.5 kg were utilized in this study. The animals were kept in individual cages with standard food and water available ad libitum. After general anesthesia was achieved with ketamine 60 mg/kg and 0.2 mg/kg acepromazine administered i.m., the hair of the scalp of each animal was shaved and the scalp prepared with a betadine scrub. Approximately 2 ml of local anesthetic (40 mg lidocaine with 0.02 mg epinephrine) was injected into the scalp subcutaneously to achieve local anesthesia and provide hemostasis. A bicoronal incision was made just behind the external auditory canals and a bicoronal flap reflected. The periosteum was incised and reflected thereby exposing the underlying calvarial bone. A 15 mm diameter full thickness calvarial defect was created on either side of the mid-sagittal suture. The outer table of the calvarium was removed using a dental # 8 round carbide bur using slow speed (<10,000 rpm), ground to a fine powder and saved to be used as a graft material alone or mixed with the Bioglass®. The inner table of the calvarium was removed in large segments without disturbing the underlying dura mater. Each full thickness calvarial defect was grafted with one of the following materials:

1. Particulate Bioglass @ (PBG), 90-710 μm.
2. PBG 90-710 μm plus 50% autogenous bone (calvarial bone powder) by volume.
3. PBG 110-310 μm.
4. PBG 110-310, μm plus 50% autogenous bone (calvarial bone powder) by volume.
5. Spherical Bioglass® particles.
6. 100% autogenous bone (calvarial bone powder).
7. Nothing was placed (control defect).

The wound was closed in layers using 3-0 chromic sutures to close the periosteum and gallea and 4-0 nylon sutures to close the skin.

Animals were sacrificed at 4, and 12 weeks using 60 mg/kg of pentobarbital sodium i.v. The calvarium of the animal was exposed by reflecting a bicoronal flap and then removed en bloc with the underlying dura mater using either a dental drill or cutting discs. The resected calvarium was then placed immediately into 10% buffered formalin. The calvarial defect closure was measured grossly and evaluated histologically for the presence of bone according to the following scale: 3 = complete fill; 2 = 50-99% fill; 1 = 25-50 % fill and 0 = < 25% fill. Results were analyzed by a Kruskal Wallis test for significance. Each calvarial specimen was decalcified in formic acid, sectioned through the center of each defect, and stained in the standard fashion with hemotoxylin and eosin for histologic evaluation.

4 weeks

2 rabbits	-	LPBG alone and LPBG + 50% autogenous calvarial bone dust
1 rabbit	-	SPBG alone and SPBG + 50% autogenous calvarial bone dust
1 rabbit	-	SPHBG alone and 100% autogenous calvarial bone dust

12 weeks

3 rabbits	-	LPBG alone and LPBG + 50% autogenous calvarial bone dust
1 rabbit	-	SPBG alone and SPBG + 50% autogenous calvarial bone dust
1 rabbit	-	SPHBG alone and 100% autogenous calvarial bone dust
2 rabbits	-	LPBG alone and control defect (nothing place in defects)
2 rabbits	-	LPBG alone and LPBG + 50% autogenous calvarial bone dust
2 rabbits	-	SPBG alone and SPBG + 50% autogenous calvarial bone dust

RESULTS

4 weeks

LPBG showed the beginning of early osteoid formation spanning less than 25% of the defect. This immature bone was seen mostly near the periosteum. The remainder of the defect was filled with dense connective scar tissue, plump fibroblasts and a scattering of inflammatory cells which surrounded particles of the glass.

LPBG + Autogenous calvarial bone dust showed new immature bone and osteoid spanning approximately 80% of the defect. In the center of the defect, dense collagen bands and fibers, similar to the scar tissue seen in the LPBG sample alone was present. The bone trabeculae were lined with metabolically active osteoblasts. Particles of the glass were seen throughout the defect.

SPBG alone showed that the glass was nearly completely resorbed. No osteoid or bone formation was present. Only dense connective tissue scar was seen with a scattering of fibroblasts and inflammatory cells.

SPBG + autogenous calvarial bone dust showed no bone formation, however, there was some early osteoid formation spanning less than 25% of the defect. The defect was mostly filled with dense connective scar tissue which surrounded some remaining glass particles.

Calvarial bone dust alone showed that the calvarial bone was nearly completely resorbed. No bone or osteoid formation was present except at margins of defect and associated periosteal layer. Dense connective tissue similar to that seen in the other samples spanned the entire defect.

SPHBG alone showed no bone or osteoid formation except at margin of defect and in the area associated with the periosteum. The spherical glass particles were completely encapsulated with dense connective tissue.

12 weeks

SPBG alone as in the 4 week sample showed little if any bone formation except at margin of defect and subperiosteally. The glass particles were encapsulated in dense connective tissue. There appeared to be loss of volume of graft and thickness of the scar tissue spanning the defect compared to the 4 week samples, indicating maturation and remodeling of the scar tissue. There were few cells present, either fibroblasts or inflammatory, and very few blood vessels.

LPBG + 50% autogenous calvarial bone dust showed near complete bone bridge spanning the defect (90-95%). The bone appeared more mature with regeneration of marrow spaces and lacunae containing osteocytes. It was difficult to determine the edge of the defect. Furthermore, we were unable to detect loss of volume or thickness of graft.

LPBG alone showed nearly 50% immature bone fill of the defect. Complete bridge of immature bone spanning the defect was present in the subperiosteal area. However, unlike the LPBG + autogenous bone samples, there was loss of thickness and volume of graft.

Autogenous bone alone showed as in the 4 week samples that complete resorption of the bone particles had occurred. Bone formation was only present at the margin of the defect. The remainder of the defect was filled with dense nearly acellular and avascular connective tissue with loss volume and thickness of the graft suggesting the presence of mature scar.

Statistical analysis of the data showed there was a significant difference between the LPBG + 50% bone ($p < .05$) and both the autogenous bone alone and the LPBG alone at both 4 and 12 weeks.

DISCUSSION

It is apparent from this study at 12 weeks that the combination of large particle Bioglass® and autogenous calvarial bone dust is superior to large particle Bioglass® alone in inducing bone formation in non-healing calvarial defects. However large particle Bioglass® alone at 12 weeks showed a bridging of the defect but the volume of the bone in-fill had not equaled the Bioglass® mixed with autogenous bone. This indicates the the repair mechanism is progressing but at a slower rate than with the addition of autogenous bone. For these studies, it will be necessary to carry out the study for a longer time period.

Small particle Bioglass® alone or in combination with autogenous calvarial bone dust and calvarial bone dust alone was completely resorbed and replaced with scar tissue. This would indicate that there is a critical size of the replacement material that is necessary for the regeneration of the calvarium. The size is possibly related to the rate of the resorption of the graft material. From these studies it would appear that there is a critical *time* that the graft must remain in place to be used as a matrix for new bone formation. This time would be directly related to the rate of resorption of the graft.

It is necessary to consider three parameters when placing a material in a bony defect: 1) the size of the defect, 2) the amount of bone stimulation hormones present (in autogenous bone or other source) and 3) the resorption rate of the graft material. Therefore when evaluating the graft material to be used it is necessary to evaluate all three parameters and select the material which will best match the defect.

The small sample size in this study necessitates confirmatory studies to further determine the effect of material parameters on the size and placement of the bony defect. Additional size ranges and longer time points would be necessary to more closely optimize the demands of the defect repair with the physical properties of the material to be used.

REFERENCES

1. Schmitz, J.P. and Rollinger, J.O., *Clin. Orthop.* 1986, 205, 229-231.
2. Fonseca, R.J., Frost, D., Zeitler, D., et. al., in *Reconstructive Preprosthetic Oral and Maxillofacial Surgery,* edited by Fonseca, R.J. and Davis, W.H., W.B. Saunders, Philadelphia 1986, 117-165.
3. LeGeros, R.Z., *Adv. Dent. Res.* 1988, 2, 164-168.
4. Wilson, J., and Low, S.B., *J. Appl. Biomat.* 1992, 123-129.
5. Wilson, J., Yu, L.T., and Beale, B.S. In *Bioceramics 5*, Kobonshi Kankokai, Inc., Kyoto, Japan, 1992, 139-146.

IN VITRO EFFECTS OF EHDP ON THE FORMATION AND OSTEOCLASTIC ABSORPTION OF BONE-LIKE APATITE FORMED ON BIOACTIVE CERAMICS

T. Nakamura* S. Yamada*, T. Kitsugi*†, S. Miyaji**, T. Kokubo**, M. Oka***

Department of Orthopaedic Surgery, Faculty of Medicine*, Department of Material Chemistry, Faculty of Engineering**, Research Center for Biomedical Engineering, Kyoto University***, deceased†

ABSTRACT

1-Hydroxyethylidene-1, 1-bisphosphonic acid (EHDP) is a potent chemical that inhibits bone absorption and is used for treatment of osteoporosis. In this study, the effects of EHDP on *in vitro* formation and osteoclastic absorption of bone-like apatite formed on A-W glass-ceramic (A-W GC) were investigated. EHDP inhibited the formation of bone-like apatite on A-W GC in simulated body fluid (SBF) at a concentration of >0.1 μg/ml. EHDP attached to bone-like apatite totally inhibited the osteoclastic absorption of the apatite. EHDP in culture medium at a concentration of 5 μg/ml decreased osteoclastic absorption partially but not totally. These results suggest that EHDP suppresses the formation and osteoclastic absorption of bone-like apatite formed on bioactive ceramics and bioactive ceramics may be a potent tool for investigation of bone metabolism.

INTRODUCTION

Bioactive ceramics are known to bind with bone through the apatite formed on their surfaces [1]. This apatite is formed *in vitro* by an inorganic chemical reaction in simulated body fluid, which contains inorganic ions like blood plasma but no organic components [2]. It has several characteristics similar to the apatite in bone tissue and is thought to be formed by a chemical reaction similar to that occurring in bone tissue. Accordingly, this apatite is known as bone-like apatite. Bone-like apatite can be used as a model material *in vitro* to evaluate the effects of drugs on the formation or resorption of apatite in bone. In this study the functions of EHDP [3] were investigated using bone-like apatite formed on A-W GC.

MATERIALS AND METHOD

Simulated body fluid (SBF) [3]

SBF with ion concentrations (Na^+ 142.0, K^+ 5.0, Ca^{2+} 2.5, Mg^{2+} 1.5, HCO_3^- 4.2, Cl^- 148.0, HPO_4^{2-} 1.0, and SO_4^{2-} 0.5 mM) nearly equal to those of human blood plasma was prepared by dissolving NaCl, $NaHCO_3$, KCl, $K_2HPO_4 \bullet 3H_2O$, $MgCl_2 \bullet 6H_2O$, $CaCl_2$ and Na_2SO_4 in distilled water. The solution was buffered to pH 7.25 at 36.5°C with 50 mM trishydroxymethyl aminomethane [$(CH_2OH)_3CNH_2$] and 45 mM hydrochloric acid (HCl) [4].

Apatite-wollastonite-containing glass-ceramic (A-W GC)

A-W GC was provided by Nippon Electric Glass Co., Ltd. (Japan). The material contained 38% oxy- and fluorapatite [$Ca_{10}(PO_4)_6(O, F_2)$], 34% wollastonite ($Ca \bullet SiO_2$) and 28% residual glass, and was synthesized by a method reported previously [5].

EHDP

EHDP was kindly provided by Sumitomo Pharmaceutal Co., Osaka, Japan. Two types of experiments were performed.

Influence of EHDP on bone-like apatite formation

Rectangular A-W GC plates (15 mm x 10 mm x 2 mm) were abraded with # 2000 alumina powder and each plate was soaked for ten days in 40 ml of SBF in a plastic centrifuge tube containing EHDP at a concentration of 0, 0.01, 0.1, 0.5, 1,10 or 100 μg/ml. After soaking, the A-W GC was dried in air. The bone-like apatite was detected by thin-layer X-ray diffraction and scanning electron microscopy (SEM).

Influence of EHDP on osteoclastic absorption of bone-like apatite [6].

Mirror-polished discs of A-W GC 14 mm in diameter were soaked for 10 days in SBF to allow bone-like apatite to form on their surface. Additionally, some discs were soaked in SBF containing 5 μg/ml EHDP for two days to allow EHDP to attach to their bone-like apatite layer. An osteoclast-containing cell fraction was obtained from long bones of 10 day old rabbits according to Tezuka et. al. [7]. The cells were washed in a centrifuge (400 rpm, 3 min) and suspended in 40 mL ∝-MEM culture medium with 10% heat-inactivated fetal bovine serum (Whittaker M.A. Bioproducts) and antibiotics (100 U/mL penicillin G, 100 μg/ mL streptomycin; Meiji, Japan). One milliliter of the cell suspension, containing 107 cells, was seeded into each well of a 4 well culture plate containing an A-W GC disc with bone-like apatite on its surface. In some wells EHDP was added at its concentration of 5 μg/ml. The experiment was done in duplicate. Ten nanomolar 1-25-dihydroxy vitamin D_3 (Dupher, USA) was then added to the cultures. The plates were incubated at 37°C in a humidified atmosphere of 5% CO_2 in air. After three days of incubation, all cells except osteoclasts were removed by incubation of the disc for 10 min in PBS containing 0.001% Pronase E and 0.02% EDTA. Then the plates were washed in PBS and fixed in 2% glutaraldehyde in 0.1 M phosphate buffer at 4°C overnight, dehydrated through a graded series of ethanol, critical point-dried in CO_2 (critical-point dryer, HCP-2; Hitachi, Japan), sputter-coated with platinum (ion coater, IB5; Eiko, Japan), and observed by SEM (S-450; Hitachi, Japan).

RESULTS

Influence on apatite formation on A-W GC

SEM and thin layer X-ray diffraction analysis of the surface of A-W GC did not show any changes after ten day soaking, when SBF contained EHDP at the concentration > 0.1

μg/ml. At the concentration < 0.1μg/ml of EHDP in SBF, bone-like apatite was detected on A-W GC by SEM and thin layer X-Ray diffraction analysis (Fig. 1).

Osteoclastic absorption of bone-like apatite

Bone-like apatite on A-W GC disc was absorbed by the cultured osteoclasts. Pits were formed around the osteoclasts. This absorption was perfectly inhibited by EHDP attached on the bone-like apatite (Fig. 2). The addition of 5μg/ml EHDP in the culture medium decreased the osteoclastic absorption of bone-like apatite partially but did not stop it completely.

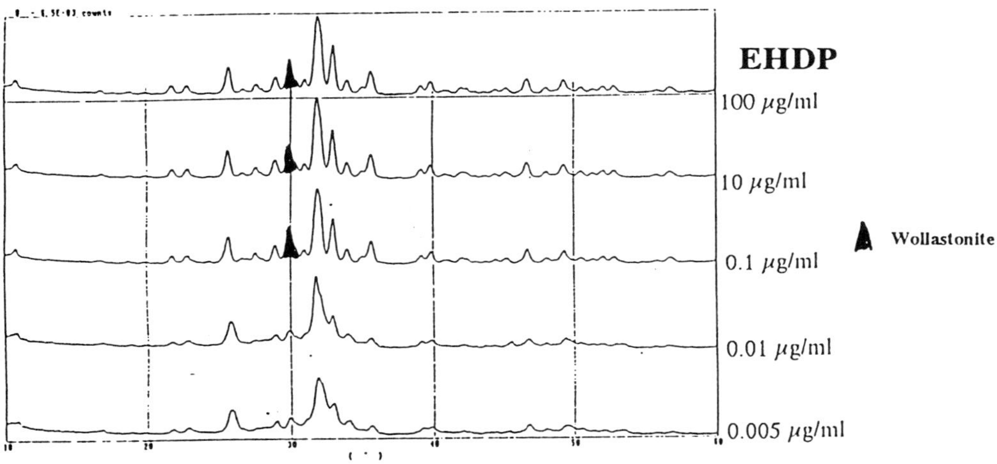

Figure 1. X-ray thin layer diffraction of A-W GC soaked in SBF for 10 days with EHDP.

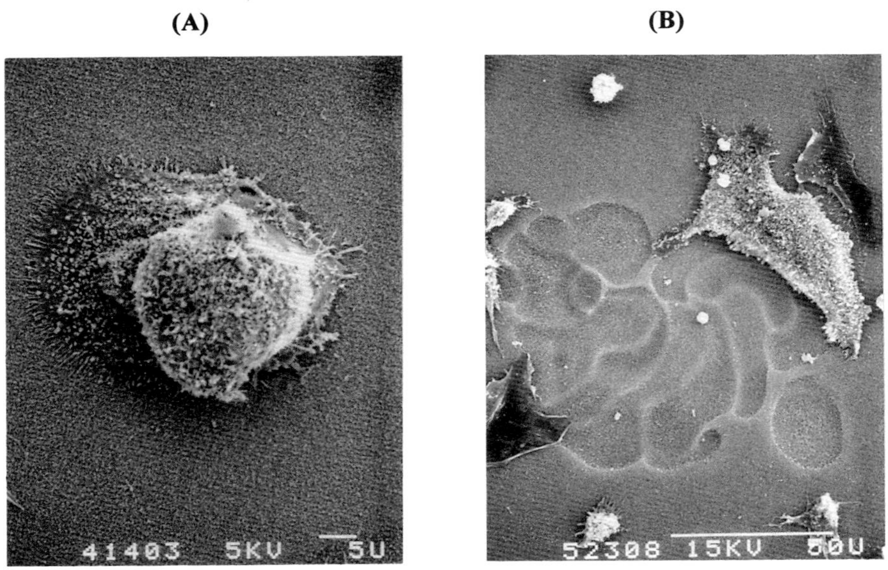

Figure 2. SEM photography of Osteoclasts cultured on Bone-like apatite with (a) and without (b) EHDP attached. EHDP inhibited osteoclastic absorption of the apatite.

DISCUSSION

Apatite formation on A-W GC in SBF was stopped by EHDP in SBF. It is known that EHDP inhibits apatite formation in bone at a high plasma concentration and this chemical is thought to bind to apatite in bone and stop the growth of apatite crystals [4]. Kitsugi et. al. reported that bonding of A-W GC to bone was inhibited in a rabbit injected with 5 mg/kg of EHDP subcutaneously every day [8] and apatite was not observed on the surface of A-W GC. These results are compatible with the present *in vitro* experiments. This same mechanism by EHDP may work to bone-like apatite on A-W GC.

Resorption lacunae and osteoclasts were clearly visible on the bone-like apatite formed on A-W GC after using pronase E to remove the stromal cells which covered the surface. Cultured osteoclasts resorbed the apatite formed on A-W GC by SBF. EHDP has a high affinity for apatite and when administrated is well known to be trapped within apatite in bone tissue [4]. The trapped EHDP is released when osteoclasts absorb bone tissue. Released EHDP enters the osteoclast to stop its activity. In this study, the effect of EHDP on osteoclasts was more obvious when it was attached to the surface of bone-like apatite previously than adding it to culture medium. This suggests that the released EHDP stops the function of osteoclasts (Fig. 3).

Recently, many kinds of bisphosphonates have been developed for treatment of osteoporosis [9]. Bisphosphonates such as EHDP have two different effects: inhibition of apatite formation and suppression of osteoclast function. The former effect is contraindicated for treatment of osteoporosis, whereas the latter effect is therapeutic. It is thus important to suppress the former effect and enhance the latter effect when using a bisphosphonate for treatment of osteoporosis. Thus, an assay of osteoclastic function is necessary in order to develop a new potent bisphosphonate for therapeutic use. Osteoclastic function has been evaluated by culture on male sperm whale dentine [10,11]. In the present study it was shown that bone-like apatite of bioactive ceramics can be used to evaluate the effects of EHDP, suggesting tha it could be a new and effective tool to assay the effects of bisphosphonates. Kokubo *et al* developed a technique for coating plastic or glass with bone-like apatite at room temperature [12]. If this system were used, it would allow observation of osteoclastic absorption using light microscopy, and easy screening for the effects of bisphosphonate on bone.

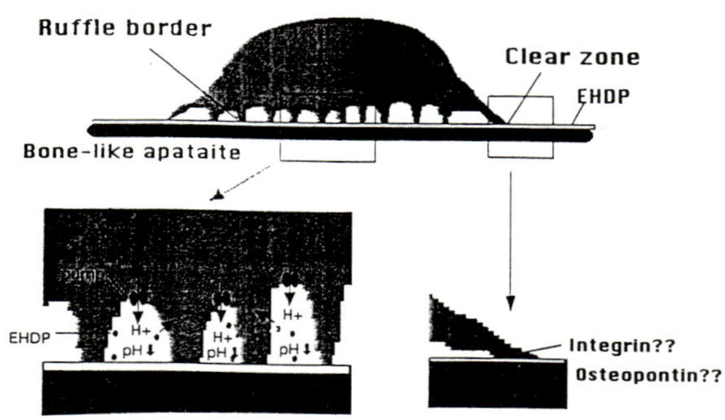

Figure 3. A model of a mechanism of EHDP to inhibit osteoclastic absorption of bone-like apatite.

REFERENCES

1. Neo M., Kotani S., Nakamura T., Ohtsuki C., Bando Y., Kokubo T. and Yamamuro T., J. Biomed. Mater. Res.,1992, 26, 1419-1432.
2. Kokubo T., Kushitani H., Sakka S., Kitsugi T.and Yamamuro T. J. Biomed. Mater. Res. 1990, 24, 721-734.
3. Fleisch, H. Recent Results in Cancer Research 1989, 116, 1-28.
4. Kokubo T., Shigematsu M., Nagashima Y., Nakamura T., Higashi S. and Yamamuro T. Bull. Inst. Chem. Res. Kyoto Univ.1982, 60, 260268.
5. Yamada S., Nakamura T., Kokubo T., Oka M., and Yamamuro T., J.Biomed. Mater. Res 1994,28,1957-1363.
6. Tezuka K., Sato T., Kamioka H., Nijweide P.J., Tanaka K., Matsuo T., Ohta M., Kurihara N., Hakeda Y., and Kumegawa M. Biochem. Biophys. Res. Commun., 1992, 186, 911-917.
7. Kitsugi T., Yamamuro T., Nakamura T., Oka M. and Kokubo T. Calcif. Tissue Int. 1993, 52,378-385.
8. Beek, E.V., Hoekstra M.H., De Ruit M.V., Lowik C. and Papapoulos S., J Bone Miner Res 1994,9,1875-1882.
9. Boyde A. Calcif. Tissue Int., 1991, 49, 65-70.
10. Kokubo T., Kushitani H., Ohtsuki C., Sakka S., and Yamamuro T. J. Mater. Sci. Mater. Med.,3, 79-83 (1992).

BONE CELL RESPONSES TO ARTIFICIALLY PRODUCED SURFACE APATITE LAYERS

J.D. de Bruijn, I. vd Brink, J. vd Meer, P. Nijweide and Y.P. Bovell

Biomaterials Research Group, University of Leiden, Professor Bronkhorstlaan 10, Bldg.57, NL-3723 MB Bilthoven, The Netherlands

ABSTRACT

By applying a "simulated body fluid" solution onto various potential bioactive substrata, a surface apatite layer was formed. Since this layer is thought to represent the intermediate entity through which bone binds to bioactive materials, we studied the responses elicited by both osteoblasts and osteoclasts. These bone cells were derived from bone marrow of either rats (osteoblasts) or chicks (osteoclasts). The mineralized matrix produced by the osteoblasts comprised a fibrillar globules that were intimately associated with the surface apatite layer, and to which collagen fibers were attached. Both large and smaller osteoclasts were capable of resorbing the produced apatite layer, while secreted osteoblast-derived factors were shown to significantly increase the number of osteoclast-like cells.

INTRODUCTION

Bioactive, bone bonding materials such as hydroxyapatite, glass-ceramics, Bioglass® and Polyactive®, are thought to bind with bone through the generation of a surface carbonate-apatite layer. Besides possible biological processes, the formation of this layer is at least partially the result of physico-chemical reactions at the material surface. Kokubo et al. (1992) [4] and Li et al. (1992) [5] have reported that, by using a so-called "simulated body fluid" (SBF), the formation of the surface reactive carbonate-apatite layer can be mimicked in an *in vitro* environment. In a model in which hydroxyapatite and A-W glass ceramic were soaked in a SBF solution, Yamada et al. (1994) [7] have recently reported the resorption of both the surface apatite layer and the underlying bioceramic substrata by rabbit osteoclasts. We have recently shown that osteoclastic resorption of calcium phosphates is potentiated in post-osteogenic culture conditions (de Bruijn et al. 1994) [2], although it could not deduced whether the osteoclast-activating factors were material related or cell mediated. The aim of the present study was therefore (i) to examine the elicited responses of osteoblasts and osteoclasts to surface apatite layers that have been produced on a variety of substrata, and (ii) to examine the effect of osteoblast-derived factors on osteoclast resorptive activity.

MATERIALS AND METHODS

Preparation of the substrata

Five substrata, including hydroxyapatite produced at either 600°C (HA600) or 1250°C (HA1250), tricalcium phosphate (TCP), dentin and heat-treated dentin (8h at 600°C; dentin-HT), were used. The production and characterization of HA600, HA1250 and TCP is described elsewhere [2]. The dentin was heat treated at 600 C to remove the organic phase [3], or was left untreated to act as a control for determining osteoclast resorptive activities.

Formation of a surface apatite layer

All substrata were incubated in 8ml sterile SBF1.5 [3,4] at 37°C, for up to 2 weeks. The SBF was refreshed every 48 hours and collected for calcium-uptake measurements with atomic absorption spectrometry (AAS) [1]. Following this incubation period, the samples were thoroughly washed in distilled water and soaked in culture medium prior to the osteoblast or osteoclast cultures. To examine the effect of osteoblast-derived factors on osteoclast resorptive activities, some SBF treated samples were soaked in conditioned medium of osteoblast cultures prior to the osteoclast cultures. Substrata that had not been immersed in SBF were used as a control for the osteoclast cultures.

Cell culture and specimen evaluation

Rat bone marrow cells were either obtained from rat femora [1], or embryonic chick femora [6]. Approximately 100μl droplets of the primary cell populations were inoculated onto the various substrata. After two hours, culture medium comprising alpha-MEM, 15% FCS and antibiotics was added, and the cells were grown under specific culture conditions to facilitate the differentiation of progenitor cells to either the osteoblast or osteoclast lineage. For the osteoblast cultures, the medium was supplemented with freshly prepared 10mM ß-glycerophosphate, 50μg/ml ascorbic acid and 10^{-8}M dexamethasone, while for the osteoclast cultures 10^{-6}M prostaglandin E2 was added. Cultures were maintained at 37°C in a humidified atmosphere of 10% CO_2. Osteoblast cultures were refed three times weekly and maintained for 3 weeks, while the osteoclast cultures were terminated after 48 hours of culture. After fixing the cells with Karnovsky's fixative, the osteoclast cultures were stained for tartrate-resistant acid phosphatase (TRAP) [2], examined with light microscopy (LM), and both osteoclast and osteoblast cultures were processed for scanning electron microscopy (SEM). Additionally, transmission electron microscopy (TEM) was performed on the osteoblast cultures to examine the elaborated tissue/apatite layer interface.

RESULTS AND DISCUSSION

Substrate immersion in simulated body fluid

Following incubation of the different substrata in SBF, AAS showed a clear difference in the amount of calcium uptake between HA600 and the other materials. As can be deduced from Table 1, approximately 30% calcium uptake was seen for HA600 after two days, while only 0-5% for the other materials. With SEM, an apatite layer was formed on all materials, except for HA600 that showed an increase in grain size after the SBF treatment (Figure 1).

Table 1. Accumulative uptake of calcium from SBF 1.5, by various materials.

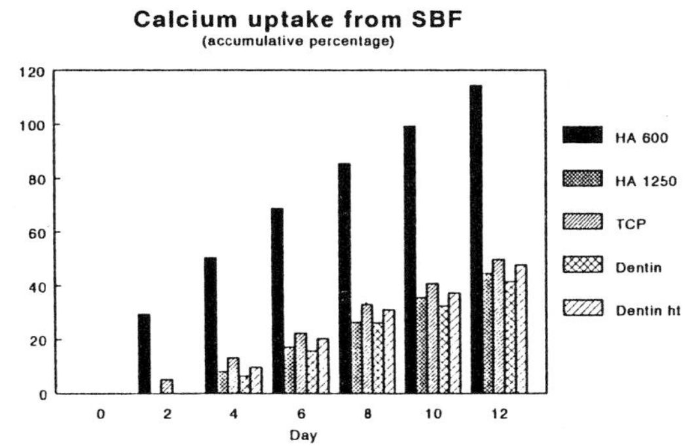

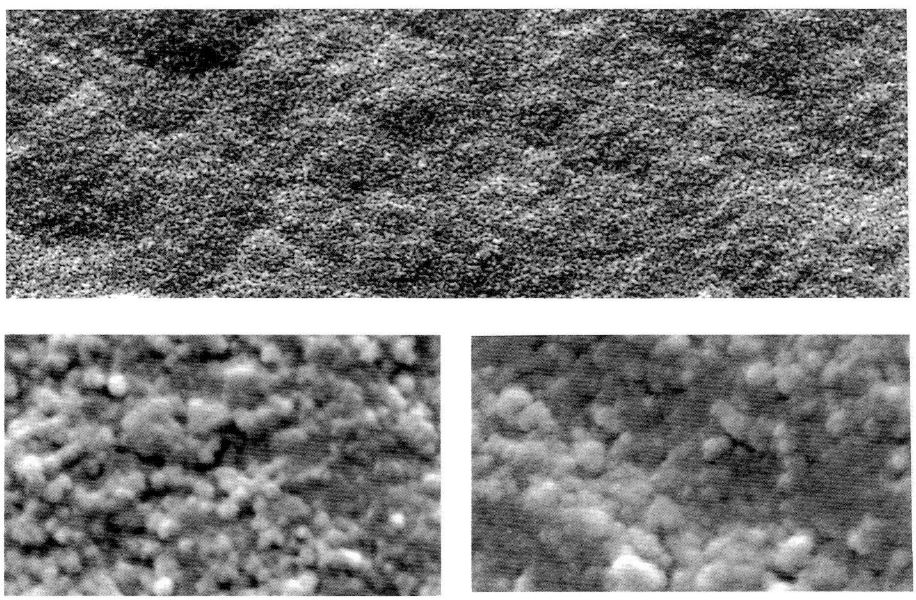

Figure 1. Scanning electron micrographs of (A) an example of an apatite layer formed on dentin, (B) the surface of HA600 prior to, and (C) after immersion in SBF. Field widths: (A) 39 μm; (B,C) 4.8μm.

Osteoblast culture

A cell multilayer had formed and its partial removal revealed a mineralized matrix on the surface of the apatite layer. This matrix comprised small globules to which collagen fibers were attached (Figure 2a). The apatite layer had a thickness of approximately 3μm and was intimately associated with the associated with the mineralized matrix. TEM revealed that the apatite had a layered structure (Figure 2b), which has also been observed at the bone-bioactive material interface [1], and that is probably due to the stages of formation of this layer. Both the mineralized ECM and the apatite layer comprised needle-shaped crystals that were intimately associated.

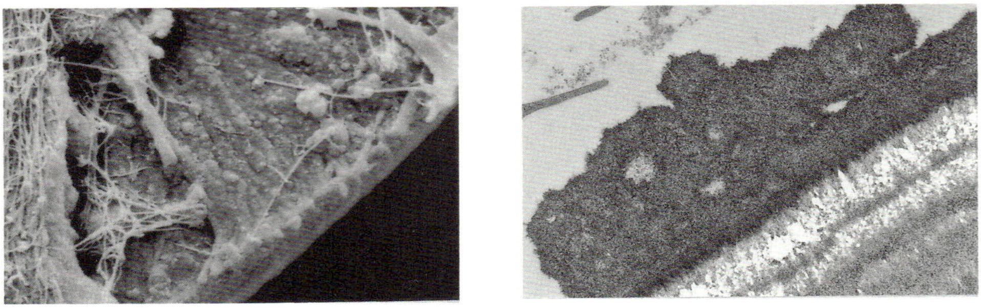

Figure 2. Scanning (A) and transmission (B) electron micrographs showing close approximation between the mineralized extracellular matrix produced by osteoblasts and the apatite layer formed on tissue culture plastic. Field widths: (A) 28.8μm; (B) μm.

Osteoclast culture

Numerous TRAP positive cells were observed on all substrata, irrespective of the presence of an apatite layer. From the control samples, that had not been immersed in SBF, only dentin showed clear scalloped resorption lacunae, while the other substrata were not resorbed by the osteoclasts. Resorption of the apatite layer that had been formed on all substrata after their immersion in SBF, except HA600, was clearly evident. Both small, but also large osteoclasts with a flat appearance, were seen in the resorption lacunae. SEM examination often showed groups of osteoclasts that were associated with a large resorption lacunae, although single osteoclasts were also seen in smaller resorption lacunae. From the underlying substrata, only dentin and TCP showed signs of resorption (Figure 3), while most resorption lacunae were seen on dentin. Neither of the other substrata were resorbed by the osteoclasts.

Effect of conditioned medium on osteoclasts

When samples were soaked in conditioned medium from osteoblast cultures, significantly more TRAP positive cells were present (Table 2). It could, however, not be concluded whether the cells were also more resorptive-active.

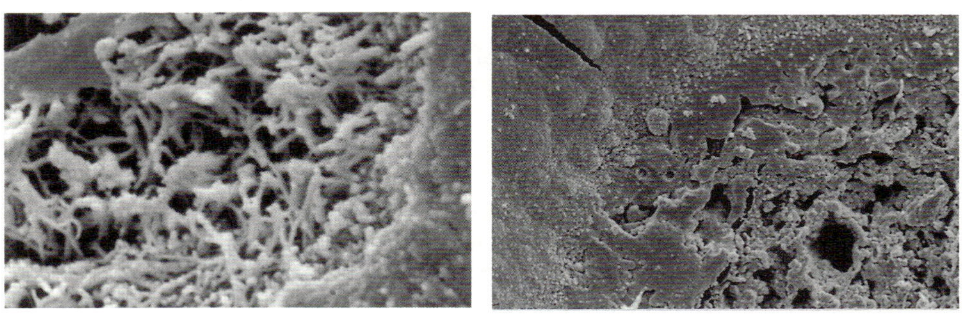

Figure 3. Scanning electron micrographs of osteoclasts resorbing dentin (A) and TCP on which an apatite layer is present (B). Field widths: (A) 18μm; (B) 48μm.

Table 2. Graph showing the number of TRAP-positive cells grown in the presence (+) or absence (-) of osteoblast-derived conditioned medium.

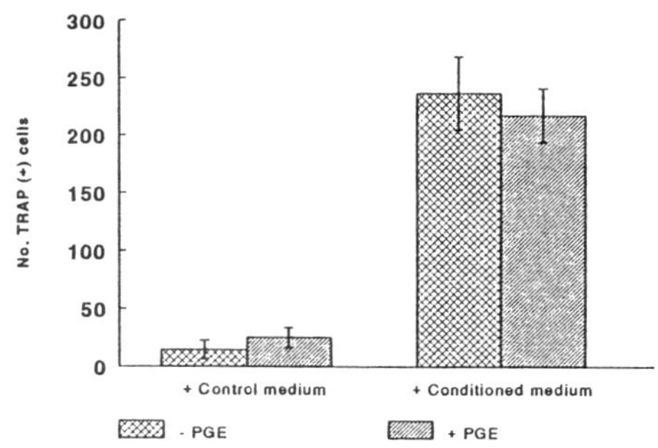

The results of this study show that an intimate interface is formed between the artificially produced apatite layer and newly formed bone tissue. The a fibrillar globular mineralized accretions, seen with SEM, are similar to our previous observations [1,2] and are suggested to represent the early stages of bone formation. This cementing substance was intimately integrated with the artificially produced apatite layer, to form a homogenous interface (see Figure 2b). The results of the osteoclast cultures show that the bone-like surface apatite layer can be resorbed by osteoclasts and might act as a stimulant for osteoclastic resorptive activity. This was deduced from the observation that TCP on which an apatite layer was present, was resorbed by osteoclasts, whereas pure TCP substrata were not. The presence of bone-like apatite is however not the only stimulant for osteoclastic resorption, because HA600 that had been soaked in SBF was not resorbed by osteoclasts in these experiments. This observation is substantiated by results from earlier experiments [2], in which HA600 was resorbed by osteoclasts after osteoblasts had been grown on the substrate surface. The influence of osteoblast-derived proteinaceous substances on osteoclastic activities is therefore expected to play an important role. The absence of resorption on heat-treated dentin, from which all organic material was removed, is an illustration of this hypothesis. The significant increase in the number of osteoclasts after treatment of the substrates with osteoblast-conditioned medium (see Table 2), is another example. Future studies will be directed towards examining the role of specific proteins and other substances (e.g. ions) in their influence on osteoclastic activities.

REFERENCES

1. de Bruijn, J.D., Flach, J.S., de Groot, K., van Blitterswijk, C.A. and Davies, J.E., *Cells and Materials* 1993, 3, 115-127.
2. de Bruijn, J.D., Bovell, Y.P., Davies, J.E. and van Blitterswijk, C.A., *J. Biomed. Mater. Res.* 1994, 28, 105-112.
3. de Bruijn, J.D., Bovell, Y.P., vd Meer, J., Nijweide, P. and Li, P., in *Trans. 21st Ann. Soc. Biomater.*, San Francisco, 1995, p 152.
4. Kokubo, T., in *Bone-bonding Biomaterials*, Reed Healthcare Communications, Leiderdorp, 1992, 31-46.

5. Li P., Ohtsuki, C., Kokubo, T., Nakanish, K., Soga, N., Nakamura, T. and Yamamuro, T., *J. Am. Ceram. Soc.*, 1992, 75, 2094-2097.
6. Ravesloot, J.H., *Proc. Natl. Acad. Sci. USA,* 1989, 86, 6821-6825.
7. Yamada, S., Nakamura, T., Kokubo, T., Oka, M. and Yamamuro, T. *Cells and Materials*, 1994, 4, 347-356.

BEHAVIOR OF BIOACTIVE GLASS IN HUMAN BONE

J.T. Heikkilä[1], K.T. Mattila[2], Ö.H. Andersson[3], J. Knuuti[2], A. Yli-Urpo[4], A.J. Aho[1]

[1]Departments of Surgery and [2]Diagnostic Imaging, Turku University Hospital, Kiinanmyllynkatu 4-8, 20520 TURKU. [3]Turku Centre for Biomaterials, Lemminkäisenkatu 2, 20520 TURKU and Department of Chemical Engineering, Åbo Akademi University, 20500, TURKU, FINLAND. [4]Institute of Dentistry, University of Turku, 20500 TURKU, FINLAND.

ABSTRACT

A prospective, randomized study was conducted to compare bioactive glass (BG) with autogenous bone (AB) as a filler in benign bone tumor surgery. The patients selection was made by the Turku University Bone Tumor Group. Preoperative examinations and postoperative follow-up included plain films, computed tomography (CT), magnetic resonance imaging (MRI) and single photon emission computed tomography (SPECT). The mean follow-up period for the 12 patients was 15 months (range 4 to 24). No complications related to the filler materials were observed. All wounds healed well without signs of infection. The repair of the defects filled with BG granules started from the periphery and advanced into the deeper parts of the defects during the follow-up. Plain films and CT revealed no resorptive changes at the BG-bone interface. Bony sclerosis appeared both at the bone margins and outer part of the bone defect. Contrast enhanced MRI indicated ingrowth of fibrovascular tissue into the spaces between the granules. In radioisotope examinations using SPECT a centripetal activation of the defects was observed. One defect was explored one year postoperatively and the retrieved specimen analysed using histology, scanning electron microscopy and energy dispersing X-ray analysis.

INTRODUCTION

The routine practice for benign bone tumor has been curettage and filling of the defect with autogenous bone chips. Since 1889 [1] the search for bone substitutes has been carried out. Boiled xenograft bone, allogenous bone, demineralized bone, tricalciumphosphate, hydroxylapatite, calcium carbonate, coralline based hydroxylapatite, bioactive glass and bioactive glass-ceramics have been proposed for clinical use as bone substitutes.

Bioactive glass is biocompatible, bone bonding [2], non-toxic [3] and osteoconductive [4,5]. Good results in animal experiments have been achieved with these materials [4,5,6]. A randomized double-blind controlled clinical study was conducted to compare bioactive glass granules (BG) with autogenous bone (AB) in reconstruction of cystic bone tumors after curettage.

MATERIALS AND METHODS

The study protocol has been approved by the local ethical committee and the patients have been chosen by the Turku University Bone Tumor Group. Until now 12 patient have been operated, 9 in the BG and 3 in the AB group. The patient and tumor data is summarized in Table 1. A cortical fenestration was performed and the tumor was visualized. A biopsy of the tumor was taken to confirm the preoperative clinical and radiological diagnosis. The tumor was evacuated by meticulous curettage. The edges and corners of the defect were carefully drilled with a special drill to remove the tumor capsule and to refresh the bone surface. The defect was filled either with autogenous bone harvested from iliac crest or with bioactive glass (S53P4) granules (Ø 630 - 3150 μm). The composition of the bioactive glass given in weight percentage is: SiO_2 53 %, Na_2O 23 %, CaO 20 % and P_2O_5 4 %. The preparation of the glass has been published earlier [7]. Autogenous bone was harvested from the iliac crest through fenestration of the crest. Only cancellous bone was used. The cortical piece of bone, turned aside during the fenestration, was fixed into its original site with absorbable sutures. The wound was closed anatomically in layers.

Table 1. The patient data. Ench. = enchondroma, ABC = aneurysmal bone cyst.

ID	age/sex	fil	tumor	vol cm^3	site	follow up	compl
1.	18/male	gr	ABC	136	prox. humerus	24	-
2.	34/fem	gr	enhc.	2,6	dig.manus	23	-
3.	44/fem	gr	ench.	3,3	dig.manus	23	infl. of scar
4.	23/male	ab	ench.	4	dig.manus	20	-
5.	43/male	ab	ench.	1	dig.manus	18	-
6.	18/fem	gr	non-oss. fibroma	270	dist.tibia	18	-
7.	29/fem	gr	recid. ench.	1	dig.manus	13	bending reoper
8.	33/male	gr	ench.	1.1	dig.manus	14	-
9.	37/fem	gr	cysta	2	navic.pedis	13	-
10.	16/male	gr	non-oss. fibroma	5	dist.tibia	7	fissure
11.	21/fem	ab	cysta	3	patella	6	fracture
12.	45/fem	gr	ench.	5,6	dig.manus	4	-

Preoperative and postoperative examinations at 2 weeks and 3, 8, 12, 18 and 24 months included laboratory tests for general welfare of the patients, liver function and inflammatory reaction; plain films, computed tomography (CT), magnetic resonance imaging (MRI) with and without contrast enhancement. The patients underwent bone scintigraphies 3, 8, 12 and 24 months postoperatively. Three hours after injection of ^{99m}Tc-DPD (^{99m}Tc dicarboxypropane diphosphonate) anterior and posterior static images were acquired. To estimate the activity of metabolic process a ratio of counts obtained from the operated and the reference (normal bone region) was calculated. In the large defects (Ø > 3 cm) also single photon emission computed tomography (SPECT) was performed [8]. One defect in the middle phalanx of finger needed exploration and was biopsied. The undecalcified biopsy specimen was embedded in methacrylate, sectioned, ground and finally polished with 4000 grit SiC- paper [9]. The specimen was coated with carbon and studied by scanning electron microscopy (SEM) and energy dispersive x-ray analysis (EDXA). After this histological sections were prepared and stained with toluidine blue, van Gieson and von Kossa methods.

RESULTS

Clinical results

No tumor recurrence nor wound infections have been observed in either group. In the BG group postoperative bending of the middle phalanx occurred and was explored. One longitudinal fissure of tibia in the BG group was diagnosed two months postoperatively and one fracture of the patella occurred in the AB group while dancing Finnish polka 4 weeks postoperatively. The tibial fissure healed untreated, whereas the patellar fracture needed casting for 4 weeks. In laboratory tests no signs of inflammatory reactions or elevated liver function levels were observed.

Radiological findings

On plain films the cortical callus appeared at 2 months, surrounding the postoperative cortical defect. The callus increased and the cortex thickened thereafter (Fig. 1). On CT there was full bony union at the fenestration site at 8 months (Fig. 2). No signs of resorption at the interface between BG granules and host bone was detected. At 8 months the granules appeared somewhat unsharp, but still clearly more dense than the host bone. A sclerotic rim appeared at the margins of the defect at 12 months. On MRI (Fig. 3) the outer part of large cavities (Ø > 3 cm) had marked contrast enhancement at three months. The enhanced area increased towards the center of the lesion with time. The narrow edematous ring at the margins of the defect disappeared after 3 months.

Scintigraphy and SPECT

In all patients increased metabolic activity was detected in the operation region during the follow-up period. The preliminary results obtained from these patients suggest, that in the AB-group the metabolic activity of the defect was highest at the first examination at 3 months and decreased gradually during the healing phase thereafter. In contrast to this, more variable findings were detected in the BG-group. The metabolic activity in the operated region was still increasing 3 months postoperatively, suggesting a prolonged healing process.

In patients with large defects the first bone SPECT at 3 months after operation showed moderately increased tracer uptake at the borders of the filled cavity. No activity was seen in the center of the cavity. In the following examinations at 8 and 12 months

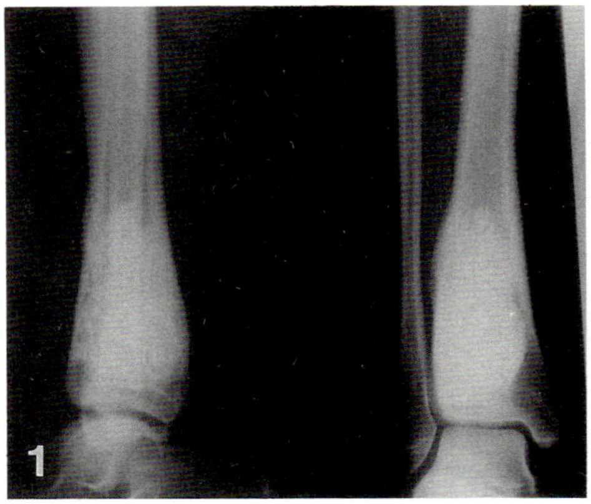

Figure 1. Postoperative defect in the distal tibia filled with BG granules (Patient #6). Plain films show the callus formation and thickening of the cortex. (12 months postoperatively)

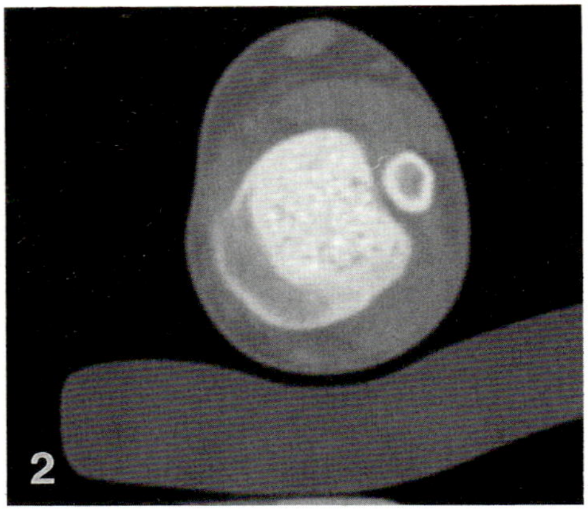

Figure 2. CT slice. (Patient #6) granules still clearly visible in the defect, but somewhat unsharp. (12 months postoperatively)

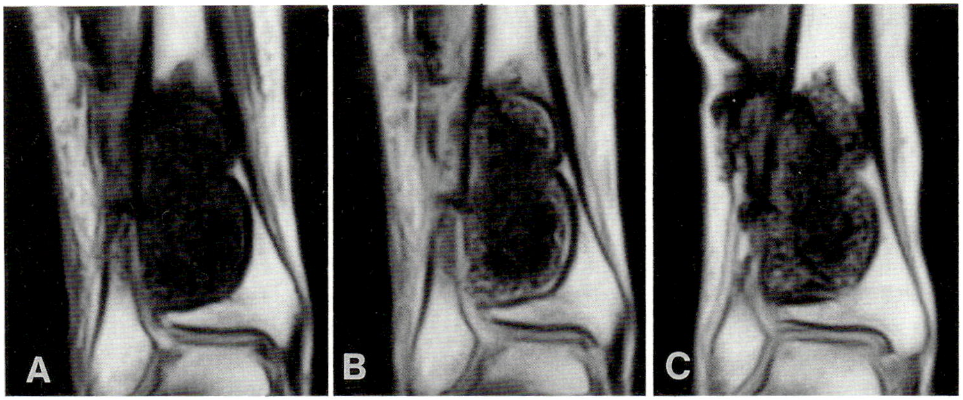

Figure 3. MRI image without contrast enhancement at 3 months (A). The same image at 3 months with contrast enhancement (B). The contrast enhancement is stronger at the margins of the defect, and proceeds inwards into the defect at 8 months (C). (Patient #6)

after operation the tracer uptake was further enhanced and the metabolic activity gradually increased inside of the cavity (Fig. 4).

Histology

During the exploration, the defect in the middle phalanx of the finger was found consolidated throughout. The sample broke into small pieces during removal. In histology using a toluidine blue staining method, an occasional inflammatory reaction was observed as lymphocytes and some granulocytes. The spaces between the granules were filled with lamellar bone, unmature bone, fibrous tissue and some areas of cartilage. Using van Gieson staining method, in areas where the tissue sample remained intact during

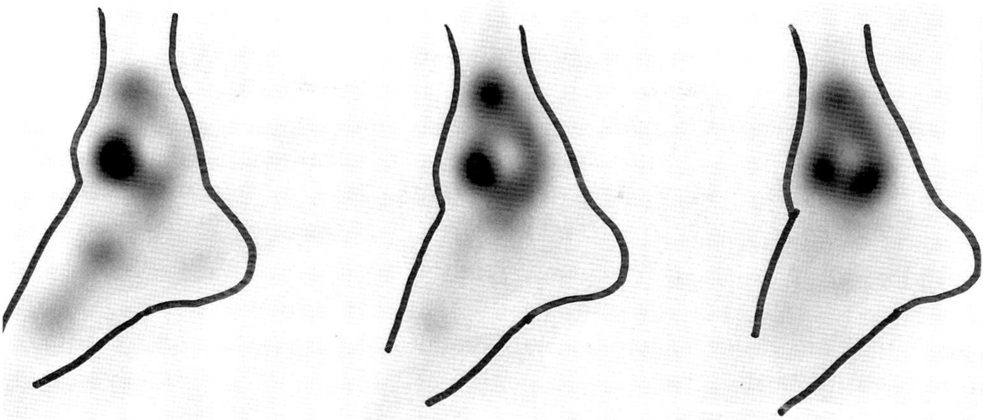

Figure 4. The coronal SPECT slice from the distal tibial region at 3 months (left), 8 months (middle) and 12 months (right) postoperatively. In the later images the tracer uptake is seen also inside the cavity. (Patient #6)

exploration, the granules were seen incorporated partly with bone and in some areas with fibrous tissue. At the surface of a few granules resorptive-like changes were observed.

EDXA and SEM

In SEM a large amount of mineralized tissue was observed. All granules showed a characteristic Ca,P-rich surface layer. EDXA showed that the Ca,P-rich layer corresponded to about half the thickness of the total reaction layer.

DISCUSSION

Clinically BG granules were well accepted without any adverse effects. All defects consolidated in 2 - 3 months. The one reoperation was due to inadequate splinting during the consolidation phase. All laboratory tests used were within the normal range during the follow-up.

Previously granular deproteinized bone, tricalcium phosphate, porous and interporous hydroxylapatite have been used with good clinical results in reconstruction of benign bone tumors after curettage [10,11,12,13,14]. No biopsies have been published in these reports.

On plain films the margins of BG granules became unsharp at 3 months. This does not however indicate bone bonding as shown by Morti et al. [15]. Nevertheless, the same observation was made on CT. There was consolidation between the host bone and granules at the margins of the defect. The sclerotic union appeared between the outer part of the granules and host bone at 12 months. No resorptive changes or signs of edema were noted on MRI after 3 months. Contrast enhancement in MRI indicates ingrowth of vascularized tissue from the margins of the defect. The reaction increased and proceded inwards to the defect as observed earlier with other bone substitute materials by microangiography [16]. In nuclear medicine studies technetium labelled DPD has been shown to bind to osteoblasts, and it can be regarded as an osteoblast-marker. The activity increase seen in SPECT was very similar to the one seen in MRI with contrast enhancement. It is normally not possible to obtain postoperative biopsies from these patients. The exploration provided us a sample of a finger phalanx almost totally filled with bioactive glass granules.

Clinically it was consolidated at the time of exploration. During the operation, solid material was curettaged from the defect. The solid bone at the margins of the defect remained untouched. In the retrieved specimen fibrous tissue, cartilage-like tissue and bone was observed. The specimen included only the tissue component which could be curettaged from the defect. Lamellar bone at the margin of the defect was not included in the specimen. All these observations together indicate bone formation in clinical bone defects filled with bioactive glass granules. The results demonstrate that bioactive glass alone can be used as a filler in bone defects.

REFERENCES

1. Senn N. Amer J Med Sci 1889;98:219.
2. Hench LL, Splinter RJ, Allen WC, Greenlee TK. J Biomed Mater Res 1972; Symp.2:17-41.
3. Wilson J, Pigott GH, Schoen FJ, Hench LL. J Biomed Mater Res 1981;15:805-17.
4. Schepers E, DeClercq M, Ducheyne P, Kempeneers R. J Oral Rehab 1991;18:439-52.
5. Heikkilä JT, Aho HT, Yli-Urpo A, Happonen R-P, Aho AJ. Acta Orth Scand 1993;64:678-82.
6. Wilson J, Yu LT, Beale BS. Abstract book of the 19th Annual Meeting of the Society for Biomaterials, Birmingham, USA.
7. Andersson ÖH, Liu G, Karlsson KH, Niemi L, Miettinen J, Juhanoja J. J Mater Sci, Mater Medicine 1990;1:219-27.
8. Fogelman I. Bone scanning. In: Maisey MN, Britton KE, Gilday DL (Eds.) Clinical Nuclear Medicine. Chapman et Hall, London 1991.
9. Donath K, Breuner G. J Oral Pathol 1982;11:318-26.
10. Hallén LG. Acta Orthop scand 1966;37:1-19.
11. Nicholas RW, Lange TA. Clin Orthop 1994;306:197-203.
12. Inoue O, Ibaraki K, Shimabukuro H, Shinkagi Y. Clin Orthop 293:287-92.
13. Bucholz RW, Carlton A, Holmes RE. Clin Orthop 1989:240,53-62.
14. Bucholz RW, Carlton A, Holmes RE. Orthop Clin NA 1987;18:323-34.
15. Morti T, Koshino T, Odaka T, Negami S. In Ceramics in Clinical Applications, pp.361-8. Ed. P Vincenzini. Materials Science Monographs, 39. Elsevier, 1987.
16. Viikari SJ, Aho AJ. Ann Chir Gyn Fenn 1963;52:665-78.

IN-VIVO STUDY OF THE DEGRADATION OF 4 DIFFERENT-COMPOSITION ACTIVE GLASSES

A.M. Gatti, L. Hench*, E. Monari, L. Chiarini, S. Bulgarelli and D. Tanza

Centro dei Biomateriali. Dip. Chirurgia, Univ. Modena, Italy
*Bioglass® Research Center, Univ. Florida, Alachua, Florida, USA

ABSTRACT

The present study investigates the behavior of 4 different glasses, used as granules for bone repair, to understand the influence of the composition in bone stimulation and their degradation in a biological environment. The glasses were implanted in dorsal muscles of 2 rabbits and in mandibular pockets of a sheep. After 1 and 3 months in rabbits and 40 days in sheep the biological tissues containing the granules were explanted and the sections observed under scanning electron microscope with an x-ray microprobe for elemental evaluations.

The results showed the difference of behavior of the glasses against soft and hard tissues.

INTRODUCTION

In implantology many different materials are used as prostheses to replace tissues. Inert or materials when placed, for instance, in a bone defect, give no chemical interaction with the biological surroundings, but only a physical one. In contrast, active biomaterials can interact with tissues through a degradation of the materials and a consequent ion release [1-6]. These ions released can interact with the cellular metabolism, for example by speeding up some reactions, or, when they are biological by-products, they are catabolized. The present work deals with some active glasses used for bone repair. These glasses, used as granules to fill bone defects, can increase the velocity of the bone growth and develop a chemical bond with bone. The aim of the work is the evaluation of the behavior of 4 different compositions implanted in soft and hard tissues.

MATERIALS AND METHODS

Four glasses were developed by Prof. L. Hench (AMRC, Univ. of Florida, USA). The first was similar to the well-known Bioglass® [7,8]; the others differ by having an increasing silicon content in Table 1. The glasses are designated by their silicon content.

Table 1. Composition in mole per cent (%) of the 4 glasses.

	SiO_2	CaO	Na_2O	P_2O_5
45S	46.1	26.9	24.4	2.6
52S	52.1	23.8	21.5	2.6
55S	55.1	22.2	20.1	2.6
60S	60.1	19.6	17.7	2.6

The glasses were obtained by melting and crushed into granules by means of a ball-mill. The selected fractions, ranging from 300 to 500 mm, were EtOx sterilized.

The experiment was divided into two parts:

a: implantation of the granules in pockets surgically created in 2 rabbits' dorsal muscles for 1 and 3 months;

b: implantation in 4-mm-diameter holes surgically drilled in a sheep's mandible for 5 months.

After sacrifice, the bone or the biological tissues containing the granules were explanted, fixed in 4% paraformaldehyde, dehydrated in increasing concentrations of ethanol and embedded in methylmethacrylate resin. Thin (90mm) and thick (200mm) sections were cut with a diamond saw (Accutom, Struers, Germany), polished with silicon carbide papers and diamond paste. The thick sections were coated with carbon film to be observed under a Scanning Electron Microscope (SEM, Philips 500, The Netherlands) in secondary emission and back-scattered (BSE) mode with an Energy Dispersion System (EDS, EDAX 9900,The Netherlands) for x-ray microanalyses of materials and biological interfaces. Through this system it is possible to detect sodium and inorganic elements with atomic weights higher than sodium. In the same way, the original glass granules were also observed to check the homogeneity in morphology and in distribution of the elements inside the granules before implantation. Thin sections were ground to 20-30 m thickness, dyed with basic fucsin and observed by optical microscopy (Zeiss, Germany).

RESULTS

First, the original glasses were studied under SEM and EDS to determine the homogeneity of the distribution of the elements present, i.e. silicon, sodium, calcium and phosphorus.

After implantation, the granules of each composition lose their homogeneity from a morphological and a compositional point of view. From a histological point of view, the granules implanted in rabbits' muscles and in sheep's bone dyed with basic fuchsin and methylene-blue show an outer layer. The thickness of this layer decreases with the increase of the silicon. In 60S glass this layer is almost absent. Some macrophages are seen around the granules with low Si, but only few around the 60S glass. The sharp edges took up more dye than the flat surfaces. The granules appear crossed by fractures. The SEM observations reveal that the original homogeneity of the elemental distribution is lost. Figure 1 shows some granules of 52S in rabbit after 1-month implantation in back-scattered mode and the x-ray dot maps for Si, P, K and Ca. Sodium is immediately released and is, therefore, absent. On the other hand potassium, which is not included in

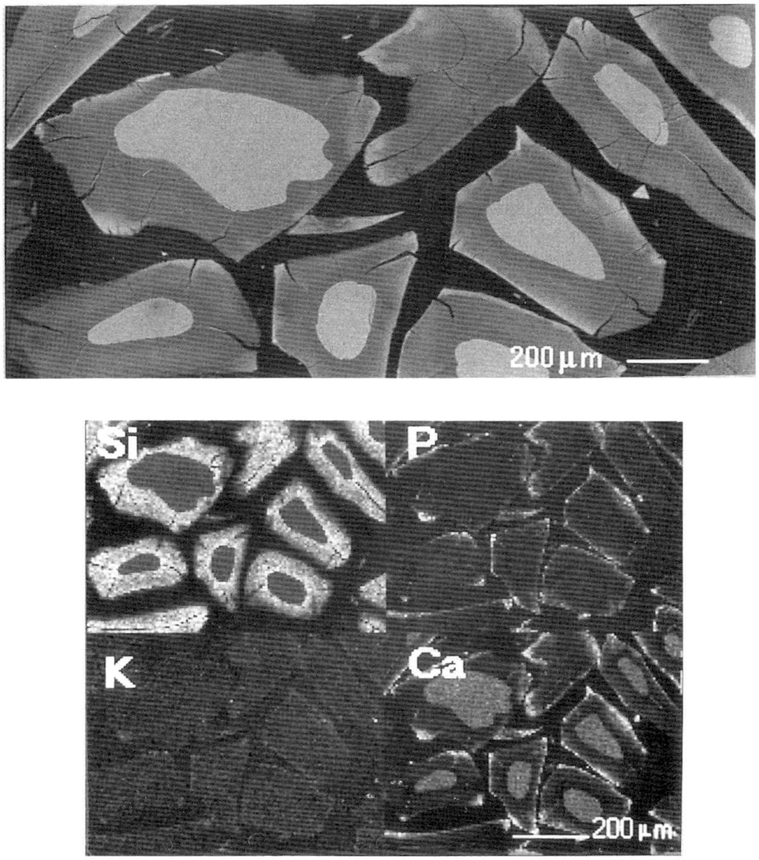

Figure 1. Microphotograph in back-scattered mode of 52S granules after 30 days' implantation in rabbit's muscle, with x-ray dot maps for Si, P, K and Ca.

the original composition, appears in the outer layer. This appearance was noted for other glasses after implantation [9]. The external layer is rich in Ca and P. Close to that there is a Si-rich layer. After a three-month implantation the 45S granules appear exhausted, i.e. the core is void and only the outer layer remains, completely transformed into a Calcium-phosphate layer.

The behavior of the glasses is similar with respect to degradation, but occurs with different velocities, so for the same time of implantation, the morphology and thickness of the interfaces are different. After 3-months' implantation, the 60S glass granules present a thick undegraded core and a degraded external part without the Ca,P-rich layer.

A behavior similar to degradation occurs in the granules implanted in mandibular bone, but other phenomena are observed as well. All the glasses develop a close contact with bone, even if at such a short implantation time no substantial differences are seen. The 45S granules (Fig. 2) appear fragmented and few of them have an intact core with the original composition.

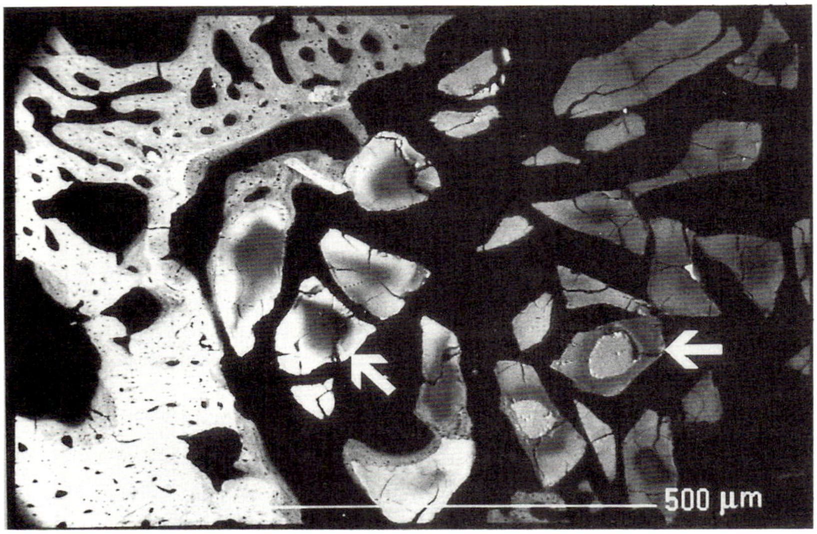

Figure 2. Microphotograph in back-scattered mode of 45S granules implanted in mandibular bone. The white arrows indicate the difference among the granules close to the bone and those far from it.

Some granules have the central part darker than the external layer. That means that no heavy elements are present. In the particles near the bone and surrounded by it, it is difficult to distinguish the border line of the granules, since the outer layer has the same electronic density of bone.

For the 53S, 55S and 60S glasses, small, needle-shaped crystals of calcium-phosphate appear on the surface of the granules (Fig. 3). The EDS analyses reveal that the P content of these precipitates is greater than that in bone, so the Ca/P is about 1.2 instead 1.9 found in bone, as it is possible to see from spectra of Figure 4.

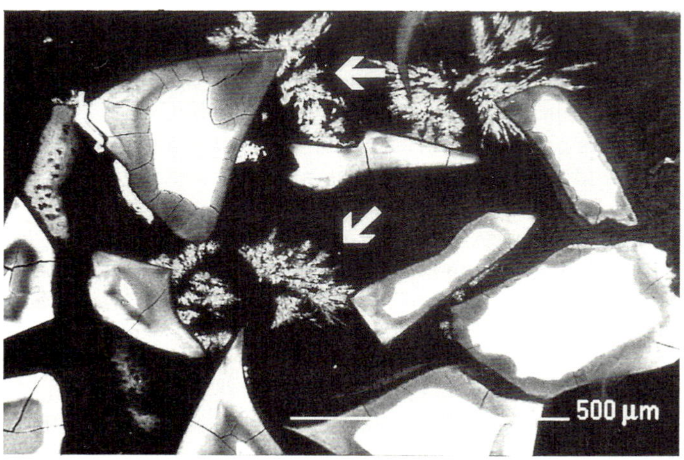

Figure 3. Microphotograph of 55S granules in the middle of the drilled hole in the mandibular bone. The arrows indicate the presence of crystals near the granules.

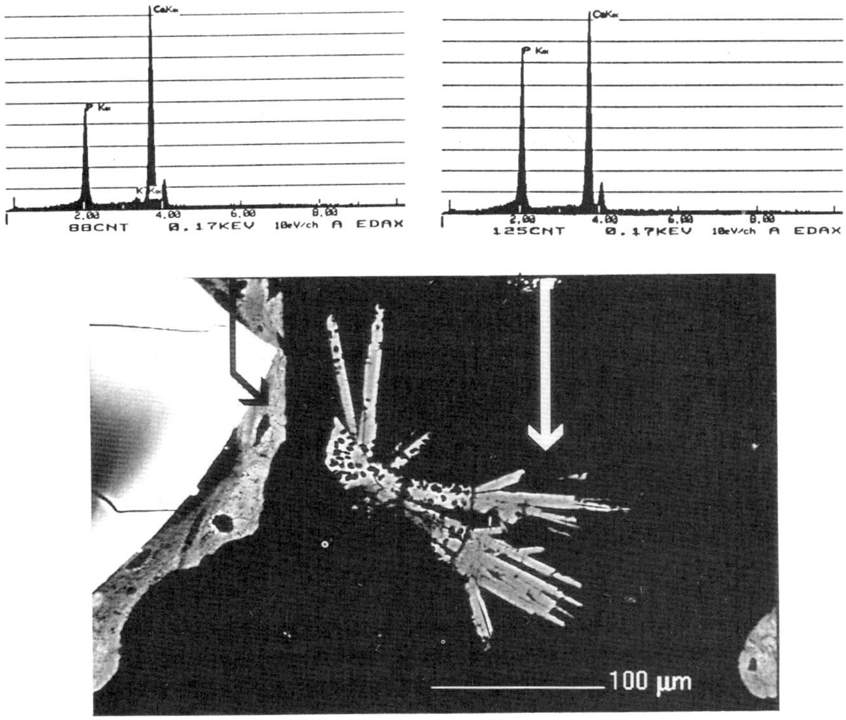

Figure 4. Microphotograph of a crystal with the EDS spectra detected in bone (black arrow) and in the crystal (white arrow).

CONCLUSIONS

The study showed that implantation in rabbits' muscles is a good means to study degradation of active glasses in a short time, but it cannot substitute for implantation in bone since other phenomena can occur in bone. In bone, in presence of 52S and 55S glass granules (less with 60S) there is the precipitation of calcium-phosphate crystals near the granules with higher percentage of silicon. The crystals probably can be formed by the ions released from the glasses combined with those present in the environment. Thus, a substrate in which the bone cells can proliferate is developed. That was the theoretical base for the development of the active glasses.

The 52S and 55S compositions seem more suitable than 45S for stimulation of bone formation in the bone defects, but other tests of implantation in sheep bone for a longer time are necessary to check the long term behavior of these compositions.

REFERENCES

1. Hench, L.L., Splinter, R.J., Allen, W.C. and Greenlee, T.K., *J. Bio. Mater. Res. Symp.* 1971, 2, 117-141.
2. Gatti A.M., Zaffe, D. and Andersson, Ö.H., in *Bioceramics and Human Body*, Elsevier, New York 1992, 402-407.
3. Gross, U. and Strunz, V., *J. Biomed. Mater. Res.* 1980, 14, 607-618.

4. Hench, L.L. and Wilson, J., in *Ciba Foundation Symposium* Volume 121, J. Wiley & Sons, New York 1986, 231-246.
5. Wilson, J., Low, S., Fetner, A. and Hench, L.L., in *Biomaterials in Clinical Applications* Elsevier, Amsterdam, 1987, 223-228.
6. Andersson, Ö.H. and Karlsson, K.H., *J. Non-Cryst. Solids* 1991, 129, 145-151.
7. Hench, L.L. and Paschall, H.A., *J. Biomed. Mater. Res.* 1977, 4, 25-42.
8. Clark, D.E., Ethridge, E.C. and Hench, L.L., *Phys. and Chem. of Glasses* 1979, Vol 20, 2, 35-40.
9. Gatti, A.M. and Zaffe, D., *Biomaterials* 1991a, 12, 345-350.

ANALYSIS OF OSTEOBLASTIC ACTIVITY AT THE SURFACE OF B-TCP USING *IN SITU* HYBRIDIZATION

M. Neo[1], C. Voigt[2], H. Herbst[1], and U. Gross[1]

[1]Institute of Pathology and [2]Department of Traumatology and Reconstructive Surgery, University Hospital Benjamin Franklin, Free University, Hindenburgdamm 30, D12200 Berlin, FRG

ABSTRACT

To assess the effects of β-tricalcium phosphate (β-TCP) on osteoblasts an *in vivo*, *in situ* hybridization technique was applied. A hole was drilled in rabbit femurs, and a β-TCP cylinder was implanted or, as a control, the hole remained empty. Specimens were collected at 3, 7, 14, 28 days after operation and hybridized with a procollagen $\alpha 1$ (I) RNA probe. Temporal and spatial expression of collagen I mRNA in osteoblasts around β-TCP was comparable to that of the control, suggesting that β-TCP had no remarkable acceleration or suppression of the bone-forming activity of osteoblasts.

INTRODUCTION

Bioactive materials differ in bioactivity, that is, the rate and the velocity of bone formation on the surface of the materials differ [1]. However, it is poorly understood whether bioactive materials stimulate bone formation or not. It is generally considered that bioactive materials only provide a biocompatible surface and bone formation on them is osteoconductive. However, some investigators have reported that bioactive materials had some positive effects on bone formation. Ohgushi et al. have demonstrated that some bioactive materials could differentiate stromal bone marrow cells into osteoblasts on their surface, whereas non-bioactive materials did not [2]. Hench speculated that only class A bioactive materials (such as Bioglass®) could stimulate osteoblasts, owing to the release of soluble silicon [3].

In the present study, a new experimental method using an *in situ* hybridization technique has been developed in order to investigate the effects of a bioactive material on bone formation. *In situ* hybridization with non-radioactive cRNA probe for procollagen $\alpha 1$(I) visualized activated osteoblasts clearly. As the first step, β-TCP implanted bones were investigated chronologically, and were compared with bones with an empty hole as a control.

MATERIALS AND METHODS

Materials

Cylinders of β-TCP 4 mm in diameter and 8 mm in length were provided by Mitsubishi Material Co., Ltd. They were sintered at 1150 °C for 1 hour. The porosity was 1.5 % and average surface roughness was 1.12 ± 0.09 μm. No other Ca-P phase was detected by X-ray diffraction. They were sterilized by autoclaving.

Surgery

A hole 4 mm in diameter was drilled in both epiphyses of the distal femurs of female chinchilla rabbits in an antero-postero direction. Drilling was done under a constant flow of physiological NaCl solution. In 7 rabbits, the β-TCP cylinder was implanted into the hole of both femurs in press-fit manner. In the other 7 rabbits the holes remained empty without implantation (control). Two rabbits of each group were sacrificed 3, 7, 14 days after operation respectively and one rabbit in each group was sacrificed 28 days after operation.

The specimens were fixed by perfusion of 4% paraformaldehyde solution at the sacrifice, were further fixed in the same solution for 1 day, and then decalcified for 10 days by EDTA. After being embedded in paraffin, sections of 4 μm thickness were cut.

In situ hybridization

For the preparation of digoxygenin labeled RNA probe, pα1R1 was used, which encodes 1.3 kb fragment of rat $\alpha 1$(I) procollagen cDNA and subcloned into plasmid pGEM 1 [4]. The plasmid was linearized and transcribed with digoxygenin-UTP appropriately to generate antisense or sense strands.

In situ hybridization was done according to the method of Milani et al. [5] with some modifications. Briefly, the sections were deparaffinized, immersed in 0.2N HCl and treated with pronase. Then the sections were fixed by paraformaldehyde and acetilated in acetic anhydride diluted 0.1 M triethanolamine. 25 μl of hybridization mixture containing 1-2 μl/ml digoxygenin-UTP labeled probe was applied to each section for about 18 hrs. at 52 °C. After hybridization, the sections were washed for 3 hrs. at 54 °C in a washing solution and treated with RNAse-A. Then the sections were further rinsed in 2 x SSC/0.1 % SDS and 0.1 x SSC/0.1 % SDS respectively. Digoxygenin was then detected using an anti-digoxygenin-AP Fab fragments. Positive signal was detected as red and the counterstaining was performed with haemalaun.

RESULTS

The positive red signal was observed only in the specimens hybridized with the antisense probe and was not detected in the specimens hybridized with sense probe. Both osteoblasts and fibroblasts showed positive signal although the signal in the osteoblasts was stronger. Discrimination between these two kinds of cell was made based on the differences in location, shape and size of cells and structure and stainability of extracellular matrix.

Control bone

In 3-day specimens, the holes were filled up with red blood cells and fibrin clots, and debris of the bone was observed around the holes. Many trabeculae adjacent to the hole were devitalized perhaps because of the impaired circulation. Few osteoblasts lining the trabeculae around the hole showed positive signals.

In day-7 specimens, new bone was formed actively towards the center of the hole. Osteoblasts lining the newly formed trabeculae and osteocytes encased in them showed positive signals (Fig. 1). At the innermost part of the bone formation, positive cells colonized, which suggested further inward new bone formation. Fibroblasts in the hole also showed weak signals.

In day-14 specimens, the number of positive osteoblasts around the hole decreased, although many osteoblasts still showed positive signals. The colonization with positive cells, which was observed in the day-7 specimens, was not demonstrated. In some areas, fibrosis at the center of the hole with weakly positive fibroblasts, was observed.

In day-28 specimens, many of the osteoblasts around the hole, especially those facing the hole, were no longer positive.

β-TCP-implanted bone

In day-3 specimens, the devitalized trabeculae and bone debris were observed around the material. Few osteoblasts showed positive signals.

In day-7 specimens, active new bone formation around the material was observed. Osteoblasts lining the newly formed bone and osteocytes encased in them showed positive signals (Fig. 2). New bone formation seemed to have begun from originally existing trabeculae or bone debris. Although osteoblasts with positive signals were observed on the material surface in some regions, they were always near the sites of new bone formation. A layer of negative cells was sometimes seen between positive osteoblasts and the material. Fibroblasts with weaker signal were also observed on the surface of the material between bone forming areas.

In day-14 specimens, more areas of the β-TCP surface were surrounded by bone in direct contact. Osteoblasts with a positive signal were fewer than those in day-7 specimens. No positive fibroblasts were observed.

In day-28 specimens, most parts of the β-TCP were surrounded by newly formed bone. The surface of the material was resorbed and replaced by the bone in places. Positive osteoblasts were observed near the material resorbing sites, suggesting intimate material resorption-bone formation relationship. On the contrary, many osteoblasts lining the surface of newly formed bone which surrounded the material were negative (Fig. 3).

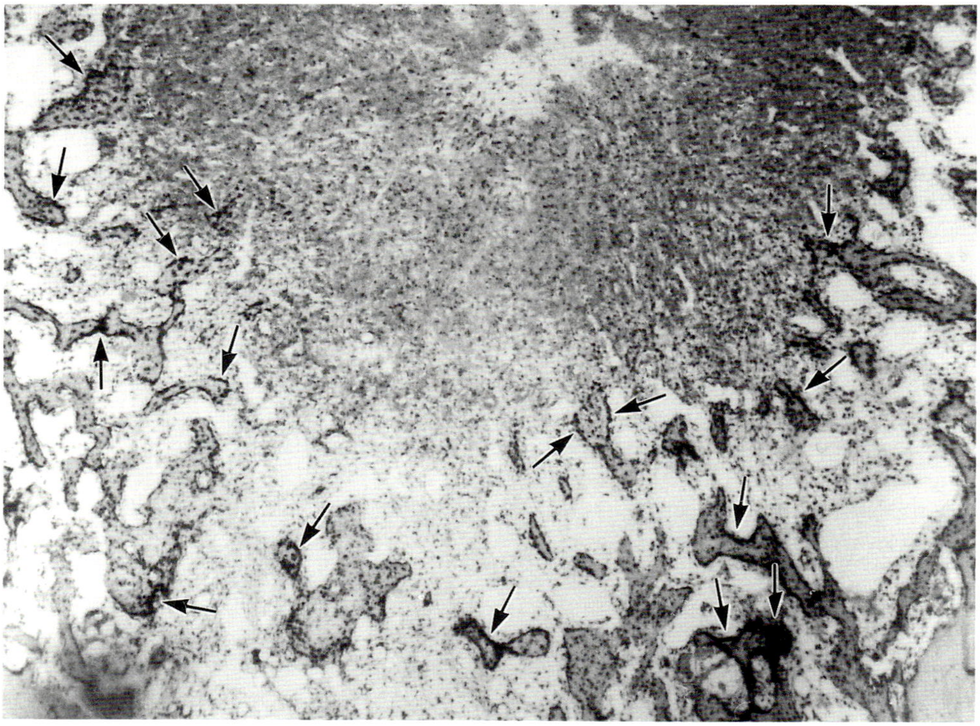

Figure 1. Localization of procollagen $\alpha 1$(I) RNA in a control specimen at day-7. Newly formed bone is growing towards the center of the hole (top). Almost all osteoblasts lining the trabeculae and almost all osteocytes encased in the bone show positive signals (arrows). (It is difficult to distinguish the red positive signal from blue nuclei of cells in the black-white photograph.)

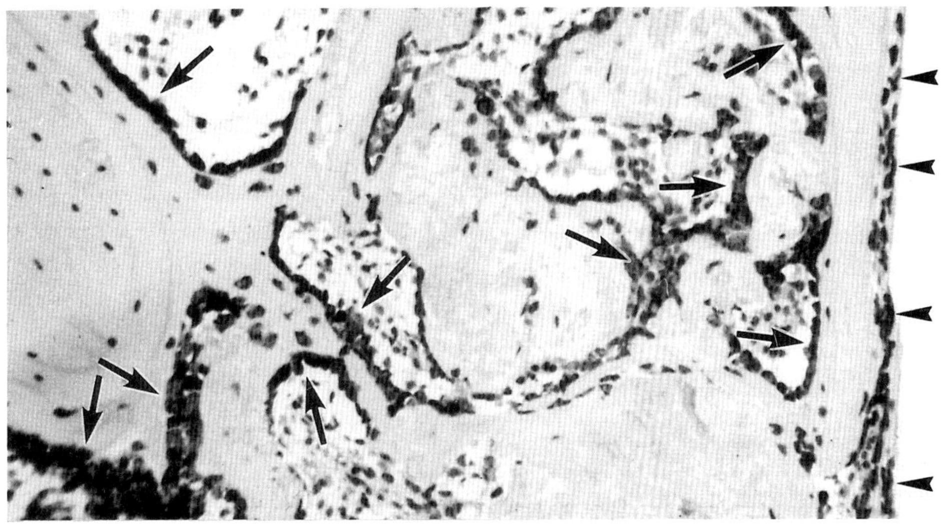

Figure 2. Localization of procollagen α1(I) RNA in β-TCP-implanted bone at day -7. New bone is actively formed around the originally existing trabeculae with positive osteoblasts (arrows) and osteocytes. Cells adjacent to the implant surface (right) also show positive signals (arrowheads).

DISCUSSION

When osteoblasts are activated or differentiated several mRNAs are expressed in a predetermined order [6,7] and the *in situ* hybridization technique visualizes the expression of these RNAs spatially and temporally at cellular level. This technique was successfully applied in order to investigate the biological effects of β-TCP on bone formation.

A procollagen $\alpha 1(I)$ non-radioactive probe was used as a marker for activated osteoblasts. Although collagen I is not osteoblast-specific, mRNA for collagen I is expressed at an earlier stage of differentiation of osteoblasts than mRNAs for alkaline phosphatase or osteocalcin, which is osteoblast-specific [6]. Therefore, the activated osteoblasts could be seen in their early stage of differentiation. Some flat osteoblasts, which were thought to be in the resting stage from purely morphological observation, showed positive signals, suggesting that they had been activated and would form new bone.

The digoxygenin labeled probe used in this study provided a clear positive signal localized in the cytoplasm, with little background. Although the sensitivity of non-radioactive probes is lower than that of radioactive probes, the higher resolution of the non-radioactive probes were useful in investigating the osteoblasts on the material surface at an individual cellular level.

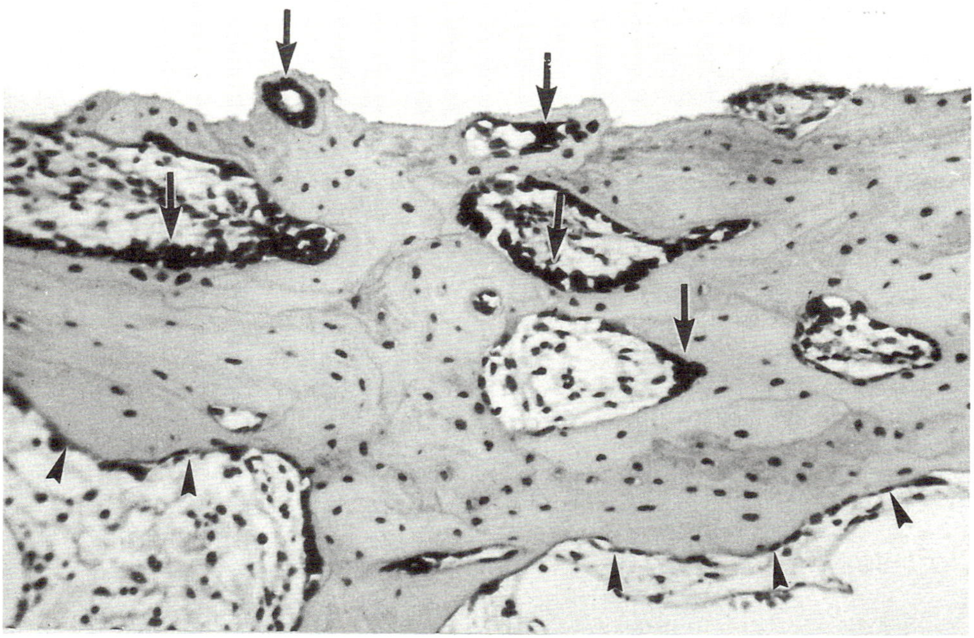

Figure 3. Localization of procollagen $\alpha 1(I)$ RNA in β-TCP-implanted bone at day -28. The implant surface (top) is resorbed and replaced by bone. Many osteoblasts lining the surface of the bone are negative (arrowheads).In contrast, osteoblasts in the remodeling canals and those adjacent to the resorption sites are positive (arrows).

In the control specimens, the osteoblasts around the hole were negative at day-3, whereas they showed active bone formation towards the center of the hole with many positive osteoblasts at day-7. This activity of osteoblasts weakened at day-14, and many osteoblasts facing the hole were negative at day-28, suggesting that inward bone formation was finished. In the β-TCP specimens, the results were comparable to these findings. That is, osteoblasts adjacent to the material were negative at day-3, showed active bone formation with strongly positive osteoblasts at day-7, and were less active at day-14. At day-28, many osteoblasts lining the surrounding bone were already negative whereas those in the remodeling canals and those adjacent to the material resorption sites were positive, suggesting that the bone formation was finished and the bone was in the remodeling stage.

These findings demonstrated that β-TCP did not affect the temporal expression of collagen I mRNA remarkably. Furthermore, most of the newly formed bone with positive signals seemed to originate in existing bone trabeculae. Some osteoblasts observed on the β-TCP surface were always near the new bone forming sites. These findings strongly suggested osteoconductive bone formation on β-TCP.

In conclusion, activated osteoblasts were clearly visualized at individual cellular level by using *in situ* hybridization technique. Application of this method to β-TCP demonstrated osteoconductive bone formation at an early stage of implantation and intimate material resorption-bone formation relationship at a later stage.

REFERENCES

1. Hench, L.L. In: *The Bone-Material Interface*, University of Toronto Press, Toronto 1991, 33-48.
2. Ohgushi, H., Okumura, M., Yoshikawa, T., Tamai, S., Tabata, S. and Dohi, Y. In: *Bone-Bonding Biomaterials*, Reed Healthcare Communications, Leiderdrop 1992, 47-56.
3. Hench, L.L. In: *Bioceramics* Volume 7, Butterworth-Heinemann, Oxford 1994, 3-14.
4. Genovese, C., Rowe, D. and Kream, B. *Biochemistry* 1984, 23, 6210-6216.
5. Milani, S., Herbst, H., Schuppan, D., Hahn, E.G. and Stein, H. *Hepatology* 1989, 10, 84-92.
6. Pockwinse, S.M., Wilming, L.G., Conlon, D.M., Stein, G.S. and Lian, J.B. *J. Cell. Biochem.* 1992, 49, 310-323.
7. Sandberg, M.M., Aro, H.T. and Vuorio, E.I. *Clin. Orthop. Rel. Res.* 1993, 289, 292-312.

SURFACE REACTIVITY OF BONE MINERAL CRYSTALS, A MODEL FOR BIOACTIVE ORTHOPAEDIC MATERIALS

C. Rey and A. Hina

Laboratoire des Materiaux - Physico-Chimie des Solides,
38, Rue des 36 ponts, 31400 Toulouse, France.

ABSTRACT

Bone mineral exhibits a high reactivity and could constitute a model for the development of bioactive orthopedic materials. The surface reactivity of bone mineral crystals was related to the existence of non-apatitic environments of phosphate and carbonate ions. These species were found to be rapidly and easily exchangeable and to interact with the binding and release of proteins. The formation and stabilization of these surface species were studied on synthetic preparations, in simulated body fluids and in cell culture media. The conditions for developing surface characteristics analogous to those of bone mineral were analysed.

INTRODUCTION

Most osteoconductive materials have the ability to nucleate carbonate apatite crystals from supersaturated body fluids [1-4]. The analogy between these neoformed crystals and bone mineral is considered to be a crucial step in the integration of biomaterials in living tissue. Bone mineral however, cannot be considered as an homogeneous compound due to constant turn-over and remodeling and the ability of its tiny, very reactive crystals to mature [5]. Thus the similarity between the neoformed crystal and bone mineral is rather ambiguous. Nevertheless bone mineral despite its heterogeneity, complex structure and composition might be a model to consider for the design of bioactive biomaterials. The aim of this report is to describe the main aspects of bone mineral reactivity, especially surface reactivity, and to determine the physico-chemical conditions for the the development of mineral crystals with characteristics similar to those of bone mineral.

MATERIALS AND METHODS

Carbonate apatite samples analogous to bone mineral were prepared by double decomposition at room temperature and pH 7.4, between a calcium nitrate solution and an ammonium phosphate solution containing sodium bicarbonate. The excess of phosphate and carbonate ions maintained pH buffering. The calcium solution (Ca $(NO_3)_2$, $4H_2O$: 17.7 g in 250 ml. of deionized water) was rapidly poured, in the phosphate-carbonate solution ($NaHCO_3$: 20g and $(NH_4)_2$ HPO_4: 40 g in 500 ml. of deionized water. The precipitate was left to mature in the mother solution at room temperature, for various periods without agitation.

Bone samples for exchange experiments were obtained from scapulae of 6 month old calves. The bones, cleaned of soft tissue, were lyophilized, ground at liquid nitrogen temperature and sieved (100 μm mesh). For ion exchange experiments 5 g of bone were immersed in 25 ml of 0.8 M sodium bicarbonate solutions or 0.8 M ammonium phosphate solution at room temperature for 30 mn. The samples were filtered, washed with deionized water and lyophilized.

FTIR spectra were obtained on a Perkin Elmer 1700 spectrometer from KBr pellets. Resolution enhancements were made using the constructor software, the enhancement parameters are reported in the figure legends.

RESULTS AND DISCUSSION

The reactivity of bone mineral can be assigned to its deficient apatitic structure and a formation process which gives at early stage of precipitation a very reactive compound rich in labile non-apatitic species, besides due to its enormous specific surface area (150 to 200 m^2/g), it can be calculated that about 20 % of the atoms of bone mineral are within a unit-cell of the surface of the crystals. Although the existence of non-apatitic phases in bone mineral has long been debated [6-9] (amorphous Ca-P, Octacalcium phosphate: OCP, Dicalcium phosphate dihydrate: DCPD, or even whitlockite), it is now accepted that bone mineral does not contain, even at the earliest stage, any appreciable amount of foreign phase. The major constituent is a non-stoichiometric carbonate apatite [10-11]. However, several investigations of the short-range organization of atoms, using spectroscopic techniques have evidenced the existence of non-apatitic environments. Studies by ^{31}P-Magic Angle Sample spinning Nuclear Magnetic Resonance (MAS-NMR) [12] have revealed that in addition to an apatitic phosphate, embryonic bone mineral contained also high amounts of HPO_4^{2-} ions exhibiting the chemical shift of OCP and the chemical shift anisotropy of DCPD. Similarly, Resolution Enhanced Fourier Transform Infrared spectroscopy (RE-FTIR) studies of early mineral deposits in several tissues have revealed the presence of non-apatitic environments [13-15] (see Figure 2) attributed to PO_4^{3-}, HPO_4^{2-} and CO_3^{2-}. Like in MAS-NMR, the spectroscopic characteristics of these environments showed some similarities with those of well crystallized non-apatitic phosphates but also significant differences. As long range order investigations excluded the existence of foreign phases, it has been suggested that these environments, related to local atomic arrangements, can not develop in three dimensions. The non-apatitic environments of bone mineral have been shown to participate in the reactivity of bone mineral crystals, especially their maturation and dissolutio properties. Thus, the relative amount of non-apatitic environment decreases in bone of aging animals, and also during dissolution of crystals.

Owing to the large specific surface area of bone crystals, one may wonder if some of the labile non-apatitic environments are located on the surface of the crystals and how they influence the apatite reactivity.

Surface Groups in Bone Mineral

The distinction between surface and bulk reactivity in crystals as tiny as those of bone mineral might seem difficult. However several reactions involving ions exchange suggest a strong surface reactivity. Such reactions can be conveniently followed by RE-FTIR due to the high specific surface area of bone mineral. The existence of surface carbonate and HPO_4^{2-} groups, especially, can be shown by exchange experiments in suspensions with a high solid/solution ratio, to minimize the dissolution phenomenon. Thus, bone crystals immersed in a carbonate-containing solution show a decrease of the amount of non-apatitic HPO_4^{2-} and an increase of the labile carbonate ions, but the other species do not appear to be affected (Figure 1). A

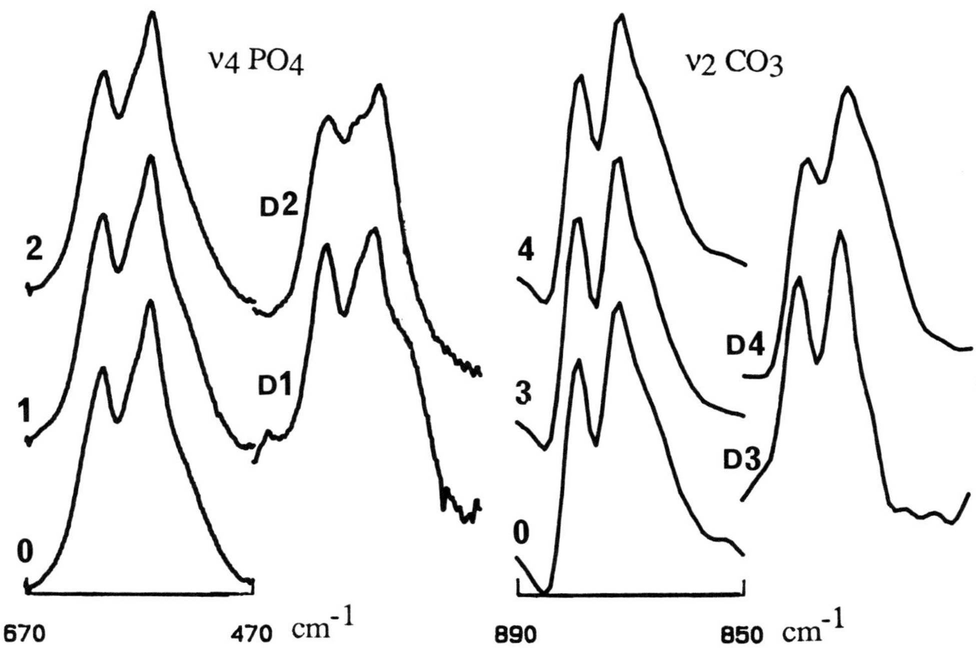

Figure 1: FTIR spectra of calf bone mineral in the ν_4 PO_4 and $\nu 2_2CO_3$ domains (resolution enhancement: band width: 10 cm^{-1}; sensitivity factor: 2). The arrows show the position of non-apatitic environments. 0- original bone sample. 1 and 3 - bone treated in a phosphate solution; the difference spectrum D1 shows an increase of the non-apatitic HPO_4 band, whereas the non-apatitic carbonate band decreases (spectrum D3). 2 and 4 - bone treated in a bicarbonate solution; the difference spectra show an increase of the non-apatitic carbonate content (D4) and a decrease of non-apatitic HPO_4 (D2).

similar experiment made with ^{13}C carbonate showed that apatitic carbonates were not affected by the reaction and thus that the crystals themselves were not altered [16]. Conversely, when bone crystals were soaked in a solution containing phosphate ions the amount of labile carbonate decreased whereas that of labile HPO_4^{2-} increased (Figure 1). These reactions are reversible and these species can be easily exchanged depending on the composition of the solution which the crystals are in equilibrium with. Such a reactivity influences the properties of the mineral, especially its interactions with proteins and its ion reservoir function.

These exchange reactions have been related to the release of non-collagenic proteins from bone [17]. This phenomenon can be compared to the desorption of acidic proteins from HA chromatographic columns. Here also phosphate (or carbonate) solutions produce a release of the adsorbed protein [18]. Inversely, it has also been shown that the adsorption of acidic proteins on HA surfaces was related to a release of phosphate ions [19]. By analogy, it may be suggested that adsorbed proteins, labile non-apatitic carbonate ions and hydrogenophosphate ions are competing for the same sites on the crystal surface. The more preponderant these labile species, the higher the capabilities of adsorption of the material are. Thus, precipitated apatites analogous to bone mineral, and very rich in labile non-apatitic environments, were seen to be able to adsorb more albumin per square meter than stoichiometric HA (3.8 mg/m^2 versus 1.1 mg/m^2). Analogous results have been found for the uptake of several growth factors, VEGF and TGFβ [20]. The amount adsorbed appeared here 10 times higher on crystals analogous to bone mineral than on stoichiometric HA. It seems then that the labile phosphate and carbonate ions are related to the reactivity of the apatite surface and could possibly determine the binding of proteins and also cell attachment and activity.

Bone mineral constitutes an exchange surface of several square kilometers, apparently easily accessible to mineral ions. Labile phosphate and carbonate ions on the bone crystal surface may then play a regulatory role. Labile carbonates, for example, have been involved in rapid re-equilibration of body fluids following acidosis [21].

Not all non-apatitic phosphate environments seem to be involved in surface reactions. The IR band at 615 cm^{-1} especially, is not affected by exchange experiments. The corresponding non-apatitic species belong to the first formed, poorly crystalline, unstable mineral phase that precipitates at early stages of biological mineralization in enamel, cartilage and bone. The amount of this non-apatitic environment decreases during maturation of the tissue as the apatitic environments and the crystallinity increase. It has also been shown to belong to easily soluble domains of the mineral. Although these species do not participate in the surface exchange, they seem to be related, to the amount of labile surface groups which decreased with the maturity of the tissue. Thus the non-apatitic species represented by the band at 615 cm^{-1} are indirectly involved in the surface reactivity of the mineral.

Controlling surface groups in synthetic analogues of bone mineral

Several methods have been proposed to prepare synthetic analogues to bone mineral [22-24]. It seems that all of them allow the formation of poorly crystalline apatite. However depending on the precipitation conditions the characteristics of the mineral may vary strongly. Non-apatitic environments formed when the precipitations were performed at low temperatures (0 to 40°C) at nearly physiological pH (7-8) and for short maturation periods. Like mineralized tissues, the non-apatitic species were essentially related to the first stages of precipitation of a mineral phase. As the precipitate was maturing in the mother solution, the non-apatitic environments progressively disappeared (Figure 2). This evolution was accelerated as the temperature increased. Minor ions such as carbonate, and Mg^{2+} were found to participate in the regulation of the amount of non-apatitic phosphates, although they were not necessary for their occurrence [25]. When they were present in the precipitation solution, carbonate ions did not seem to be incorporated into the apatite lattice of the first precipitate formed, they were bound essentially at surface positions, but as maturation proceeded, more and more ions occupied site A (OH sites) and site B (phosphate sites) of the apatite structure in the same ratios as in bone mineral (Figure 2). This ratio seems, in fact to be dependent only on the conditions of maturation of the initial precipitate, and has been observed for a wide range of pH and composition. The carbonate ions delay the maturation process and favor the persistence of non-apatitic environments, especially the phosphate environment characterized by the IR band at 615 cm^{-1}. The Mg^{2+} ions exhibit the same properties and produce an increase of the IR band at 530 cm^{-1} assigned to surface HPO_4^{2-} [25]. Thus, the amount of ions in labile environments may be controlled through adequate synthesis and maturation conditions and apatities close to young bone mineral or old bone mineral can be easily produced.

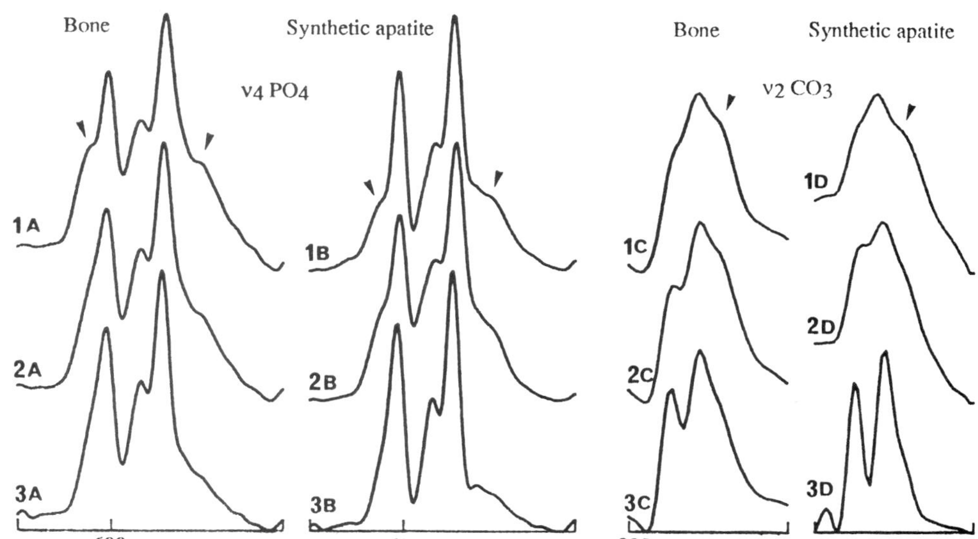

Figure 2. RE-FTIR spectra of bone mineral and poorly crystalline apatites in the ν_4 PO_4 (Resolution enhancement: width 22 cm^{-1}, sensitivity factor 2) and the ν_2 CO_3 domains (Resolution enhancement: width 10 cm^{-1}, sensitivity factor 2). 1A and C, embryonic chicken bone (14 days); 2A and C 2-week old chicken; 3A and C, 70-week old chicken. 1B and D, poorly crystalline apatite as precipitated; 2B and D, maturation time 3 days; 3B and D, maturation time 1 month.

The characteristics of bone mineral may be compared to those of neoformed apatites obtained in cell culture media or in simulated body fluids [24]. These apatites can be very close to bone mineral, however the effect of maturation is also in this case predominant. Besides, as the rate of formation of the apatite crystals depends on the substrate and the solid/solution ratio, compositional variations may be observed. Thus on different substrates, but in the same experimental conditions, the characteristics of the neoformed layer may vary.

CONCLUSION

Bone mineral crystals show a high surface reactivity related to the existence of labile non-apatite environments of phosphate and carbonate ions. These environments form at the first stages of precipitation of apatites at low temperature and they appear strongly dependent on the conditions of synthesis, especially maturation time. The surface reactivity of apatite can be monitored by controlling the occurrence of these environments. The adaptation of the surface reactivity of apatites could be particularly interesting for the attachment of bioactive proteins or the preparation of composite materials.

REFERENCES

1. Hench, L. *et al.,* G.P. In: *Bioceramics,* Volume 4, Butterworth-Heinemann, London, 1991, 155-162.
2. Daculsi, G. *et al., Calcf. Tiss. Int.* 1990, 46, 20-27.
3. Kokubo, T. *et al., J. Biomed. Mater. Res.* 1990, 24, 331-343.
4. Bakker, D. *et al., J. Biomed. Mat. Res.* 1990, 24, 277-293.
5. Rey, C., Renugopalakrishnan, V. *et al., Calcf. Tiss. Int.* 1991, 49, 251-258.
6. Termine, J.D., Posner, A.S. *Calcf. Tiss. Res.* 1966, 6, 335-342.
7. Brown, W.E. *Clin. Orthop.* 1966, 44, 205-220.
8. Francis, M.D., Webb, N.C. *Calcf. Tiss. Res.* 1971, 6, 335-342.
9. Driessens, F.C., Verbeeck, R.M., Z. *Natur. Forsch. C Biosci.* 1986, 44, 468-471.
10. Glimcher, M.J. In: *Am. Ac. O S Lectures XXXVI,* Park Ridge, IL, 1987, 49-69.
11. Grynpas, M.D., Bonar, L.C., Glimcher, M.J. *Calcf. Tiss. Int.* 1984, 36, 291-301.
12. Wu, Y., Glimcher, M.J., Rey, C., Ackerman, J. *J. Mol. Biol.* 1994, 244, 423-435.
13. Rey, C., Collins, B., Shimizu, M., Glimche, M.J. *Calcf. Tiss. Int.* 1991, 49, 383-388.
14. Rey, C. *et al., Calcf. Tiss. Int.* 1990, 46, 384-394.
15. Rey, C. *et al., Calcf. Tiss. Int.* 1989, 45, 157-164.
16. Rey, C. *et al.,* In: *HA and Related Materials* CRC Press, Boca-Raton, 1994, 181-188.
17. Rey, C., Strawich, E., Glimcher, M.J. *Bull Inst Oc. Mon.* 1994, 14-1, 55-64.
18. Bernardi, G. *Methods Enzymmol.* 1971, 21D, 95-139.
19. Pearce, E.I.F. *Calcf. Tiss. Int.* 1981, 33, 395-402.
20. Midy, V. These, *Institut National Polytechnique de Toulouse,* 1994.
21. Blitz, R.M., Pellegrino, E.D., Letteri, J.M. *Miner. Electrolyte Metab.* 1981, 5, 1-7.
22. Bachra, B.N. *et al., Arch. Biochem. Biophys.* 1963, 103, 124-138.
23. Posner, A.S. *et al., J. Dent. Res.* 1975, 54, B88-93.
24. Li, P. *et al., J. Mater. Sci, Mater, Med.,* 1993, 4, 127-131.
25. Apfelbaum, F. *et al., J. Cryst. Growth,* 1994, 144, 304-310.

BONE INDUCTION ON THE SURFACE OF HYDROXYAPATITE CERAMICS

H. Ohgushi, M.Okumura, K. Inoue, S. Tamai, Y.Dohi*, M. Murata** and Y.Kuboki***

Department of Orthopedics and Public Health*, Nara Medical University, Kashihara City, Nara, Japan. Department of Oral Pathology**, School of Dentistry, Okayarna University, Okayama, Japan. Department of Biochemistry***, School of Dentistry, Hokkaido University, Hokkaido, Japan

ABSTRACT

Composites of bone morphogenetic proteins (BMP), collagen and porous hydroxyapatite ceramics (HA) were implanted at rat subcutaneous sites. Small areas of cartilage followed by endochondral ossification were detected outside of the HA at 1 and 2 weeks post implantation. Extensive bone formation was found inside of the pore regions after 3 weeks. The cascade of bone formation in the pore regions was exclusively intramembranous ossification initiated on the HA pore surface. Undecalcified histological section and scanning electron microscopy showed direct contact between thus formed bone and the HA surface. All of these results proved that the surface of HA can support BMP induced osteogenic differentiation resulting in firm bone bonding.

INTRODUCTION

We have reported that the composites of marrow stromal stem cells and bioactive porous hydroxyapatite ceramics (HA) showed *de novo* bone formation after subcutaneous implantation of the composites, whereas marrow cells or HA themselves did not show bone formation [1-6]. Thus, the composites were osteogenic materials at ectopic sites. Histological [2,3] studies showed that the bone formation primarily occurred on the ceramic surface and analysis of bone specific markers by biochemical [4] and gene expression study [5,6] demonstrated the osteogenic differentiation of marrow stromal stem cells. Therefore, the surface of bioactive materials can support cell mediated osteogenic differentiation which results in firm bone bonding. In contrast to these findings, surface of non-bioactive materials such as alumina ceramics can not support the osteogenic differentiation and fibrous tissue formation occurs between bone and materials surface [5].

Concerning the ectopic bone formation, it is also well known that intramuscular or subcutaneous implantation of demineralized bone matrix results in endochondral bone formation [7]. Recent molecular biological technology [8] identified the nature of the osteoinductive signal as a protein termed bone morphogenetic protein (BMP).The composites of BMP and porous ceramics also showed *de novo* bone formation [9-14].

However, an important question is whether the surface of materials can support the protein induced osteogenic differentiation or not. In the present paper, we focus on the question by analyzing the BMP/HA composite at rat subcutaneous sites.

MATERIALS AND METHODS

Preparation of bone morphogenetic protein (BMP)

Partially-purified BMP was obtained from 4M guanidine extract of bovine bone powders as reported [13]. The extract was purified by a three-step chromatographic procedure using hydroxyapatite, heparin-sepharose and sephacryl S 300 HR(Pharmacia, Japan) columns. The eluted fraction which contained all of the bone inducing activity was pooled and used for experiment [13]. This fraction (S-300 BMP fraction) was proved to contain at least BMP-2,3 and 4 determined by Western blot using respective antibodies, and assumed to contain all other active BMPs. Three hundred microgram of S-300 BMP was mixed with 0.12 mg (0.3% in 0.1 M acetic acid) of pepsin-treated bovine skin collagen (Celgen, Koken Co. Japan) and loaded on one disc of HA to make BMP/HA composite.

Porous hydroxyapatite ceramics(HA) and implantation

Disk shape of HA(5 mm in diameter and 2 mm in thickness: Interpore 200, Interpore International, CA., USA) were used [l-4]. The BMP/HA composites were implanted in rat (4 week-old Wister King rat) subcutaneous sites and harvested 1 to 4 weeks post implantation. Control ceramics (collagen/HA composites without BMP) were also implanted. Total implants used were 20, most of them were stained with toluidine blue after decalcification and some were used for undecalcified histological section as well as scanning electron microscopical observation.

RESULTS

All the BMP/HA composites showed *de novo* bone formation after 2 weeks post implantation (Table 1). Some areas showed cartilage formation at 1 week post implantation (Fig. 1). However, the most cartilage area was restricted outside of the HA and followed by endochondral ossification. Majority of the bone formation occurred on the pore surface by a process of intramembranous bone formation. Undecalcified histological sections (Fig. 2) showed that there was no intervening fibrous tissue between thus formed *de novo* bone and the HA surface (direct contact between the bone and ceramic). Scanning electron microscopy (Fig. 3) also demonstrated the contact. Electron probe microanalysis showed continuous high counts of calcium and phosphorus across the bone/HA interface. To observe bone dynamics, tetracycline and calcein were injected 8 days and 2 days before sacrifice, respectively. The fluorochrome labeling study showed tetracycline was detected near the surface of HA and calcein was detected away from the surface. Therefore, the bone formation was so called bonding osteogenesis (bone formation starts on the ceramic surface then proceeds in a centripetal manner). As we already reported, the same pattern of bone formation (bonding osteogenesis) was observed when marrow cell/HA composites were implanted at rat subcutaneous sites [2]. These findings confirm that bone formation by BMP/HA and marrow/HA composites were HA surface dependent phenomena and imply that the HA surface supports osteoblastic differentiation which results in firm bone bonding.

Table 1. Bone and cartilage formation after subcutaneous.

Post trans-plantation	BMP/HA composite		Collagen/HA composite		Marrow/HA composite**		HA alone**	
	bone	cartilage	bone	cartilage	bone	cartilage	bone	cartilage
1 week	1/2	1/2	0/2	0/2	0/4	0/4	0/4	0/4
2 weeks	2/2	1/2	0/2	0/2	0/4	0/4	0/4	0/4
3 weeks	3/3	0/3	0/3	0/3	2/4	0/4	0/4	0/4
4 weeks	3/3	0/3	0/3	0/3	6/6	0/4	0/4	0/4

*Number of implants showing bone or cartilage/total number of implants.
**Data are obtained from reference [3].

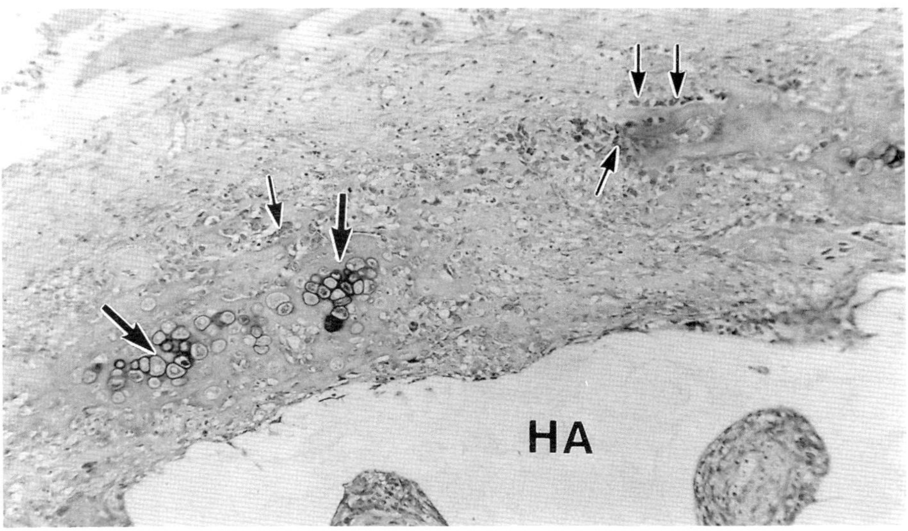

Figure 1. Decalcified histological section of BMP/HA composites at 1 week post implantation. Cartilage foci (large arrows) and bone formation by osteoblastic cells (small arrows) are seen outside hydroxyapatite (HA). Toluidine blue stain (x 100).

DISCUSSION

A difference of the bone formation by BMP/HA composite compared with bone formation by marrow/HA composites was that cartilage foci and bone formation were detected not only in the pore regions but also outside of the BMP/ceramic composites, thus some areas of bone formation induced by BMP was independent on the ceramic surface. However bone formation by marrow/HA composites was exclusively a surface dependent phenomenon (bone formation always initiated on the HA pore surface) and cartilage was not detected in the marrow/HA composites [1-6]. Interestingly, the bone induced by BMP appeared much faster than the bone formed by marrow cells. As shown

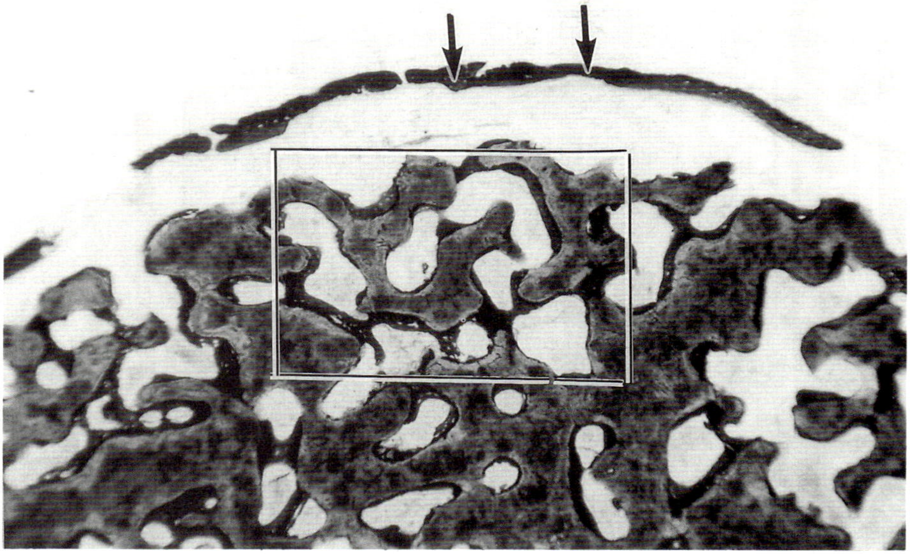

Figure 2a. Undecalcified histological section of BMP/HA composite at 3 weeks post implantation. Black areas indicate *de novo* bone and gray areas indicate HA. Though the figure shows the bone (arrow) which locates away from the ceramic outer surface, majority of bone formation is seen inside the pore areas of the HA (Toluidine blue stain, X 40).

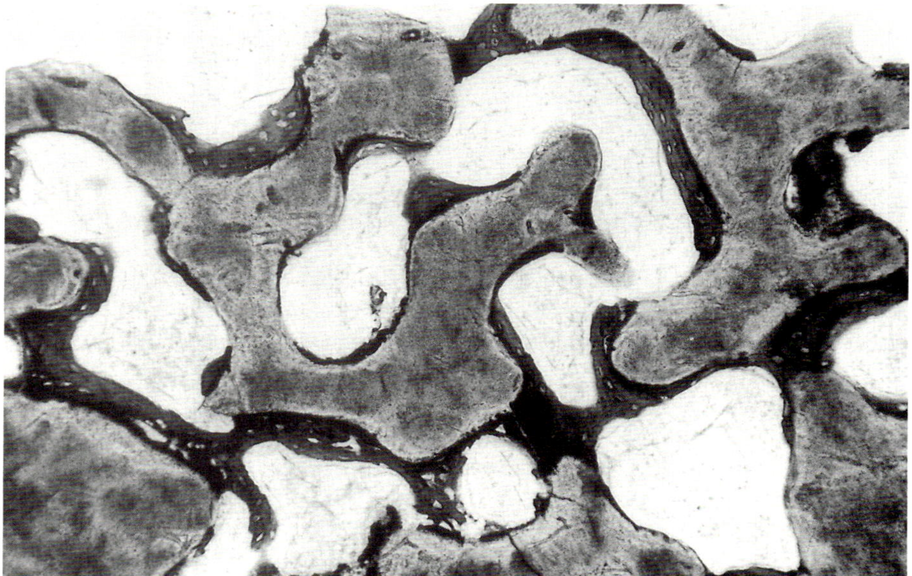

Figure 2b. Higher power magnification of the rectangular area of Figure 2a. Bone (black area) is in contact with HA (gray area).

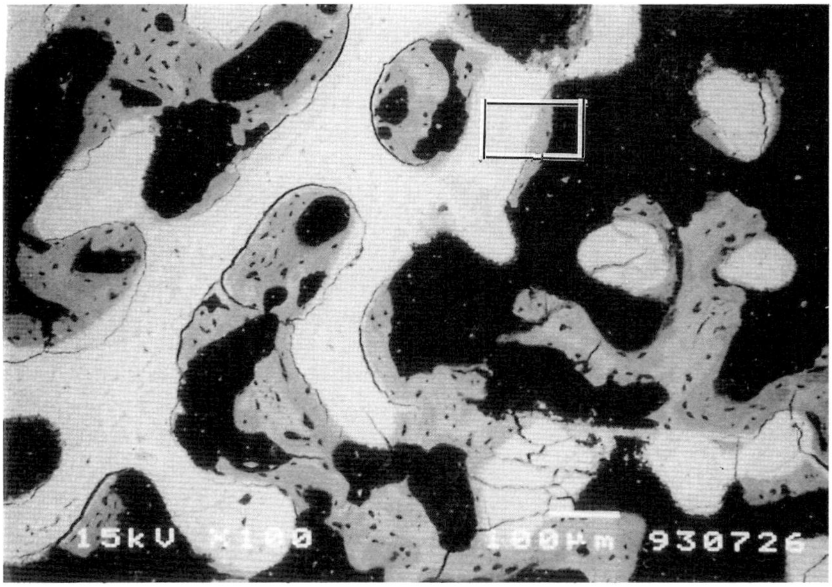

Figure 3a. Scanning electron microscopical observation (back scattered electron image) of BMP/HA composite at 3 weeks post implantation. Gray and white areas indicate *de novo* bone and HA, respectively.

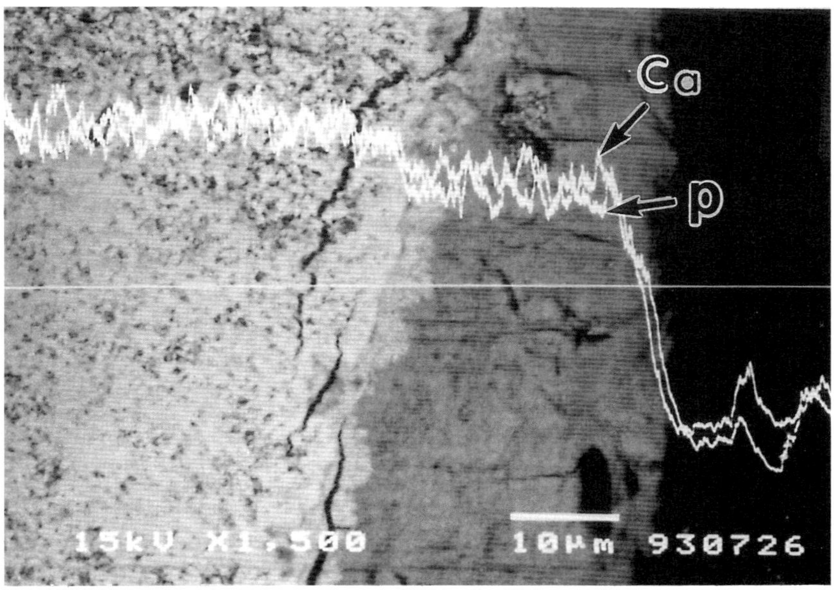

Figure 3b. Higher power magnification of the rectangular area of Figure 3a. Electron-prove microanalysis shows the continuous high counts of Calcium (Ca) and Phosphorus (P) across the interface between bone (gray area) and HA (white area).

in Table 1, some areas of BMP/HA composites showed bone and cartilage formation started at 1 week post implantation whereas marrow/HA composite showed bone formation after 3 weeks post implantation. The rapid bone formation was confirmed by the evidence of extensive bone formed in many pore areas of BMP/HA composites at 3 weeks post implantation. The marrow/HA composites showed extensive bone formation after 4 weeks post implantation. Thus, the bone formation of BMP/HA composites was at least 1 week earlier than that of marrow/HA composites. Our recent study of biochemical analysis of bone formed in BMP/HA composite showed high Alkaline phosphatase activity (ALP) at 1 week and significant amount of bone specific bone Gla protein (BGP) at 2 weeks post implantation. The ALP is localized on osteogenic cells and BGP is the most abundant non-collagenous protein in bone matrix, thus the ALP activity reflects the osteoblastic activity and the amount of BGP parallels the bone volume. Our previous study [4] found that high activity of ALP began to appear at 2 weeks post implantation of marrow/HA composites and that of BGP at 3 weeks post implantation. Again these biochemical analyses confirmed the rapid bone formation of BMP/HA composites compared with marrow/HA composites. In contrast to the osteogenic capacity of BMP/HA and marrow/HA composites, ceramic alone or collagen/ceramic composite did not show bone and cartilage formation (Table 1). Thus, marrow and BMP are definitely osteogenic or osteoinductive.

CONCLUSIVE REMARKS

Present results demonstrate that BMP induced bone formation was exclusively initiated on the ceramic surface and direct contact between thus formed bone and ceramic surface was observed. Therefore, the surface of hydroxyapatite ceramics can support the protein induced bone formation through the cascade of osteoblastic differentiation. Our previous findings using marrow cell/ceramic composites, clearly showed that surface of bioactive materials (calcium phosphate ceramics and glass-ceramic) could support the osteoblastic differentiation whereas surface of nonbioactive ceramics such as alumina could not support the differentiation and fibrous tissue intervened between the bone and the ceramic surface. All of these results support our hypothesis [5,6] that bioactive materials have the capability to support cell differentiation, and cause the expression of its specific phenotype on the materials surface. Such cellular events finally result in the integration of the material with surrounding new tissue.

REFERENCES

1. Ohgushi, H.,Okumura, M.,Tamai S.and Shors,E.C. *J. Biomed. Mat. Res.* 1990,24,1563-1570
2. Okumura, M., Ohgushi H. and Tamai, *S,Biomaterials* 1991,12, 411-416
3. Ohgushi, H., Okumura,M., Yoshikawa, T., Inoue, K., Senpuku, N. and Tamai, S., *J. Biomed. Mat. Res.* 1992,26,885-896
4. Yoshikawa, T., Ohgushi, H. Okumura, M., Tamai, S., Dohi, Y. and Moriyama, T., *Calcified Tissue International* 1992 50,184-188.
5. Ohgushi, H., Okumura, M. Yoshikawa, T. Tamai, S. Tabata, S and Dohi, Y. in *Bone bonding Biomaterials,* Helthcare Comm. Publ, the Netherlands, 1992,pp.47-56.
6. Ohgushi, H.,Dohi, Y.,Tamai, S.and Tabata,*S.J.BiomedMat. Res.* 1993.27,1401 1407.
7. Urist, M.R., Science 1965,150, 893-899

8. Wozney, J.M., Rosen, V., Celeste, A.J., Mitsock, L.M., Whiters,M.J.,Kriz, R.W. Hewick, R.M. and Wang, E.A. Science 1988, 242, 1428-1534
9. Urist, M.R., Nilsson,O.,Rsmussen, J., Hirota, W., Lovell, T., Schmalzred, T. and Finerman ,G.A. *Clin. Orthop.* 1986, 214, 295-304.
10. Takaoka, K., Nakahara, H., Yoshikawa, H.,Masuhara, K., Sugamoto, K., Tsuda T., Aoki, Y., Ono, K. and Sakamoto, Y. *Clin. Orthop.* 1988, 244, 258-264
11. Ripamonti, U. and Reddi, A.H., *Matrix* 1992, 3, 202-212
12. Ono, I., Ohura, T., Murata, M., Yamaguchi, H., Ohnuma, Y. and Kuboki, Y. *Plast. Rec. Surg* 1991, 90, 870-879
13. Kuboki, Y., Saito, T., Murata, M., Takita H., Mizuno, N. and Nagai, N. *Connect. Tis. Res.,* in press
14. Ijiri,S., Yamamuro, T., Nakamura, T., Kotani, S., Shibuya, T., Notoya, K. and Sato, Y., in *Bioceramics* Volume 6, Butterwort-Heinemann, Oxford 1993, 15-20.

HISTOLOGICAL ANALYSIS OF BIOGLASS® -FILLED RADIUS DEFECTS

D.L. Wheeler, D.C. Senft, M.D. Scott, J.J. Prescott, K.E. Stokes, J.O. Hollinger and H.M. Park

Oregon Health Sciences University, Department of Surgery, Divisions of Orthopaedics and Plastic Surgery, 3181 SW Sam Jackson Park Rd., L477, Portland, OR 97201

ABSTRACT

The repair of comminuted bone fractures and orthopaedic reconstructions require autograft, allograft, or other synthetic graft materials to promote healing. Due to donor site morbidity and infection risks, there is a strong clinical need to develop alternatives to autograft and allogenic bone grafts. Bioglass® provides a promising alternative synthetic graft material to be used in orthopaedic applications and has been successfully used in oral surgical applications.

The objective of this study was to determine the ability of Bioglass® particles to promote healing of a 20 mm defect created unilaterally in the radius of a rabbit. The amount of bone within the defect was assessed after 4 and 8 weeks histologically. The Bioglass® filled defects (BG) were compared to untreated defects (CTL).

Active mineralization was apparent throughout the BG defect with the greatest mineralization occurring adjacent to the host bone. Mineralization of CTL defects occurred only adjacent to the host bone. The amount of bone within the BG-filled defect was greater than the CTL animals at both 4 and 8 weeks, yet only significant at 4 weeks ($p=0.04$). The amount of bone within the defect at 4 weeks for the BG-treated animals was equivalent to the bone ingrowth of the CTL animals at 8 weeks. With improvements in Bioglass® placement and retention in the defect, this material is a promising bone graft substitute for use in orthopaedic applications.

BACKGROUND

The repair of comminuted bone fractures, orthopaedic reconstruction following *en bloc* osseous tumor resection, and primary and revision total joint reconstructions often require the use of autograft, allograft, or other synthetic graft materials to promote healing and to fill gaps between host bone or between the host bone and the adjacent implant [1]. Between 100,000 and 200,000 bone grafts are performed annually in the United States [2]. The most common graft material is autologous bone. However, the morbidity (blood loss, pain, and wound healing complications) and moderate success rate associated with autologous bone grafts make this option less appealing [3]. The overall failure rate of autologous bone grafts is between 13 and 30%, while allograft failure rate is much higher [4]. Allogenic bone has a lower overall success rate, requires longer to incorporate into the surrounding host bone, and has a potential for disease transmission [2,5]. Neither autograft nor allograft provide the patient with ideal bone graft material. Consequently, there is a strong clinical need to develop alternatives to autograft and allogenic bone grafts [6,7].

Materials such as polymers, ceramics, and hydroxyapatite derivatives have been investigated as possible synthetic bone graft materials [1,8-12]. New biodegradable polymers and hydroxyapatites have been used in conjunction with growth factors to promote healing and filling of defects [12]. Polymers, spiked with allogeneic and xenogeneic bone morphogenic protein, have not been successful in regenerating bone within cranial defects in monkeys [13] or in long bone defects in dogs [14]. Additionally, many of these biodegradable polymers resorb prior to bone formation leaving a mechanical unstable void. Recent work with ceramics, particularly Bioglass®, as a synthetic bone graft material prove to be promising [9,15-17]. Bioglass® has been shown to be superior to other graft materials in regeneration of osseous tissue in the treatment of periodontal disease in monkeys [16,18] and to maintain alveolar ridge after dental extraction in pigs [19] and humans [15]. The bioactive nature of Bioglass® stimulates bone formation [20]. The bone uses the glass substrate as a template and for constituents of the newly formed bone matrix. The Bioglass® is slowly degraded and replaced by bone. Bioglass® does not resorb, as with polymers, but is replaced by new bone making this material an excellent candidate for synthetic bone grafts.

OBJECTIVE

The objective of this investigation is to determine the ability of Bioglass® particles to promote healing of a 20 mm defect created unilaterally in the radius of a rabbit. Bone formation within the defect will be quantified histomorphometrically at 4 and 8 weeks. The Bioglass® filled defects (BG) will be compared to untreated defects (CTL).

MATERIALS AND METHODS

Transcortical osteotomies (20 mm) were surgically created, unilaterally, in the radial diaphysis of anesthetized, skeletally mature New Zealand white rabbits (2-4 kg) with an oscillating bone saw. This defect measures approximately 6 times the diaphyseal diameter of the radius and provides a critical gap between the host bone in which complete osseous filling is unlikely without the aid of bone graft material. The osteotomy opening was stabilized by internal splinting of the intact ulna adjacent to the radius.

The osteotomy site was either left unfilled (CTL) or packed with Bioglass® particulates (BG). Twenty-four animals were randomly assigned to treatment groups (BG and CTL) and two euthanasia periods (4 and 8 weeks), with 6 animals in each group.

Following sacrifice, radii were be harvested, stripped of soft tissue, and fixed in 70% ETOH. Following dehydration, the radial segments were embedded in Technovit 7200 plastic (Kulzer & Co., Dammwold, Germany) using standard methods. Thin longitudinal cuts were taken through the defect using an Exakt Bone Saw and MicroGrinder (Exakt Corp., Hamburg, Germany). Sections were either left unstained for evaluation of fluorescent label or stained using both a modified Von Kossa and Goldner's Trichrome.

Fluorescent labels were qualitatively assessed to identify areas of active mineralization. Stained section were quantitated using a Leitz Aristoplan microscope (Leica Corp, Cambridge, U.K.), a Sony 3CCD color video camera (Sony Corp., Montvale,

NJ) and Optimas image analysis software (Optimas Corp., Edmonds, WA). The amount of bone within the radial defect relative to defect size (% bone) was measured for both the BG and CTL animals. Statistical comparisons were made using a Student's T-test (SAS, Cary NC).

RESULTS

Active mineralization was apparent throughout the BG defect with the greatest mineralization occurring adjacent to the host bone. Mineralization of CTL defects only occurred adjacent to the host bone at 4 weeks. By 8 weeks active mineralization was occurring in mid-defect for both BG and CTL animals.

Table 1 summarizes the mean, standard deviation, minimum and maximum values for percent bone at both time points. The amount of bone within the BG-filled defect was significantly greater than for the CTL animals ($p=0.04$) at 4 weeks but not at 8 weeks ($p=0.23$). These results are also displayed in Figure 1.

Table 1. Percent Bone within Radial Defects

	Mean ± SD (%)	Minimum (%)	Maximum (%)
BG, 4 weeks	64.5 ± 20.1	43.7	95.2
CTL, 4 weeks	43.9 ± 17.8	18.4	66.4
BG, 8 weeks	83.3 ± 15.1	58	99.8
CTL, 8 weeks	68.4 ± 24.4	33.4	93.3

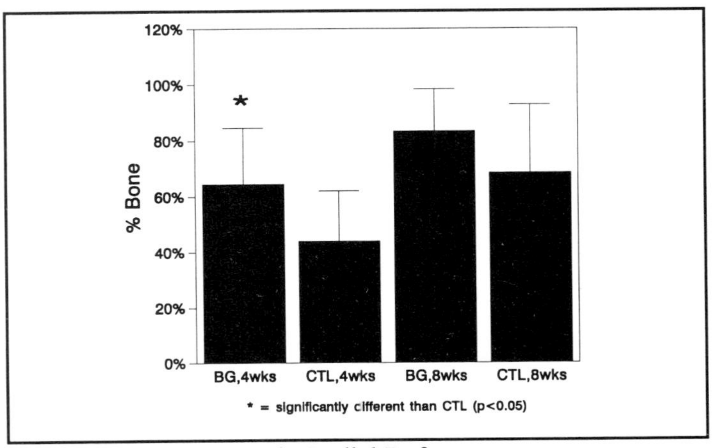

Figure 1. Percent Bone in Radial Defects

DISCUSSION

Bioglass® stimulated greater bone formation than unfilled defects at both 4 and 8 weeks post-grafting. The short-term (4 week) effects of Bioglass® produced significantly greater mineralization than untreated defects. By 8 weeks, the amount of bone within the untreated defects was equivalent to the percent bone within the BG-treated defects at 4 weeks. It appears from these results that the bioactive nature of Bioglass® enhances early mineralization and graft incorporation. The bone formation within the BG-treated defects was more consistent than the untreated defects. This inconsistency in the CTL animals is reflected in the large standard deviations in the percent bone measurements at 8 weeks tabulated in Table 1.

The Bioglass® particles within the defect had a characteristic pattern of mineralization. The fluorescent labels were incorporated into the Bioglass® particle in rings from the periphery to the inner core. Mineralization occurred from the outside to the inside rather than typical mineralization patterns "growing" from the surface of the graft material. This may be an indication that the constituents of the Bioglass® are being used to form the bone matrix rather than resorbing. The areas of high fluorescent activity (mineralization) were confirmed with incorporation of bone stain, both VonKossa and Goldner's, around the periphery of the Bioglass® particles. It is possible that the bone stain is picked up by compositional changes in the Bioglass® particles due to the placement of the particles in a physiological environment. Additional analyses, including osteoblast surface and surface analysis using a Kevex x-ray diffraction probe, will be performed to confirm the presence of bone versus compositional changes on the periphery of the Bioglass® particles.

Malformed radii were noted in the BG group which may have resulted from stray Bioglass® particulates adjacent to the bone promoting osteoblast activity and creating an irregular, atypical bone geometry. Structural inadequacies at the graft site could potentially adversely affect bone strength. Biomechanical analyses will be performed on 24 additional animals to test the mechanical integrity of the graft site.

Bioglass® stimulated greater bone formation than unfilled defects. With improvements in Bioglass® placement and retention within the defect, this material is a promising bone substitute graft material for use in orthopaedic procedures.

ACKNOWLEDGMENTS

The authors would like to thank U.S. Biomaterials Corporation for their support of this research. We would also like to acknowledge Ms. Barbara Kochevar for her patience and clerical support in preparation of this abstract and manuscript.

REFERENCES

1. Prolo, D. J. and Rodrigo, J.J. *Clin. Orthop.* 1985, 200,322-342.
2. Buck, B. E. and Malinin, T. I. *Clin. Orthop.* 1989, 260, 129-136.
3. Glancy, G. L., Brugioni, D. J., Eilert, R. E., and Chang, F. M. *Clin. Orthop.* 1991, 262, 28-33.
4. Enneking, W. F. and Mindell, E. R. *JBJS* 1991, 73A, 1123-1142.
5. Tomford, W. W., Starkweather, R. J., and Goldman, M. H. *JBJS* 1981, 63A, 244-248.
6. Goldberg, V. M. and Stevenson, S. *Clin. Orthop.* 1987, 225, 7-16.
7. Lane, J. and Sandhu, H. *Orthop. Clin. N. Am.* 1987, 18, 213-225.
8. Bostman, O. M. *JBJS* 1991, 73A, 148-152.

9. Hollinger, J. O. and Battistone, G. C. *Clin. Orthop.* 1986, 207, 290-305.
10. Holmes, R. E., Bucholz, R. W., and Mooney, V. *J. Orthop. Res.* 1987, 5, 114-121.
11. Hulbert, S., Young, F., Mathews, R., Klawitter, J., Talbert, C., and Stelling, F. *J. Biomed. Mater. Res.* 1970, 4, 433-442.
12. Takaoka, K., Nakahara, H., Yoshikawa, H., Mashuhara, K., Tsuda, H., and Ono, K. *Clin. Orthop.* 1988. 234, 250-254.
13. Hollinger, J. O., J. P. Schmitz, D. E. Mark, and A. E. Seyfer. *Surgery* 1990, 107, 50-54
14. Heckman, J. D., Boyan, B.D., Aufdemorte, T.B. and Abbott, J.T. *JBJS* 1991, 73A, 751-763.
15. Stanley, H. R., Hall, M.B., Colaizzi, F. and Clark, A.E. *J. Pros. Dent.* 1987, 58, 607-613.
16. Wilson, J. and Low, S. B. *J. Appl. Biomat* 1992, 3, 123-129.
17. Wilson, J., Yu, L.T., and Beale, B. S. *Bioceramics* 1993, 5, 139-146.
18. Wilson, J., Low, S., Fetner, A., and Hench, L. L. *Biomat.Clin. Appl.* 1987, 5, 223-228.
19. Oguntebi, B., Clark, A., and Wilson, J. *J. Dent. Res.* 1993, 72(2), 484-489.
20. Hench, L. L., Andersson, O.H. and LaTorre, G. P. *Bioceramics* 1991, 4, 156-162.

MECHANICAL ASSESSMENT OF POROUS HYDROXYAPATITE IMPLANTS BEFORE AND AFTER OSSEOINTEGRATION

K.A. Hing, S.M. Best, K.E. Tanner, P.A. Revell* and W. Bonfield

IRC in Biomedical Materials, Queen Mary Westfield College, University of London, London. E1 4NS. *IRC in Biomedical Materials, Royal Free Hospital School of Medicine, University of London, London. NW3 2QG.

ABSTRACT

Porous hydroxyapatite (HA) implants offer the potential of osseous defect repair and much work has been carried out on both the *in* vivo and *in vitro* response of this material. However, in conjunction with the biological assessment of a material it is also important to fully characterise its physical, chemical and mechanical properties to aid understanding and control of any exhibited bio-response. In this study cylinders of porous hydroxyapatite with apparent densities between 0.4 and 1.3 Mg m^{-3} underwent chemical, physical and mechanical characterisation. Three groups of specimens with mean apparent densities of 0.61, 0.90 and 1.2 Mg m^{-3} were then implanted into cancellous bone for a period of 5 weeks before being studied histologically and mechanically. Before implantation the material behaved as an elastic, brittle foam and the ultimate compressive stress (UCS) was highly dependent on apparent density. After implantation the amount of bone ingrowth was found to vary with apparent density, the least amount of ingrowth being in the high density specimens. The osseointegrated, low density specimens exhibited mechanical behaviour similar to trabecular bone while the high density implant, which had a higher UCS than the cancellous bone, still behaved as a ceramic. These results suggest that implants may be selected for different applications using porosity as a guide to mechanical competence, and that the matching of mechanical properties to the host tissue results in a more compatible implant.

INTRODUCTION

The biocompatibility [1,2] of hydroxyapatite ($Ca_{10}(PO_4)_6(0H)_2$) and the similarities between the crystal structure of HA and bone mineral [3] has led to great interest in the potential of dense HA as a material for the augmentation of osseous defects. The use of low density HA, with highly interconnected porosity, has also been advocated as a viable alternative to bone grafts without the sterilization, infection, rejection and supply complications often associated with bone grafts. Furthermore, this porous structure invites the ingrowth of bone into the implant leading to a more securely fixed and integrated repair, particularly in cancellous bone where the structure closely mirrors that of the host. However, although the morphology of biomedical implants has been of interest since the use of a porous ceramic was described in 1963 [4], there has been no thorough study of the effects of physical properties such as macro-pore size and apparent density on (HA) implants before and after integration.

MATERIALS AND METHODS

Endobon® specimens, with a broad range of apparent densities (0.4 - 1.3 Mg m^{-3}), were supplied by E. Merck in the form of 4.5 mm diameter cylinders with a length of 6.5 mm. Endobon® is produced via the hydrothermal defatting and calcination of bovine cancellous bone in a manner which preserves the trabecular macro-structure and converts the bone mineral into hydroxyapatite.

Physical characterisation

The specimens were physically characterised using a number of techniques, the bulk or apparent density was calculated from specimen dimensions and weight, while gas porosimetry was used to determine the real density, i.e., the density of the specimen "struts". In order to study the microstructure, specimens were vacuum embedded in epoxy resin, polished (Struers Abramin™), and where appropriate etched with 10% phosphoric acid, prior to viewing using a Joel™ 6300-F scanning electron microscope. Macrostructure was assessed using a Zeiss™ Axioscope light microscope to study the embedded, polished specimens.

Chemical analysis

For chemical analysis, specimens were ground down using a mortar and pestle. X-ray fluorescence was performed to determine the Ca:P ratio and detect any impurities, while X-ray diffraction using a Siemens™ D-5000 yielded information about the phase purity of the material. Any carbonate substitution in the apatite lattice was then determined using a Nicolet™ 730 infra-red spectroscopy unit.

Biological performance

Three groups of specimens with mean densities of 0.62, 0.93 and 1.17 Mg m^{-3} were selected to be implanted in the distal end of the right femur of six month old New Zealand White rabbits. Defects were generated in the sub patella bone with the use of a saline cooled diamond tipped trephine. After removal of the bone plug implants were press fit into the defect and care was taken to ensure that the implants were flush with the surface of the bone. Any loose ceramic particles were then rinsed away with saline and the wound stitched internally with Viacryl™ and externally with PDS monofilamen™. Specimens were left *in vivo* for 5 weeks. Integration of bone within the specimens was studied histologically, two fresh integrated specimens from each of the three density groups were fixed in formal alcohol and embedded in Technovit™ resin and slices from each specimen were ground down to approximately 10 μm and stained with toluidine blue for examination.

Mechanical testing

Mechanical testing was performed in compression on both as-received specimens and osseointegrated implants with a cross head velocity of 0.001 mm s^{-1} using an Instrono™ 4464 testing machine. Specimens were tested in Ringer's solution at 37°C (Fig. 1a) to maintain continuity. Test pieces of the integrated implants were prepared by extracting a plug using a 6.5 mm inside diameter trephine. The surplus ends of the plugs were then carefully removed before testing (Fig. 1b). Plugs of trabecular bone were also removed from identical positions on the contra lateral femurs as control specimens.

RESULTS AND DISCUSSION

Physical characterisation

All specimens exhibited the same basic structural characteristics of a foam, with a 3 dimensional interconnecting network of struts and pores (Fig. 2a). However specimens also exhibited varying degrees of anisotropy which was particularly marked in low density specimens. Specimens selected for the *in vivo* work had minimal anisotropy variation. Macrostructure varied considerably with apparent density as can be seen in Fig. 2b and c. This is reflected in the variation in pore size and a thickening of the ceramic "struts" whereas the microstructural features were similar in all specimens (Table 1).

Chemical analysis

The X-ray fluorescence results indicated that Endobon® did not contain significant quantities of impurities, although there were some traces of Mg, Na, Al and Si (Table 2). These results were also used to determine the Ca:P ratio, calculated from the data as 1.68, hich is close to the theoretical value of 1.67 for stoichiometric hydroxyapatite. This

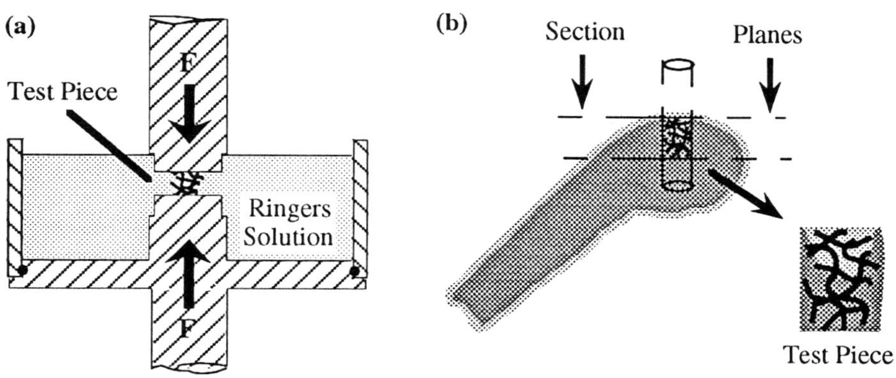

Figure 1 (a) Compression testing jig and (b) integrated test piece preparation.

Table 1. Summary of physical characteristics.

Apparent Density Mg m^{-3}	Macro-Pore Size Length μm	Real Density Mg m^{-3}	Micro-Pore Size μm	Grain Size μm
0.61±0.04 0.90±0.03 1.19±0.06	1380±810 760±240 460±290	3.039±0.004	0.856±0.418	1.38±0.70

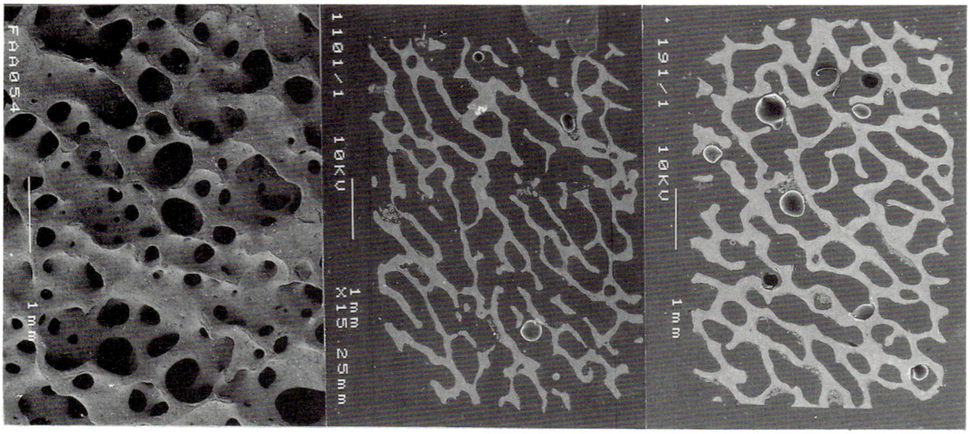

(a) (b) (c)

Figure 2. Examples of Endobon® macrostructure: (a) Surface view. Longitudinal sections of specimens with apparent densities of (b) 0.65 and (c) 1.11 Mg m^{-3}.

slight discrepancy in Ca:P ratio may be due to phase impurity such as traces of CaO or substitution of carbonate for phosphate groups. The X-ray diffraction patterns obtained for Endobon®, matched the ASTM standard for hydroxyapatite, and did not indicate the presence of any significant quantities of secondary phase, demonstrating phase-purity. However, there was some peak shifting of about 0.1° and refinement of the structural data indicated that the lattice was severely distorted in the region of the phosphate tetrahedra. Moreover, the infra-red spectra detected the presence of carbonate, which coupled with the lattice distortion indicates B-type carbonate substitution. Thus the slight discrepancy in Ca:P ratio is likely to arise from carbonate substitution, a consequence of either the stage in production when organic material is reduced to carbon before pyrolysis, or direct conversion from the bone mineral. Allhough it is still possible that traces of CaO, not detectable using XRD, are present as a result of the pyrolysis of the organic material and subsequent oxidisation of any unstable calcium salts present in the bone mineral.

Biological response

Endobon® displayed a highly osseoconductive surface as a result of the B-type carbonate substitution which also occurs in natural bone mineral. Integration within all the implants was good with direct apposition of bone on the implant surfaces and no fibrous encapsulation (Fig. 3a). Cellular response was favourable with cells such as osteoblasts and osteocytes observed in close proximity to the implant surfaces exhibiting normal activity (Fig. 3a and b). Integration tended to proceed predominately from the bottom with some ingrowth from the walls of the defect. However the amount of integration varied with apparent density, with the least being in the high density specimens (Fig. 3c and d).

Table 2. Results of X-ray fluorescence.

Oxide	CaO	P_2O_5	MgO	Na_2O	Al_2O_3	SiO_2
Weight %	55.4	41.7	0.85	0.58	0.20	0.18

Mechanical testing

Specimens exhibited similar behaviour to an elastic brittle foam, where linear elastic deformation at low stresses is followed by a collapse plateau due to the failure of the individual struts (Fig. 4a). The ultimate compressive stress (UCS) was found to be highly dependent on the apparent density (ρ) with a relationship similar to those previously postulated for cancellous bone and porous HA [5,6] (Fig. 4b):

$$\text{UCS} = 5.87\ \rho^{1.99} \tag{1}$$

The mechanical behaviour of the low and medium density specimens altered significantly after implantation (Fig. 4c), will behaviour closer to that of the cancellous bone removed from the contra lateral femur (Fig. 4d), than the elastic-brittle behaviour displayed before implantation. The mechanical behaviour of the higher density material was less affected (Fig. 4c) by the bone ingrowth. This may be a result of the increased content of ceramic (thickening of struts) in the higher density material dominating the behaviour, where as the failure of the lower density material is controlled by the Large volume of bone ingrowth, which is less brittle.

CONCLUSIONS

These findings suggest that Endobon® is highly biocompatible. It acts as a support for new bone and encourages bone growth on its surfaces. The amount of bone ingrowth

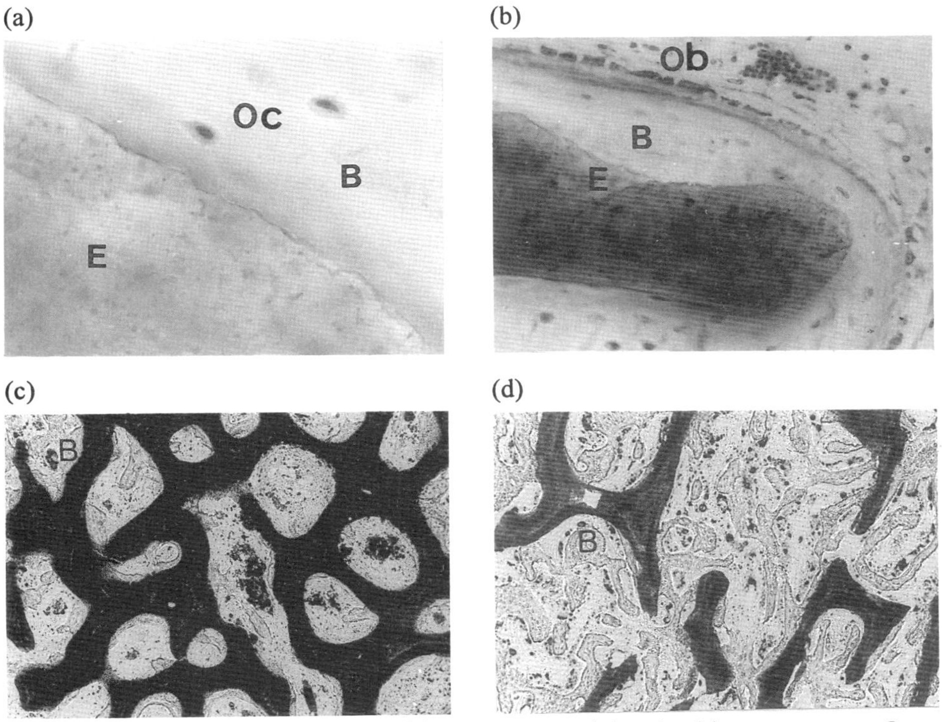

Figure 3. (a) Direct apposition of bone, **B**, containing healthy osteocytes, **Oc**, on Endobon®, **E**, (x 1000). (b) Osteoblastic activity, **Ob**, around an Endobon® strut, (x 400). Bone ingrowth within (c) high density and (d) low density Endobon®, (x 100).

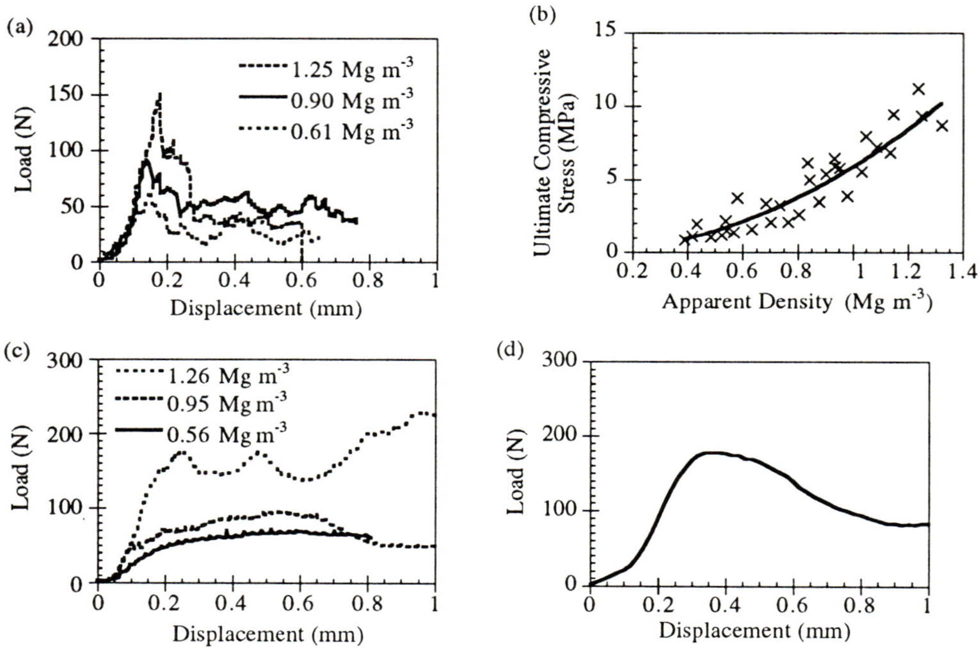

Figure 4 (a) Compression behaviour of as-received specimens. (b) Dependence of ultimate compressive stress on apparent density (r^2 = 0.865). (c) Compression behaviour of explanted specimens during compression. (d) Compression behaviour of trabecular bone.

varied with apparent density, with the least ingrowth in the high density specimens. Before implantation the material behaved as an elastic brittle foam and the ultimate compressive stress (UCS) was highly dependent on apparent density. After implantation the osseointegrated low density specimens exhibited behaviour similar to trabecular bone while the high density material, which had a higher UCS than the cancellous bone, still behaved as a brittle material. These results suggest that implants may be selected for different applications using porosity as a guide to mechanical competence, and that the matching of mechanical properties to the host tissue results in a more compatible implant.

ACKNOWLEDGEMENTS

The support of E. Merck GmbH., and of EPSRC are gratefully acknowledged.

REFERENCES

1. Denissen H.W., Van Dijk H.J.A., De Groot K., Klopper P.J., Vermiden J.P.W. and Gehring A.P. *Mechanical Properties of Biomaterials* John Wiley & Sons Ltd. 1980, 489-505.
2. Eggli P.S., Muller W. and Schenk R.K. *Clin. Orthop. Rel. Res. 1988,* 232, 127-138.
3. PosnerA.S. *Physiological Reviews* 1969, 49, 760-792.
4. Smith J.W. J. *Bone* J. *Surg.* 1963, 45-B, 761.
5. Rice R.W. J. *Am. Ceram. Soc.* 1993, 79, 1801-1808.
6. Gibson L.J. and Ashby M.F. *Cellular Solids Structure and Poperties* Pergamon Press, 1980, 316-331.

COMPARATIVE PROPERTIES OF BIOACTIVE BONE GRAFT MATERIALS

R.Z. LeGeros, C. Bautista, D. Styner, J.P. LeGeros, T.V. Vijiayaraghavan, M. Retino, and A. Valdecanas

New York University College of Dentistry, 345 East 24th Street, New York, New York

ABSTRACT

This study compared some physico-chemical properties of commercial and experimental bone-graft materials belonging to the following categories: (1) synthetic hydroxyapatite (Calcitite®, Bioroc®, Osteogen®, BCP); (2) bone-derived materials (BioOss®, Osteograf®/N, 'BonAP'); (3) coral-derived materials (Biocoral® and Interpore®); and (4) a bioactive glass (Perioglas®).

SEM analyses showed differences in surface morphology, porosity and crystal sizes. X-ray diffraction and Infrared absorption analyses showed differences in composition and difference in crystallinities among materials of the same category or of similar, but not identical composition. The comparative extent of dissolution in Tris buffer after one hour was as follows: Biocoral® > > Perioglas® > > BioOss® > > 'BonAP' > Osteogen® > Bioroc® > BCP> Osteograf®/N > Interpore® > Calcitite®.

This study demonstrated that the bioactive bone graft materials investigated differed in composition between categories and in crystallinity and composition within each category. All the materials exhibited the following: (1) release calcium and/or phosphate ions to the microenvironment; (2) formation of carbonate apatite by the processes of dissolution and precipitation.

INTRODUCTION

Materials (not including autogeneous or banked bones) presently used as particulates, blocks or as coatings on dental and orthopedic implants for bone repair, augmentation and substitution differ in origin, methods of preparation, composition and therefore in differ in properties and host response [1-9,11-13,15-23,25-27]. They are described either as bioinert (e.g., metals, polymers) or bioactive (e.g., special glasses, ceramics, calcium phosphates) materials. Bioactivity was initially used to describe the ability of glasses of special formulations (e.g., Bioglass®) to form an intimate and uniquely strong interface with host bone [10] . Bioactivity has subsequently been associated with calcium phosphate materials (e.g. hydroxyapatite, HA; tricalcium phosphate, TCP; biphasic calcium phosphate, BCP), including bone- and coral-derived materials [2-9,12,18,21-27]. Recent studies speculate that bioactivity maybe related to the formation of carbonate apatite crystals *in vitro* [11,12,18-20]; which may be related to biodegradation, which in turn, may be related to solubility [18-20]. The carbonate apatite crystals, similar to bone apatite [14], are believed to become subsequently incorporated in the mineralization of collagen during the formation of the new bone at the material/host bone interface [11,20].

Previous studies compared some physico-chemical properties of ceramic hydroxyapatite, HA; tricalcium phosphate, ß-TCP; biphasic calcium phosphate, BCP (of varying ß-TCP/HA ratios); coralline HA; bovine-derived material; special glass ceramics and polymethylmetacrylate polymer beads [1,2,6,11,13,15-18]. In the present study, the bioactive materials investigated belong to the following general categories: (1) synthetic hydroxyapatite and related calcium phosphates; (2) bone-derived materials; (3) coral-derived materials; and (4) special glasses.

MATERIALS AND METHODS

Commercial and experimental materials studied for each category were: (1) synthetic hydroxyapatite (Calcitite®, Bioroc®, Osteogen®); (2) bone-derived materials (Bio-Oss®, Osteograf®/N, 'BonAP'); (3) coral-derived materials (Biocoral® and Interpore®); and (4) special glasses (Perioglas®). Some of the materials were purchased for this study, others were donated.

X-ray diffraction analyses using Philips APD 3520 were made on powdered materials (200 mesh). Infrared (IR) analyses using Perkin-Elmer 983G Spectrometer were made on KBr pellets prepared by mixing 1 mg sample with 300mg KBr (IR grade) pressed at 12,000 psi. Scanning electron microscopy (SEM) analysis were made using a JEOL SEM. For chemical analyses, calcium, Ca; magnesium, Mg; and strontium, Sr, were analyzed using atomic absorption spectrophotometry; phosphorus, P, by colorimetric method; fluoride, F, by ion-selective electrode.

Dissolution experiments were made by suspending material particulates in Tris buffer, pH 7.3, at 37°C; solid/solution ratio was 25 mg/50 ml; stirring at 500 rpm. Ca ions released to the buffer with time (up to 3 hrs) were monitored using a calcium ion selective electrode.

Reactivity in serum of some of the materials was investigated by incubating 100 mg in 5 ml calf serum in a shaking water bath maintained at 37°C for two weeks. Calcium and phosphate concentrations of the serum were analyzed before and after suspension. The materials before and after suspension were analyzed using SEM and IR. Transformation to carbonate hydroxyapatite, CHA, was also compared for some of the materials.

RESULTS AND DISCUSSION

X-ray diffraction (Fig. 1) and IR (Fig. 2) analyses showed similarities and differences in composition (Table 1) and crystallinities which may be attributed to the differences in preparation methods and origin (synthetic vs. natural). Apatite materials differed in crystallinity (reflecting crystal size): Calcitite® > Bioroc® > Osteograf®/N > BonAP > Interpore® > > Osteogen® > BioOss®.

The extent of dissolution (reflected by the amount of calcium ions released to the Tris buffer after one hour (Figs. 3, 4) is presented below in the decreasing order:

Biocoral® > > Perioglas® > > Bio-Oss® > Osteogen® > BCP* >
Bioroc® > Osteograf®/N > Interpore® > Calcitite®.

Fig. 1

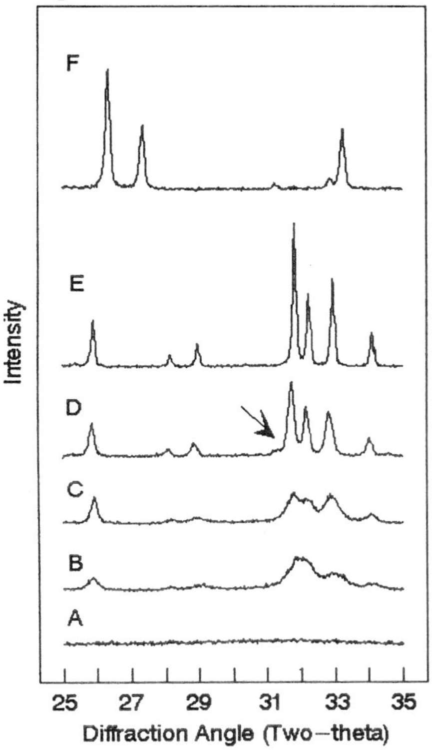

Fig. 2

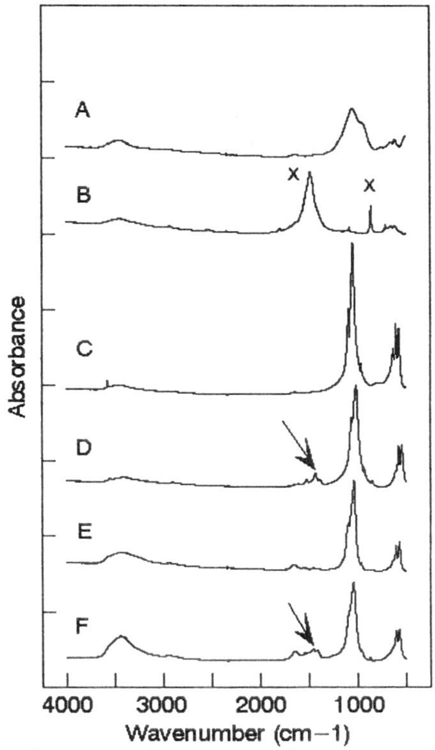

Fig. 1: X-ray diffraction (XRD) patterns: (A) Perioglas ^{R}; (B) BioOss^{R}; (C) Osteogen^{R}; (D) Interpore^{R}; (E) Calcitite^{R}; and (F) Biocoral^{R}. (A) is amorphous; (B) and (C) are apatite of poor crystallinity as shown by broad diffraction peaks compared to (D) and (E); (D) includes β-TCMP (Mg-substituted β-TCP), arrow; (E) calcium hydroxyapatite; (F) $CaCO_3$, aragonite form. XRD patterns of Osteograf^{R}/N, Bioroc^{R} and 'BonAP' are similar to that of Calcitite^{R} (E).

Fig. 2: Infrared absorption (IR) spectra: (A) Perioglas ^{R}; (B) Biocoral^{R}; (C) Calcitite^{R}; (D) Interpore^{R}; (e) Osteogen^{R}; (f) BioOss^{R}. CO^3 incorporated in the apatite structure is shown (arrow) in (D) and (F); contrasted to CO_3 (arrow) in $CaCO_3$, aragonite (B). IR spectra of Ostegraf^{R}/N and 'BonAP' are similar to that of Calcitite^{R} (C).

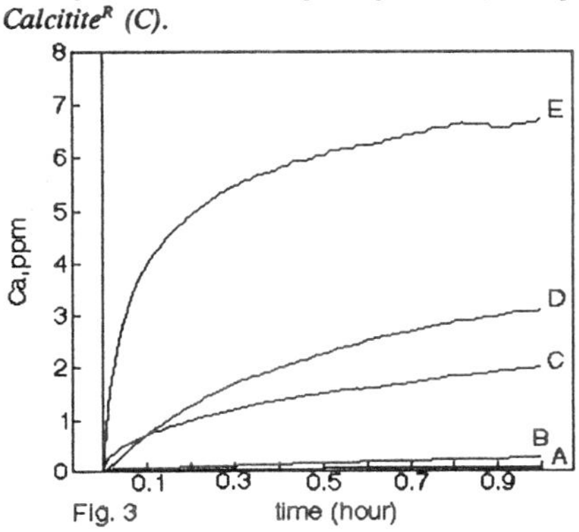

Fig. 3

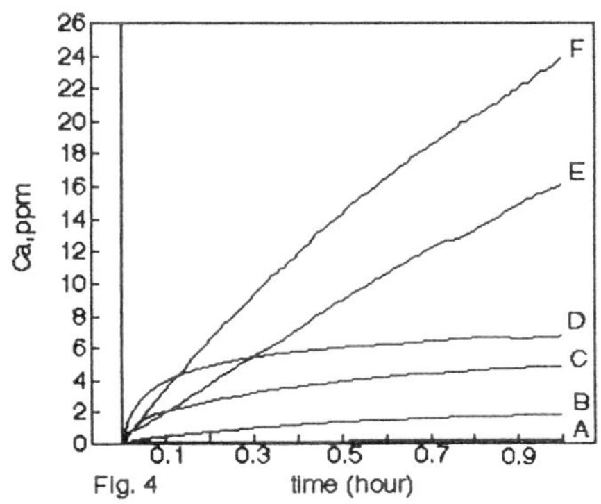

Fig. 4

Fig. 3: Comparative extent of dissolution in Tris buffer, pH 7.3, 37°C expressed as ppm Ca in buffer with time: (A) Calcitite^{R}; (B) Interpore^{R}; (C) Bioroc^{R}; (D) Osteogen^{R}; (E) BioOss^{R}.

Fig. 4: Comparative extent of dissolution in Tris buffer, pH 7.3, 37°C: (A) Interpore^{R}; (B) Osteograf^{R}/N; (C)'BonAP'; (D) BioOss^{R}; (E) Perioglas ^{R}; and (F) Biocoral^{R}. Note that while the dissolution curves of (A), (B), (C), and (D) have appeared to reached saturation after 3 hrs, (E) and (F) have not.

Table 1. Composition of Bioactive Materials

Biomaterials	*Composition*	*Origin*	*Porosity*
Perioglas®(US Biomaterials)	Ca, P, Si, Na	synthetic	nonporous
Biocoral® (Inoteb)	$CaCO_3$ (aragonite)	coral	macroporous
Interpore (Interpore)	'CHA$^{(1)}$' + ß-TCP	^{h}coral	macroporous
Calcitite® (Calcitek)	HA	*synthetic	dense
Bioroc® (Bioland)	HA	*synthetic	micrporous
Osteogen® (Impladent)	Ca-deficient AP	synthetic	microporous
BCP	HA + ß-TCP	synthetic	m/m
BioOss® (EdGeitslich)	'CHA$^{(2)}$'	bovine bone	macroporous
BonAp (HiMed)	'HA'	*bovine bone	microporous
Osteograf®/N (Ceramed)	'HA'	*bovine bone	microporous

HA - calcium hydroxyapatite, $Ca_{10}(PO_4)_6(OH)_2$; ^{h}coral - corraline HA, hydrothermally converted [24]; 'CHA$^{(1)}$'- carbonate hydroxyapatite, $(Ca,X)_{10}(PO_4,CO_3)_6(OH,Z)_2$, where X=Na, Sr, etc; Z = Cl, F; 'CHA$^{(2)}$' - bone apatite obtained by removing organic phase of bone; ß-TCP - pure tricalcium phosphate, $Ca_3(PO_4)_2$; ß-TCMP-Mg-substituted, $(Ca,Mg)_3(PO_4)_2$; Ca-deficient apatite - calcium deficient apatite, unsintered, cortains HPO_4, maybe prepared by precipitation of hydrolysis of $CaHPO_4.2H_2O$ or $CaHPO_4$ [17]; 'HA' - HA with other substituents (e.g., Mg, Na), sintering process removes CO_3 from bone apatite and increases crystallite size [14,17]; BCP - varying ß-TCP/HA ratios; *sintered (sintering temperature may differ).
All materials are crystalline excent for Bioglass® and Perioglas®, which are amorphous (Fig. 1A).

SEM analyses showed differences in surface morphology, porosity, particle and and crystal sizes (Fig. 5). The comparative extent of dissolution for time periods 5, 30 and 60 min is summarized in Table 2. Extent of dissolution is influenced by composition: (e.g., Biocoral > > Perioglas® > > BioOss®; or particle size for materials of the same type (e.g., Bioroc® > > Calcitite®). For BCP materials, dissolution increases with increasing ß-TCP\HA ratio.

Initial studies on the amount of calcium uptake from the serum after incubation showed variability: BiosOss > > coralline HA > > ceramic HA. Partial transformation of the biomaterials to CHA similar to bone apatite [14,18,19] also differed in degree: coralline HA > > ceramic HA.

SUMMARY AND CONCLUSION

Bioactive bone graft materials differ in composition between categories and in crystallinity and composition within each category. Dissolution properties are influenced by particle size, crystallinity and composition. Bioactive materials release calcium and/or phosphate ions to the microenvironment and forms carbonate hydroxyapatite (CHA) through the processes of dissolution and precipitation.

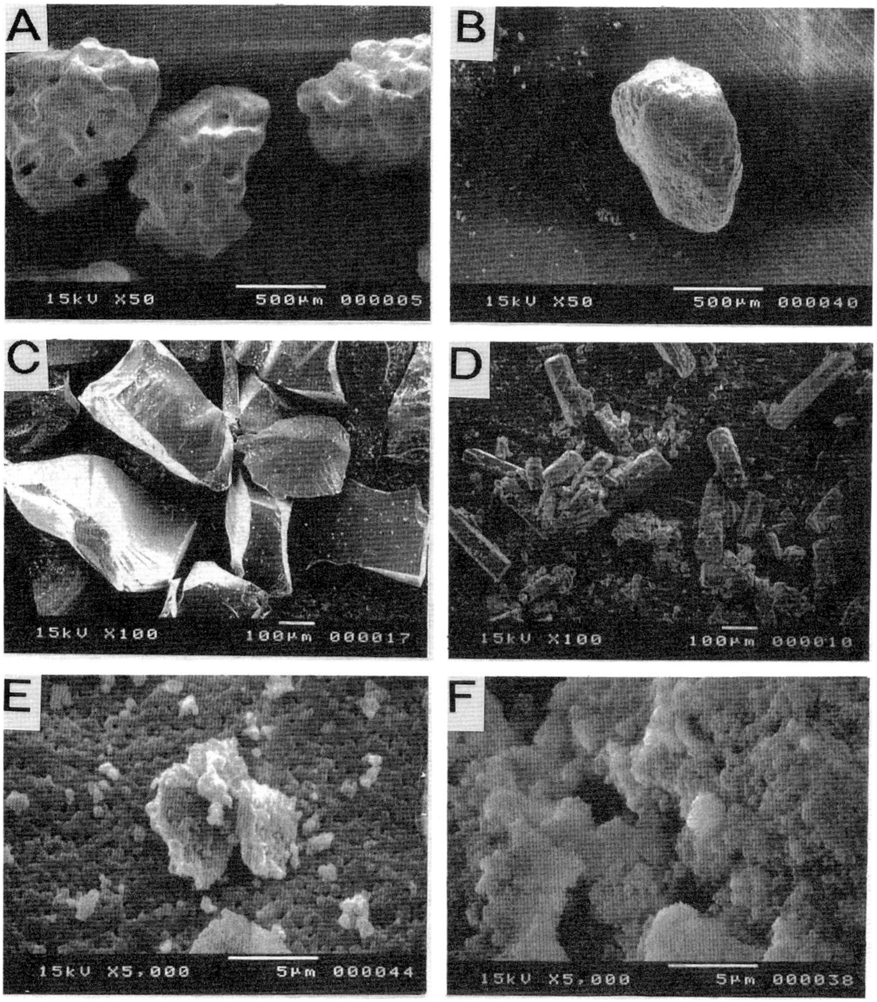

Fig. 5: Scanning electron micrographs (SEM): (A) Biocoral^{R}; (B) Calcitite^{R}; (C) Perioglass^{R}; (D) Osteogen^{R}; (E)'BonAP' and (F) Osteogen^{R}. Macroporosity of Interpore^{R}, BioOss^{R} are similar to Biocoral^{R}(A). HA crystal of Calcitite^{R} and Osteograf^{R}/N are larger than those of 'BonAp' (E).
The large crystals of Osteogen^{R} shown in (D) consists of apatite microcrystals shown in (F).

Table 2. Comparative Extent of Dissolution in Tris Buffer

Biomaterials	*Particle Size, µm*	*ppm Ca 5 min*	*ppm Ca 30 min*	*ppm Ca 60 min*
Calcitite®	425-850	0.03	0.05	0.07
Interpore®	425-1000	0.07	0.16	0.26
Bioroc®	80-160	0.67	1.52	2.02
Osteogon®	300-400	0.61	2.28	3.11
Ostegraf®/N	250-425	0.44	1.42	1.86
'BonAP'	180-250	1.96	3.96	4.88
BioOss®	250-1000	3.73	6.03	6.73
Perioglas®	106-425	1.73	8.97	16.41
Bioglass®	106-355	2.53	10.40	18.21
Biocoral®	450-850	2.94	14.34	23.80

ACKNOWLEDGEMENTS

We acknowledge the generosity of the following in providing materials used in this study: Drs. E. Garofalo (HiMED); D. Greenspan (US Biomaterials), L. Machi; P. Seebag; E. Shors (Interpore); A. Tofe (Ceramed); W. Tozzi (Osteohealth Co); and W. Wagner (Calcitek);

REFERENCES

1. Amler, M.H. and LeGeros, R.Z., *J. Biomed. Mat. Res.* 1990, 24, 1079-1089.
2. Aoki, H., Kato, K., Ogiso, M. and Tabata, T., *J. Dent. Enz.* 1977 ,18, 86-89.
3. Boyne P.J., *J. Long-term Effects Med. Impl.* 1993, 3, 143-159.
4. Callan, D.P. and Rohrer, M.D., *J. Periodontol* 1993, 64, 575-582.
5. Daculsi, G., LeGeros, R.Z. and Deudon, C. *Scan Micros* 1990, 4, 309-314.
6. DeGroot, K., *Biomaterials* 1980, 1, 47-50.
7. Guilemin, G.J., Patat, J.L. and Fournier J., *J. Biomed. Mat. Res.* 1987, 21, 557-567.
8. Gross, U. and Strunz, V., *J. Biomed. Mater. Res.* 1985, 19, 251-271.
9. Hashimoto-Uoshima, M., Ishikawa, I., Kinoshita, A., Went, H,T. and Oda, S., *Int. J. Perio. & Resto. Dent.* 1995, 15, 204-213.
10. Hench, L.L., Splinter, R.J., Allen, W.C. and Greenlee, T.K., *J. Biomed. Mater. Res.* 1971, 2, 117-141.
11. Hench, L.L. and Andersson, Ö.H., In *An Introduction to Bioceramics,* World Scientific, London 1993, 41-62.
12. Hyakuna, K., Yamamuro, T., Kotoura, Y. and Oka, M., *J. Biomed. Mater. Res.* 1990, 24, 471-488.
13. Jarcho, M., *Clin. Orthop.* 1981, 157, 259-278.
14. LeGeros, R.Z. *Prog. Crystal Growth Charact.* 1981, 4, 1-45.
15. LeGeros, R.Z., *Adv. Dent. Res.* 1988, 2, 164-180.

16. LeGeros, R.Z., In *Biomechanics in Orthopedics*, Springer-Verlag, Tokyo 1992, 147-174.
17. LeGeros, R.Z., in *Calcium Phosphates in Oral Bioloav and Medicine Monographs in Oral Sciences* Volume 15, 1991.
18. LeGeros, R.Z. and Daculsi, G., In *Handbook of Bioactive Ceramics* Volume 2, CRC Press, Boca Raton 1990, 17-28.
19. LeGeros, R.Z., Orly, I. and Gregoire, M., *J. Dent. Res.* 1988, 67, 177: In *Apatite* Volume 1, Japanese Association of Apatite Science, Japan 1992, 229-35. (1992).
20. LeGeros, R.Z., Orly, I., Gregoire, M. and Daculsi, G., In *The Bone-Biomaterial Interface*, University of Toronto Press 1991, 76-83.
21. Nery, E.B., LeGeros, R.Z. and Lynch, K.L., *J. Periodont* 1992, 63, 729-735.
22. Osborn, F.J. and Newesely, H., *Biomaterials* 1980, 1, 108-111 (1980).
23. Ricci, J.L., Blumenthal, N.C., Spivek, J.M. and Alexander, H. *J. Oral Maxill. Surg* 1992, 50, 969-978.
24. Roy, D.M. and Linnehan, S.A., *Nature* 1974, 247, 220-227.
25. Saffar, A.L., Comlombier, M.L. and Detienville, R., *J. Periodont* 1990, 61, 209-216.
26. Shors, E.C., White, E.W. and Kopchok, G., *Mater. Res. Soc. Proc.* 1989, 110, 211-218.
27. Wilson, J. and Low, S.B., *J. Appl. Biomat.* 1992, 3, 123-129.

BONE TISSUE REACTION OF OCTACALCIUM PHOSPHATE

F. Sugihara,* H. Oonishi,** S. Kushitani,** N. Iwaki,** Y. Mandai,* K. Minamigawa,* E. Tshuji,*** M. Yoshikawa,**** and T. Toda****

*Nitta Gelatin Inc. Research Laboratory; 2-22, Futamata, Yao-shi, Osaka 581, Japan **Department of Orthopedic Surgery, Osaka-Minami National Hospital; 677-2, Kido-cho, Kawachinagano-shi, Osaka 586, Japan ***Osaka Prefectural Industrial Engineering Laboratory; 1-53, Enokozima 2-chome, Nishi-ku, Osaka 550, Japan ****Department of Endodontics, Osaka Dental University; 5-31, Otemae 1-chome, Chuo-ku, Osaka 540, Japan

ABSTRACT

The purpose of this study is to investigate the biodegradability as well as osteoconductivity of octacalcium phosphate(OCP). The OCP fine particles used were prepared by hydration of a-tricalcium phosphate in phosphate buffer solution (pH7.0). Histologically the particles conducted massive bony tissue early and were then resorbed partially by osteoclast-like cells. The result shows that OCP particles have osteoconductive and biodegradable characteristics and are useful as a component of a bone substitute material and as a filling material in bone defect area created by perforation on root canal wall or chamber floor.

INTRODUCTION

It has been suggested that precursor phases such as octacalcium phosphate [$Ca_8(HPO_4)_2(PO_4)_4 . 5H_2O$: OCP] was present and that interaction between precursor phases of apatite and organic substances occurred in the initial stage of biological mineralization [1,2,3]. Suzuki et al. have shown that OCP granules implanted subperiosteally in mouse calvariae were converted into apatitic crystals and that the OCP implantation stimulated bone formation [4]. The purpose of this study is to investigate the biodegradability as well as osteoconductivity of OCP fine particles implanted into femoral condyle of mature rabbit.

MATERIALS AND METHODS

OCP fine particles were prepared by the hydration of a-tricalcium phosphate in phosphate buffer solution (pH 7.0) at room temperature for 24hrs. The particles with particle size 10 μm were implanted into a hole of 6 mm in diameter drilled bilaterally through right femoral condyle, and as a control, an unfilled drilled hole was made through left femoral condyle of mature rabbits. The rabbits were sacrificed by intravenous injection of overdoses of *Nembutal*, one, 3, and 6 weeks after implantation of the particles. Condyles were trimmed out en bloc including the particles and fixed. Undecalcified and decalcified sections were made for light microscopic and back scattered electron imaging observations.

RESULTS AND DISCUSSIONS

After one week, the OCP particles were surrounded by fibroblasts and osteoblasts, and the spaces among the particles were penetrated by bone marrow cells and fibroblasts (Figure 1A). The control became a granulation tissue; fibroblasts penetrated from the marrow toward the granulation tissue, and bleeding and sinusoid formation were observed. No new bone formation was seen in the control. After 3 weeks, woven bone tissues of about 50-200 μm in width were formed from the defect bony wall. Many particles were incorporated into new trabecular bone. Abundant woven bone and calcification were generated at the periphery of the particles from the wall, and many osteoblasts were lining around the bone (Figure 1B).

In the control, loose fibrous connective tissue occurred; no new bone formation was present at 3 weeks..

After 6 weeks, trabecular new bone tissues were in the center of the hole (Figure 1C), and almost all the particles had been incorporated into them (Figure 2). Figure 2 also revealed that in the cavity, the trabecular bone had remodeled because of the surface irregularities which were created by resorption of the particles. Osteoclast-like cells existed adjacent to them (Figure 1C). In contrast, a very small amount of bone formation was observed in the control at 6 weeks.

It was hypothesized that OCP particles bound with osteocalcin were resorbed by the cells [5, 6] and were incorporated into trabecular new bone by osteoblasts within 6 weeks after implantation.

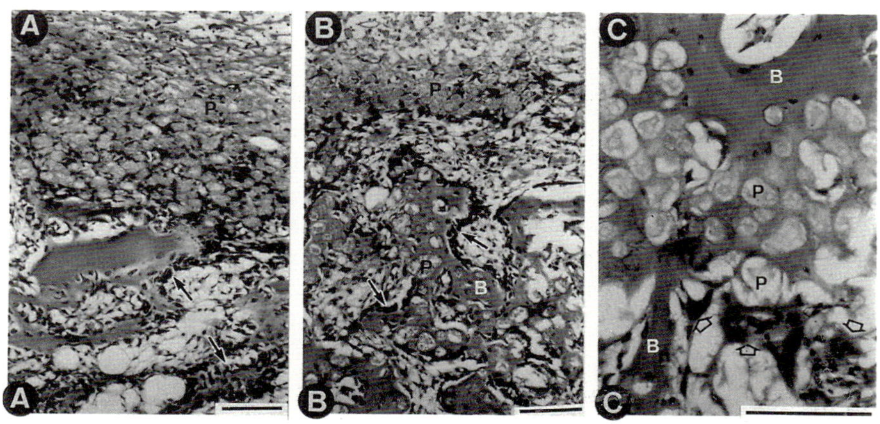

Figure 1. Micrographs of decalcified sections after one(A), 3 (B) and 6 (C) weeks ofimplantation. B: new bone, P: OCP particles, arrows: osteoblasts, arrow heads: osteoclast-like cells bar: 100 μm.

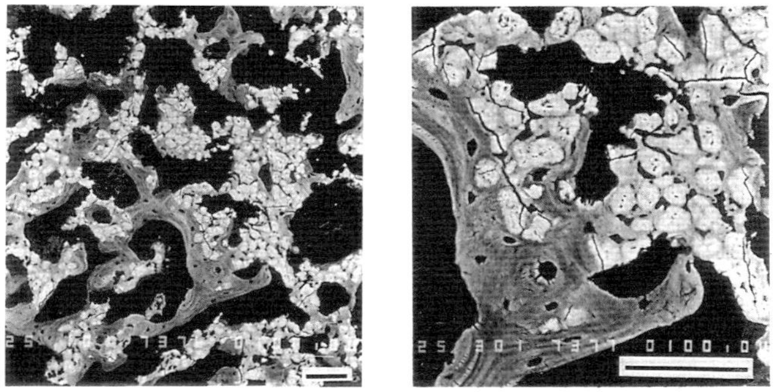

Figure 2. Back scattered image of central area implanted with OCP particles after 6 weeks. bar: 100 μm.

CONCLUSIONS

These results show that OCP particles have osteoconductive and biodegradable characteristics and is useful as a component of a bone substitute material. The particles are also useful as the filling material in a bone defect area created by a perforation on a root canal wall or chamber floor. Moreover, OCP may be useful as a component of a root canal sealer due to its osteoconductivity.

REFERENCES

1. Brown, W.E., Eidelman, N. and Tomazic, B., *Adv. Dent. Res.* 1987, 1, 306-3132.
2. Fisher, L.W. and Termine, J. D., *Clin. Orthop.* 1985, 200, 362-385.
3. Suzuki, O., Nakamura, M., Miyasaka, Y., Kageyama, M. and Sakurai, M., *Bone Miner.* 1993, 20, 151-166.
4. Suzuki, O., Nakamura, M., Miyasaka, Y., Kageyama, M. and Sakurai, M., *Tohoku J. Exp. Med.* 1991, 164, 37-50.
5. Chenu, C., Colucci, S., Grano, M., Zigrio, P., Barattole, R., Zallone, A.Z., *J. Cell Biol.* 1994, 127, 1149-1158.
6. Glowacki, J., Rey, M., Glimcher, M.J., Cox, K.A. and Lian, J., *J. Cell Biochem.* 1991, 45, 292-302.

THE PHENOMENOLOGICAL BEHAVIOR OF HUMAN BONE MARROW CELLS ON BIOGLASS® SURFACES. A CELL CULTURE STUDY

A.Wilke, H. Poenitz, J. Orth, H. Kienapfel, K. Boelte, and P. Griss

Dep. of Orthop. Surg., Philipps-University Marburg
Baldingerstrasse, D-35033 Marburg

ABSTRACT

The objective of this study was to investigate the behavior of human bone marrow cells cultivated for 2 and 12 weeks on different types of round shaped biomaterial specimens (Bioglass® 45S5, HA (Osprovit), Titanium and UHMWPE). Afterwards the cells were investigated with episcopic light microscopy, SEM and SEM-EDX.

After 2 weeks we saw many adherent cells at the surfaces of the different Bioglasses® but no signs of extracellular matrix. After 12 weeks the specimens demonstrated many cells and ECM which contained a high amount of calcium and phosphate in SEM-EDX analysis. Concerning cell adhesion, cell number and production of ECM, Bioglass® demonstrated a good biocompatibility in a human bone marrow cell culture system.

INTRODUCTION

The adherence of cells to a biomaterial surface is a prerequisite for tissue integration. New bone formation on biomaterials depends on surface structures which promote cell proliferation and production of extracellular matrix.

A cytotoxic affect of biomaterials clearly can inhibit osseointegration [1,2]. In the field of biocompatibility testing of biomaterials different cell culture systems were used. These culture systems consisted mainly of highly differentiated cells which normally had no contact to orthopedic implants in human surgery [3].

Among these studies culture systems of non-human origin and tumor cell lines were used [4]. Most cell culture systems that are used to test biomaterials for bone implants have some disadvantages. They are either of non human origin [3,5,6,7] or exploit cells which are not opposed to orthopaedic implants in situ [8,9,10].

In comparison to the cell culture systems described elsewhere the human bone marrow cell culture used here had the following advantages:

- the cells were of human origin.
- Cell populations were used which are opposed to orthopaedic implants in situ.

- Besides immunocompetent and differentiated cell populations (B- and T-cells) this culture system contains mesenchymal stem-cells (progenitor cells) which have the potential to differentiate into various cell types depending on the culture condition (e.g. type of biomaterial) [10,11]. The description and the quantification of cellular differentiation *in vitro* may give useful information on tissue reactions which occur after implantation of biomaterials *in vivo.*

MATERIALS AND METHODS

Human bone marrow was harvested during a patient's first total hip replacement by removing a marrow containing cancellous bone block from the side of the femoral osteotomy. The marrow cells were isolated and immediately incubated into a special medium which was originally used by Dexter [12] and modified by Kalla [13]. Kalla's medium contains: Iscoves Modified Dulbeccos Medium (IMDM) with a fetal calf serum (12,5%), horse serum (12,5%), Hydrocortisone (2,4 ng/ml), Certomycin (50 mg/L), L-Glutamin (292,3 ng/ml), $NaHCO_3$ (0,3%) and Aqua dest. Afterwards ten million cells were seeded directly onto each biomaterial sample. The following growth factors were added: Interleukin III and Granulocyte-Macrophage-Colony-Stimulating-Factor (0,625 ng/ml medium). Fourteen days thereafter the following techniques were used to investigate the adherent cells: Episcopic light microscopy, transparent light (fluorescence) microscopy, SEM and SEM-EDX. The following materials were tested: A)Polymeres: Polyethylene (UHMWPE). B) Ceramics: HA (Osprovit ®). C) Metals: Pure titanium (Ti). D) Bioglass® 45S5.

The biomaterial samples were disc like (20mm in diameter, 2mm thick). To study the surface qualities all samples were investigated by SEM and energy dispersive X-ray analysis (SEM-EDX).

The cell parameters on the different surfaces were evaluated by different methods:

- cell adherence and matrix production by SEM,
- cell vitality after Acridine-Orange (4min.) with episcopic light (fluorescence) microscopy (520nm),
- cell numbers after hematoxylin staining by episcopic light microscopy with the help of an image analysis system (OPTIMAS).

RESULTS

The SEM-EDX analysis revealed the surface morphology and local concentrations of elements at the surface of biomaterials.

In case of the Bioglass® specimens we saw a cracked surface after contact with medium and especially after preparation for SEM which limited the analysis of the local concentrations of elements at the surface.

By SEM-analysis we could observe well attached spread cells, which showed the morphological signs of extracellular matrix production in case of HA-ceramics, titanium specimens and Bioglass® 45S5. With UHMWPE as a substrate we could observe only a few adherent cells and practically no ECM production (Figs. 1, 2, 3 and 4).

The long term bone marrow culture demonstrated on the Bioglass® surfaces many cells with ECM which contained a high amount of calcium and phosphate in the SEM-EDX.

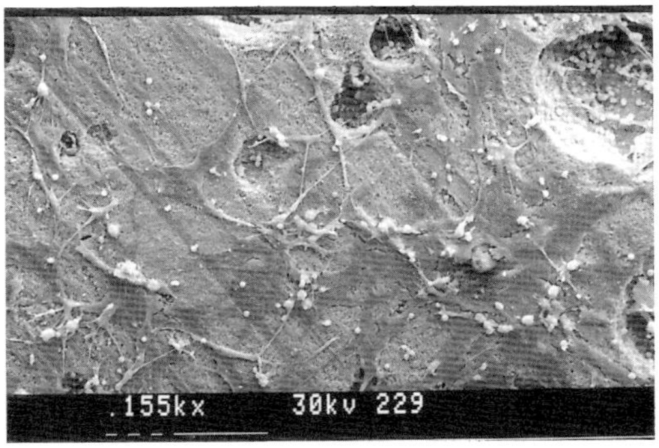

Fig. 1. Ha-Ceramic (Cerasiv®) with well attached spread cells and ECM-Production (2 weeks culture, SEM x 155)

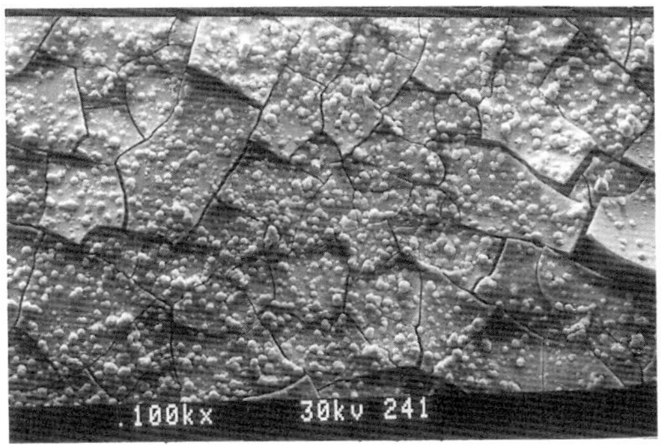

Fig. 2. Many cells on the Bioglass® surface, no signs of ECM. The surface was broken during preparation for SEM as a sign of instability (2 weeks culture, SEM x 100)

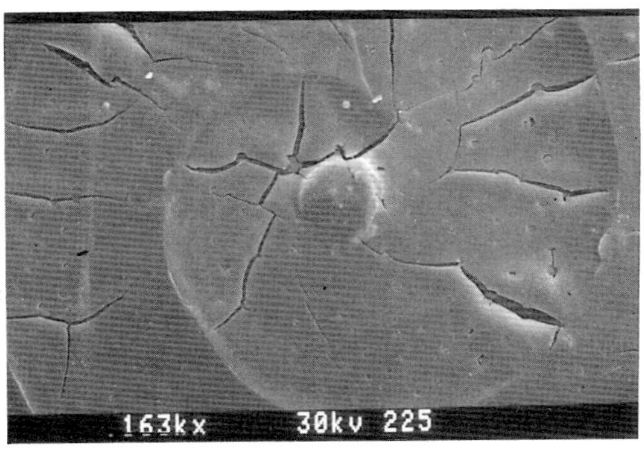

Fig. 3. Only a few cells and no ECM on UHMWPE (2 weeks culture, SEM x 163)

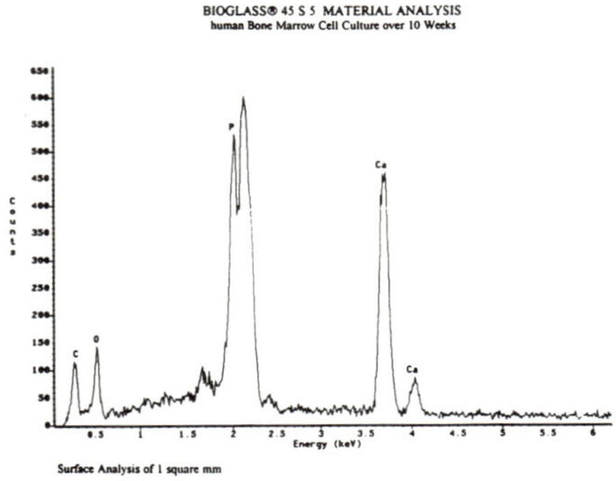

Surface Analysis of 1 square mm

Element	Element Wt %
C	40,43
O	22,13
Ca	25,52
P	11,92

Fig. 4. A high amount of calcium and phosphate is shown on a sample of Bioglass® 45S5 after being in cell cuture for 10 weeks

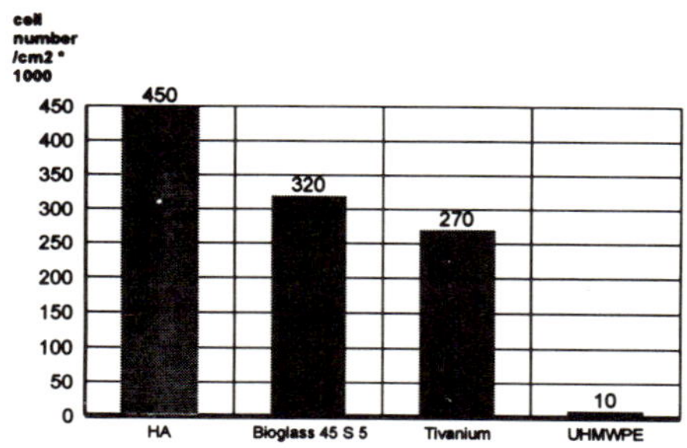

Fig. 5. The chart demonstrate the average cell number of ten experimental runs on the biomaterials

Figure 5 shows the results of cell counts with the help of an image analysis system (OPTIMAS) after staining with hematoxylin. Highest cell density was found on the HA-ceramics. There were less cells on Bioglass® and Ti-specimens. Only a few cells were on the PE-substrate.

Evaluation of the cell differentiation with both the Pappenheim staining and immunostaining of CD-antigens revealed no differences between cells on ceramics, on Ti-specimens and on the glass controls.

Visualization of the cytoskeleton in cells on these biomaterials demonstrated filament networks and stress fibers similar to cells *in situ.*

Concerning the indicative parameters cell adherence, cell number and cell proliferation, our results demonstrated striking differences between the tested materials. The best results were demonstrated in case of HA, followed by Bioglass® and titanium

DISCUSSION

Human bone marrow cells can be grown on suitable biomaterials. There is a general agreement that growth enhancing surface properties of biomaterials are a prerequisite for a sufficient long-term performance [1,2] of an implant. As was shown here, biomaterials could influence cells to react differently, indicated by characteristic cell activities like cell adhesion, proliferation and ECM production.

In control cultures as well as on HA, Bioglass® and titanium we saw cell growth with proliferation and ECM production. These results seem to be in concordance with the pathophysiological processes seen in patients and in many animal experiments [14,15,16, 17].

Cells on PE were reduced in number and often showed a conspicuous cell shape. This again was demonstrated in animal experiments [18,19,20].

Comparing all our results we could demonstrate great differences between the biomaterials with respect to cell number and ECM production.

In future we want to look for the cell differentiation of human bone marrow cells in contact to Bioglass® 45S5, especially in case of long-term bone marrow cell cultures (FACS analyses).

We hope that in the future the mechanisms of osseointegration of biomaterials can be understood by revealing the cellular and molecular processes involved.

REFERENCES

1. Weiss, R.E. and Reddi, A.H., *J. Cell Biol.* 1981, 88, 630-636.
2. Stutzmann, J. and Petrovic, A., In: *Factors and Mechanisms Influencing Bone and Growth*, NY, USA, 1982, 29-42.
3. Uchida, A.; Nade, S.; McCartney, E.; and Ching, W., *J. Biomed. Mater. Res.*, 1987, 1-10.
4. Goshima, J., Goldberg, V.M. and Caplan, A.J., *Clin. Orthop.*, 1991, 262, 298-311.
5. Hench, L. L. and Ethridge, E. C., *Adv. Biomed., Eng.*, 1975, 5, 35-150.
6. Maroudas, N. G., *Cell Res.*, 1973, 16, 104-110.
7. Bgambisa, F. B. and Joos, U., *Biomaterials*, 1990, 50-56.
8. Folkman, J. and Maskona, A., *Nature,* 1978, 273, 345-349.
9. Schachtschnabel, D. O. and Blencke, B. A., *Europ. Surg. Res.*, 1976, 8, 71-80.
10. Wilsnack, R. E. and Smith, F. J., *Biomat., Med. Dev., Art. Org.*, 1973, 543-562.
11. Wilke, A., Orth, J., Lomb, M., v. Hirschheydt, S., Schröder, G., Griss, P. and Franke, R. P., *Trans. 2nd annual conference of the European Orthopedic Research Society,* Varese, Sep. 27-30. 1992, 50.
12. Dexter, T. M., Spooncer, E., Simmons, P. and Allen, P., *Long Term Culture*, 1984, 57-96.
13. Kalla, P., Hintz-Obertreis, P., Wilke, A., Griss, P., Seiler, F. R., Rüde, E. and Krummwieh, D., *Behring Inst. Mitteil.*, 1991, 90, 93-98.
14. Cook, S. D., Thomas, K. A., Kay, J. F. and Jarcho, M., *Clin. Orthop.*, 1988, 230, 303-312.
15. Geesnik, R. G. T., de Groot, K. and Klein, C. P. A. T., *J. Bone Joint Surg.* 1988, 70-B, 17-22.
16. Osborne, J. F., *Implantatwerkstoff Hydroxylapatit: Grundlage und klinische Anwendung*. Quintessenzverlag, Berlin, Chicago, Rio de Janeiro und Tokyo, 1985.
17. Hench, L. L., Stanley, H. R., Clark, A. E., Hall, M. and Wilson, J., *Bioceramics*, Vol. 4, Butterworh-Heinemann, 1991, 231-238.
18. Wilke, A., Orth, J., Kienapfel, H., Schröder, G. and Griss, P., *Trans. 4th World Biomaterial Congress*, April 24.- 28., 1992, Berlin, 1992, 162.

19. Orth, J., Kautzmann, J.and Griss, P., *Clinical Implant Materials, Advances in Biomaterials*, Vol. 9, G. Heimke, U. Soltesz and A. J. C. Lee (eds.), Elsevier Science Publishers, B. V., Amsterdam, 1990, 283-287.
20. Mathiesen, E. B., Lindgren, J. U., Reinholt, F. P. and Sudmann, E., *J. Biomed. Mater. Res.*, 1987, 21, 459-466.
21. Wilke, A., v. Hirschheydt, S., Orth, J., Kienapfel, H., Griss, P. and Franke, R. P., Die humane Knochenmarkszellkultur: Eine sensitive Methode zur Beurteilung der Biokompatibilität von Materialien, die in der Orthopädie verwendet werden. Z. Orthop.

MEASUREMENT OF INTACT BONE GLA PROTEIN CONTENTS IN POROUS HYDROXYAPATITE

K. Inoue, H. Ohgushi, T. Yoshikawa, S. Tamai, Y. Dohi*, K. Hosoda** and T. Ohta**

Department of Orthopaedic Surgery and Public Health*, Nara Medical University, Kashihara city, Nara, JAPAN; Teijin Institute for Bio-Medical Research**, Teijin Ltd., Tokyo, JAPAN

ABSTRACT

Bone Gla protein(BGP) is synthesized by osteoblasts and is a reliable marker of bone formation. We measured the N-terminal region of BGP(N-BGP) and intact BGP(I-BGP) in the composites of rat marrow cells and bioactive hydroxyapatite(HA) ceramics which showed bone formation after subcutaneous implantation. The amounts of these BGP molecules were compared with that measured by conventional radioimmunoassay(RIA). Levels of these BGP molecules in the composites determined by three different methods were observed in a similar pattern over the experimental period. These results indicated that most BGP molecules in the bone formed in porous HA were intact. Therefore, the surface of HA can support a natural process of osteoblastic differentiation which results in mature bone formation.

INTRODUCTION

Previously, we reported that suboutaneous implantation of various biomaterials with rat bone marrow cells showed bone formation in the back of syngeneic Fischer rats [1]. The bone formation started at about 2 to 3 weeks post implantation and the significant amount of BGP could be detected by conventional RIA [2]. The RIA was done using polyclonal antibody against purified rat BGP [9]. It is also known that the degradation of intact BGP molecules showed immunochemical heterogeneity. Recently, we established the methods to measure intact rat BGP using anti N- and anti C-terminal rat BGP monoclonal antibodies raised against a N-terminal 20 residues peptide and a C-terminal 10 residues peptide of rat BGP, respectively [3,4]. This report analyzes these BGP molecules in the bone formed in porous hydroxyapatite.

MATERIALS AND METHODS

Materials

The discs of porous hydroxyapatite ceramics (Interpore International) were used in this experiment. It is made by conversion of the calcium carbonate skeletal structure of reef building sea corals into pure hydroxyapatite by means of hydrothermal chemical exchange reaction [10]. The solid and porous components of the microstructure are completely interconnected. The average pore size of this implant is 200 μm in diameter and the average void volume is 60%. In this study, we used disk-shaped coralline hydroxyapatite with 5 mm in diameter and 2 mm thick. The total number of ceramics used was 54.

Marrow cell preparation

The detailed procedure was already reported [2]. Briefly, both ends of the femora and tibiae of male Fischer 344 rat were cut away from the epiphysis. The rats were 8 weeks old. The marrow plugs were taken from the prepared bone shafts and disaggregated by sequential passage through 18-G and then 21-G needles. The cells were concentrated by centrifuge, resulting in 5 X 10^8 nucleated cells/ml.

Implantation of ceramics

Six ceramics were implanted subcutaneously in the back of each rat. Three ceramics soaked in the marrow cell suspension were implanted in the left side, and the other three without marrow cell suspension were implanted in the right side.

Measurement of BGP contents

Ceramics were harvested 1 to 4 weeks after implantation. Each ceramic was immediately crushed, homogenized in 0.2% Nonidet P40 containing 1 mM $MgCl_2$ and centrifuged at 13,000 rpm for 10 minutes at 4°C. BGP was extracted from the sediment by shaking in 1 ml of 20% formic acid at 4°C for 2 weeks. An aliquot (500μl) of the formic acid extract was then applied to a column of Sephadex G-25 (fine) and eluted with 10% formic acid. Protein fractions were collected, lyophilized and used for measurement of BGP by three different methods.

Conventional radioimmunoassay(RIA) for BGP (C-BGP)

One of the methods was our previously reported conventional RIA[2] and thus measured contents were represented as C-BGP. Lyophilized protein fractions were dissolved in assay buffer composed of 0.01M phosphate buffer saline(PBS), 0.14M NaCI, 0.025M EDTA, 0.1% gelatin and 0.1% Tween 20. All assays were performed with rabbit antiserum to rat BGP and purified rat BGP was used for standard. Briefly, the assay system consisted of 100 μl of sample dissolved in assay buffer, 100 μl of a 1: 1600 dilution of antiserum, 15,000-20,000 cpm ^{125}I-BGP, and a dilution of normal rabbit serum in a final volume of 400 μl. This was incubated for 20 h at 25°C and then 200 μl of goat anti-rabbit IgG coated immunobeads suspension (Bio-Rad Laboratories) were added to precipitate rabbit antibody. Finally, the mixture was incubated at 37°C for 2 h. Assays were linear between 3.9 and 1000 ng/ml BGP.

Sandwich immunoassay for rat n-terminal BGP(N-BGP)

Detail procedures are to be represented [3,4]. Briefly, a peroxidase conjugated with a rabbit $F(ab')_2$ fragment of the anti-N-terminal 20 residues peptide antiserum(anti-N-20) was prepared according to the method of Fujiwara et al [5]. Polystyrene balls were dipped in anti-N-20 monoclonal antibody (MAb) in PBS and incubated at 4°C overnight. Immobilization was terminated by rinsing the balls three times with PBS, followed by coating with 1% BSA-PBS at 4°C for 2 days. Standard solutions of purified rat BGP were prepared at concentrations of 0-5 ng/ml. Two hundreds μl of standard solution and 200 μl of peroxidase-labeled anti-N-20 $F(ab')_2$ solution with the anti-N-20 MAb-fixed balls were placed in glass tubes. After incubation for 1.5 h at 37°C, each ball was washed three times with saline, then 0.4 ml of tetramethylbenzidine and 0.017% hydrogen peroxide were added to the tube, and finally the mixture was incubated at 37°C for 30 min. The enzymesubstrate reaction was terminated by adding 1 ml of 1 NH_2SO_4 and the absorbance was measured at 450 nm.

Sandwich immunoassay for rat intact BGP(I-BGP)

Intact rat BGP levels were measured by using the anti-C-10 IgG-fixed balls. Standard solution and washing steps were the same as described above.

RESULTS AND DISCUSSION

Previously, we reported the bone forming capability of the composites of porous hydroxyapatite and bone marrow cells by histological analysis (Fig. l). However, no bone formation was seen in porous hydroxyapatite without bone marrow cells. BGP is a prominent non-collagenous protein in bone matrix, which is synthesized particularly by osteoblasts and is considered to play an important role in bone formation. In fact, we demonstrated the extensive amount of BGP in the HA/marrow composites and only traces of BGP in HA without marrow.

The immunoassay for human BGP was first devised by Nishimoto and Price [6]. Their system utilized an antibody that recognized the C-terminal sequence of human BGP. In recent years, various improved methods have been reported, such as the sandwich immunoassay systems for human BGP by Koyama [7] and intact human BGP by Hosoda et al [8]. More recently, we developed a sandwich enzyme immunoassay system for the intact rat BGP molecule using monoclonal antibodies raised against N-terminal and C-terminal synthetic peptides [3,4]. A monoclonal antibody against the N-terminal sequence of BGP was selected to characterize its epitope and species specificity. We have also utilized conventional RIA for measurement of rat BGP using polyclonal antibody [9]. However, a polyclonal antibody may recognize more than one epitope. Therefore, broad cross-reactivity could appear between polyclonal antibody and proteins which have epitopes of similar structure. In view of this, the method of using a monoclonal antibody is reliable.

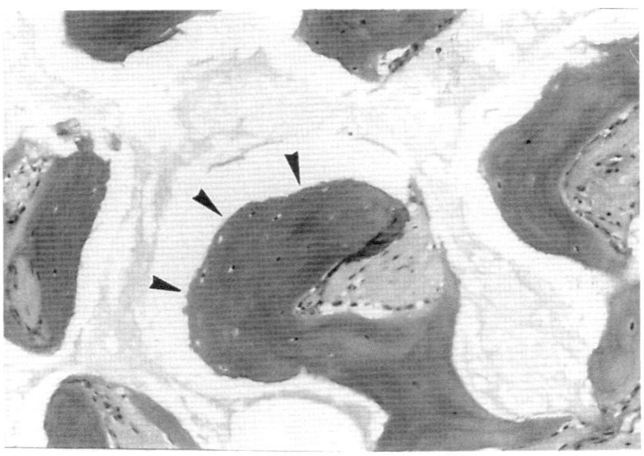

Figure1. Four weeks after subcutaneous implantation of HA with marrow cells. (Decalcified section, X150) White area shows the ghost of HA produced by decalcification procedures, and arrow heads show bone formed in the HA pore regions.

Table 1. Average BGP contents (μg/implant) in the HA with marrow cells (data are mean ± SEM).

	1W	2W	3W	4W
N-BGP	0.088±0.013	0.224±0.051	0.186±0.027	0.521±0.139
I-BGP	0.072±0.012	0.218±0.061	0.165±0.023	0.588±0.165
C-BGP	0.045±0.013	0.159±0.032	0.289±0.098	1.083±0.117

In our conventional radioimmunoassay, samples were maintained at 4°C for about 3 weeks. If BGP of our samples was destroyed partially through the process of measurement, value of the measurement may be less than real value. However, as shown in the Table 1, three different methods showed the similar pattern of BGP appearance in the porous HA. The amounts of N-BGP and I-BGP were very comparable. These results indicate the reliability of our previous reports of BGP measurements in HA/marrow composites and also imply that most BGP molecules in bone formed in porous HA seem to be intact. These results together with our previous reports [11,12] indicate that surface of bioactive HA can support natural process of osteoblastic differentiation which results in mature bone formation.

REFERENCES

1. Ohgushi, H., Goldberg, V.M. and Caplan, A.I. J. *Orthop. Res.* 1989, 7, 568-578.
2. Yoshikawa, T., Ohgushi, H., Okumura, M., Tamai, S., Dohi Y. and Moriyama, T.: Calcif: Tissue Int. 1992, 50, 184-188.
3. Eguchi, H., Hosoda, K., Kurihara, N., Nakamoto, T., Kobayashi, S., Hasegawa, R., Ohta, T., Kiyoki, M., Yamaji, T. and Shiraki, M.: manuscripts in preparation.
4. Ohta, T., Azuma, Y., Kiyoki, M., Eguchi, H., Hosoda, K., Tsukamoto, Y. and Nakamura, T.: manuscripts in preparation.
5. Fujiwara, K., Yasuno, M. and Kitagawa, T., *CancerRes.* 1981, 41, 4121-4126.
6. Nishimoto, S.K. and Price, P.A. J. *Biol. chem.* 1980, 255, 6579-6583.
7. Koyama, N., Ohara, K., Yokota, H., Kurome, T., Katayama, M., Hino, F., Kato, I. and Akai, T. J. *Immunol. Methods* 1991,139, 17-23.
8. Hosoda, K., Eguchi, H., Nakamoto, T., Kubota, T., Honda, H., Jindai, S., Hasegawa, R., Kiyoki, M., Yamaji, T. and Shiraki, M. *Clin. Chem.* 1991, 38, 2233-2238.
9. Dohi, Y., Ohgushi, H., Tabata, S., Yoshikawa, T., Dohi, K. and Moriyama, T. *J. Bone Min. Res.* 1992, 7, 1173-1180.
10. Shors, E.C., White, E.W. and Kopchok, G. *Mat Res. Soc. Symp. Proc.* 1989, 110, 211-218.
11. Okumura, M., Ohgushi, H. and Tamai, S. *Biomaterials 1991,* 12, 411-416.
12. Ohgushi, H., Dohi, Y., Tamai, S. and Tabata, S. *J. Biomed. Mat. Res.* 1993, 27, 1401- 1407.

BONE REMODELING AROUND IMPLANTED CERAMICS

M. Oka, Y.S. Chang, T. Nakamura, M. Kobayashi, T. Kitsugi

Department of Artificial Locomotive Systems, Research Center for Biomedical Engineering, Kyoto University, Kyoto, Japan

ABSTRACT

Bone formation and remodeling around implanted materials is influenced by the kind of material, its surface properties and the anatomical site of implantation. In this study, any differences in bone formation around the various kinds of ceramics, depending on their location in the rabbit tibia, were investigated. By implanting three kinds of ceramics, alumina, zirconia and hydroxyapatite (HA), either into the medullary cavities, or transcortically, the time-dependent formation of bone around the materials were histologically examined until 24 weeks postoperatively. The most abundant bone formation was found around the materials, the rank order being adjacent to the periosteum > endosteum > bone marrow in the approximate ratio of 70%, 40%, and 10%, respectively.

INTRODUCTION

Recently, loosening has been frequently encountered at the bone-cement interface after total joint replacement using bone cement. To solve these cement-related problems, various types of cementless total arthroplasties have been developed. In this respect, one of the most important problems is how securely and rapidly is the implant fixed to the bone.

Previous studies have shown that fixation between the bone and implant can be divided into chemical bonding [1] and mechanical interlocking. The chemical bonding is related to osteoconductivity of the materials and osteogenic potency of the tissues where the materials are implanted. In other words, bone formation and remodeling around implanted materials is influenced by the kind of materials, their surface properties and also by the anatomical site of implantation in the bone.

In this study, we have investigated whether bone formation differs with the site of implantation, in addition to any differences between bioactive and bioinert ceramics.

MATERIALS AND METHODS

Three kinds of materials were used in the experiments: (1) dense hydroxyapatite ceramic, (2) alumina ceramic and (3) zirconia ceramic. The test pieces of bioactive and bioinert materials were manufactured into rectangular shapes (diameter 1.5 x 3.0 x 10.0 mm) by Kyocera Corporation, Japan. All the surfaces of the test pieces were smooth.

For the first experiment, 78 Japanese adult rabbits were allocated randomly to three groups of 26 each. Two test pieces of each ceramic was implanted into the medullary cavities of the upper ends of both tibiae. In the second experiment, 30 rabbits were used and they were allocated randomly to three groups of 10 each. Using a dental barr, two holes were made from medial to lateral cortex of the upper end of each side tibiae. Two test pieces were then placed transcortically in a state of press-fit into the holes of tibiae.

The rabbits were killed at intervals of 2, 4, 6, 8, 12 and 24 weeks after the operation. Two weeks before sacrifice, 30 mg/kg body weight of tetracycline was given intravenously. All the specimens taken from the animals were examined using soft X-ray and histologically.

RESULTS

Neither superficial nor deep infection was observed macroscopically in these two experiments. The following were histological findings of the bone formed around the implants in experiments 1 and 2.

Four weeks after the operation, good new bone formation was observed in contact with endosteum even with zirconia. However, In some cases of HA, there was much more new bone formation around the implants, not only in contact with endosteum but also in the center of the bone marrow. At 6 weeks postoperatively, abundant new bone formation can be seen around both bioactive and bioinert materials, even with zirconia. Under fluorescent tetracycline labeling, abundant new bone could be differentiated clearly from the old. Quantitative computerized analysis of new bone formation around the implant surface showed that 65% of zirconia, 68% of HA and 70% of alumina implant surfaces were covered by new bone at eight weeks. At 12 weeks postoperatively, the fact that bone formation around the implants was influenced more by the implanted site than by the kind of material used can be seen in Figure 1 in which the bone around the three types of ceramics is compared by CMR.

At 24 weeks postoperatively, the bone around HA and zirconia which were implanted in the center of the medullary cavity was resorbed according to Wolff's law which indicated that mechanical stress influence the bone remodeling process, leaving very little bone around the sample. On the other hand, however, much more bone remained surrounding the alumina which was implanted in contact with endosteum. Quantitative computerized analysis showed that 12% of zirconia, 28% of HA and 72% of alumina implant surfaces were covered by new bone at 24 weeks.

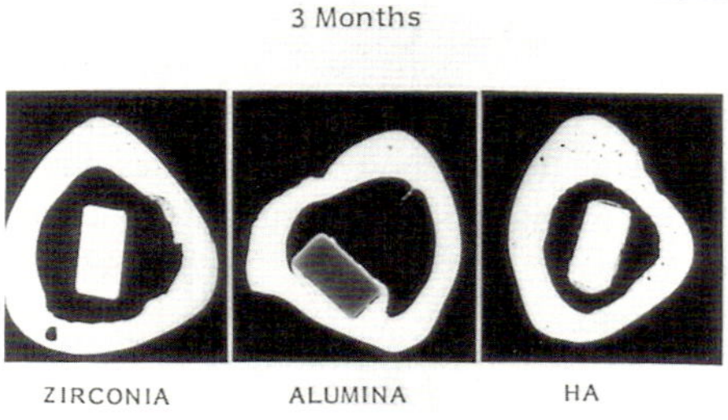

Fig. 1. Less bone were formed around HA and zirconia implanted in the center of bone marrow than that around alumina located in contact with endosteum. (12 weeks P.O. CMR x 10)

In the second experiment, quantitative computerized analysis of new bone formation at the different sites 8 weeks postoperatively showed that the ratio of new bone formation around the three kinds of ceramic was almost same, that was 10% in the center of the bone marrow, 40% in contact with the endosteal surface and 70% when in contact with cortical bone and the periosteal surface. From 12 to 24 weeks, between the cortex and the ceramic surface, newly formed bone was remodeled into lamellar bone. A small amount of newly formed bone remained at the ceramic surface in the bone marrow.

DISCUSSION

Many reports about the bonding behavior of various types of ceramics to bone have been published [2].

Our findings show that at an early stage, until 6 weeks after the operation, new bone formation around the materials follows the biological process of fracture healing irrespective of the kind of material used. These findings coincide well with Brunski's result in which the bone-biomaterial interface was influenced by biomechanical factors, such as micromotion, but was independent of the biomaterial [3]. In the present study, the quantity of new bone around the materials at eight weeks after implantation was not less than that at 24 weeks after implantation, the difference being only in the degree of bone maturation. These findings are supported by the result of Bunte's study with Ceravital [4]. In addition, quantitative computerized analysis of new bone formation around these three ceramics showed that some difference existed, but more marked difference depending on the different sites of implantation was revealed. In other words, the new bone formation around the materials is not so strongly influenced by the osteoconductivity of the materials in contrast to the osteogenic capacity of the tissues.

Schmitz and Hollinger [5] demonstrated the large effect of anatomical location upon bone growth around an implant. Histologically, the periosteum contains many more blood vessels and osteoblasts than the endosteum. Thus, after implantation bone formation is more abundant in the periosteum than in the endosteum. With regard to the bone marrow, it is well known that stromal stem cells also exist in the marrow, and under specified conditions, they can proliferate and differentiate into osteoblastic cells resulting in the formation of bone. Inoue et al. [6] reported that when bone marrow cells were combined with porous HA ceramics and implanted in subcutaneous tissues, the cells induced osteogenesis 4 to 6 weeks after implantation; additionally, regenerated bone marrow capable of hemopoiesis was also observed in the composite. These composites maintained osteogenic activity one year after implantation, even if the activity was very low. Our experiments showed that new bone formation around the materials is influenced by their location within the bone. When the implants were completely embedded in the medullary cavity and did not contact the endosteum, some new bone formed around the materials at an early stage, but at 24 weeks postoperatively, only a little bone remained probably due to the remodeling process. Most new bone around the surface of the material in the bone marrow, if present, seem to be continuous with new bone formed in the endosteum. Our results would also suggest that bone marrow has osteogenic activity but that it is very low in contrast with periosteum and endosteum.

Finally, turning the discussion to the process of bone remodeling, after eight weeks, the bone formed on the surface of the implants in contact with the cortex remodelled into lamellar bone. However, as a result of resorption, only a little bone remained around the implants in the medullary cavity where there are no loading stresses. These findings indicate that the bone remodeling process follows Wolff's law once the bonding between the surface of the bone cortex and the implants has been completed.

CONCLUSIONS

(1) The new bone formation around the materials is more strongly influenced by the osteogenic capacity of the tissues than the osteoconductivity of the materials.

(2) Bone marrow has osteogenic activity but it is very low in contrast with those of periosteum and endosteum.

(3) The difference between bioactive and bioinert ceramics does not lie in the amount of bone formed but in the interface between material and bone, that is, direct or indirect.

REFERENCES

1. Hench, L.L., Splinter, R.J., Allen, W.C. and Greenlee, T.G. J. Biomed. Mater. Res. Symp. 1971, 2, 117-141.
2. Kotani, S., Yamamuro, T., Nakamura, T., Kitsugi, T., Fujita, Y., Kawanabe, K. and Kokubo, T. Clin. Orthop. Rel. Res. 1992, 278, 226-234.
3. Brunski, J.B. In: The Bone-Biomaterial Interface, Toronto, 1990, 391-405.
4. Bunte, N., Strunz, V., Gross, U.M., Bromer, H. and Deutscher, K. Dtsch. zahnarztl. Z. 1977, 32, 825-828.
5. Schmitz J.P. and Hollinger, J.O. Clin. Orthop. Rel. Res. 1986, 205, 299-308.
6. Inoue, K., Ohgushi, H., Yoshikawa, T., Okumura, M., Tamai, S. and Dohi, Y. In: Bioceramics Volume 5, Kyoto, 1992, 125-129.

BONE GROWTH INTO SURGICALLY CREATED CAVITIES IMPLANTED WITH GLASS GRANULES

N.C.Lindfors*, P.Slätis**, K.H.Karlsson***, Ö.H.Andersson***

Orton Research Institute, Invalid Foundation, Tenholantie 10, 00281 Helsinki, Finland*
Invalid Foundation, Helsinki, Finland**
Åbo Akademi University, Department of Chemical Engineering, Turku, Finland***
Turku Centre for Biomaterials, Turku, Finland***

ABSTRACT

Recent reports have indicated that the reactions and biological behaviour of bioactive glass granules depend on granule size, the ratio of surface area to solution volume (SA/V). In this study the effect of granule size and glass composition on bone growth and calcium phosphate formation was investigated. Glass granules of three different compositions and two different sizes were implanted in rabbit femur. After 8 weeks the animals were killed and the implants with surrounding bone were prepared with routine histological methods for light microscopy and SEM/EDX-analysis. The results show that glasses which according to the literature should be inactive when implanted as bulk may show bioactivity when implanted as granules. This phenomenon is most likely explained by differences in the SA/V ratio.

INTRODUCTION

Bioactive glasses form a chemical bond with living tissue [1,2]. In contact with body fluids, the surface of a bioactive glass is transformed to a Si-rich layer. The appearance of the bond between the implant and the tissue is related to development of a hydroxy carbonate apatite reaction layer on the surface of the implanted material [1-5].

The bioactivity of glasses has been shown to be composition dependent [1,2,7]. In a SiO_2-Na_2O-CaO system with a constant P_2O_5 content of 6 wt-%, glasses with a silica content of 60 mol-% or more have been reported not to be bioactive [2]. Many of the bioactive glasses show a high solubility which may reduce their long-term reliability. The solubility of glasses can be controlled by addition of Al_2O_3. A problem with addition of alumina is that it disturbs the mineralization of osteoid [8]. It also affects the surface reactions of the implanted glass. For glasses of relatively low solubility alumina additions may stabilize the structure of the glass surface and completely inhibit Ca,P-formation [7]. In glasses with higher solubility a partial stabilization may take place [7].

Bioactive glasses also have an osteoconductive ability i.e. they conduct bone growth along their surfaces [4,6]. The osteoconduction is important particularly considering the case of filling bone defects with granules. Recent reports have indicated that the reactions of bioactive glass granules depend on granule size and surface area to solution volume (SA/V) ratio [9]. This means that results obtained for bulk specimens are not necessarely valid for granules. The aim of this study was to investigate the effect of granule size on bone response.

MATERIALS AND METHODS

Three different glasses were used in this study (Table 1). In the preparation of the glasses, the raw materials were SiO_2, Na_2CO_3, $CaCO_3$, $CaHPO_4.2H_2O$, H_3BO_3 and Al_2O_3. The glasses were melted in a platinum crucible at 1360°C for 2.5 hours. The melt was annealed, crushed and sieved to two different sizes of 200-250 um and 630-800 um.

Ten nine week old rabbits whose weight ranged from 1.6 to 1.9 kg were used. The operations were performed with the animals under general anesthesia using intramuscular fentanylfluanisone.

A channel with a diameter of 3.2 mm was surgically created intra-articularly in the distal femur with an Astra Meditec 6124SPS drill. The sterilized glass granules were pushed into the bone channel and the channel was closed with ethoxiethylmethacrylate wound glue (Nobecutan,Astra Tech). Five different combinations of glass compositions and sizes of granules were used (Table 2). The combinations were chosen by the Plackett and Burman [10] method for minimizing the number of experiments. For each combination three parallel experiments were performed.

After the operation one single doze of 0.5 ml procain penicillin was injected subcutaneously to prevent infections. The animals also got the analgesic buphrenorphin for three days. After 8 weeks the animals were killed. The bones containing the glass granules were explanted and fixed in buffered formaldehyde. The samples were dehydrated in increasing concentrations of ethanol and methylmethacrylate for 2 months and finally embedded in methylmethacrylate (Technovit, Kulzer GmbH, Wehrheim, Germany). Sections were prepared with cutting grinding technic [11]. After preparation of the histological sections, the remaining blocks were studied using scanning electron microscopy (SEM) and energy dispersive X-ray analysis (EDXA).

RESULTS

Glass S53P4 showed extensive bone growth between the granules. All the granules had developed the characteristic Ca,P-rich layer (Fig. 1). For glass S52P3 and glass S59.7P2.5 the bone formation between the granules was considerably smaller.

Table 1. Glass composition in wt-%.

Glass	Na_2O	CaO	P_2O_5	B_2O_3	Al_2O_3	SiO_2
S53P4	23.00	20.00	4.0	0.00	0.00	53.00
S59.7P2.5	25.50	11.00	2.5	1.30	0.00	59.70
S52P3	18.00	24.00	3.00	0.00	3.00	52.00

Table 2. Combination of glass and granule size.

Experiment	Granule size (um)	Glass
1	200-250 + 630-800	S52P3
2	200-250	S59.7P2.5
3	630-800	S59.7P2.5
4	630-800	S52P3
5	200-250	S53P4

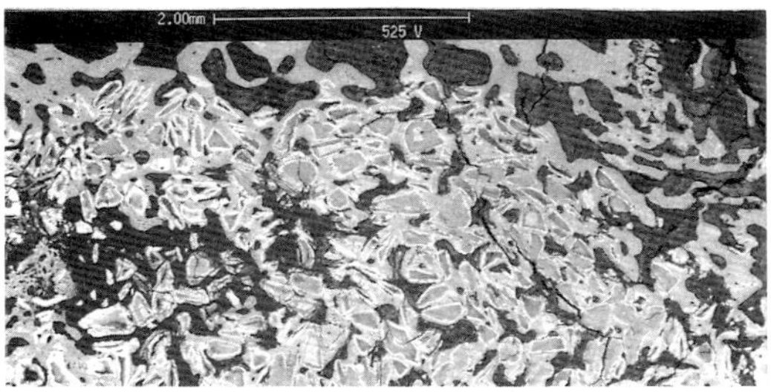

Figure 1. SEM image of glass S53P4, granule size 200-250 um.

Bone bonding could be seen for both granule sizes of glass S59.7P2.5 (Fig.2). Granules to which bone had bonded showed a Ca,P-rich surface layer of 10 to 15 um. Granules without bone contact showed less, if any, calcium phosphate formation. A larger network formation of bone growth could be seen between the granules of 630-800 um than between the granules of 200-250 um.

Glass S52P3 which was implanted both as granules of 630-800 um and as a 1:1 mixture of granules of 200-250 um and 630-800 um showed good bone contact, possibly even bone bonding. Granules of 630-800 um size showed bone contact both alone and in the mixture, whereas granules of 200-250 um size showed hardly any bone contact at all. The bone formation for the mixture was smaller than for the 630-800 um granules.

EDX-analysis of S52P3 granules of 630-800 um size showed a slightly different behaviour for granules with and granules without bone contact. The granules with bone contact had approximately 4.5-6.5 weight-% Al_2O_3 in their reaction layer and calcium phosphate had accumulated within the Si-rich layer (Fig. 3a,b). Granules without bone contact had more than 10 weight-% Al_2O_3 at the surface and no Ca,P-rich layer (Fig. 3c).

DISCUSSION

Glass S53P4 which from previous experiments is known to be bioactive both as bulk and as granules, behaved as expected. It therefore serves as a reference for a highly bioactive glass.

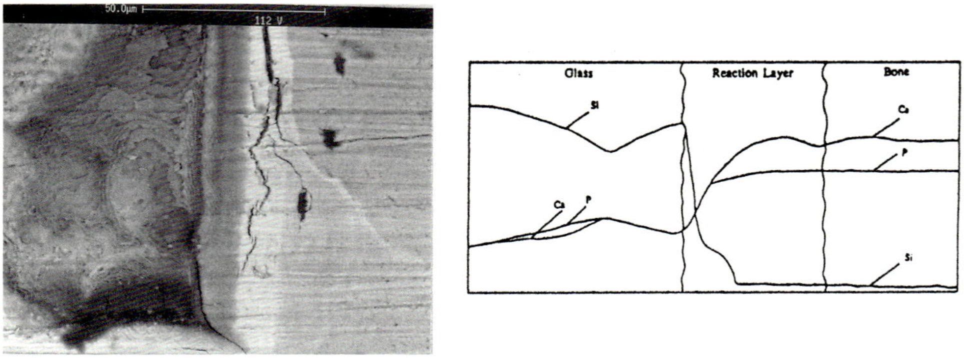

Figure 2. (a) SEM image and (b) corresponding composition profiles of glass S59.7P2.5, granule size 200-250 um.

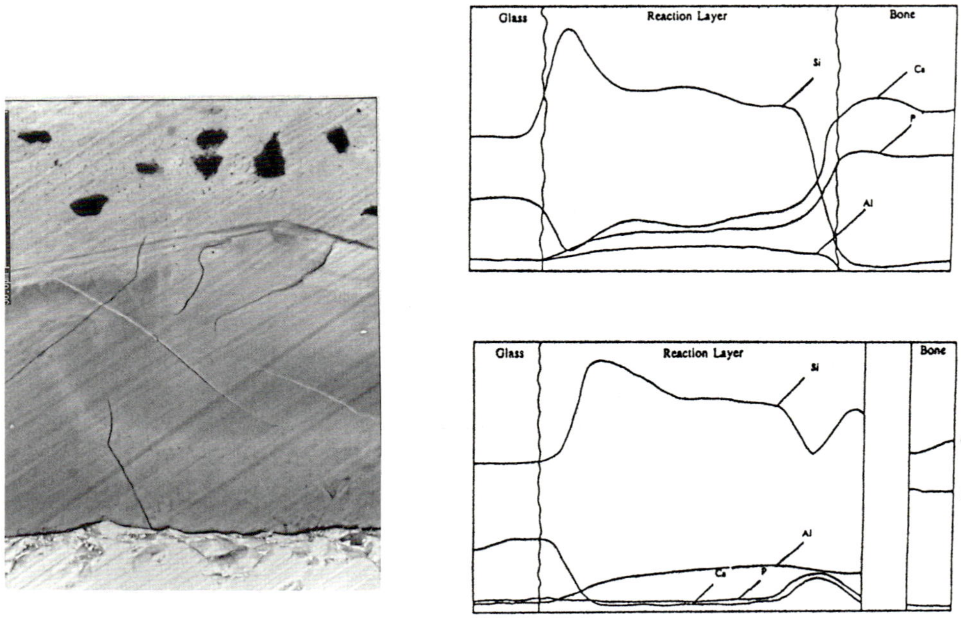

Figure 3. (a) SEM image and (b) corresponding composition profile of glass S52P3 with bone contact. (c) Composition profile at the surface of glass S52P3, no bone contact. Granule size 630-800 um.

Glass S59.7P2.5 has not previously been implanted. Despite its high Si-content the results showed bone bonding for both granule sizes. No difference between the bone bonding ability could be seen between the two sizes but the network of growing bone was greater between the bigger granules than between the smaller ones.

bone contact and osteoconduction only for the granules of 630-800 um size. The bone formation was also greater between the granules of 630-800 um size than in the mixture.

These results indicate that the small granules have a negative influence on the bone growth in the bone defect. It seems like there would be an optimum size between bulk and small granules where different glasses show most bone growth and osteoconduction. This is most likely related to differences in the SA/V-ratios. This study also shows that results for bulk glasses cannot always be used for granules. This emphasizes the importance of studying the effect of SA/V ratios.

REFERENCES

1. Hench, L.L., Paschall, H.A. *J.Biomed.Mater.Res* 1973, 4, 25-42.
2. Hench, L.L. *Ann.N.Y.Ac.Sci* 1988, 523, 54-71.
3. Andersson, Ö.H., Karlsson, K.H., Kangasniemi, K. *J.Non.Cryst.Solids* 1990, 119, 290-296.
4. Gatti, A.M., Yamamuro, T., Hench, L.L., Andersson, Ö.H. *Cells and Materials* 1993, 3, 283-291
5. Neo, M., Nakamura, T., Ohtsuki, C., Kokubo, T., Yamamuro, T. *J.Biomed. Mater.Res* 1993, 27, 999-1006.
6. Oonishi, H., Kushitani, S., Yasukawa, E., Hawakami, H., Nakata, A., Koh, S., Hench, L.L., Wilson, J., Tsuji, E., Sugihara, T. *Bioceramics* Vol. 7, Butterworth-Heinemann, Oxfors 1994, 139-144.
7. Andersson, Ö.H., Liu, G., Karlsson, K.H., Niemi, L., Miettinen, J., Juhanoja, J. *J.Mater.Sci*: Mater in Medicine 1990, 1, 219-227.
8. Andersson, Ö.H., Karlsson, K.H., Kangasniemi, K., Yli-Urpo, A. *Glastech.Ber.* 1988, Vol. 61, 300-305.
9. Greenspan, D.C., Zhong, J.P., La Torre, G.P. *Bioceramics* Vol 7, Butterworth-Heinemann, Oxford 1994, 55-60.
10. Montgomery, D.C., *Design and Analisis of Experiments*, 2nd edd., New York, Wiley 1984.
11. Donath, K. *EXAKT-Kulzer-Publication*, Norderstedt 1990.

SPINAL RECONSTRUCTION

BIOMECHANICS OF THE SPINE - A MATERIALS PERSPECTIVE

Vijay K. Goel

Iowa Spine Research Center
Departments of Biomedical Engineering and Orthopaedics,
College of Engineering
University of Iowa, Iowa City, IA 52242

ABSTRACT

The need for man-made devices to restore spine function from a biomechanical view point is reviewed. Examples of the artificial devices used are presented. The biomechanical characteristics of these devices are very briefly discussed, and materials on the horizon for spinal surgery are presented.

INTRODUCTION

In a young healthy person numerous spinal components function in unison to provide trunk flexibility, support the upper body weight, and protect spinal cord and nerve roots that pass through the spinal canal. In an abnormal state (e.g., tumors, disc herniation, scoliosis), trauma (e.g., vertebral body fractures), and/or with age (e.g., disc degeneration, spondylolisthesis), the quality of life may be compromised due to improper functioning of the spinal components. Interventions become essential to restore spinal function. In most cases, people respond favorably to conservative treatments (e.g., bed rest, medication, braces, manipulation). Surgery may be indicated for those who do not respond to conservative treatment. The basic principle underlying surgery, from a biomechanical view point, is to either dissect or remove the impinging structures. However, these procedures depending upon the amount of bony and soft tissue decompression achieved, may lead to spinal instability. Fusion of the spinal segment with and without spinal instrumentation may be indicated. Procedures like subtotal discectomy and interbody fusion with autologous bone graft have been used extensively for the treatment of discogenic pain in the absence of any other obvious symptom/pathology.

SURGICAL PROCEDURES

Surgical procedures technically allow for complete exposure and visualization of all portions of the spinal segment.[1] Under most circumstances, the choice of approach should be dictated by the site of the primary pathologic condition. Disease or deformities that primarily involve the vertebral bodies may be approached directly from the anterior. Posterior elements may be approached directly through a vertically oriented posterior incising in the midline. A posterolateral approach provides direct access to the transverse processes and pedicles, as well as limited exposure to the vertebral bodies themselves.

Laminectomies, facetectomies, foraminotomies, etc. involving one or more spinal segments are performed through the posterior approach (Figure 1). Cervical laminoplasty is an established technique for spinal cord decompression. Bone grafts are used to keep the lamina open. In the lumbar and thoracic regions, partial and total discectomies are also amenable to the posterior approach. In the cervical spine region, discectomies are best performed through the anterior approach.

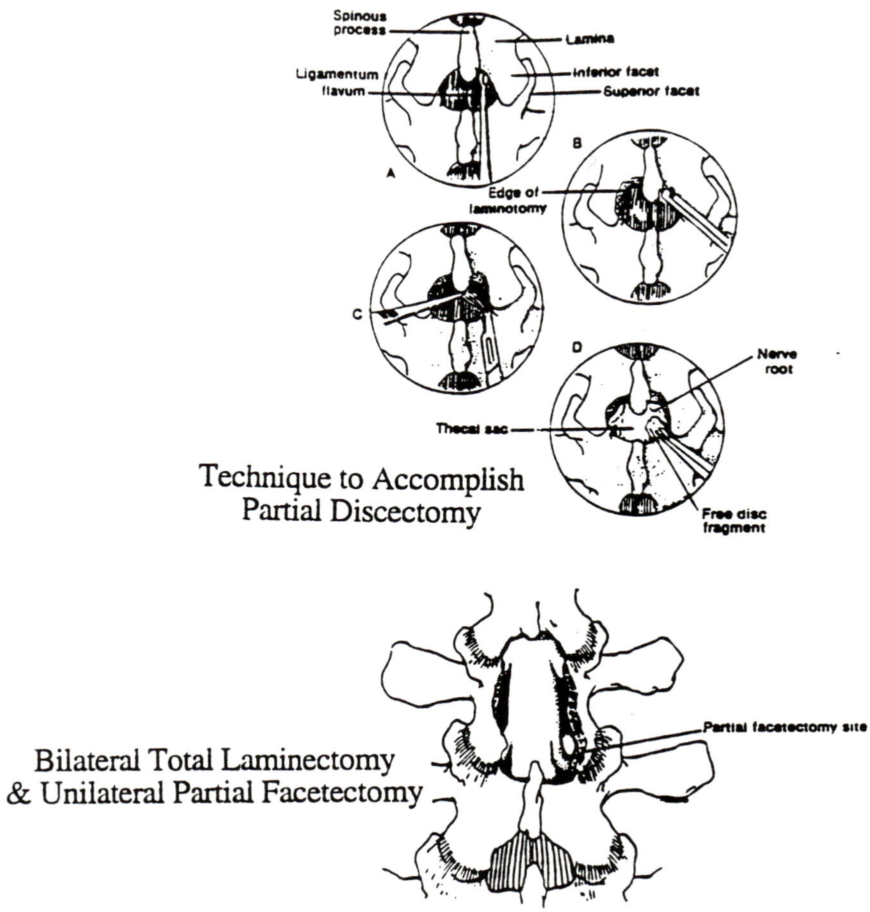

Figure 1: Some of the surgical procedures depicting the spinal elements that are discected.

The anterior surgical approach, although demanding, enables one to perform total discectomy, removal of the vertebral bony fragments, insertion of the graft and further stabilization of the segment using spinal instrumentation. The anterior approach has been utilized for spondylolisthesis, for tumors, and for pseudoarthrosis following failed posterior surgery.

From the above description it becomes clear that almost all of the spinal components (e.g., ligaments, disc annulus, nucleus, vertebral bodies, facets, laminae) are liable to be dissected at surgery, depending upon the pathology or deformity. To restore spinal stability, alignment and function, it often becomes necessary to fuse segments. Internal fixation with instrumentation often accompanies surgical fusion to augment spinal stability and enhance postoperative mobilization (Figure 2). Three classes of materials,--metals, plastics and ceramics, are currently used as spinal implants. These span a range of properties diverse enough to meet the desired needs. As the materials science develops, composites, biodegradable materials and the like will be investigated.[2] The following paragraphs describe the biomechanics of several surgical procedures, to highlight the application of the artificial devices used to restore function.

BIOMECHANICS OF SPINE SURGERY

Interpositional Barriers: Surgical procedures like laminectomy and foraminotomy are undertaken to relieve pressure on the spinal cord or the nerve roots. These procedures invariably lead to scar (granulation) tissue. It is not entirely clear whether the scar tissue regresses or progresses with time and how this relates to patient symptomatology and response to treatment.[3,4] As an example, reoperation on a scar may lead to a poor surgical result. Unsuccessful efforts have been made to place gel foams or fat grafts to prevent scar tissue formation. Is there a place for the use of a photochemically driven material to inhibit scar tissue growth and formation?

Interbody Spacers: Total disc removal alone, or in combination with other surgical procedures, invariably leads to a loss of disc height, and an unstable spinal segment.[1] Both allo- and autologous grafts have been used as a interbody spacers. Associated with the use of bone grafts are several complications: pain, dislodgement of the anterior bone graft, pseudoarthrosis, fracture, collapse of the bone graft, loss of alignment, etc. Recently, the use of cages (titanium alloy with and without hydroxypatite bioactive coating, ceramic or polysulphone), and solid or porous HA blocks, implanted through an anterior or posterior approach, have gained popularity to enhance stabilization of the segment, prevent postoperative collapse and supplement autologous bone graft.[5,6] Glass-ceramic spacers, in place of the bone graft, have been used in conjunction with laminoplasty in the cervical spine region with success.[7]

Intervertebral Disc Arthroplasty: A recent concept to restore spine function following disc removal is not to provide a solid fusion across the vertebral bodies but restore the space to normal. The goal is to restore function and comfort an otherwise degenerated or painful intervertebral disc. Such can be done for most of the other joints of the body. Why not the disc?[8] Of course, this concept becomes feasible only when the rest of the spinal components are normal, i.e., are not affected by the pathology. A number of artificial disc prostheses have been designed. The concepts vary from the bearing prostheses, fillable flexible bladder, springs, a sandwich of porous metal plates and elastomeric cushion, plates with hinges, and ceramic ball and sockets. Hydrophilic material based artificial discs (prosthetic nucleus) have also been

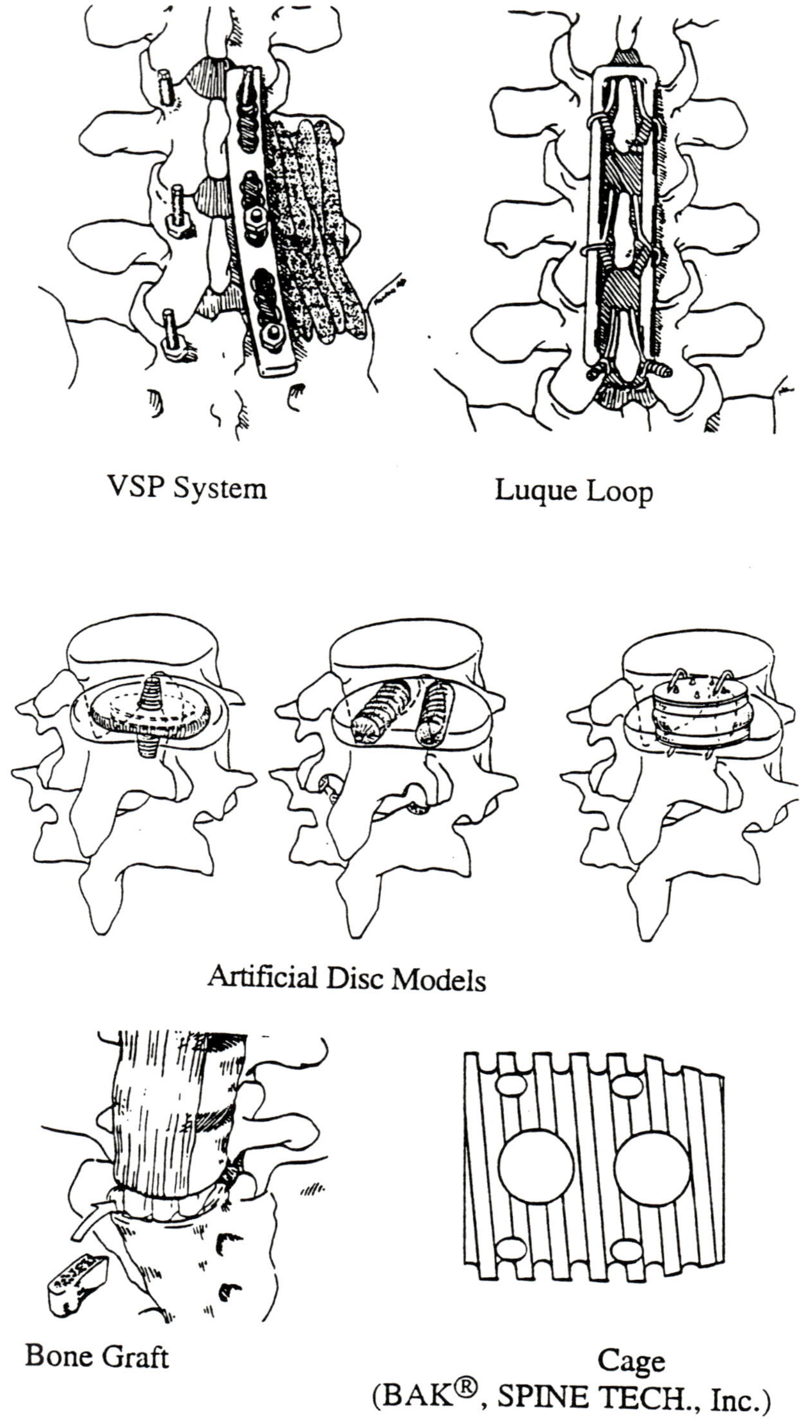

Figure 2: Examples of the devices used to restore spine function.

tested. This material absorbs water which is squeezed out when loads are applied slowly, similar to a normal nucleus.[7,8] The flexible disc spacer has been tested to 20 million cycles with minimal wear. The device can be easily implanted within the disc. Many problems need to be resolved before an artificial disc prosthesis becomes a viable solution, at least from a biomechanical perspective -- mechanical failure modes include fatigue response, attachment to the bone, resistance to expulsion, tissue compatibility, etc.

Wires: Arthrodesis of a single or multiple spinal segment is also facilitated by wires. The most commonly used wire material is 316L stainless steel. After the procedure, however, the diagnostic capabilities of magnetic resonance images are limited by wire-induced artifact.[9] To reduce artifacts, a number of alternative materials have come on the market. Biomechanical testing has shown that titanium alloys, such as Ti6Al4V in its present form, may be a poor choice for fixation because of its decreased fatigue resistance due to notch sensitivity. Thus, titanium alloy wires are brittle and harder to bend. Although pure titanium wires are ductile and easy to bend they do not possess adequate strength.[10] Cobalt chrome alloys have an ultimate strength higher than stainless-steel, while having less MRI artifacts. It may be an appropriate choice for fixation from imaging point of view.

Wires are also used to secure metallic loops/rods (e.g., Luque rods or loop) to the vertebral bodies. Since surgeons cannot see within the canal, wires may damage the spinal nerves or cord and lead to scar tissue formation and irritation of the *dura mater*.[1] Malleable 'wires' (fabricated from mersilene tape, knitted fabrics, polymeric braided cable, etc.), have come on the market.

Pins and Screws: In recent years stainless steel tongs and pins have been replaced by an MRI-compatible graphite tong and titanium pin system.[11] Mechanical testing has revealed that titanium alloy pins fail because of pin tip deformation with subsequent slippage along the skull surface. The stainless steel pins fail because of skull fracture at the skull-pin interface, which eventually leads to pull-out of tongs from the skull. Furthermore, the MRI-compatible pins have an average strength of 75 pounds and the MRI-incompatible (stainless steel) pins fail at an average of 225 pounds. Accordingly, the low strength titanium MRI-compatible pins may fail during reduction of a dislocated cervical spine itself. Co-Cr alloy wires of comparable size will be able to withstand over 250 pounds of force.[12]

Internal fixation with one or two screws (ordinary or compression type) to obtain a direct fixation of the dens fracture is recommended to avoid the limited motion.[12] Screws are also used to obtain fusion across the facets (e.g., in the lumbar region) of a motion segment.[13] The screws, when placed into the pedicles or the vertebral bodies themselves, act as anchor points for the rods/plates to restore spinal 'function'. Strength across the screw and bone interface influences the success of the fixation. This becomes especially vital if the spine is osteoporotic and the screw is subjected to cyclic loads.[14] As such, failure of screw fixation following instrumentation of the lumbosacral spine is a challenging clinical problem. The use of PMMA and other grouting agents has been shown to improve the bone-screw interface strength especially in osteoporotic vertebral bodies.[15] The screw strength can be enhanced through surface treatment such as with nitrogen-ions.

Plates and Rods: The use of plates or rods, secured to the vertebral bodies with the aid of screws and wires (as described above), or hooks secured to the laminae, can material choice (e.g., from stainless steel to titanium), or the stiffness of the plate/rod itself. If the system is too rigid, it becomes difficult to bend and twist to provide the normal curvature of the spine (e.g., appropriate lordosis in the lumbar region) and may lead to stress induced osteopenia of the vertebral bodies and spinal degeneration of the adjacent normal segments.[16-21] Several designs that are somewhat more flexible have come on the market.[21] These devices have been developed on the premise that the undesirable iatrogenic effects of using rigid devices will decrease with the use of semirigid devices. However, the optimum rigidity of the device is hard, if not impossible, to predict. Furthermore, clinical and animal based biomechanical studies have shown that a rigid system promotes and accelerates the solid fusion process. These observations dictate that one should design a system whose rigidity decreases with time; being very rigid until fusion occurs and thereafter diminish. In one such design, viscoelastic polymer washers are inserted between the plate and the nuts of the conventional VSP system.[16] This provides rigid fixation immediately after surgery and decreasing rigidity with time, due to the viscoelastic behavior of the polymer washers. This, in turn, imposes higher loads/stresses over time on the vertebral bodies across the stabilized segments. Biomechanical investigations have lent support to this concept; the system was found to decrease in rigidity with time and was effective in providing stability and lessen stress-induced osteopenia. Biodegradable washers have been proposed as a substitute, to reduce polymer debris, since the debris can be absorbed by the body. It is also possible that one may design bioabsorbable/ biodegradable devices (e.g., PLA or PGA).[2] Currently, these materials lack the necessary bending and torsional strength. Wear and wear debris may be a source of complications. At present, these designs have not gained acceptance from manufacturers or surgeons.

When plates/rods with screws, wires, hooks or combinations thereof are used to restore spinal deformity (e.g., in scoliosis surgery), the viscoelastic effects of the involved tissues become an important factor.[1] A decrease in the corrective forces takes place with time following surgery as a result of the viscoelastic effects of the spinal tissue. In order to sustain spinal alignment following surgery, devices based on shape memory alloy have been proposed.[22] Manipulation of the forces following surgery becomes feasible with such devices.

CONCLUSIONS

A wide variety of man-made materials is currently being used to help the natural bone to heal and restore 'function' across the spinal segments. Revolutionary new concepts (e.g., artificial discs and devices fabricated out of shape memory alloy) are on the horizon. One may see the introduction of bioactive materials, including bioactive coatings applied to conventional substrates, intelligent or interactive and cooperative materials. It also appears that in the future the design and selection of devices based on biomechanical principles alone may take a back seat to chemistry based materials that will promote healing, primarily at the cellular level.

ACKNOWLEDGEMENTS

Work supported in part by an NIH grant (AR 40166-4) and Sofamor-Danek, Inc. The suggestions and critical comments of several individuals (J. B. Park, University of Iowa, T. Oxland, Spine-Tech, Inc, L. Boyd, Sofamor-Danek, Inc.) during the preparation of this manuscript are also gratefully acknowledged.

REFERENCES

1. Goel, V.K. and Weinstein, J. *Biomechanics of the Spine: Clinical and Surgical Perspective* CRC Press Inc. Boca Raton, Florida, 1990.
2. Hastings, G.W. In: *Proc. of 8th International Conference on Biomedical Engineering,* National University of Singapore, Dec. 7-10, 1994, 83-85.
3. Modic, M.T., Ross, J.S. In: *Clinical Efficacy and Outcome in the Diagnosis and Treatment of Low Back Pain.* Weinstein JN (ED.), Raven Press, 1992, 57-66.
4. Abitbol, J-J., Lincoln, T.L., Lind, B.I., *et al. Spine,* Volume 19, 1994, 1809-1814.
5. Brantigan, J.W., Steffee, A.D., Geiger, J.M. *Spine,* Volume 16, 1991, S270-S276.
6. Passuti, N., Daculsi, G., Martin, S., Deudon, C. In: *Handbook of Bioactive Ceramics,* Vol. II, Yamamuro, T., Hench, L.L., and Wilson, J. (Eds.), CRC Press, Inc., Boca Raton, Fl., 1990, 345-354,.
7. Yamamuro, T. In: *Bioceramics 8,* Wilson, J., Hench. L.L., and Greenspan, D. (Eds.) Elsevier Science, 1995.
8. Ray, C.D. *et al.*, In: *Clinical Efficacy and Outcome in the Diagnosis and Treatment of Low Back Pain.* Weinstein JN (ED.), Raven Press, 1992 205-280.
9. Scuderi, G.J. *et al., Spine,* Volume 18, 1993, 1991-1994.
10. Park, J.B. and Lakes, R.S. In: *Biomaterials - An Introduction.* 2nd Edition, Plenum Pub., NY, 1992, 79-93.
11. Blumberg, K.D., Catalano, J.B., Cotler, J.M., Balderston, R.A. *Spine,* Volume 18, 1993, 1895-1896.
12. Chang, K.W., Liu, Y.W., et al. *J. Spinal Disorders* Volume 7, 1994, 62-69.
13. Heggeness, M.H. and Esses, S.I. *Spine,* Volume 16, 1991, S266-S269.
14. Okuyama, K. *et al., Spine,* Volume 185, 1993, 2240-224.
15. Liu, Y.K., Njus, G.O., Bahr, P.O., Geng, P. *Spine,* Volume 15, 1990, 311-317.
16. Lim, T.H., Goel, V.K., Winterbottom, J.M. *et al., J. Spinal Dis.,* Volume 7, 1994, 1-11.
17. Goel, V.K., Kim, Y.E., Lim, T.H., Weinstein, J.N. *Spine,* Volume 13, 1988, 1003-1011.
18. Goel, V.K., Lim, T-H., Gilbertson, L.G., Weinstein, J.N. *Seminars in Spine Surg.,* Volume 5, 1993, 29-41.
19. Goel, V.K., Lim, T-H., Gwon, J., Chen, J-Y., Han, *J. Spinal Stenosis,* Mosby 1992, 403-414.
20. Goel, V.K., Lim, T.H., Gwon, J. *et al., Spine,* Volume 16, 1991, S155-161.
21. Pfeiffer, M. *et al.*, American Society of Mechanical Engineering, IMECE - WAM, Chicago, Ill., Nov. 6-11, 1994.
22. Haasters, J., v.Salis-Solio, G., Bensmann, G. In: *Engineering Aspects of Shape Memory Alloys,* Butterworth-Heinemann, London, 1990.

AW GLASS-CERAMIC IN SPINAL REPAIR

Takao Yamamuro

Biomaterials Research Laboratory, Research Institute for Production Development, 15 Morimoto-Cho, Shimogamo, Sakyo-Ku, Kyoto, 606 Japan

ABSTRACT

AW glass-ceramic has been used for the spinal repair in the form of vertebral prostheses (1,070 cases since 1983), laminoplasty spacer (778 cases since 1987), and intervertebral spacer (1,000 cases since 1989) in Japan. Neither breakage nor dislocation has been experienced to date. Their complete bone bonding was observed on radiographs within one year of the operation in most of the cases, and late collapse of the spinal segment has been well prevented.

INTRODUCTION

In the past, when bone structure of the vertebrae was extensively damaged by tumor, trauma, or degenerative changes, its reconstruction had been attempted by the use of autograft or allograft in combination with metals, PMMA cement, or alumina ceramic. However, autograft and allograft have certain limits in their availability, and long-term durability of the non bone-bonding implants was often unsatisfactory, due to their loosening and/or dislocation. Therefore, in attempts to make strong, bone-bonding vertebral replacements, we used AW glass-ceramic which has greater mechanical strength as well as higher bioactivity than synthetic hydroxyapatite.[l] This paper deals with an overview of 2-8 year results of the patients who underwent reconstruction operations of the vertebrae by the use of vertebral prostheses (Figure 1) and spacers made of AW glass-ceramic (Figure 2).

VERTEBRAL PROSTHESIS

The vertebral prosthesis made of AW glass-ceramic is a quadrangular pillar in different sizes. In many cases, it is inserted through an anterior approach to replace the affected vertebrae and fixed to the adjacent vertebrae with a Kaneda device.

However, in a few cases where a posterior total en bloc spondylectomy [2] is performed, the prosthesis is inserted posteriorly and fixed with an Isola instrument. The vertebral prosthesis has good indications for primary and secondary bone tumors, burst fracture, compression fracture, and fracture dislocation of the thoracic and lumbar vertebrae. During the period from 1983 to 1994, 1,070 cases underwent the prosthetic replacement operation of the thoracic or lumbar spine in Japan Except in a few cases with malignant tumor metastasis who passed away in the few months after the operation,complete bone-bonding of the prosthesis was observed on radiographs usually within one year of surgery. Neither breakage nor dislocation of the prosthesis has been experienced to date. Advantages of the vertebral prosthesis made of AW glass-ceramic are 1) less morbidity because of no additional surgical intervention for harvesting bone graft, 2) any size of implant is available, 3) late collapse of the implant does not occur because of its persisting high mechanical strength, and 4) late dislocation or loosening of the prosthesis does not occur because of its bone-bonding character.[3]

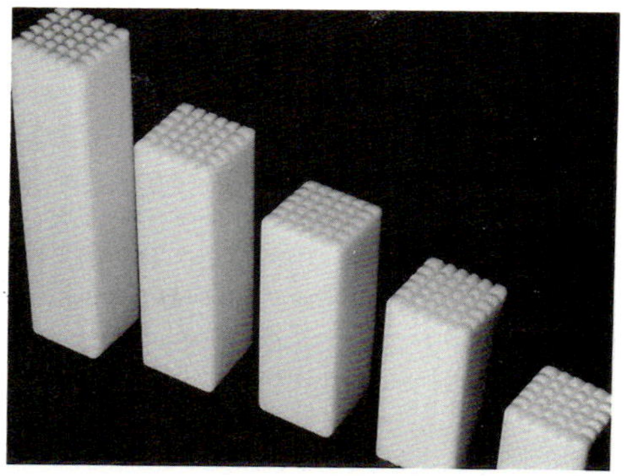

Figure 1. Vertebral prosthesis.

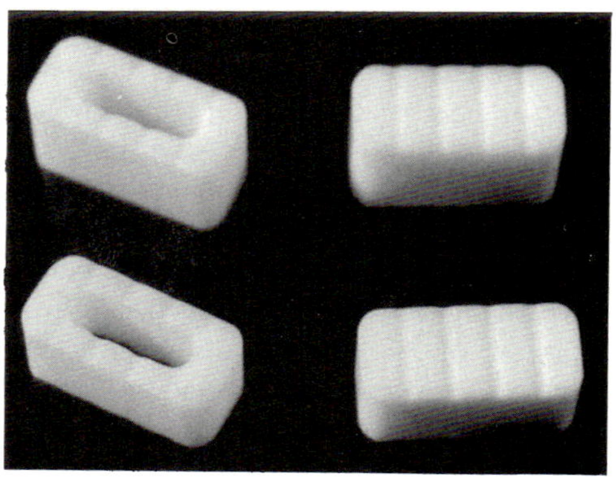

Figure 2. Intervertebral spacer.

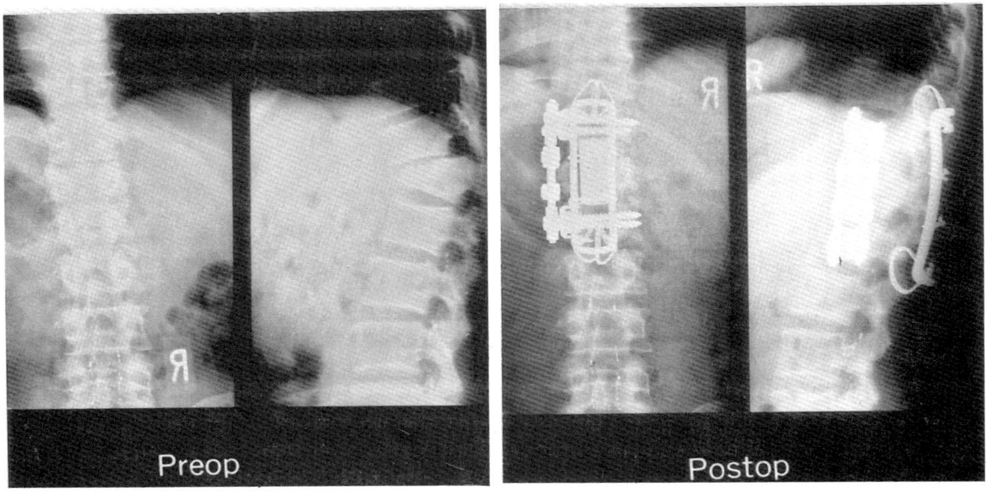

Figure 3. A 45 year old male, vertebral prosthetic replacement for T12 fracture dislocation with a Kaneda device anteriorly and Luque rods posteriorly.

In cases of burst fracture and compression fracture, the prosthetic replacement of the affected vertebra is accomplished with minimal surgical intervention when this vertebral prosthesis is used, (Figure 3) and blood transfusion is not necessary in most cases. The vertebral prosthesis is particularly useful in cases of multilevel tumor metastasis which require a large implant and in cases of compression fracture due to osteoporosis that do not provide an autograft with good bone quality.

INTERVERTEBRAL SPACER

Intervertebral spacers are made of AW glass-ceramic to be used for postero-lateral interbody fusion of the lumbar spine. For interbody fusion in cases of spinal canal stenosis, degenerative spondylolysis and spondylolisthesis, and postdiscotomy syndrome, the intervertebral disc and annulus fibrosus are removed after laminectomy, and two spacers are inserted into one intervertebral space together with some autogenous bone graft. They are securely fixed with Steffee's instruments posteriorly (Figure 4). Multiple spondylolysis and spinal instability are also treated by the same method. Recently, we performed a follow-up study on 28 patients who were operated on with the intervertebral spacers 2 to 5 years ago.[4] We found that bone union with spacers occurred in all cases, accompanied by improvement of clinical symptoms. It was observed on radiographs that the spacers not only bonded to the adjacent bone but promoted new bone generation around them. During the period from 1989 to 1994, the intervertebral spacer made of AW glass-ceramic was used in 1,005 cases in Japan. Advantages of using this spacer for interbody fusion are less morbidity because of no additional surgical intervention in other bones for harvesting grafts, and prevention of late narrowing of the intervertebral space, which often occurs when autograft or allograft are used for the interbody fusion.

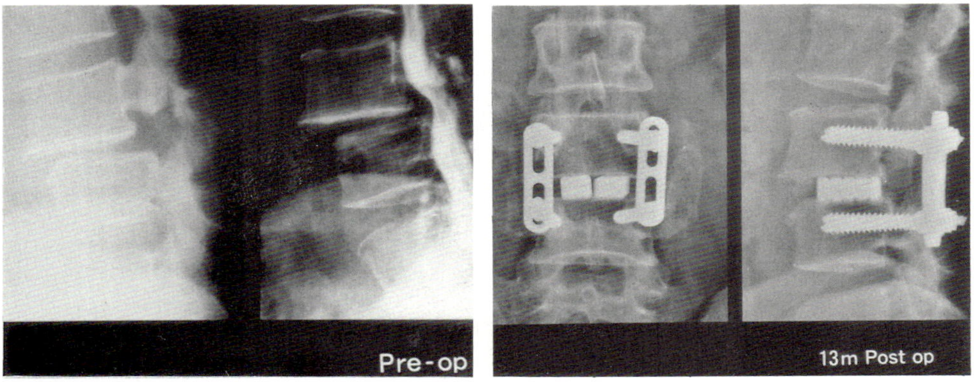

Figure 4. A 40 year old male, posterior interbody fusion for isthmic spondylolisthesis between L3 and L4 by the use of two intervertebral spacers which are fixed with Steffee's instruments.

LAMINOPLASTY SPACER

Laminoplasty spacers are made of AW glass-ceramic (Figure 5) to be used for laminoplastic enlargement in cases of multilevel spinal canal stenosis of the cervical spine. There are two sizes, but the spacer of small size is usually used. The approach to the cervical spine is made posteriorly and multilevel laminae are exposed. A fine gutter is created longitudinally near the facet joint in the bilateral sides. Spinous processes are split vertically and both split surfaces are gradually opened with a spreader to enlarge the spinal canal. Usually, four or five laminae are enlarged, and the bone defect remaining in each lamina is filled with the spacer. Good indications for this operation are the continuous type of ossification of the posterior longitudinal ligament and multi-level spondylotic myelopathy of the cervical spine. Enlargement of the spinal canal in 20-60% is obtained by the operation, and bone-bonding of the spacer to the lamina is observed on radiographs within six months after the operation in most cases (Figure 6.). During the period 1987 through 1994, the laminoplasty spacer made of AW glass ceramic had been used in 778 patients in Japan. The number of spacers is about 3,500. Stability of the spacer at an average follow-up of three years was 100% and there have been no complications. Improvement of neurological symptoms after the operation was significant, although complete recovery from the symptoms did not take place in one third of the patients.

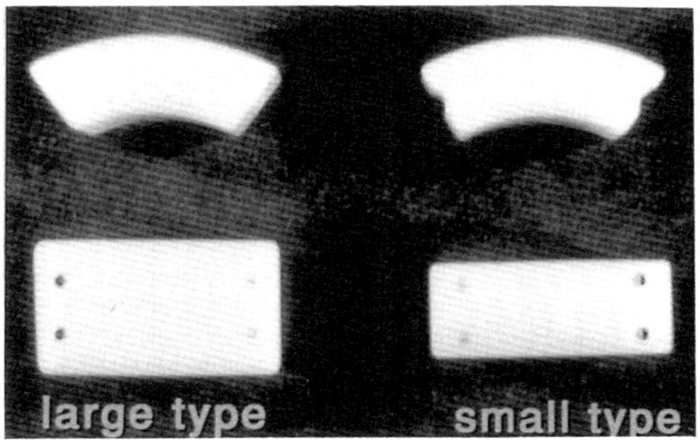

Figure 5. Laminoplasty spacers.

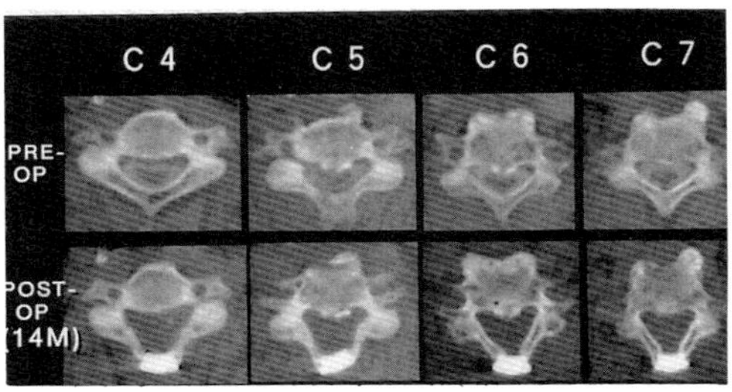

Figure 6. A 75 year old male, ossification of the posterior longitudinal ligament treated with an A/W spacer.
(Courtesy Dr. Y. Takemistu, Asahikawa Medical College)

REFERENCES

1. Kokubo, T., Ito, S., Shigematsu, M., Sakka, S., Yamamuro T. *J Mater Sci* 1985, 20, 2001-2004.
2. Tomita, K., Nakahara, N., Baba, H., Tsuchiya, H., Nagata, S., Toribatake, Y. *Internat Orthop* 1994, 18, 291-298.
3. Yamamuro, T. In: *Handbook of Bioactive Ceramics* Volume 1, CRC Press, Boca Raton 1990, 343-351.
4. Shimizu, K., Iwasaki, R., Matsushita, M., Yamamuro, T. In: *Bioceramics 5*, Kobunshi Kankokai, Kyoto 1992, 435-441
5. Kamo, H., Takemitsu, Y., Hamada, 0., Yamaga, S. *Clin Orthop Surg*, 1992, 27, 1115-1122.

ANTERIOR COLUMN SUPPORT OF THE SPINE: THE LINK BETWEEN BIOMECHANICS, BIOLOGY AND BIOMATERIALS

Gary L. Lowery

Research Institute International, Inc., 1034-C NW 57th Street, Gainesville, Florida 32605 U.S.A.

ABSTRACT

To maximize spinal fusion success rates, both spine surgeons and bioceramics researchers must understand the importance of: (1) the biology of bone formation, (2) the biological and biomechanical environments, and (3) differences between the anterior and posterior environments. Based on a review of these factors, this paper concludes that the anterior column is the optimal biological and biomechanical environment for fusion.

INTRODUCTION

There have been many elegant studies performed to elucidate the mechanisms of fracture healing [1,2,3,4]. As in fracture healing, the biology of bone formation should always be of paramount importance when a spinal fusion is considered. This not only requires meticulous technique but also an understanding of the appropriate biological and biomechanical environments in which the bone grafts will be placed for maturation. Too often, surgeons are enamored with the instrumentation for stabilization rather than the biological and biomechanical events that must occur for successful fusion. The aim of this paper is to provide insight into certain philosophies of spinal fusion.

HISTORICAL SPINAL FUSION LITERATURE

This review organizes the spinal fusion literature from the perspective that the anterior column is the optimal biological and biomechanical environment for fusion.

Although the early literature reports single-level uninstrumented autologous bone fusions as 95% successful [5,6,7], most recent papers are less optimistic. Reported fusion successes of 70-80% are more common, even with rigid posterior instrumentation [8,9]. However, several well-documented randomized prospective studies have shown that posterior spinal instrumentation and autologous bone grafting yield the best results [10,11,12,13].

Posterior lumbar interbody fusions (PLIF) have also met with varying success [14,15,16,17], but more recent articles on instrumented PLIFs have come up to the success range of 95-98% fusion [18,19]. The instrumented PLIF technique appears to be successful irrespective of confounding constitutional factors (i.e., smoking, diabetes, osteoporosis); and similar excellent results are achieved even in revision fusion cases. The intradiscal space is a well-vascularized area for bone graft consolidation.

Instrumented anterior lumbar interbody fusions (ALIF) also share excellent fusion success[20]. However, 95% fusion reported for instrumented ALIFs falls to 80% for uninstrumented ALIFs [21,22]. Since stabilizing the intradiscal fusion environment leads to better results, the important question arises that perhaps ALIF should be the primary operation and not simply a "salvage" surgery to repair failed posterior surgery.

With regard to bone graft material, autograft is the "gold standard" for all bone fusions. However, donor site morbidity--including infection, cosmesis, fracture, and chronic debilitating pain--have led surgeons to seek alternative means for bone fusion [23,24,25]. Allograft used in posterior spinal fusions has been uniformly noted to be inferior to autograft [10,26]. Although osteoconductive surface area is present, the osteoinduction process fails to be elicited in most cases.

Of special interest, however, is the use of allograft anteriorly. Its fusion success rivals that of autograft when coupled with posterior instrumentation, thus, becoming a likely replacement in the armamentarium of most surgeons [27,28]. Allograft anteriorly under compression can fuse to host vertebrae. When the cancellous allograft is in the posterior fusion bed primarily undergoing tension forces, the process of fusion falls short. When evaluating bioactive compounds, as with allograft, one must understand the areas that need to be addressed, since these are different for the anterior spinal column and posterior spinal column.

Like fracture healing, a successful spinal fusion can be modulated both by the surgeon and the environment. A stable biomechanical environment which allows controlled motion must be established. Micromotion will stimulate microvascular invasion, which provides the "osteoprogenitor cells" as well as other local and systemic factors, thus modulating fracture healing. Obviously, the surgeon plays an extremely important role by meticulous preparation of the fusion site as well as by providing postoperative stability, either in the form of internal fixation and/or external immobilization. However, the donor graft, whether autologous or allogenic, must be able to induce a bone-healing response. This response usually is a combination of osteoinduction and osteoconduction. Autologous bone remains the "gold standard" for bony fusion in spite of significant failure rates, especially in posterior spinal fusions [8,9]. Allograft alone or in combination with autograft has led to even more dismal results [10,26].

The spinal surgeon is often led to "salvage" procedures to achieve a successful vertebral bony union. These salvage procedures are intradiscal fusions, both via the anterior and posterior interbody techniques [19,28,29]. I propose that intradiscal fusions should be considered the optimal grafting technique and a primary rather than a "salvage" procedure. This philosophy has its basis in biomechanics as well as biology and will be discussed further.

CONCEPT OF ANTERIOR COLUMN DEFICIENCY

One can understand the concept of weakened bony structures when one thinks of fractures, tumors, and infections. The bony architecture no longer functions in the same manner as it did before the pathologic event. Post-traumatic deformity and kyphoscoliosis are other examples of deficiencies in the bony anterior column leading to the sequelae of deformity.

The surgeon must also appreciate that there can be intradiscal deficiencies in the anterior column. Isthmic spondylolisthesis is a prime example. Slippage of the spine (L5 on S1) would not occur if the disc were capable of counteracting the shear forces acting at this functional spinal unit (FSU). Upright stance alone produces axial compressive forces of 800-2500 N and a bending moment of 10-25 N. Repetitive bending torsional movements and loading of the disc will lead to deterioration. Slipping occurs when the posterior elements (lamina, facets, facet capsules, ligaments, and posterior musculature) no longer aid in providing the adequate tension band. The only way to counteract the shear forces is to reconstruct the anterior column integrity and provide adequate posterior stabilization via compression and tension. A structural anterior intradiscal graft can be stabilized (neutralized) by application of a posterior compressive force. An exemplary fusion environment (intradiscal) is thus provided, both from a biomechanical and biological viewpoint. Other examples of monosegmental intradiscal deficiencies include degenerative spondylolisthesis, isolated disc resorption, and recurrent disc herniation. Multisegmental deficiencies are seen in degenerative scoliosis and stenosis and the "cascading" spine, usually iatrogenic in origin.

RELEVANT BIOMECHANICS AND ANTERIOR COLUMN DEFICIENCY

Many authors have demonstrated that 80% of the axial forces are directed through the anterior column of the spine, especially the last three lumbar discs [30,31,32]. The anterior column consists of anterior longitudinal ligament, intervertebral disc (nucleus pulposus and annulus), vertebral bodies, and posterior longitudinal ligament. The posterior column receives 20% of the axial forces and consists of the posterior bony elements, facets and facet capsule, ligaments, and posterior spinal musculature. The normal physiologic state, therefore, is one of "load-sharing," a concept which has been promoted widely by surgeon-philosophers such as Drs. Jürgen Harms and Arthur Steffee. Loads are shared proportionately by the anterior and posterior columns and have passive restraints (i.e., disc, ligaments, facet capsules) and active restraints (i.e., posterior spinal musculature).

When one looks at the blood supply to the spine, several obvious features are noted. Of prime importance is the vascularity to the vertebral bodies. The cancellous nature of the vertebral bodies demonstrates the trabeculae, which are marrow channels of blood and osteoprogenitor cells. Indeed, Arthur Steffee, MD, has coined the term "the optimal living bone graft" as it applies to the vertebral bodies [33]. The intervertebral disc supports two living vascularized bone grafts known as the vertebral bodies. Compression across the anterior column graft promotes communication between these two autologous vascularized bone grafting surfaces. The blood supply to the posterior bony elements is not as extensive and has to be stripped when one is performing a posterior or intertransverse process fusion. Repeat fusion attempts posteriorly, even with instrumentation, do not meet the same success as intradiscal fusions. The neovascularization in this environment of "scar" should be likened to direct surface bone grafting procedures of tibial nonunion. The best results are achieved by approaching this nonunion by a posterior route (tibia-profibula grafting) where the vasculature environment is pristine.

ROLE OF BIOACTIVE SUBSTANCES

The scope of this paper is not to exhaust the potential applications of bioactive substances in their ability to promote spinal fusions. The general role of bioactive substances can be subdivided by actions in the two distinctive areas for bony fusion. Again, the posterior elements and intradiscal areas differ, both in their biology and biomechanical influences on the fusion mass.

Bioactive substances have to have the ability to enhance and/or extend the biological events occurring posteriorly. These substances can be osteoinductive, having a direct effect on the cellular activity which leads to the production of new bone. Their inductive activity can be linked also to promotion of microvascular invasion to bring in osteoprogenitor cells and to help bring in humoral or local factors which can modulate the fusion process. Osteoconductive properties are beneficial, since they can be an actual bone extender, serving as a lattice for the fusion front to move forward. The surface of bioactive substances can even be resorbed as the fusion mass continues to mature and respond to "Wolff's Law."

Biomechanically, the posterior environment is one which routinely is reflected in tension forces. There is evidence to suggest that there is stress-shielding by posterior transpedicular instrumentation which leads to a weakened bone mass [34,35]. The forces are transferred to the rigid posterior implants, and this "load transferring" phenomenon may decrease the ultimate bone strength. We do know that posterior spinal instrumentation has led to an increase in the percentage of successful fusions when compared to uninstrumented fusion and spine instrumented with semi-rigid devices [10,11,12,13].

The different role of bioactive substances anteriorly is also reflected in the differences in biology and biomechanics of the anterior column. The bioactive substances are placed in an optimal biomechanical environment: compression. When posterior (or anterior) stabilization is employed, constant compression is maintained. In addition, there is neutralization of flexion, extension, and torsional forces. Biologically, the bleeding subchondral endplates provide the ideal osteoinductive environment. Again, each endplate is a "vascularized living autologous bone graft." Bioactive substances, however, have to have supportive strut characteristics or be placed in a conduit which is in itself supportive and not stress-shielding. Routinely, the surgeon uses hybrid grafts, such as carbon fiber or titanium cages, together with autograft [33,36,37,38]. Obviously, an important extrapolation will be the use of bioactive substances that are supportive, induce bone to form, and will in themselves be eventually resorbed and replaced by host bone.

Anteriorly, AWG ceramic and hydroxyapatite blocks have been used with varying degrees of success [39,40]. Fusion or endplate annealing to the ceramic surfaces occurs, but total reincorporation or replacement by host bone has not been demonstrated. These bioactive ceramics, however, recreate the appropriate biomechanical conditions as they reconstruct the anterior column and compressive forces (80%) that normally occur in the spine.

CONCLUSION

In conclusion, an optimal biological and biomechanical environment for bony reconstruction and fusion exists in the anterior column of the spine. Animal models and investigative clinical studies have demonstrated that posterior spinal fusions using allograft or bioactive compounds do not achieve the same fusion success as these materials do in the anterior spinal column. Ultimate spinal stabilization is in the form of bony union, not metallic implantation. The spinal surgeon should better understand the events around spinal fusions to improve results and enhance the clinical outcome.

REFERENCES

1. Goldberg, V.M., Stevenson, S. and Shaffer, J.W. In: *Bone and Cartilage Allografts: Biology and Clinical Applications*, American Academy of Orthopaedic Surgeons, Park Ridge 1991, 3-12.

2. Schenk R.K. and Hunziker E.B. In: *Bone Formation and Repair*, American Academy of Orthopaedic Surgeons, Rosemont 1994, 117-146.

3. Friedlander G.E. *J. Bone Joint Surg.* 1987; **69A**, 786-790.

4. Glowacki J. In: *Bone and Cartilage Allografts: Biology and Clinical Applications*, American Academy of Orthopaedic Surgeons, Park Ridge 1991, 55-74.

5. Boucher H.H. *J. Bone Joint Surg.* 1959, **41B**, 124-259.

6. Wiltse L.L. et al. *J. Bone Joint Surg.* 1968, **50A**, 919-926.

7. Dawson E.G., Lotysch M. and Urist M.R. *Clin. Orthop.* 1981, **154**, 90.

8. Bernhart M., Swartz D.E. and Clothiaux P.L., et al. *Clin. Orthop.* 1992, **284**, 109-115.

9. McGuire R.A. and Amundson G.M. *Spine* 1993, **18**, 1662-1672.

10. Wood G.W., Boyd R.J., and Carothers T.A., et al. *Spine* 1995, **20**, 819-830.

11. Zdeblick, T.A. *Spine* 1993, **18**, 983-91.

12. Lorenz M., Zindrick M. and Schwaegler P., et al. *Spine* 1991, **16**, S455-468.

13. Bridwell K.H., Sedgewick T.A. and O'Brien M.F., et al. *J. Spinal Disorders* 1993, **6**, 461-472.

14. Zuckerman J.F., Selby D. and Delong W.B. In: *Lumbar Spine Surgery*, C.V. Mosby, St. Louis, 1987.

15. Lee C.K., Vessa P. and Lee J.K. *Spine* 1995, **20**, 356-361.

16. Simmons J.W. *Clin. Orthop.* 1985, **193**, 85-89.

17. Ma G.W. *Clin. Orthop.* 1985, **193**, 57-63.

18. Steffee A.D. and Sitkowski D.J. *Clin. Orthop.* 1988, **227**, 99-102.

19. Enker P. and Steffee A.D. *Clin. Orthop.* 1994, **300**, 90-101.

20. Holte D.C., O'Brien J.P. and Renton P. *Eur. Spine J.* 1994, **3**, 32-38.

21. Selby D.K., Henderson R.J., Blumenthol S. and Dosset D. In: *Lumbar Spine Surgery*, C.V. Mosby, St. Louis, 1987.

22. Watkins R.G. In: *Lumbar Spine Surgery*, C.V. Mosby, St. Louis, 1987.

23. Banwart J.C., Asher M.A. and Hassanein R.S. *Spine* 1995, **20**, 1055-1060.

24. Kurz L.T., Garfin S.R. and Booth R.E. *Spine* 1989, **14**, 1324-1331.

25. Younger E.M. and Chapman M.W. *J. Orthop. Trauma* 1989, **3**, 192-195.

26. Jorgenson S.S., Lowe T.G. and Sabin J., et al. *Spine* 1994, **19**, 2048-2053.

27. Young W.F. and Rosenwasser R.H. *Spine* 1993, **18**, 1123-1124.

28. Kozak J.A., Heilman A.E. and O'Brien J.P. *Clin. Orthop.* 1994, **300**, 45-51.

29. Watkins R.G. In: *Lumbar Interbody Fusion*, Aspen Publishers, Rockville, 1989, 107.

30. Harms J. and Stoltze D. *Eur. Spine J.* 1992, **1**, 142-151.

31. Matthias H.H. and Heine J. *Clin. Orthop.* 1986, **203**, 34-44.

32. Nachemson A. *Clin. Orthop.* 1966, **45**, 107.

33. Lehmer S.M. et al., *Spine* 1994, **19**, 2060-2067.

34. Heggeness M.H. and Esses S.I. *Spine* 1991, **16S**, S449-454.

35. Craven T.G., Carson W.L., Asher M.A. and Robinson R.G. *Spine* 1994, **19**, 1664-1673.

36. Lowery G.L., Harms J., Biedermann L. Paper presented: First International Meeting on Self-Contained Instrumented Interbody Fusions. Minneapolis, Minnesota, October 19, 1994.

37. Lowery G.L. Paper to be presented: Tenth Annual Meeting of National Association of Spine Surgeons. Washington, D.C., October 18, 1995.

38. Lowery, G.L., Harms, J. In: *Manual of Internal Fixation of the Spine*, Raven Press, New York (in press).

39. Tsuji H., Hirano N. and Katoh Y., et al. *J. Spinal Disorders* 1990, **3**, 77-86.

40. Pintar F.A., Maiman D.J. and Hollowell J.P., et al. *Spine* 1994, **19**, 2524-2528.

ORTHOPAEDIC APPLICATIONS

COMPARATIVE BONE FORMATION IN SEVERAL KINDS OF BIOCERAMIC GRANULES

H. Oonishi[1], S. Kushitani[1], H. Iwaki[1], K. Saka[1], H. Ono[1], A. Tamura[1], T. Sugihara[2], L.L. Hench[3], J. Wilson[3] and E. Tsuji[4]

Dept. of Orthopaedic Surgery, Artificial Joint Section and Biomaterial Research Laboratory, Osaka-Minai National Hospital, 677-6, Kido-Cho, Kawachinagano-Shi, Osaka, 586 JAPAN[1]
Nitta Gelatin Inc. Research and Laboratory Center, 2-22, Futamata Yao, Osaka 581, JAPAN[2]
Bioglass® Research Center University of Florida,Gainesville, FL. 32611, U.S.A.[3]
Osaka Prefectural Industrial Engineering Research Institute, 1-53, 2-Chome, Enokoshima, Nishi-Ku, Osaka, 550, JAPAN[4]

ABSTRACT
Several kinds of bioceramic materials were implanted into 6 mm diameter holes made in the femoral condyles of mature rabbits. Bioceramics were both bioinert ceramics (Alumina), and bioactive ceramics (HAp and Bioglass®), and resolvable bioactive ceramics (TeCP, a-TCP, b-TCP, DCPD, DCPA, wet with unsintered HAp and OCP). Granule sizes of 100-300 μm and 10 μm were used. Bone growth behavior varied with the kind and size of bioceramic used.

INTRODUCTION

Bioceramics can be divided in to three categories:
1) Bioinert ceramics, such as alumina and zirconia.
2) Surface bioactive ceramics, such as sintered hydroxyapatite (HAp), Bioglass® and A-W glass ceramics .
3) Resorbable bioactive ceramics, such as wet HAp, α-tricalcium phosphate, β-tricalcium phosphate, tetracalcium phosphate, and octacalcium phosphate.

When granules of these bioceramics are implanted in bone, bone growth behavior and reaction to the bone are expected to be different due to the variation in composition and in granule sizes.

In this study, bone reaction to granules in several sizes of several different bioceramics are compared.

MATERIALS

The following materials were used.

Alumina,
Hydroxyapatite (HAp) sintered at 1200°C (HAp,$Ca_{10}(P0_4)_6(OH_2)$,
Bioglass®,
Wet Hydroxyapatite,
α-Tricalcium Phosphate (α-TCP,$Ca_3(PO_4)_2$),
β-Tricalcium Phosphate (β-TCP, $\beta Ca_3(PO_4)_2$), Tetracalcium Phosphate (TeCP, $Ca_4O(PO_4)_2$),
Octacalcium Phosphate (OCP, $Ca_8H_2(PO_4)_6°5H_2O$),
Dicalcium Phosphate Dihydrate (DCPD, $CaHPO_4°2H_2O$)
Dicalcium Phosphate Unihydrate (DCPA, $CaHPO_4$)

The granule size was 100-300 μm in diameter. The porosity of the bioactive ceramics was near 65%. Mature rabbits were used for the animal model.

METHOD

Holes 6 μm in diameter were drilled bilaterally in the femoral condyles of mature rabbits and sufficient hemostasis was achieved by filling and compressing the holes with gauze for five minutes. Immediately following, granules of prepared bioceramics were placed in sufficient amounts to fill the holes. Three animals were used for each time.

The animals were killed at intervals; non-decalcified specimens were observed by light microscopy and backscattered electron imaging, and decalcified specimens by light microscopy. Unfilled drilled holes were used as controls.

RESULTS AND DISCUSSION

Control

Drilled holes were made in the femoral condyles of mature rabbits and left vacant. At three weeks and also at six weeks, the density of bone formation in the unfilled hole was very low. By twelve weeks, cancellous bone formation in the cavity returned to normal. No changes were observable on surface cross sections by the naked eye.

Bioinert Ceramics

1) Alumina granules of 100 μm diameter

At one week, bone grew close to the alumina granules. However, bone never contacted the granules. At four weeks, new bone ingrowth between alumina granules to the center of the hole was seen. The new bone growth never directly contacted the alumina granules [1].

Surface Bioactive Ceramics

1) Sintered Hydroxyapatite granules of 100-300 μm diameter.

When sintered HAp granules of 100-300 μm were implanted, at one week new trabecular bone grew into spaces between granules from the surrounding bone and reached the outermost layer of HAp granules.

At three weeks, new bone tissue reached the sixth and seventh layers of HAp granules while at the same time enclosing HAp granules to a depth of 1000 μm.

At six weeks, spaces less than 20 μm at initial implantation were almost completely filled with new bone. Spaces larger than 100 μm had no new bone growing from surrounding bone and were not filled with new bone. New bone reached the 15th and 16th layers from the circumference, to a depth of 2500 μm. Generally, no new bone was seen where HAp granules were more than 100 μm apart [1] (Fig. 1).

Bioglass® Particles of 100-300 μm diameter

Two days after implantation of the 45S5 Bioglass® particles the periphery of Bioglass® in the outermost layer became silica-rich, and in some areas new bone had formed. New bone reaching the Bioglass® was observed in back scattered electron images. At five days, new bone penetrated most of the first two layers of Bioglass® which was bound directly to bone.

Twelve days after implantation, new bone entered and surrounded most surfaces of Bioglass® particles as far as the eighth and tenth outer layers. In comparison, by the third week, bone growth into HAp granules had only reached the fourth and fifth layers and surrounded surfaces of the first and second outer granule layers.

At six weeks, bone growth between Bioglass® particles continued to increase in density, all particles were enveloped with thick new trabecular bone and very few spaces remained unfilled (Fig. 2). In contrast with HAp at the sixth week, only granules of the outer three layers had been entirely encompassed. At deeper layers new trabecular bone only partially surrounded HAp granules, and only a few of these spaces were filled with new bone.

In summary, the speed of bone growth around Bioglass® particles was much faster and the new bone was much denser than bone growth associated with HAp [2, 3, 4].

Resorbable Bioactive Ceramics

In this category, TeCP, α-TCP, β-TCP, OCP, DCPA, DCPD and wet HAp (not sintered) were used in animal experiments.

1) TeCP, DCPD, DCPA granules of 100-300 μm

TeCP, DCPD and DCPA showed almost the same reactions (they will be noted together as Ca-P in this section). One week after implantation, bone tissues grew close to the Ca-P and replaced some of it, if even only to a very small extent. At three weeks, new laminar bone formed from the bone base. Ca-P in the vicinity of this new bone began to be slowly replaced by more new bone from the periphery (Fig. 3). Ca-P gradually diminished in amount with time. At twelve weeks, most of the Ca-P was replaced by new trabecular bone.

Backscattered electron images at high magnification showed that, at the edge of these Ca-P crystals, new bone was slowly replacing the Ca-P implanted three weeks earlier.

In close observation of these crystal remnants, it was noted that they gradually changed color from white to black from their peripheries. Furthermore, the configuration of some crystals was unclear, while others were hardly distinguishable from the new surrounding bone after twelve weeks [5] (Fig. 4).

2) α-TCP and β-TCP granules of 100-300 μm diameter.

α-TCP and β-TCP showed almost the same reactions (they will be noted together as α-/β-TCP in this section).

At three weeks, new laminar bone 100-200 μm wide formed from the host bone. The laminar trabecular new bone developed to the center of the hole that had been filled with the α-/β-TCP granules. The density of distribution of the trabecular bone was high (Fig. 5). No inflammatory reactions were observed. Bone growth behavior of

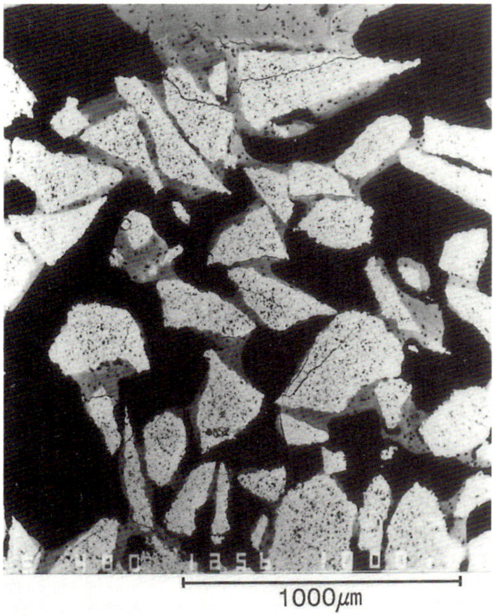

Fig. 1. HAp (100-300 μm), 6 weeks at the tibia periphery. Backscattered electron image

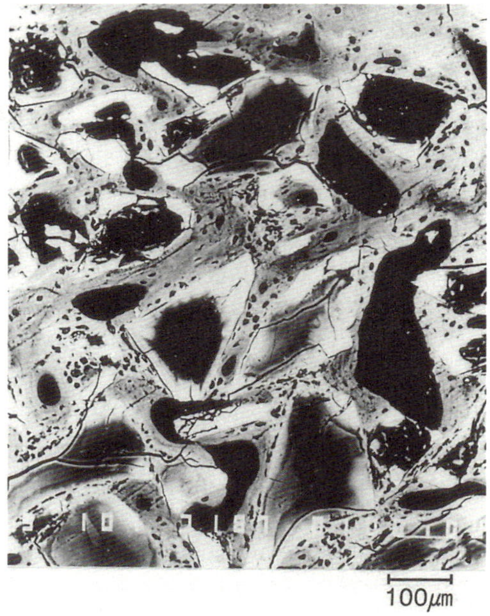

Fig. 2. Bioglass® (100-300 μm), 6 weeks at the tibia periphery

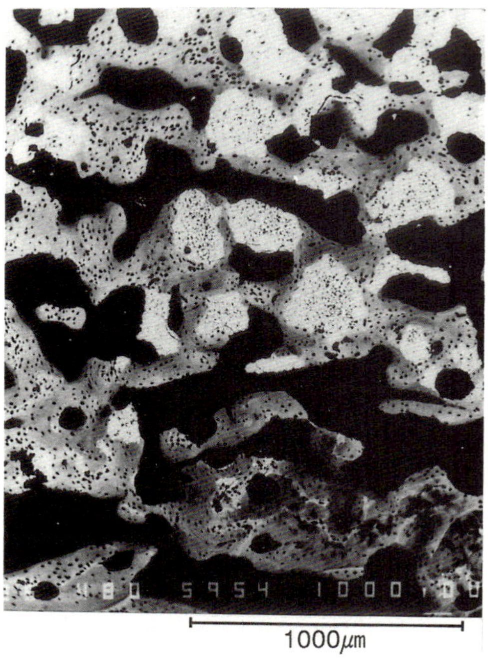

Fig. 3. DCPA (100-300 μm), 6 weeks at the tibia periphery

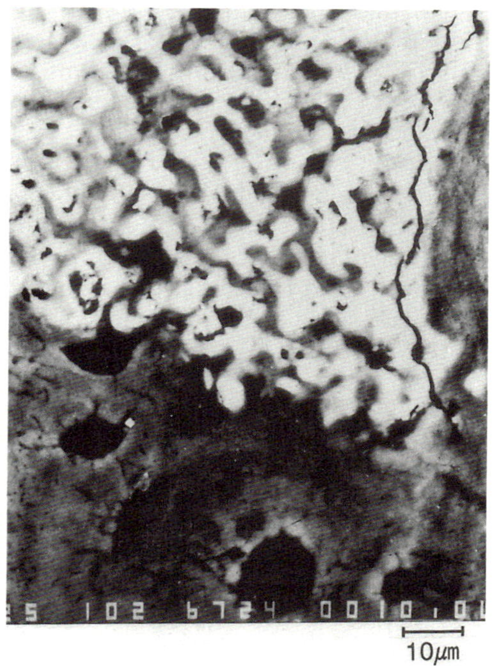

Fig. 4. DCPD (100-300 μm), 12 weeks at the tibia periphery

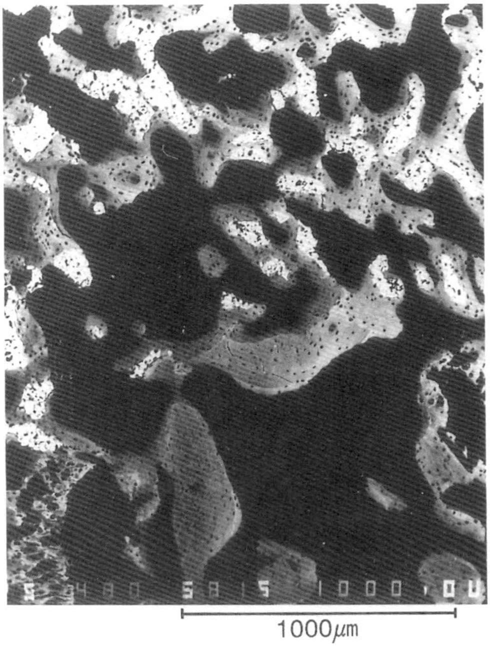

Fig. 5. α-TCP (100-300 μm), 3 weeks at the tibia periphery

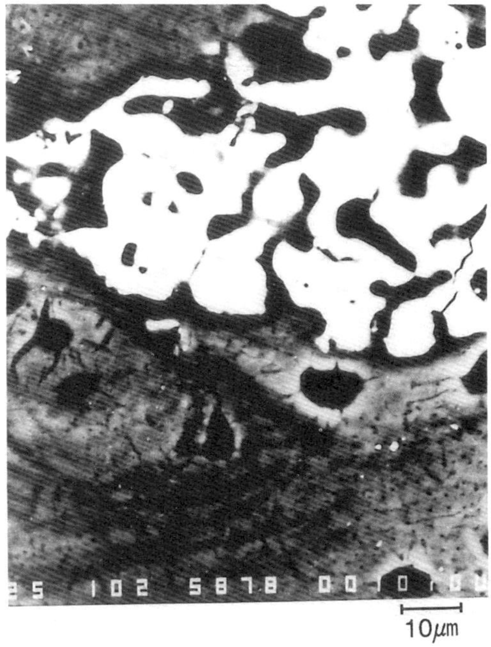

Fig. 6. β-TCP (100-300 μm), 6 weeks at the tibia periphery

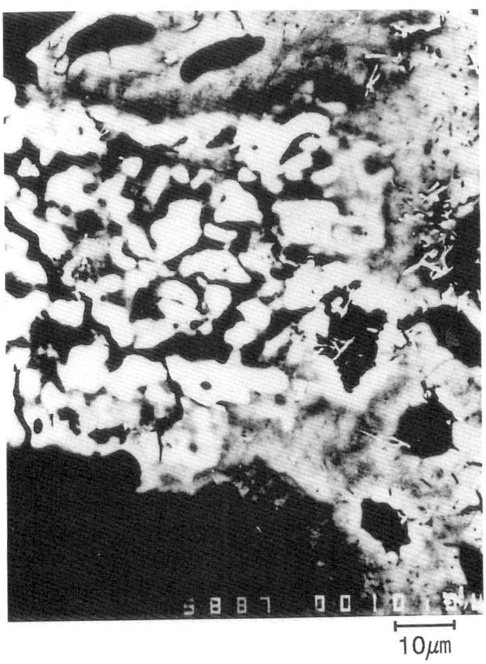

Fig. 7. TeCP (10 μm), 3 weeks at tibia periphery

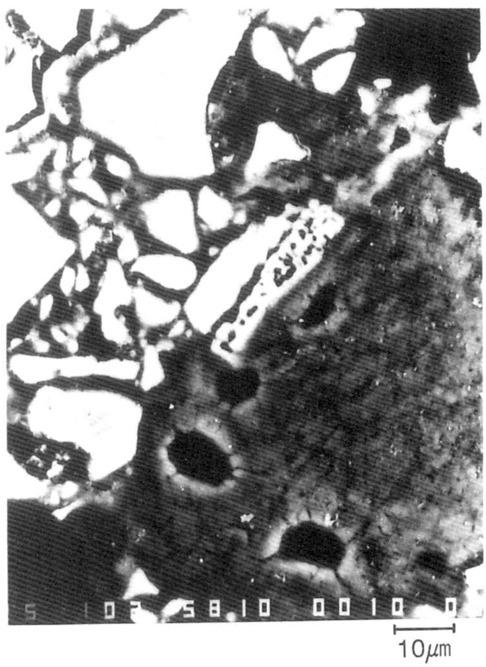

Fig. 8. α-TCP (10 μm), 3 weeks at tibia periphery

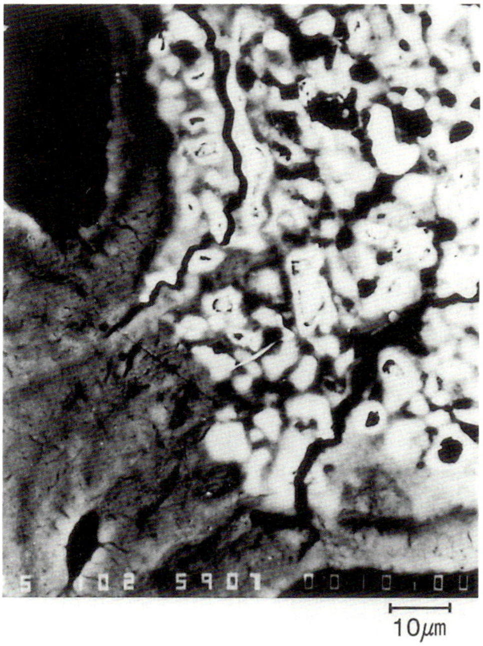

Fig. 9. TeCP (10 μm), 6 weeks at tibia periphery

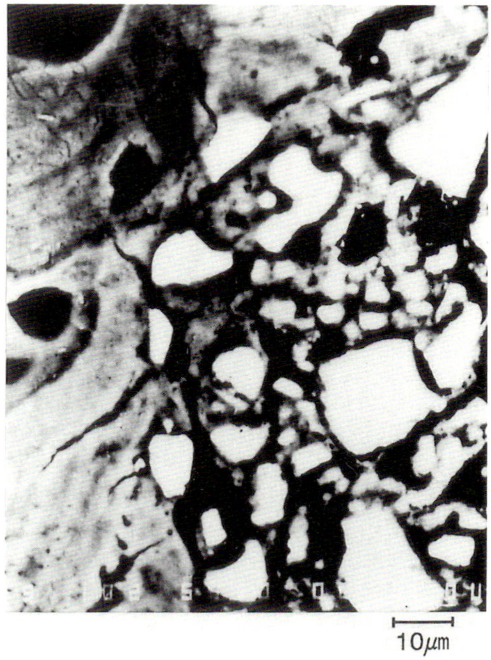

Fig. 10. α-TCP (10 μm), 6 weeks at tibia periphery

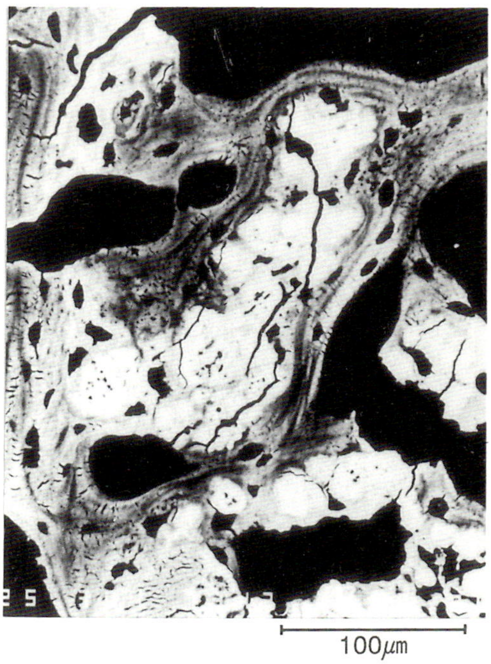

Fig. 11. Wet HAp not sintered (10 μm), 3 weeks

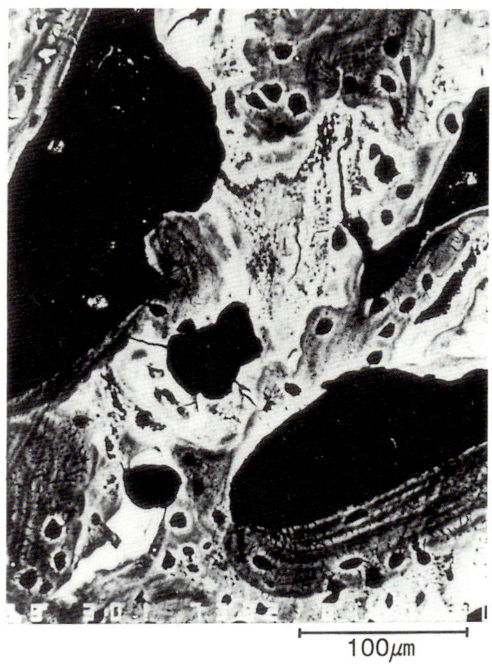

Fig. 12. Wet HAp not sintered (10 μm), 6 weeks

HAp, and α-/β-TCP of 100-300 μm diameter were very different. In the HAp, new bone entered the spaces between granules, however, the laminar trabecular new bone forming with α-/β-TCP granules showed results very similar to TeCP granules. At six weeks, over half the mass of the α-/β-TCP granules was resorbed, and the density of distribution of the trabecular bone became lower. At twelve weeks, the size of the granules became smaller, only small amounts of α-/β-TCP granules remained. The trabecular bone remodeled and returned to its normal structure. The interface between α-/β-TCP granules and bone was rather distinct, which was different from the changes of TeCP (Fig. 6).

3) TeCP, α-TCP, β-TCP, DCPD and DCPA granules of 10 μm diameter.

TeCP, α-TCP, β-TCP, DCPD and DCPA of 10 μm diameter showed similar reactions (they will be noted together as Ca-P in this section).

At three weeks, little bone growth into the spaces of theCa-P granule was seen (Fig. 7, 8). At six weeks, bone growth into the spaces of Ca-P granules was seen only around the mass, however, new bone surrounding the Ca-P mass increased (Fig. 9, 10). Slight inflammation and congestion were observed with β-TCP.The degree of inflammation in β-TCP powder was higher than that of α-TCP powder.

TeCP, DCPD and DCPA showed behavior little different from α-TCP and β-TCP. TeCP, DCPD, and DCPA powders of 10 μm diameter were being resorbed gradually by the trabecular bone surrounding theCa-P mass, and are being replaced by new trabecular bone (Fig. 7, 9). TeCP, DCPD and DCPA granules of 100-300 μm diameter also showed different behavior from α-TCP and β-TCP.

From these phenomena, is assumed that TeCP, DCPD and DCPA may have a higher bioactivity or may be more resorbable than α-TCP and β-TCP.

4) Wet HAp non-sintered and OCP resorbable granules of 10 μm diameter.

Wet HAp and OCP granules of 10 μm diameter showed similar behavior (they will be noted together as Ca-P in this section).

At one week, new bone reached a depth of one or two layers, surrounded some Ca-P granules, and bonded to others. However, on the whole, large spaces were observed between the Ca-P border and original bone. At three weeks, laminar new bone tissue of 50-150 μm width had begun to form. The trabecular new bone formed with these Ca-P granules just as on the HAp granules of 10 μm (Fig. 11). At six weeks, new bone developed on Ca-P granules to the center of the hole. Granules were being replaced by the new bone from the periphery of the granules, and the number of granules diminished (Fig. 12).

TeCP, α-TCP, β-TCP, DCPD and DCPA also showed very different behaviors from wet HAp and OCP. The former granules as a mass, were surrounded by new bone, and only a few granules in the periphery of a mass were taken into the trabecular bone.

From these observations we suppose that sintered HAp, being surface active with low reactivity and non-resorbable, by six weeks was surrounded by trabecular bone. The wet, non-sintered HAp and OCP were more bioactive but at the same time were resorbable and were replaced by new bone. It appears that wet HAp and OCP are more bioactive and probably more resorbable than TeCP, α-TCP, β-TCP, DCPD and DCPA.

CONCLUSION

Bone growth behavior varied with the kind and size of bioceramics used. In surface bioactive ceramics, Bioglass® was more bioactive than HAp. In resorbable bioactive ceramics, the probable order of higher bioactivity and more resorbability might be as follows; first, wet HAp and OCP, second, TeCP, DCPD, DCPA, and third, α-TCP and β-TCP. In terms of biocompatibility, α-TCP was better than β-TCP.

ACKNOWLEDGEMENTS

The authors gratefully acknowledge receiving the Bioglass® particulate from U.S. Biomaterials Corp. Alachua, Florida, and receiving TeCP, α-TCP, β-TCP, DCPD, DCPA, wet HAp and OCP from Nitta Gelatin Inc. Osaka.

REFERENCES

1. Oonishi, H., Tuji, E., Kushitani, S., Aono, M., Minami, K. and Hidaka, T. *Bioceramics, 5,* Kobunshi Kankokai, Japan, 1992, 149-153.
2. Wilson, J. and Low, S. *J. Appl. Biom.* 1992, 3, 123-129.
3. Wilson, J., Yu, L.T., Beale, B.S. *Bioceramis, 5,* Kobunshi Kankokai, Japan, 1992, 139-146.
4. Oonishi, H., Kushitani, S., Yasukawa, E., Nakata, A., Koh, S., Hench, L.L., Wilson, J., Tsuji, T. and Sugihara, T. *Bioceramics, 7,* Butterworth-Heineman, Oxford 1994, 139-144.
5. Oonishi, H., Tsuji, E., Mizukoshi, T., Kushitani, S., Aono, M., Minami, K., Watanabe, A., Ogino, A. and Fujisawa, N. *Bioceramics, 4,* Butterworth-Heineman, Oxford 1991, 191-197.

WEAR DEBRIS AND INFLAMMATORY RESPONSE IN TISSUES AROUND FAILED ALUMINA CERAMIC-ON-CERAMIC HIP PROSTHESES

S. Lerouge,[1,2] L'H. Yahia,[2] O. Huk,[3] L. Sedel[1]

[1]Orthopaedic Research Laboratory, Lariboisiere Saint Louis Faculty of Medicine, 10 av. Verdun, 75 010 Paris, France,
[2]Biomechanics / Biomaterials Research Goup, Biomedical Engineering Institute, Ecole Polytechnique, Station Centre Ville, CP Box 6079, Montreal H3C 3A7
[3]Division of Orthopedic Surgery. McGill University, 3755 Chemin de la Cote Sainte Catherine, Montreal, Canada

ABSTRACT

Semi-quantitative comparative histology of pseudomembranes (PM) from aseptic loosened ceramic-ceramic (CC) and metal-polyethylene (MPE) hip prostheses was performed and isolated wear debris from CC pseudomembranes were characterized by SEM. Ceramic-ceramic PM presented a less intense cellular reaction than MPE although grades of presence of debris were not significantly different. Titanium alloy and alumina debris were isolated from CC PM, as well as zirconia debris from PMMA bone cement, where it served as a contrast agent. There were different foreign body cellular reactions to alumina and zirconia debris. Zirconia debris could play a significant role in loosening of CC prostheses.

INTRODUCTION

Aseptic loosening remains the principle etiology responsible for long term failure of total hip arthroplasties (THA). Biologic response to wear debris has been recognized as the main loosening mechanism of metal-polyethylene (MPE) hip prostheses [1,2]. As a response to problems related to UHMWPE wear, the alumina ceramic on ceramic (CC) load-bearing couple has been used as an alternative to MPE for more than 20 years in France. Our results showed a 90% survival rate at 10 years in patients less than 50 years of age [3]. Failure was mostly due to cup loosening, and stem loosening was very rare. To date, the mechanism of loosening of CC prostheses has not been understood or investigated. The average wear rate *in vivo* of this CC prosthesis is more than a thousand times less than that of MPE THA [4]. Based on ceramic wear rate and alumina biocompatibility, our working hypothesis is that there should be less debris and less cellular response in periprosthetic tissue around failed CC than failed MPE prostheses. The aim of our study was to compare the histology of pseudomembranes (PM) harvested around loosened MPE and CC THA, and to identify and characterize wear debris found in the CC pseudomembranes.

MATERIALS AND METHODS

A total of 47 PM were harvested at revision surgery for aseptic loosening at Hospital Saint Louis in Paris. Since CC THA never failed by stem loosening alone, and to permit comparison between groups, we excluded 8 specimens of PM from MPE THA that were revised for stem loosening. Of the 39 PM retained for study, 17 cases involved a CC and 22 a MPE load-bearing couple. All membranes studied were harvested at the cup-bone interface. The average patient age at revision surgery was 64 and 61 years, respectively and duration of implantation was 7.2 and 9.6 years respectively. There was no significant demographic difference between groups. In the CC group, 16 revisions were for cup loosening and one for the cup and stem. In the MPE group, only 4 cases were revised for cup loosening and 18 for both cup and stem.

Histology

PM stained with H&E underwent light and polarized microscopy. The presence of each type of debris particle and foreign body inflammatory cell (macrophages, giant cells) was graded according to the method of Willert and Semlitsch [5] on a scale from 0 to 3 to permit a semi-quantitative comparison between groups. Presence of fibroblasts, lymphocytes, and necrosis was also evaluated. Ten fields in each histologic section were evaluated by a single observer.

Debris characterization

Debris from CC pseudomembranes was isolated by tissue digestion using collagenase and formic acid, followed by ultracentrifugation on a sucrose gradient. Because of tissue heterogeneity, care was taken to get as representative a sample as possible.The CC PM was sectioned into small pieces, mixed and 1 g of tissue then taken for digestion. Isolated debris was washed and dispersed by ultrasonification in solution. A known volume of this solution was filtered though a 0.2 μm filter and the deposited debris was observed by Scanning Electron Microscopy (SEM) in association with Energy Dispersive X-ray Analysis (EDXA) and image analysis. As metal and ceramic particles in the CC PM have approximately the same density ($d=4.5$), separation of debris could not be achieved by ultracentrifugation. We therefore used backscattered electron microscopy and grey level contrasts to distinguish between the various particle compositions.

RESULTS

Cellular reaction

Mean counts of macrophages, giant cells and sum of cell types for each group are reported in Figure 1. The mean grade of cellularity was less in the CC group than the MPE group. The difference was significant for giant cells and the sum of both cell types (Anova $p < 0.05$).

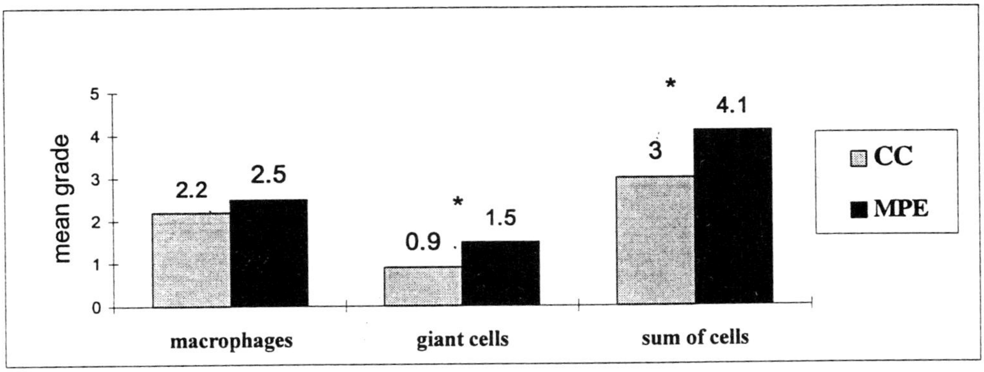

Figure 1. Mean grade of macrophages, giant cells, and sum of both cell types in PMs from ceramic-ceramic (CC) and metal-polyethylene (MPE) THA (* $p<0.05$)

Debris characterization

Light microscopy allowed the differentiation of 3 types of debris particles: titanium, ceramic and PMMA. Titanium alloy (TiAIV) particles were found in 9 specimens of CC PM. These TiAIV particles originated from either the stem or metal-back cup fixation system and were recognized by their black colour under light microscopy. Ceramic particles were found in almost every case (15 of 17). They were small (mostly under 0.5 μm), yellow-amber in colour, with brown outlines. Because of their small size, a magnification of 1000 was necessary to distinguish them from metallic particles. Empty vacuoles corresponding to PMMA cement debris, dissolved during histologic preparation, were seen in 10 specimens.

Mean grades of each type of debris and of the sum of debris for each group are shown in Figure 2. Surprisingly, no difference was found between groups. The average amount of ceramic particles in the CC group was not significantly lower than UHMWPE in the MPE group.

Scanning Electron Microscopy permitted further identification of the particles. Table 1 summarizes the three types of debris obtained by tissue digestion from CC pseudomembranes. EDXA identified 2 types of ceramic particles: alumina and zirconia.

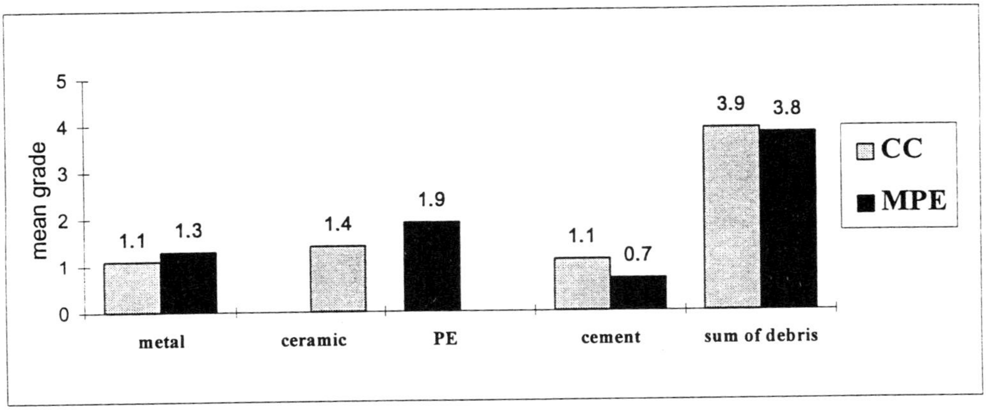

Figure 2. Mean grade of each type of debris in pseudomembranes of ceramic-ceramic (CC) and metal polyethylene (MPE) THAs

Alumina debris was of prosthetic origin and zirconia debris was from cement. The majority of ceramic particles that we observed were zirconia. Zirconium oxide has been and is still used as a contrast agent in some PMMA bone cement products, instead of barium. Free zirconia particles were found dissociated from PMMA, well dispersed in the tissue, and mostly phagocytozed by macrophages. Statistical tests showed that the mean amount of foreign body cells was significantly lower ($p<0.01$) in PM containing a prevelance of zirconia particles when compared to those with mostly alumina.

Alumina particles tended to be polygonal in shape and had a more variable size distribution(0.2-1.0μm) than zirconia particles, which had a more rounded morphology, and narrower size distribution (0.1-0.5μm). Light microscopy did not allow differentiation between alumina and zirconia particles for the following reasons: (1) similar colour; (2) both particles sizes were at the limit of light microscopic resolution; and (3) overlapping size distributions.

Figure 3 shows a SEM field with a majority of alumina particles.

DISCUSSION

Comparative histologic grading of periprosthetic tissue has shown a less intense cellular reaction in pseudomembranes retrieved from failed CC hip prostheses than from MPE prostheses. This is in agreement with *in vivo* and *in vitro* studies from other investigators. Qualitative observations of pseudomembranes from retrieved ceramic-ceramic implants showed very weak foreign body reactions to ceramic particles in well fixed prostheses [6] as well as a lower cellular reaction in loosened prostheses when compared to metal-polyethylene THA [7, 8, 9]. This is believed to be related to the lower reactivity of alumina debris, which may be due to the material inertness, the small and uniform size, or the morphology of alumina particles. Indeed, *in vitro* culture of macrophages and fibroblasts with alumina powder have found no cytotoxic effect and a lower level of cell stimulation than metal or polyethylene particles [10, 11].

Nevertheless in our study, most ceramic debris was not alumina of articular origin, but zirconia originating from the cement. Furthermore, we identified a different reaction to alumina and zirconia particles. Where zirconia was the prevailing debris,

Composition	Source	colour under light microscopy	size (µm)	morphology
ZrO_2	cement contrast	yellow-amber	0.1 - 0.5	rounded
TiAlV	femoral stem or cup fixation system	dark	0.3 - 4.0	irregular
Al_2O_3	load bearing couple	yellow-amber	0.2 - 1.0	polygonal

Table 1. Composition and properties of the three main types of debris isolated from CC pseudomembranes

the cellular reaction was more intense than when it was alumina, suggesting that reactivity of zirconia may be more intense than of alumina. Previous biocompatibility studies on zirconia of high purity have shown controversial results [12]. Zirconia used as contrast agent is not as pure as that used for ball manufacturing; it is radioactive [13] and its reactivity could be higher than that of zirconia used in hip arthroplasty. Zirconia particles may play a significant role in the loosening mechanism of those prostheses. To our knowledge, this is the first report on the importance of contrast material on aseptic loosening. This result will be further investigated.

In contrast to zirconia containing cement, THA fixed with barium sulphate containing cement did not have a large quantity of barium sulphate in the tissue. The lower hardness and smaller quantity of barium added to those cements are two possible explanations.

The subdued reaction observed in this study is even more evident for foreign body giant cells. This is probably due to the absence of polyethylene: the presence of giant cells in pseudomembranes is usually associated with UHMWPE cement debris, or with large metallic particles, but not with ceramic particles.

CC PM exhibit a less intense cellular reaction than MPE PM. Previous studies had demonstrated a significantly lower level of PGE_2 in CC PM [14]. Biological response to wear debris, which leads to periprosthetic osteolysis, may be less intense with CC hip prostheses. Loosening mechanisms of CC prostheses may involve mechanical factors, directly related to the modulus mismatch between alumina, bone and cement, which leads to microfractures in the cement. The presence of zirconia particulate from the cement suggests that cement fragmentation had occurred at the cup-bone interface and may have initiated loosening.

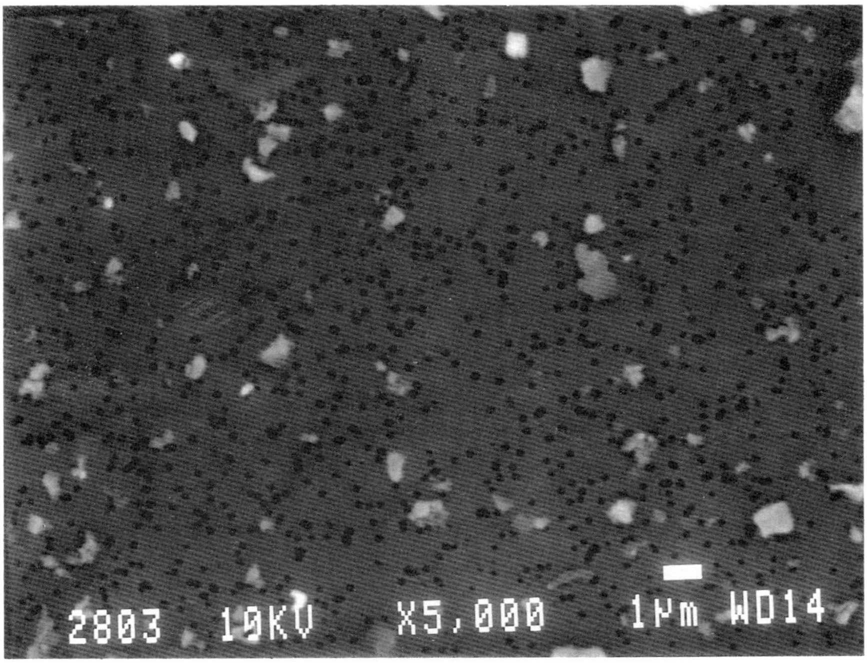

Figure 3. SEM field of isolated debris of a CC PM with a majority of alumina particles.

REFERENCES

1. Spector M *et al., Clin. Orthop. Relat. Res* 1991, 261, 140.
2. Howie DW. *J Arthroplasty* 1990, 5(4):337-348
3. Sedel L., Nizard R., Kerboull L. and Witvoet J. *C.O.R.R. 1994,* 298, 175-183
4. Dorlot JM, Christel P and Meunier. J *Biomed. Mater. Res: Applied Biomaterials* 1989, 23, 299-310
5. Willert H .G. and Semlitsch R. *Sulzer Tech Rev 1975,* 119- 133
6. Boutin P, Christel P, Dorlot JM *et al.,* J. *Biomat Mat Res* 1988, 22, 1203-1232
7. Plitz W and Griss P. In *Implant Retrieval: material and biological analysis,* NBS special publication 601, Weinstein, Gibbons, Brown & Ruff (Eds), 1981, 131-156
8. Pizzoferrato, V. Stea S, Sudanese A, Toni A *et al., Biomaterials,* 1993, 14 (8), *583-587*
9. Boynton E, Waddel JP, Morton J., Gardiner GW. *Can. J. Surg.* 1991, 34, 599-605
10. Kuroki Y. In *Bioceramics 1 (1989), 308-313*
11. Hann;s J, Mausle E. J *Biomed Mater. Res.* 1979, 13, 67-87
12. Li J., Liu Y, Hermansson L and Soremark R. *Clinical Materials* 1993,12,197-201
13. Hopf T.W. and Globel B. J. *Applied Biomaterials* 1990,1, 215-216.
14. Sedel L, Simeon J, Meunier A, *et al., Arch Orthop Trauma Surg* 111 :255-258, 1992.

EVALUATION OF THE EFFECT OF STRESS CORROSION ON ZIRCONIA FEMORAL HEADS

M.G.S.Murray[1], M Newman[1], R. Morrell[2], W.P. Byrne[2]

[1] Morgan Matroc, Ltd, Rugby Division, Rugby, UK, CV21 3QR
[2] National Physical Laboratory, Teddington, Middx., UK, TW11 0LW

ABSTRACT

The successful development and clinical use of high-strength zirconia ceramics for orthopaedic use, such as in femoral heads has allowed the range of head designs to be extended with a modular approach to component selection. To analyse the stress generated in heads, as a function of design, a strain gauge analysis during loading and unloading is described. Permanent strains are developed in heads after unloading, sometimes greater than those during loading. To investigate their effect on head life, different designs were forced onto titanium spigots at loads corresponding to 40%, 60% and 80% of the short-term fracture load. These heads were aged in simulated body fluid at 37°C for months to simulate in-service conditions. The delayed failure results have allowed risks from high loading in different geometries to be determined.

INTRODUCTION

The clinical advantages of ceramic femoral heads compared with metallic heads are reduced wear and hence reduced formation of wear debris, recognised as a cause of stem loosening and short prosthesis life [1]. The development of zirconia ceramic heads with higher intrinsic strength has resulted in a degree of design modularity such as smaller diameter heads and heads with greater neck length, to suit the individual patient. However, a key element in the effective use of ceramic heads is to ensure that the in-patient stress levels defined by the geometry of spigot contact and forces applied are well inside the limits for the ceramic material. These limits derive from the scatter of strengths of ceramic components, and the phenomenon of subcritical crack growth which can occur at high stresses, leading to lifetime limitations in both static loading and in fatigue.

In FE modelling, many assumptions have to be made concerning the contact condition and elastic/plastic effects in the spigot [2,3] and to account for long-term behaviour. Two series of experiments have been performed to investigate the potential stress levels in and lifetimes of various head/spigot geometries. In the first, heads have been strain-gauged on the spherical surface and axially loaded titanium spigots, recording the strains during both loading, unloading and cyclically reloading to progressively higher applied forces. In the second series, following from the behaviour in the first series, heads and spigots loaded to various fractions of the mean ultimate failure load have been immersed for up to 450 days in simulated body fluid at 37 °C, and times to failure recorded in comparison with dry controls.

EXPERIMENTAL

For the strain gauging experiments, a series of pairs of Zyranox™ zirconia ceramic femoral heads were used, each pair with different geometry summarised as follows: diameter 28 mm (except type A1 = 32 mm), spigot angle 4° (except type A8 = 5° 43′ 30″), spigot geometry standard (except type A3 = + 3 mm: extended position and A4 = ±5 mm: short position design). Previous work by Kleer et al. [4] suggested that the regions of highest hoop stress would be in the lower hemisphere of the head, especially around the mouth. Accordingly, 2 mm strain gauges were placed on the equator, at about -45° latitude, on the as-fired chamfer near the mouth, and on the flat base near the mouth (Figure 1, not on types A3, A8). The gauges had a nominal resistance of 120 Ω, a gauge factor of 2, were compensated for use with aluminium, and were bonded with a cyanoacrylate adhesive to measure hoop strain. The gauges were wired into a multichannel data logger which also recorded the force applied by the Instron testing machine used to force the heads onto the spigots. The loading was performed in a jig in accordance with to ISO 7206/5 [5] using a brass loading ring. Heads for long-term testing were similarly prepared. The loaded heads were placed individually into labelled polyethylene bottles containing freshly prepared simulated body fluid, the cap sealed, and then placed in the tank attached to trays. Dry controls were similarly placed in bottles containing silica gel. The tank contents were inspected at regular intervals, daily at first, then weekly and then monthly.

STRAIN GAUGING EXPERIMENTS

A series of tests was performed, monitoring strain at the three or four strain gauges as the load was increased or decreased at costant crosshead speed. In summary, it has been shown that:

1. High applied forces leave the ceramic head permanently stressed by the spigot to a level determined by the applied force, and varying with design and position.
2. The externally measured strains are highest near the mouth, and these increase on unloading the head (Figure 2 (left), type A2 head). Strain levels of typically 0.1% represent stress levels which are comfortably within the mechanical strength criteria defined in FDA approval testing [6].
3. Some stress relaxation occurred initially on load holding, but within the available time frame of the strain gauge experiments, the strains did not relax significantly in the unloaded condition (Figure 2 (right) type A2 head).
4. On reloading, when the force reaches the level from which the previous unloading took place, there is an abrupt change in slope, and loading continues along the

original line (Figure 3, type A3 head). This is indicative of elastic/plastic effects in the spigot material.

5. For the different 28 mm diameter head designs, the residual strains for a given initial force increase as the spigot contact position is moved away from the head centre towards the mouth. Thus the extended position designs are subject to higher strains.

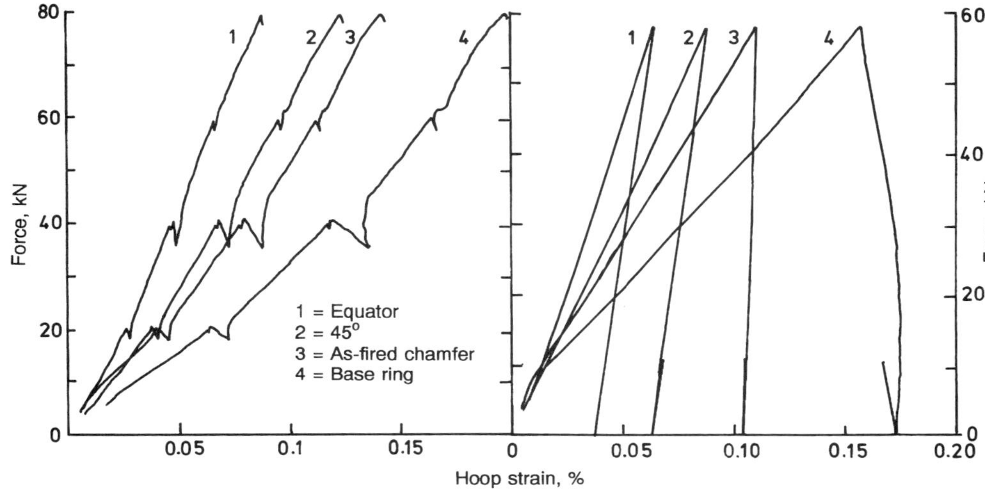

Figure 2. Force vs hoop strain for: (left) type A2 head, each kink being a 5 min hold with load relaxation but strain increase; (right) type A2 head in a loading and unloading cycle. Note mouth strain increases on unloading and no strain relaxation during 5 min hold at zero load.

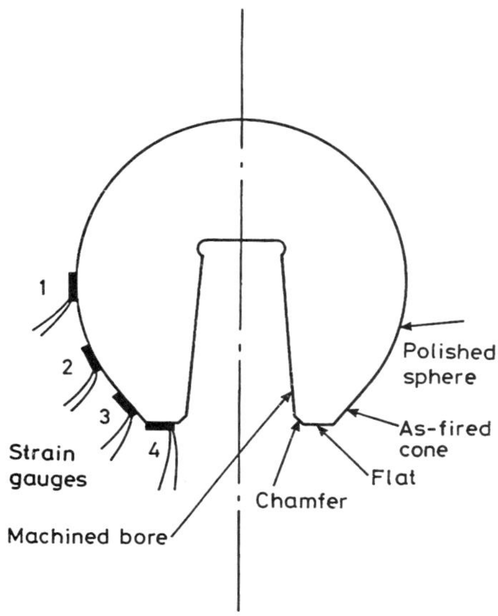

Figure 1. Location of strain gauges on head (sometimes not enough space for gauge 4)

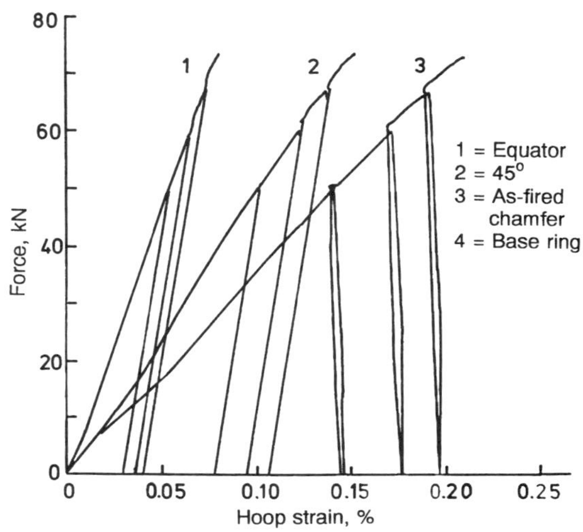

Figure 3. Force versus hoop strain femoral for a type A3 head with three unloading /reloading cycles. The residual strain increases with increasing applied force.

Table 1 - Ageing Programme

Head type	Short term UCS, kN, (No. tested)		Long-term pre-load, kN, (No. tested)		
	Mean	Std. dev.	80% of UCS	60% of UCS	40% of UCS
A1	121.9 (10)	15.6	-	73.1 (22)	-
A2	96.7 (10)	11.0	77.4 (30)	58.0 (30)	38.7 (30)
A3	83.7 (10)	6.4	-	50.2 (17)	-
A4	132.6 (10)	13.4	106.1 (18)	79.6 (30)	53.1 (18)
A2 (dry)	96.7 (10)	11.0	-	58.0 (30)	-

This overall strain behaviour may be explained by consideration of the elastic/plastic behaviour of the spigot. The yielding of the spigot material means that the spigot stress cannot greatly exceed the yield stress. The higher the applied force, the greater is the volume of the spigot which is yielding, and this changes the stress distribution applied to the ceramic head. The permanent deformation in the spigot means that the stresses in the head cannot relax to zero when the load is removed. This has been demonstrated by FEA by Andrisano *et al.* [3,4], and has now been shown experimentally in these tests.

LONG-TERM EXPERIMENTS

The matrix of Zyranox™ experiments defined by available materials is shown in Table 1. Since the heads of different geometry are manufactured in the same way, but had different ultimate compression strengths (UCS), the most valid examination of the long-term effects is to pre-stress them at different percentages of UCS rather than at the same force level. In this way there should be some equivalence in the long-term behaviour. The forces applied are much higher than those ever anticipated in service, and were designed to understand the ultimate performance rather than simulate clinical behaviour.

Particularly with those heads loaded to 80% of their UCS, some premature failures were encountered, either during loading, or during unloading, or while in their individual bottles awaiting placement in the tank. To examine the failure statistics, it is necessary to take these failures into account in each batch, not only those placed in the tank. Furthermore, to compare behaviour between different sized batches, it is necessary to normalise the failure probability, P_f. This was done by using the simple ranking estimator $P_f = (i - 0.5)/N$ where i is the rank number and N is the total in each batch. In the plots of $P_f = \log (t_f)$ where t_f is the time to failure, the premature failures have been arbitrarily assigned a time to failure of 0.001 d, which was shorter than any failure time resulting from inspection of the tank (the shortest was 5 min). At the time of writing these experiments are on-going, and the results reported at this stage represent approximately 16 months of exposure. No failures occurred in the dry control batch A2, either during loading or in the tank up to 450 days.

Figure 4 shows a plot of cumulative probability of failure against log (t_f, days) for type A2 heads at the three pre-load levels. There is a marked trend of increased failure rate with increased pre-load, a significant number failing prematurely at the 80% UCS pre-load, whereas at 40% UCS pre-load, the first failure occurred only after 160 days. Figure 5 shows a similar plot comparing failures at the 60% UCS level for all head types. They clearly indicate that the least strong design in short-term testing, type A3, is also the shortest lived during long-term testing, while the strongest, type A4, has fewest failures. The 32 mm type A1 heads pre-loaded at 60% UCS appear to behave similarly to the 28 mm type A2 heads of the similar design and percentage pre-load. In reviewing these results, it has to be borne in mind that it is risky to draw too many conclusions from this relatively small number of failures, but the test method offers potential for discriminating between different designs on a statistical basis.

DISCUSSION AND CONCLUSIONS

The strain-gauging experiments have shed light on strain distributions arising during loading and unloading of a ceramic femoral head on to a titanium spigot, and reveal that high residual strains exist in the head after a loading cycle resulting from the spigot's elastic/plastic behaviour. During unloading the residual strains increase near the bore mouth, and this explains the phenomena of failures during unloading. The residual stresses did not relax in the short-term, demonstrating that the strains developed *in vivo* will depend on the loading history, including during surgery. The maximum strains developed are also determined by the position of contact between the spigot and the bore, and this correlates with the observed UCS values for different designs. Moving the contact region further into the ball increases strength, while moving out from the standard position reduces strength by increasing the strains for a given applied load. In normal clinical use the forces applied to the head/spigot are

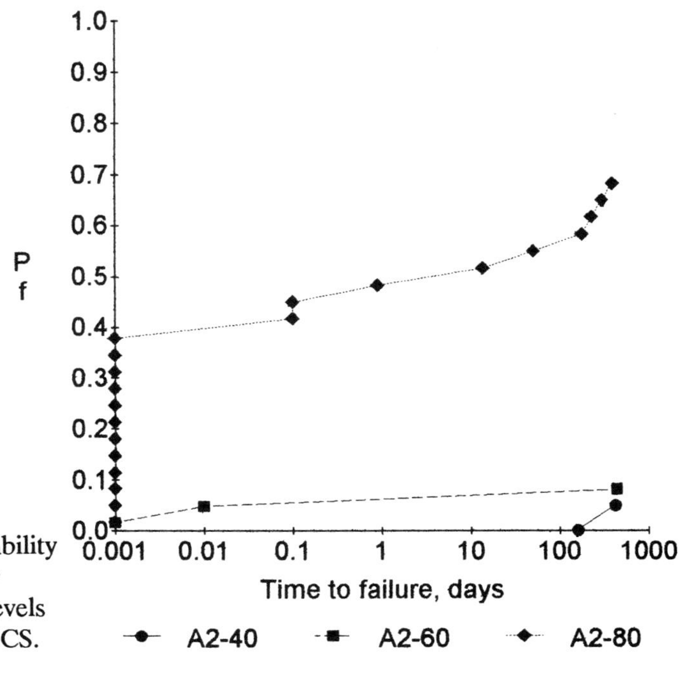

Figure 4. Cumulative probability of failure against log (t_f) for type A2 heads at pre-load levels of 40%, 60% and 80% of UCS.

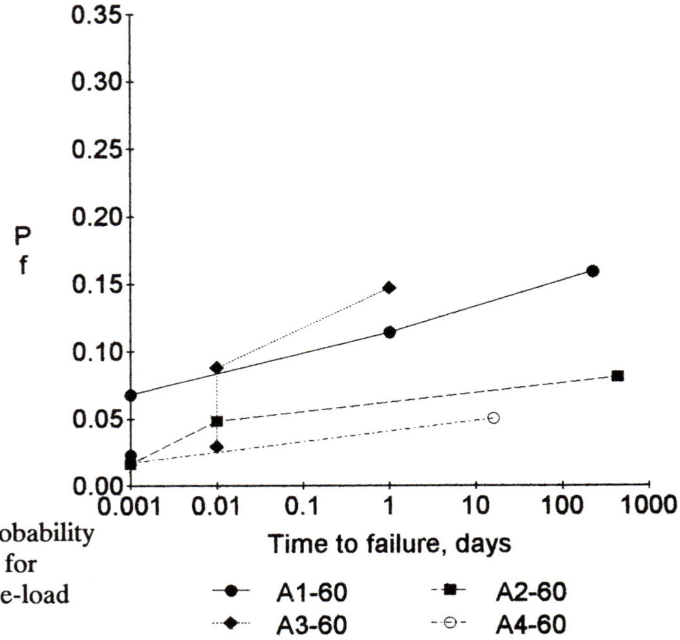

Figure 5. Cumulative probability of failure against log (t_f) for for all head types at a pre-load of 60% UCS.

less than 10 kn [7], representing a small fraction of those used in these experiments and based on a Young's Modulus of 200 GPa, would produce stresses in the range 30-50 MPa and well within the materials's capacity for high reliability. These results assist in the design of head systems.

The initial results of the long term experiments confirm the mechanical stability of Y-TZP zirconia *in vitro* at low stresses. This is in-line with the recent findings *in-vivo* that show there is no degradation of properties after implantation. Although there is an in-built assumption in these tests that the pre-loading strains are retained indefinitely in the head, which has yet to be proved conclusively, for long-term reliability against residual stresses *in vivo* it appears desirable to keep the clinical service loads below 40% of the short-term UCS. Zyranox™ heads examined comfortably meet this criterion.

REFERENCES

1. Pazzagili, U.E., Ceciliani, L., et al. *Arch. Orthop. Traumat. Surg.* 1985, 104, 164-74.
2. Andrisano, A., Dragoni, E., Strozzi, A. *Proc. I. Mech. E.* 1990, 204, 157/67.
3. Dragoni, E., Andrisano, A., Bertuzzi, F. *Exp. Mechanics.* ed. Little, G.E., Elsevier Science Publ. BV, Amsterdam, Neth. 1992, 23-34.
4. Kleer, G., Siegele, O., Soltész, U. *Proc. 4th Eur. Soc. Biomechanics*, Davos, Switz., 1984, ed. Perren, S.M., Schneider, E., Martinus Nijhoff, Dordrecht 1985, 353-8.
5. ISO 7206/5, 1992E.
6. US Food and Drugs Adminstration Doc. CER736, June 1994.
7. Willmann, G. *Proc. Conf. Bioceramics 7* Türkü, Finland, 1994, 359-64.
8. Pryce, A. and Murray, M.G.S. To Be Presented at Fourth ECERS Conf., Oct., 1995.

LONG TERM CLINICAL RESULTS OF USING HAp IN REVISION OF TOTAL HIP REPLACEMENT INVOLVING MASSIVE BONE DEFECTS IN THE ACETABULUM

H. Oonishi, S. Kushitani, H. Iwaki, K. Sakai and H. Ono

Department of Orthopeadic Surgery, Artificial Joint Section and Biomaterial Research Laboratory Osaka-Minami National Hospital 677-2, Kido-Cho, Kawachinagano-Shi, Osaka, 586, JAPAN

ABSTRACT
Hydroxyapatite (HAp) granules of 100-300 m, 1-2 mm and 4-5 mm, mixed at a ratio of 10:45:45, were over-filled into massive acetabular defects during revision of total hip arthroplasty. This was done in 40 joints since March 1986. Sockets remained mobile in three joints, and in two joints, spaces between HAp granules appeared in the area next to the bone. In other joints, no morphological changes, no decrease in volume and direct bonding of HAp to bone was observed radiographically.

INTRODUCTION

Freeze-preserved allografts have been used during revision surgery in cases involving massive bone deficiencies and excellent results have been reported in Europe and the U.S.A. [1, 2, 3]. Cases using allografts have also been reported in Japan [4], although material, other than femoral heads from osteoarthritis cases, is still very difficult to obtain.

Increasing interest in bioactive ceramics, particularly in hydroxyapatite (HAp), during the past ten years, has resulted in a significant increase in its clinical application during this period [5, 6, 7].

We have obtained good results when performing bone grafting in revision and repeat revision of femoral bone defects in three cases during 1984 by placing fine HAp granules (300-500 μm) between the bone cement and the bone [6, 7, 8]. In addition, since 1986 we have been filling massive bone defects, at the time of revision, with small HAp granules [8, 9].

MATERIALS AND METHODS

Reconstruction procedures using HAp for massive acetabular bone deficiencies.

The soft tissue and necrotic tissue adhering to the acetabulum are completely scraped. At the site of a bone defect, only the necrotic and inflamed tissues are removed. HAp granules (Bone Ceram P. Sumitomo Cement Co.) are prepared for defect filling. Granules of 100-300 m (G-1), 1-2 mm (G-4) and 4-5 mm (G-6) are mixed in the ratio of 10:45:45. Physiological saline is added to mix and, due to their porous characteristic, facilitates the adhesion of granules one to another. This results in better adhesion of the mix and more stable shape. The acetabulum is then filled with the mixture. At this time, a previously determined space for the socket installation is left open. A hemispherical compressor 3 mm larger than the outer diameter of the socket is then inserted into this space and firmly struck into the acetabulum using a plastic hammer, while determining proper location (Figure 1-I, II).

When cementing the socket, a 2-3 mm thickness of cement in a paste-like consistancy is placed on the entire surface of the acetabulum immediately after aspirating liquid completely from the acetabulum. The cement is then compressed with a compressor 1 mm larger than the outer socket diameter, and time is allowed for polymerization to take place. The paste-like consistancy of the cement makes handling easy.

If the margin of the acetabulum has not been sufficiently filled with HAp granules, it can be easily filled with HAp at this time. When a bone defect extends over a large area on the superior part of the acetabulum or iliac bone, HAp granules are placed in this region and fixed using a 1-2 mm thickness of cement (Figure 1-III).

Before the socket is cemented, the hardened cement surface is dried and the socket is fixed with viscous cement which contains extra monomer (Figure 1-IV). This procedure facilitates the socket insertion and allows the hardened and viscous cement to polymerize and bond solidly.

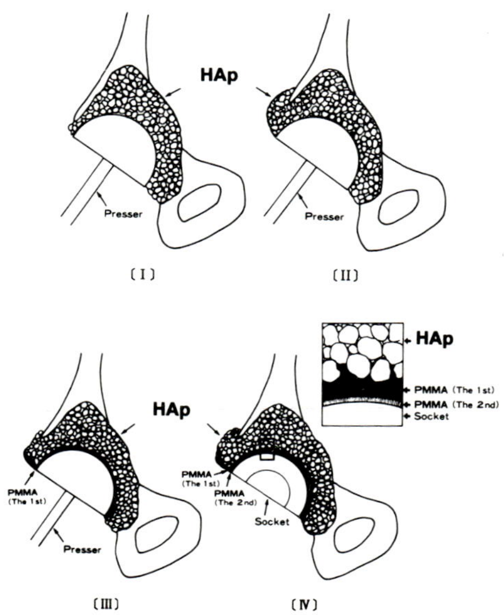

Figure 1. (I, II, III, IV) Reconstruction procedures using hydroxyapatite for massive bone deficiencies in the acetabulum due to loosening after total hip replacement.

Clinical Cases

We have performed revision THR for large acetabular defects using HAp on 40 joints in 40 patients since 1986. The AAOS Committee classification for acetabular deficiencies was used (Table 1) to grade the deficiencies. Whole peripheral deficiencies were found in 11 joints (28%), and cavities with absent medial walls were found in 18 joints (45%). These are very unstable cases after revision surgery (Table 2.).

Clinical follow-up ranged from 3 to 9 years after surgery. The study group included 2 males and 38 females. Age at surgery ranged from 35 to 81 years. The post-operative period ranged from 9 years to 8 years in one joint, from 8 to 7 years in three joints, from 7 to 6 years in five joints, from 6 to 5 years in nine joints, from 5 to 4 years seven joints, and 4 to 3 years in fifteen joints. Revision THR was performed because of osteoarthritis in thirty three joints, rheumatoid arthritis in five joints, ANF in one joint, and SLE in one joint.

Revision, second and third revisions were respectively performed on 36 joints, three joints, and one joint. None of the patients underwent repeat or third revision after revision with HAp. Repeated revisions were performed only on patients with osteoarthritis.

For radiographic evaluation, the interface between bone and HAp, the interface between bone cement and HAp, changes in volume and shape of HAp granules, absorption of HAp, and movement of component were carefully observed.

RESULTS

Filling is stable when HAp granules are very firmly packed. Our radiographic evaluation showed that sockets moved in three joints where spaces in the HAp beneath the bone was seen. In other joints neither morphological changes nor decrease in volume were seen. Although occasional spaces were observed in parts of the interface between HAp granules and bone immediately after operation, these gradually disappeared within 3 months and it was supposed that HAp granules then connected with the bone directly, probably due to new bone tissue entering the spaces among HAp granules in the vicinity of the interface, and then binding with the HAp granules (Figure 2, 3).

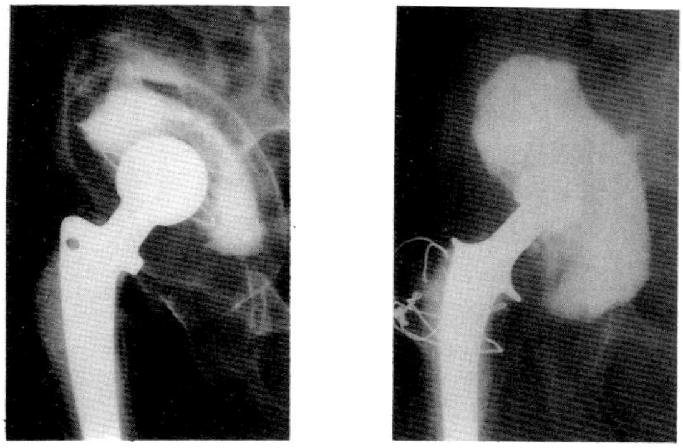

a b

Figure 2. O.A. Female 8-1/2 years after revision surgery. 72 years old at revision surgery. Osteoporosis is a very high grade. She walks with a slight limp because the other side hip had THR surgery. However, she is pain free. (a) Before surgery (b) 8-1/2 years after surgery

Table 1. Classification of acetabular deficiencies (from AAOS Committee)

Type I segmental deficiencies
- **A Peripheral**
  - **1 superior**
  - **2 anteiror**
  - **3 posterior**
- **B central (medial wall absent)**

Type II Cavitary deficiencies
- **A Peripheral**
  - **1 superior**
  - **2 anteiror**
  - **3 posterior**
- **B central(medial wall intact)**

Type III Combined deficiencies

Type IV Pelvic discontinuity

Type V Arthrodesis

Table 2. Grade of acetabular massive deficiencies in which revision THR was performed using HAp granules.

states of Acetabular Deficiency		Joints	(%)
Type I A1		2	(5%)
Type I A1.2.3		3	(8%)
Type I B		1	(3%)
Type II B		2	(5%)
Type III	(Type I A1.2.3 / Type II B)	7	(18%)
	(Type I B / Type II A1.2.3)	18	(45%)
	(Type I A1.2.3 / Type II A1.2.3)	1	(3%)
	(Type I B / Type II A1)	1	(3%)
	(Type I A1 / Type II B)	5	(13%)
	Total	40	

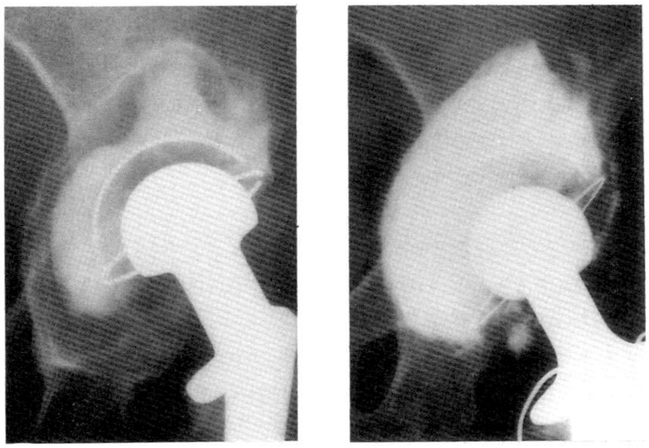

a b

Figure 3. O.A. Female 7 years after revision surgery. 59 years old at revision surgery. She walks normally and without pain. (a) Before surgery (b) 7 years after surgery.

DISCUSSION

Several reports have been published on allografts for revision THR involving massive bone deficiencies however, ours was the first group to do so. The advantages of HAp are that immunoreaction can be completely ignored, post-operative morphological changes and volume decreases do not occur if adequate amounts of granules are packed densely and firmly during surgery, post-operative HAp absorption, if any, is minimal and very slow and cement fixation on HAp prevents the harmful influence of osteolysis by polyethylene wear particles on cement interfaces.

We believe that the reasons for the marked pain relief noted is due to the lack of change in the shape of packed HAp granules and lack of movement of the component. This can be attributed to the HAp granules, which were packed firmly and stably and also fixed with bone cement, which physicochemically bonds to the bone. Since HAp granules were not apparently absorbed even 9 years after operation, the packed HAp granules are expected to be stable for a long period of time.

In three cases, all with severe conditions, sockets moved. It is assumed that, as in all these cases, the central medial wall was absent and whole peripheral cavity deficiencies were too large for filled HAp masses to be sufficiently stable. In the first case, bone formation was very poor because of multiple revisions, in the second case HAp masses could not endure the early 60 kg load following surgery which resulted from the patient's activity and in the third case, as the central medial wall and anterior and posterior walls were absent, HAp masses were very unstable.

In two cases spaces in between HAp granules right under the bone and the rest of the HAp granules were seen. This was assumed to be the result of rather wide spaces between bone base and packed HAp granules. In some places the area around these zones was unstable immediately after surgery, and continuous micromotion most likely occurred right under the bone before sufficient bone growth into the spaces between granules was obtained.

CONCLUSION

Reconstruction using HAp granules of several sizes for massive bone deficiencies in the acetabulum due to loosening after THR is an excellent method. However, for a huge bone deficiency at the central medial superior anterior and posterior walls, stable covering with bone blocks is needed.

REFERENCES

1. Borja, F.J. and Mmaymneh, W. Bone Allografts in Salvage of Difficult Hip Arthroplasties, Clin. Orthop., 1985, 197: 123-130
2. Gross, A.E., Lavoie, M.V., McDermott, P. and Marks, P. : The Use of Allograft Bone in Revision of Total Hip Arthroplasty, Clin. Orthop., 1985, 197: 115-122
3. McGann, W. : Massive Allografting for Sever Failed Total Hip Replacements, J Bone Joint Surg., 1986, 68-A: 4-12
4. Itoman, M. and Sunabe, S. : Revision Total Hip Replacement Supplemented with Allogeneic Bone Grafting, J. of Joint Surgery (Japan), 1988, 7, 3, 83-93
5. Oonishi, H., Murata, N., Kushitani, S., and Aono M. : Application of Alumina and HAp to Massive Bone Defect and the Clinical Results, Orthop. Ceramic Implants, 1987; 7, 123-135
6. Oonishi, H., Kushitani, S., Aono, M., Ukon, Y., Yamamoto, M., Ishimaru, H., Tsuji, E. : The effect of HAp coating on bone growth into porous titanium alloy implants, The Journal of bone and Joint Surgery, 1989, 71-B, 2, 213-216
7. Oonishi, H., Kushitani, S., Aono, M., Maeda, E., Tsuji, E., Ishimaru, H. : Interface Bioactive Bone Cement by Using PMMA and Hydroxyapatite Granules, Bioceramics, 1989, Vol. 1, 102-107, Ishiyaku-Euro-America
8. Oonishi, H. : Orthopedic Applications of Hydroxyapatite Biomaterials, 1991, Vol. 12, 171-178, Butterworth-Heinman Ltd.
9. Oonishi, H. : Revision of THR for Massive Bone Defects, J. of Joint Surg. (Japan), 1988, 7, 3: 49-60

STRUCTURAL CHARACTERIZATION OF NATURAL AND SYNTHETIC BIOCERAMICS BY PHOTO ACOUSTIC - FTIR SPECTROSCOPY

I. Rehman and W. Bonfield

IRC in Biomedical Materials Queen Mary and Westfield College University of London, Mile End Road, London E1 4NS, (UK)

ABSTRACT

An understanding of the interfacial relationship between a bioceramic implant and the adjacent bone tissue is facilitated by a precise characterization of the associated structures. Therefore the structure properties of different commercial synthetic hydroxyapatite powders, a novel carbonated hydroxyapatite and natural bone mineral have been studied by using Photo-acoustic (PAS) Fourier Transform Infrared (FTIR) spectroscopy.

INTRODUCTION

Fourier Transform Infrared spectroscopy (FTIR) is a widely used analytical technique that is routinely applied to the characterization of biomaterials. Preparing samples of biomaterials for infrared spectroscopy is often a tedious process. The main sampling problem in FTIR characterization of biomaterials is that nearly all solid materials are too opaque in their normal forms for direct transmission analysis in the mid-infrared region. This problem can be solved by reducing the optical density of samples to a suitable level by employing various sampling techniques [1,2]. These procedures, however, can alter the nature of the sample and are time consuming. Various techniques, such as, diffuse reflectance (DRIFT) and attenuated total reflectance (ATR) can be employed, but are limited due to stringent surface requirements.

Photo-acoustic sampling (PAS) provides a solution to these problems. A photo-acoustic signal is generated when infrared radiation absorbed by a sample is converted into heat within the sample. This heat diffuses to the sample surface and into the adjacent atmosphere. Thermal expansion of this gas produces the PAS signal. The signal generation process isolates a layer extending beneath the sample's surface, which has a suitable optical density for analysis, without altering the sample. The technique directly measures the absorbance spectrum of this layer.

An understanding of bone function and its interfacial relationship to an implant is clearly dependent upon its associated structure and composition. Traditional technologies used for structural analysis include light microscopy, electron microscopy, X-ray diffraction, FT-Raman spectroscopy and chemical analysis [3-5].

The techniques of (FTIR) and FT-Raman spectroscopy are recognized as analytical techniques for biomedical applications [4,5], because they are non destructive techniques and a minimal amount of sample preparation is required.

Work is continuing to study the correlation between the mineral phases of bone and synthetic hydroxyapatites and only recently photo-acoustic sampling technique has made it possible to obtain good infrared spectral details. In this study, spectrochemical investigations of the inorganic phase of cortical bone, synthetic implantable hydroxyapatite and carbonated synthetic hydroxyapatite were performed and correlations between the spectra obtained were examined.

The aim of such studies is to assess the ways in which the PAS-FTIR technique can aid in the spectrochemical analysis of biological material and in particular, whether such analysis can take its place alongside traditional tools used in the investigation of bone tissue structure and composition.

MATERIALS AND METHODS

Cortical bone was obtained from the mid-shaft femoral region of human (56 year old male) and mature sheep bone. Bone samples were obtained frozen at 0°C and were deproteinated before analysis, following the procedure described elsewhere [4,5].

Synthetic hydroxyapatite (HA) powders (P120), as received from Plasma Biotal and research grade, carbonated apatite in powder form developed in the IRC were also analyzed.

SPECTROSCOPIC ANALYSIS

FTIR spectra were obtained using a Nicolet 800 spectrometer in conjunction with a MTech PAS cell. Spectra were obtained at 8cm^{-1} resolution averaging 128 scans. The sample chamber of the PAS cell was purged with helium gas and dried with magnesium perchlorate.

RESULTS AND DISCUSSION

PAS-FTIR spectroscopy of the bone samples revealed numerous peaks associated with an inorganic phase, which primarily consists of carbonated phosphate groups (a naturally existing apatite), see Figure 1 and Table 1.

The spectra of hydroxyapatite powders also provide a number of spectral details indicating similarities with naturally hydroxyapatite. Spectra of the synthetic hydroxyapatite powders are given in Figure 2 and their peak positions are tabulated in Table 1.

Hydroxyl stretch is observed at 3569 cm^{-1} in the spectra of synthetic commercial and carbonated apatite powders but not in the natural apatite's spectra (see Figures 1 & 2). The hydroxyl band at 3569 cm^{-1}, in the spectrum of carbonated apatite has a lower intensity than the P120 sample, which is also masked by broad H_2O absorptions. The hydroxyl stretch band is not observed in the spectra of bone, only a broad band of absorbed water can be seen. The large decrease in the hydroxyl band intensities of the carbonated apatite powder may be attributed to the increase in the carbonate substitution. This effect is measured by calculating the peak area of the carbonate and hydroxyl groups (Table 2). The peak area of hydroxyl stretch in the case of carbonated and P120 hydroxyapatite powders is 1.92 and 7.4, respectively, indicating that hydroxyl groups decrease with an increase in the carbonate substitution. The results obtained agree with data reported by Elliot, who suggested the carbonate replacement with the hydroxyl ions [7].

Theoretically, carbonate ions have four vibrational modes, three of which are observed in the infrared spectrum and two in the Raman spectrum [8]. The carbonate υ_4 has very low intensity and is seldom seen in the infrared spectrum [9]. Usually υ_1 and υ_4 have strong vibrational bands in the Raman spectra of bone and carbonated apatite [3,8], and

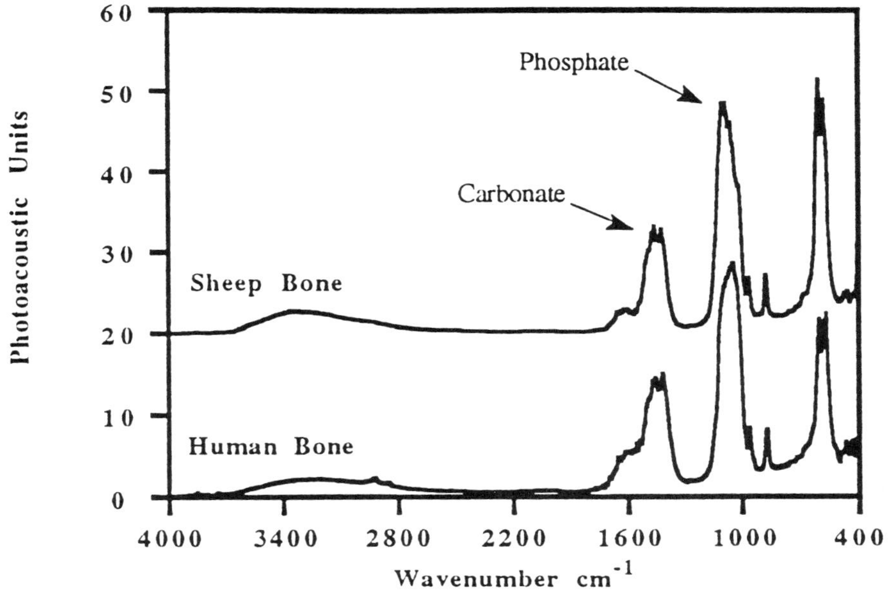

Figure 1. FTIR spectra of human and sheep bone.

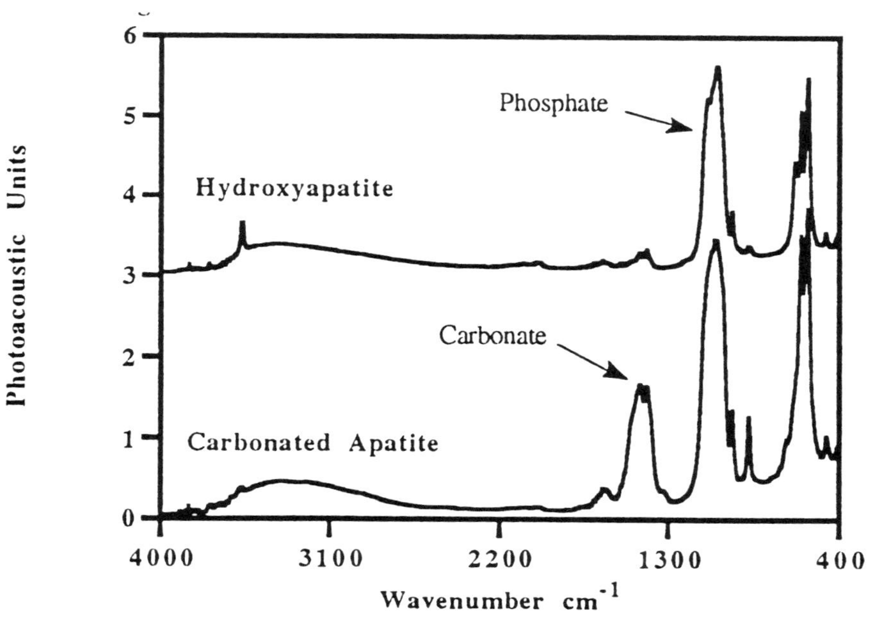

Figure 2. FTIR spectra of carbonated and hydroxy apatite.

Table 1. Observed Infrared band positions for bone and hydroxyapatite powders.

Peak Assignments cm^{-1}	Human Bone	Sheep Bone	Carbonated HA	Commercial HA (P120)	Ref.
Hydroxyl stretch	--	--	3569	3568	6.7
Carbonate υ_3	1650-1300	1650-1300	1650-1300	1650-1300	7-9
----(m)	1609	1609	1649	1648	--
----(m)	1473	1471	1470	1454	--
----(m)	1420	1419		1419	--
Phosphate υ_3	1190-976	1190-976	1190-976	1190-976	7.8
----(vs)	--	1096		1092	9
----(s)	--	1085	--	--	--
----(m)	--	1056	--	--	--
----(vs)	1046	--	--	1042	9.10
----(w)	--	1012	--	--	7
Phosphate υ_1 (m)	961	960	960	962	4.9
Carbonate υ_2 (ms)	874	873	873	874	7-10
Phosphate υ_4	660-520	660-520	660-520	660-520	--
----(m)	--	--	--	633	9
----(vs)	605	601	603	602	--
----(vs)	565	579	567	566	--
Phosphate υ_2 (w)	467	470	469	472	--
----(vw)	445	454	--	--	--

Table 2. Peak Area calculation for hydroxyl (stretch), and carbonate bands.

Peak Assignments	Human Bone	Sheep Bone	Carbonated HA	Commercial HA (P120)
Hydroxyl stretch	--	--	1.92	7.14
Carbonate (υ_3)	188.7	198.9	164.8	12.7
Phosphate (υ_3)	300.9	321	314.5	225.8
CO^{-2}_3/PO^{-3}_4	1.59	1.61	1.90	17.77

υ_2 and υ_3 vibrational modes are observed in the infrared spectra. Carbonate ion occupy two different sites in bone mineral, with peaks in the region of 1650 to 1300 cm^{-1} due to υ_3 vibrational mode carbonate ion and the peak at 873 cm^{-1} due to υ_2 vibrational mode [6]. The υ_3 peaks split into three peaks centered at 1609, 1473 and 1420 cm^{-1} and the distribution of the carbonate υ_3 sites depend on the maturation and formation of apatite crystals. Occupancy of the υ_2 sites is considered to occur competitively between the OH^- and carbonate groups at the interface of the growing crystal, whereas occupancy of the υ^3 sites depends on competition between the phosphate and carbonate ions [6,7]. The presence of υ_2 and υ_3 vibrational modes of carbonates in bone may contribute to the absence of hydroxyl ions in the bone mineral, as there is no hydroxyl band present in the spectra of the bone samples.

The spectra of synthetic hydroxyapatites also have peaks in the region of 1650 and 1300 cm^{-1}. Carbonated apatite has only two well defined peaks for υ_3 sites centered at 1649 and 1470 cm^{-1}, whereas synthetic commercial hydroxyapatite has three sites for υ_3 vibrational mode centered at 1648, 1454 and 1419 cm^{-1}. The results obtained by peak area calculation of the carbonate υ_3 band indicates that the inorganic matrix of the sheep bone has more carbonate groups than human bone (Table 2).

Theoretically, there are four vibrational modes present for phosphate ions: υ_1, υ_2, υ_3 and υ_4. All these modes are Raman and infrared-active and are observed for all the spectra of bone, carbonated apatite and commercial hydroxyapatite powders.

In the human bone spectrum, a single intense υ_3 band is present at 1046 cm^{-1}, whereas, in the sheep bone spectrum, υ_3 band has three different sites present at 1096, 1085 and 1056 cm^{-1}, (see Figure 1, Table 1). This intense υ_3 band is thought to be responsible for totally obscuring the υ_1 carbonate bands [8]. The peak area of the υ_3 band is calculated and used to derive the phosphate/carbonate ion ratio. Calculated value of phosphate/carbonate ions ratio is 1.59 and 1.61 for human and sheep bones respectively. Peak areas of the υ_3 band of carbonated and P120 type hydroxyapatites are also calculated and values obtained for phosphate/carbonate ions ratio are 1.9 and 17.8, respectively (see Table 2). This ratio increases with an increase in the phosphate content.

The phosphate υ_1 band is present at 960 cm^{-1} and can be observed in all the spectra of natural and synthetic hydroxyapatites. (Figures 1 & 2). Phosphate υ_4 band present in the region of 660 and 520 cm^{-1}, is a well defined and sharp band observed in natural and synthetic hydroxyapatites. It has two sites in the case of natural and synthetic hydroxyapatites centered at, 603 and 567 cm^{-1}, while P120 type hydroxyapatite has three sites observed at 633, 602 and 566 cm^{-1}. This splitting of the υ_4 vibrational band indicates the low site symmetry of molecules, as two and three observed bands, confirm the presence of more than one distinction site for the phosphate group [10].

Phosphate υ_2 band is observed in the region of 475 and 440 cm^{-1} and has two sites, which are not as strong as the υ_3 and υ_4 bands. In the natural hydroxyapatites and carbonated hydroxyapatite these sites are at 467 and 450 cm^{-1}, whereas in the commercial hydroxyapatite, only one site is present at 472 cm^{-1}.

COMPARISON OF NATURAL AND SYNTHETIC HYDROXYAPATITES

Both human and sheep bone provide almost identical spectra (Figure 1 & 2, Table 1). The deproteination procedure has clearly resulted in removal of the organic phase of the bone, as no organic peak was observed in either spectrum. Therefore, the PAS-FTIR spectroscopic technique may be used to monitor the deproteination process.

Spectral details of synthetic carbonated spectra provided a number of peaks similar to that of human and sheep bone. FTIR spectra of synthetic commercial hydroxyapatite and synthetic carbonated apatite powder indicate that there are number of differences between the two materials. The most apparent change in the spectrum of carbonated apatite is the large degree of decrease in the hydroxyl peak centered at 3568 cm^{-1} compared to the commercial material's spectrum, which has a well defined, sharp peak in the same position. The infrared spectrum of commercial HA has a hydroxyl band at 624 cm^{-1}, which is absent in the case of carbonated apatite.

CONCLUSIONS

The quality of the structural and compositional detail which can be revealed by this technique, combined with minimal sample preparation makes PAS-FTIR spectroscopy a very attractive tool for the analysis of natural and synthetic biomaterials. Materials can be easily analyzed by PAS-FTIR without the need to reduce the particle size or dilute with KBr. Spectra of bone samples provide valuable information which is helpful in developing equivalent implant materials.

ACKNOWLEDGEMENT

The support of EPSRC for the IRC in Biomedical Materials is gratefully acknowledged.

REFERENCES

1. Rockley, M. G., Spectrosc., 1980, Volume 34(4), 405-406.
2. Colthup N.B., Dally, L.H. and Wiberley S. E., *Introduction to Infrared and Raman Spectroscopy* 3rd. edition, 1990.
3. Martin, R. B. and Burr, D. B., *Structure, function and adaptation of compact bone*, Raven Press, New York, 1989, 127-172.
4. Rehman, I., Smith, R., Hench, L. L. and Bonfield, W., Bioceramics, Volume 7, Butterworth-Heinemann, Oxford 1994, 84-89
5. Rehman, I., Hench, L. L. and Bonfield, W., Bioceramics, Volume 6, Butterworth-Heinemann, Oxford 1993, 124-28.
6. LeGeros, R. Z., Kijkowska, G., LeGeros, J. P., Abergas, T. and Bleiwas, H., J. Dent. Res., 1987, 66, 190.
7. Elliott, J. C., Holcomb D. W. and Young, R. A., Calcif. Tissue Int., 1985, 37, 372-75.
8. Nelson, D. G. A. and Featherstone, J. D. B., Calcified Tissue Int., 34, 1982, S69-81.
9. El Feki, H., Rey, C. and Vignoles, M., Calcified Tissue Int., 1991, 49, 269-274.
10. Young, R. A., J. Dent. Res. {Suppl.}, 1974, 53, 193-203.

OXIDIZED ZIRCONIUM FOR HEMIARTHROPLASTY: AN *IN VITRO* ASSESSMENT

A.M. Patel and M. Spector

Department of Orthopedic Surgery, Brigham and Women's Hospital
Harvard Medical School, 75 Francis Street, Boston, Massachusetts

ABSTRACT

The problems of total joint replacement that have surfaced in recent years make the identification of a more conservative hip reconstructive procedure compelling. In the present study, we developed an *in vitro* test method to evaluate biomaterials for hemiarthroplasty. The tribology of a new bioceramic material, oxidized zirconium, articulating with bovine articular cartilage was investigated, with cobalt chromium alloy serving as the control. Results of this study demonstrate the suitability of oxidized zirconium as the bearing surface for hemiarthroplasty.

INTRODUCTION

Concern about the longevity of total joint replacement has renewed interest in hemiarthroplasty as a treatment for certain hip disorders. Hemiarthroplasty has been well established as a practical and beneficial treatment for elderly patients with femoral neck fractures because of low morbidity and expedient return to independence [1,2,3,4]. Young patients with avascular necrosis of the femoral head would also be good candidates for hemiarthroplasty. However, reports of gross acetabular erosion [2,3,4,5,6] have made this indication for the procedure questionable. Changes in design from unipolar to bipolar have not significantly reduced acetabular erosion while introducing concerns of polyethylene wear. Clinically, cobalt chromium is the primary material that has been employed as the bearing surface. It would clearly be beneficial to identify a biomaterial that could articulate with a lower rate of articular cartilage wear, and therefore extend the longevity of hemiarthroplasty.

Animal hemiarthroplasty models have been employed to evaluate various materials for hemiarthroplasty. Mendes *et al* [7] reported the poor performance of high density polyethylene as a femoral head replacement material. More recent studies by Cook *et al* [8,9] demonstrated differences in the wear rates of acetabular cartilage caused by cobalt chromium and titanium alloys and carbon prostheses. In general, studies employing animal hemiarthroplasty models have resulted in gross amounts of wear of the articular cartilage, regardless of the material selection [7,8,9,10,11].

Two key characteristics that affect the wear resistance and hence the performance of the hemiarthroplasty are lubricity and abrasion resistance. A material with increased lubricity could be expected to reduce friction and adhesive wear of both counterfaces in joint articulation. A material with high abrasion resistance would be less susceptible to 3-body wear and other mechanisms that intensify the wear rate of the counterfaces. Orthopedic metallic alloys possess passive oxide films which can be damaged by articulation. Interest in ceramics, such as alumina and zirconia, for orthopedic applications has arisen because of their surface characteristics. UHMWPE demonstrated greater wear resistance in articulations with zirconia than with other metallic alloys [12,13,14,15]. Results of these experiments make a strong case for the investigation of bioceramics for hemiarthroplasty.

METHODS & MATERIALS

A pin-on-disk wear apparatus (Implant Sciences Company, Danvers, MA) was used to evaluate the tribological performance of the biomaterials. Osteochondral plugs served as the pin and the biomaterials as the disk. Disks of oxidized wrought zirconium and forged and cast cobalt chromium with highly polished finish (Ra < 0.03 μm) were manufactured by Smith & Nephew Richards Inc. Memphis, TN. The apparatus was modified to maintain articular cartilage in a fluid environment while generating loaded sliding contact with the disks. The apparatus was instrumented with a Chatillon 250g force transducer (Commercial Scales) and PC based data acquisition system for real-time measurements of the friction forces.

Osteochondral Plug Preparation

Stifle joints of 1-2 week old bovine calves were obtained within four hours of slaughter (Research 87, Hopkinton, MA). The surface of the femoral condyles was isolated and kept moist with a solution of phosphate buffered saline (PBS). Osteochondral plugs were harvested with a 9 mm cannulated coring reamer (Miltex Inc.). The proximal femur was mounted in a ball-and-socket mechanical vice to facilitate perpendicular coring of the condyles. This ensured that the underlying subchondral bone was perpendicular to the surface cartilage and hence stresses were evenly distributed when the plug was loaded. When coring, the drill press was operated at low speeds and the reamer was lubricated with PBS to avoid over heating of the tissue. A 7 mm dermal punch (Miltex, Inc.) was used to provide a clean edge and to clarify the cartilage-bone interface. The thickness of the cartilage on the plugs ranged from 4 - 7mm. The plugs were mounted in polymethylmethacrylate (PMMA) to give them the mechanical strength required for stable fixation to the wear apparatus. Plugs were stored at 4 degrees Celsius in PBS for a maximum of 5 days until tested. Twelve plugs were used for a friction study of the three biomaterials. Another twelve plugs were used to evaluate the wear performance.

Friction Coefficient Determination

Coring from the femoral condyles yields a convex surface geometry. This geometry minimizes anomalous friction measurements due to abnormal edge effects. Friction analysis was performed on four disks of oxidized zirconium, cast cobalt chromium, and forged cobalt chromium. Tests were performed at speeds of under 100 mm/sec. This speed is within the maximum estimated range experienced by articular cartilage *in vivo*. In addition, staying below this speed avoids atypical high speed lubrication mechanisms such as hydrodynamic lubrication as well as an atypical thermal effect.

The articulation was lubricated with triple 0.1 μm sterile filtered bovine calf serum (Hyclone Labs, Inc.). McKellop *et al.* [14] had previously reported a build up of calcium phosphate on the surface of zirconia balls tested in a hip simulator with bovine serum as the lubricant. To investigate this possibility, we performed ESCA on tested disks of oxidized zirconium and cast cobalt chromium. We found no signs of a calcium precipitate and thus did not require chemical additives for our lubricant.

The real time measurements of the frictional forces recorded during the tests were divided by the normal load (1.5 kg) to obtain the coefficient of friction. These values were plotted against slide distance. Coefficients of friction for the materials were then determined by the asymptotic values of the real-time measurements.

Wear Analysis

Quantitative analysis of the wear was done by evaluation of the change in thickness of the cartilage due to articulation. Four disks of each material, oxidized zirconium, forged cobalt chromium, and cast cobalt chromium, were articulated with pins of calf articular cartilage. Before a plug was tested, the thickness of the cartilage was measured with calipers at four points around the circumference and then averaged to obtain an estimate for the thickness of the cartilage at the center of the plug. Normal loads of 2.5 kg were applied and tests were run for a slide distance of 9 km. Immediately after testing, the plug was stored in 10% neutral buffered formalin (Fisher Scientific, Inc.). After 24 hrs, the plug was sliced in half perpendicular to its surface and the thickness at the center of the plug was measured. This measurement was then subtracted from the initial estimate to obtain the change in thickness.

After taking the measurement, one half of the cartilage was prepared for histological evaluation. The cartilage was dehydrated in ethanol, infiltrated with catalyzed buffer, and embedded in glycol methacrylate (GMA) for histological evaluation. 3 μm cross sections were cut with a Reichert Jung microtome. These sections were stained with Masson Trichrome for collagen and Safranin O/Fast Green for proteoglycans. Histological evaluation of the specimens served two purposes: 1) It enabled us to qualify our quantitative wear measurements, and 2) it gave us insight into the mechanism by which the articular cartilage breaks down.

The other half of the cartilage was prepared for surface analysis with Environmental Scanning Electron Microscopy (ESEM). We chose to evaluate the articular cartilage surfaces with ESEM as opposed to conventional Scanning Electron Microscopy (SEM) as it allows for the examination of hydrated specimens. This is important for the evaluation of cartilage which is composed of about 80% water. Dehydration of the material for conventional SEM may compromise morphological information. Coating the specimens with a conductive film is not required for ESEM, and thus the chances of viewing artifacts is reduced [16].

Three factors thought to effect the accuracy of the quantitative analysis were investigated: 1) The accuracy of the pretest estimate of the thickness of the cartilage, 2) the amount the cartilage swells due to the damage that the collagen matrix incurs from the sliding contact, and 3) the change in thickness of the cartilage due to creep.

We used five osteochondral plugs to evaluate the accuracy of the pretest estimate. Four circumferential measurements of the thickness of the cartilage were taken for each plug. The plugs were then sliced perpendicular to their surfaces and thickness measurements at the center of the plugs were taken. These values were then compared with the average value of the circumferential measurements to evaluate the accuracy of the pretest estimate.

Six plugs were used to investigate the amount that the cartilage would swell due to damage of the collagen matrix. Circumferential measurements of each plug were taken. Surface layers ranging from 1.0 - 1.8 mm were sliced off each plug with a scalpel. The samples were stored in bovine calf serum and periodic circumferential measurements were taken for 24 hours.

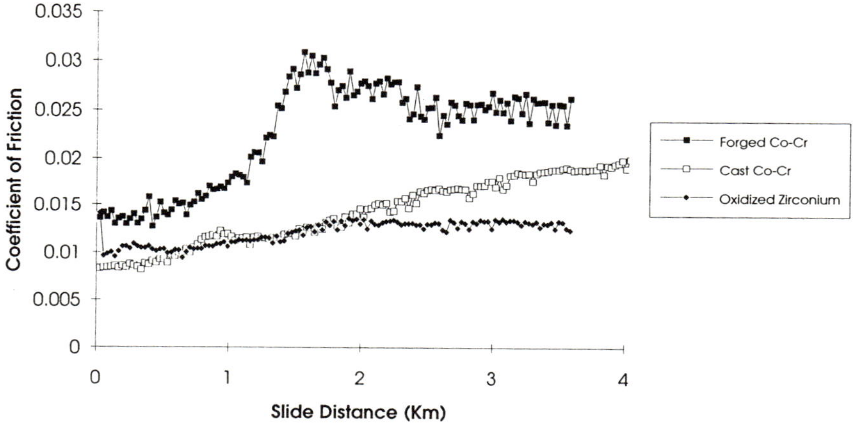

Figure 1 shows typical plots of coefficient of friction versus slide distance for the three materials.

To evaluate the effects of creep, four plugs were tested. Circumferential measurements of each plug were taken. Each plug was then loaded in an environment identical to the test environment without the sliding contact. Plugs were then stored in 10% neutral buffered formalin and periodic circumferential measurements of the thickness were taken for a period of 24 hours.

RESULTS

Coefficient of Friction

Typical plots of coefficient of friction versus slide distance started at a relatively low value and climbed to an asymptote (Figure. 1). Tests conducted with a load of 2.5 Kg for wear analysis frequently produced frictional forces that abruptly increased to a level that exceeded the maximum capacity of the 250g transducer (approximately equivalent to a coefficient of friction > 0.17). Three out of the four tests performed with each of the cobalt chromium alloys and one out of the four tests run with oxidized zirconium had to be stopped short of completion due to shear failure of the cartilage.

Using the 1.5 Kg load, the average coefficient of friction for the oxidized zirconium was 0.015 ± 0.002 (SD), n=4. This was significantly less than (P < 0.0001) the average value of cast cobalt chromium, 0.021 ± 0.003, n=4, and the forged cobalt chromium, 0.023 ± 0.003, n=4.

Wear Analysis

It was found that the pretest estimate of the thickness of the calf cartilage at the center of the plug was on average 0.1 mm ± 0.1 (n=5) greater than the actual thickness. Swelling of the cartilage due to the damaged collagen was found on average to be 0.1 mm ± 0.1 (n=6). The effects of creep were found to decrease the thickness of the cartilage 0.1 mm ± 0.0 (n=4).

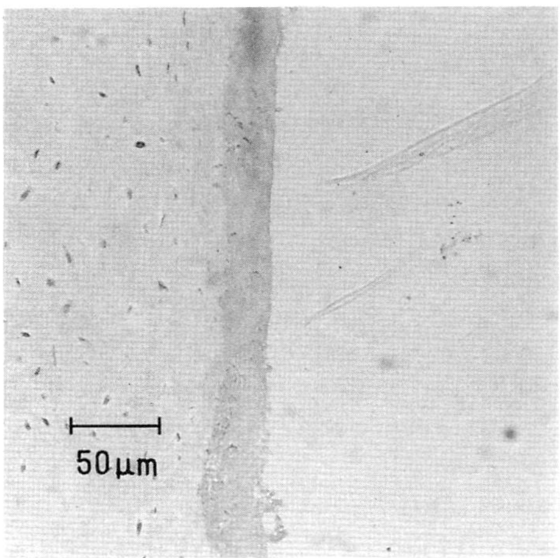

Figure 2

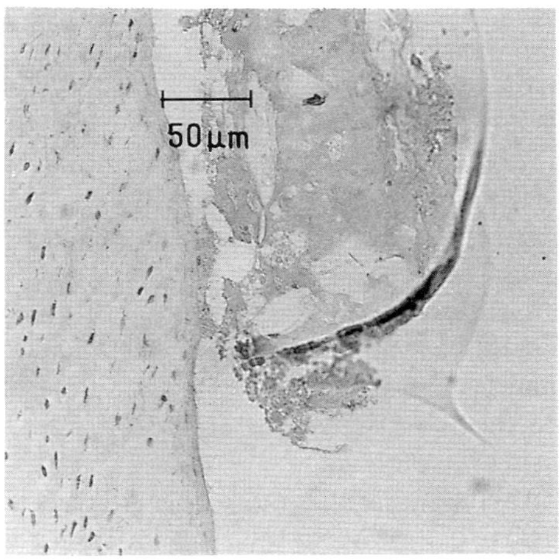

Figure 3

Figure 2 is a cross section of articular cartilage that was tested against oxidized zirconium. The formation of a wear layer on the surface is apparent. Figure 3 is a cross section tested against cast cobalt chromium. The wear layer has accumulated on one side of the plug.

Quantitative wear analysis was performed on the plugs that did not fail in shear. The average loss of cartilage thickness due to articulation with the oxidized zirconium was 0.5 mm ± 0.1 (n=3). This value was less than the values obtained for the forged and cast cobalt chromium tests, 0.8 mm (n=1) and 1 mm (n=1), respectively.

Histology

A distinct layer of material that appeared to be degraded cartilage was found on the surface of the three plugs articulated with the oxidized zirconium. This wear layer was generally uniform across the surface and was 25 - 50 μm thick (Figure 2). It was found that the plug with the 50 μm thick wear layer exhibited a higher coefficient of friction than the plug with the 25 μm thick wear layer. On the plugs that articulated with the cobalt chromium alloys, the wear layer was not uniform and appeared to accumulate on one side of the plug (Fig. 3). When stained with Safranin O/Fast Green, the degraded cartilage appeared to be deficient in proteoglycan content. This loss of proteoglycan was consistent with a failure mechanism found in an animal model of hemiarthroplasty [11].

Environmental Scanning Electron Microscopy

Analysis of the surface of untested calf articular cartilage revealed an irregular surface morphology with protrusions ranging from 15 - 25 μm in diameter. Tested specimens revealed wear tracks aligned with the direction of articulation. These tracks, characteristic of plowing wear, covered the entire surface of the cartilage. There were no significant differences observed between the wear tracks formed by articulation with the oxidized zirconium and the cobalt chromium alloys.

DISCUSSION

Oxidized zirconium's significantly lower coefficient of friction against articular cartilage should be beneficial in applications in which the material is employed as the bearing surface for hemiarthroplasty devices. This lower coefficient of friction may account for the histological finding that the wear layer remained intact on the plugs tested against oxidized zirconium. Although the mechanisms leading to the shear failures produced in this study are not fully understood, the histology suggests as a possible mechanism the accumulation of the wear layer resulting in high frictional forces. There appears to be some correlation between the wear layer thickness and the resultant coefficient of friction, however, no conclusions can be drawn until more tests are conducted.

Shear failure of the osteochondral plugs occurred only one out four times when articulated with oxidized zirconium compared with six out of eight times with the cobalt chromium alloys. This indicates that the interaction with oxidized zirconium is more favorable. This could be due to the bioceramic's greater lubricity and abrasion resistance. Although the measurements for change in thickness of the cartilage were insufficient for statistical significance, there does appear to be a trend in favor of the oxidized zirconium.

This study demonstrates the potential value of a laboratory wear apparatus for investigation of biomaterials for hemiarthroplasty. Analysis of this nature provides an accelerated screening process that should precede *in vivo* testing. Results indicate that oxidized zirconium may be a more suitable material than the currently employed cast cobalt chromium alloy for hemiarthroplasty.

ACKNOWLEDGMENT

This research was funded in part by Smith & Nephew Richards Inc.

REFERENCES

1. Eiskjaer S., Ostgard S.E., *Clin Orthop - Rel Res* 1993, 286, 206 - 211
2. LeStrange N.R., *Clin Orthop - Rel Res* 1990, 251, 7 - 19
3. D'Arcy J., Devas M., *J. Bone-Joint Surg* 1976, 58-B, 3, 279 - 286
4. Devas M., Hinves B., *J. Bone - Joint Surg* 1983, 65-B, 5, 548 - 551
5. Amstutz H.C., Grigoris P., Safran M.R., Grecula M.J., Campbell P.A., Schmalzried T.P., *J. Bone - Joint Surg* 1994, 76-B 3, 423 - 427
6. Leyshon R.L., Mathews J.P., *J. Bone - Joint Surg* 1984, 66-B, 2, 172 - 174
7. Mendes D.G., Figarola F., Bullough P.G., Loudis P., *Clin Orthop - Rel Res* 1975, 3, 274 - 283
8. Cook S.D., Thomas T.A., Kester M.A. , *J. Bone-Joint Surg* 1989, 71B, 189-197
9. Cook S.D., Anderson R.C., Kester M.A., Thomas K.A., Reynolds M.C., Haddad R.J. Jr., *Proc. 31st ORS* 1985, 92
10. LaBerge M., Bobyn J.D., Drouin G., Rivard C.H., *J. Biomed Mat Res* 1992, 26, 239 - 254
11. Cruess R.L., Kwok D.C., Duc P.N., Lecavalier M.A., Dang G.T., *J. Bone-Joint Surg* 1984, 66-B, 592 - 597
12. Davidson, J.A., *Clin Orthop - Rel. Res* 1993, 294, 361- 378
13. White S.E., Whiteside L.A., McCarthy D.S., Anthony M., Poggie R.A., *Clin Orthop - Rel Res* 1994, 309, 176 - 184
14. McKellop H., Lu B., Benya P., *Proc. ORS* 1992, 402
15. Kumar P., Oka M., Ikeuchi K., Shimizu K., Yamamuro T., Okamura H., Kotoura Y., *J. Biomed Mat Res* 1991, 25, 813 -828
16. Collins S.P., Pope R.K., Sheetz R.W., Ray R.I., Wagner P.A., Little B.J.,*Microscopy Res.-Tech.* 1993, 25, 398-405

HYDROXYAPATITE AND A-W GLASS-CERAMIC SPACER FOR KNEE JOINT SURGERY -APPLICATIONS OF BIOACTIVE CERAMIC SPACER FOR PATELLO-FEMORAL OSTEOARTHRITIS

M. Ishimura, H. Ohgushi, K. Inoue, M. Shitnaya, and S.Tatnai

Department of Orthopedic Surgery, Nara Medical University, Kashihara, Nara 634, Japan

ABSTRACT

The anterior displacement of the tibial tubercle is a popular operative procedure for patients with patello-femoral osteoarthritis of the knee. Since 1988, we have utilized a hydroxyapatite (HA) spacer for 10 patients and an A-W glass-ceramic (AW) spacer for 6 patients in this operation. During the mean follow-up period of 3.6 years, no case suffered from obvious inflammatory reaction to these materials. In all cases, patello-femoral pain decreased after this operation and daily activities have improved. Radiographic findings showed that the HA spacer was almost completely covered by new bone, although cracks in the spacer were found in 2 cases. No crack occurred in the AW spacer and good bone union was found between the spacer and base tibia bone. Regional radiolucent lines could be detected between the spacer and elevated tubercle. These findings showed the usefulness of bioactive ceramic spacers for the treatment of patello-femoral osteoarthritis.

INTRODUCTION

The operation for anterior displacement of the tibial tubercle decreases the pressure between the patella and femoral groove, resulting in relief of the anterior knee pain caused by patello-femoral osteoarthritis [1-2]. Clinical results of this procedure are largely satisfactory [3]. However, iliac autogeneous graft bone is needed as the spacer between the elevated tubercle and tibia base in this operation, and morbidity associated with autogeneous bone grafts is well known. Since 1988, we have used an HA spacer for 10 patients and an AW spacer for 6 patients instead of autogeneous iliac graft bone. This paper describes the new operation and discusses the clinical and radiological results.

MATERIALS AND METHODS

Ten patients (12 knees) were operated with an HA spacer (HA group). Nine were female and 1 was male. The average age at operation was 65.1 years (55 to 76 years).

Six patients (7 knees) were operated with an AW spacer (AW group). Five were female and 1 male. The average age at operation was 60.7 years (55 to 73 years). Except for one case each in the HA and AW groups, concomitant high tibial osteotomy (HTO) was performed because of associated femoro-tibial osteoarthritic changes. The HA spacer (APACERAM®) is a pure hydroxyapatite ceramic manufactured by Asahi Optical Co., Ltd. The porosity is 35% and the average pore radius is 200 μ m. The mechanical properties are 100 MPa bending strength, 300 MPa compressive strength, and 74 GPa elastic modulus. AW is a glass-ceramic containing oxy-fluoroapatite $Ca_{10}(PO_4)_6(OF_2)$ and β- wollastonite CaO S_1O_2, was developed in 1982 at Kyoto University in Japan [4]. AW glass ceramic (CERABONE®) is manufactured by Nippon Electric Glass Co., Ltd. The spacer has a high density of 99.3% and its mechanical properties include bending strength, 200 to 220 MPa, compressive strength, 1000 MPa, and elastic modulus, 103 GPa [5]. The shape of these two types of spacers is trapezoidal (proximal and distal height are 15mm and 9mm, respectively) and thus it is possible to elevate the proximal end of the tibial tubercle by 15 mm. Two holes are opened for screw fixation (Fig. 1).

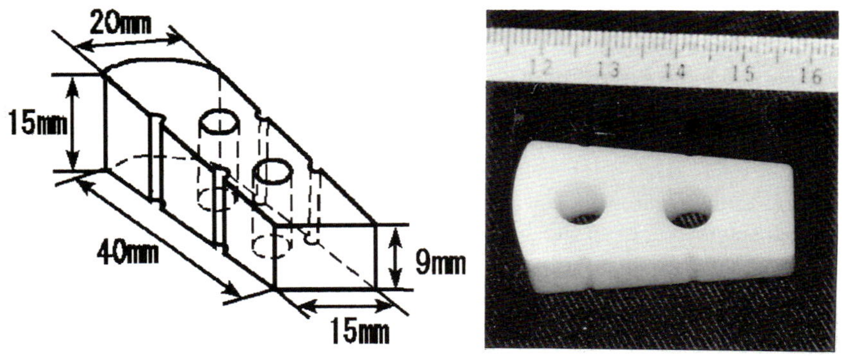

Figure 1. A spacer for tibiae tubercle elevation originally designed by us.

The operative techniques utilized for the elevation of the tibial tubercle Maquet procedure or modified Maquet procedure (Antero-Medial Displacement of the tubercle; our original method) [1, 6]. An HA or AW spacer is inserted between the elevated tubercle and tibia base, and then fixed with 2 screws. HTO was performed by barrel vault shape osteotomy, and fixed with 2 Steinmann pins and Charnley clamps (Fig. 2). Mobilization with partial weight bearing was allowed a few days after surgery. Full weight bearing was begun 6 weeks after surgery. The average follow-up period of the HA group was 4.7 years (1.8 to 6.2 years) and of the AW group was 1.7 (I to 2.4 years). Clinical evaluation was based on the JOA score: (Table 1). X ray films were examined for the purpose of assessing the bone formation around the spacer.

Table I Criteria for Evaluating Osteoarthritis of the Knee (The Committee on Assessment Criteria for Knee Disease and Treatments of the Japanese Orthopaedic Association).

Items	Points right	Points left
Pain on walking		
walking 1 Km or more usually with no pain, but without regard to mild pain, rarely felt, with certain activities	30	30
walking 1 Km or more regardless of pain	25	25
walking 500 m or more, but less than 1 Km without regard to pain	20	20
walking 100 m or more, but less than 500 m without regard to pain	15	15
walking indoors or nearby, but less than 100 m, without regard to pain	10	10
inability to walk	5	5
inability to stand	0	0
Pain on ascending or descending		
no pain	25	25
pain ; relieved by using handrails	20	20
pain with handrails, but no pain with step by step ambulation	15	15
pain with step by step ambulation ; pain relieved by using handrails	10	10
pain even with step by step ambulation and handrail use	5	5
inability to ascend or descend due to pain	0	0
Range of motion		
squatting	35	35
sideways or cross-legged sitting	30	30
flexion or arc of motion of 110 degrees or more	25	25
flexion or arc of motion of 75 degrees or more	20	20
flexion or arc of motion of 35 degrees or more	10	10
flexion or arc of motion less than 35 degrees including ankylosis or severe flexion contracture	0	0
Joint effusion		
no edema, no swelling	10	10
occasional puncture required	5	5
frequent puncture required	0	0

Note : a normal subject's score is 100 points

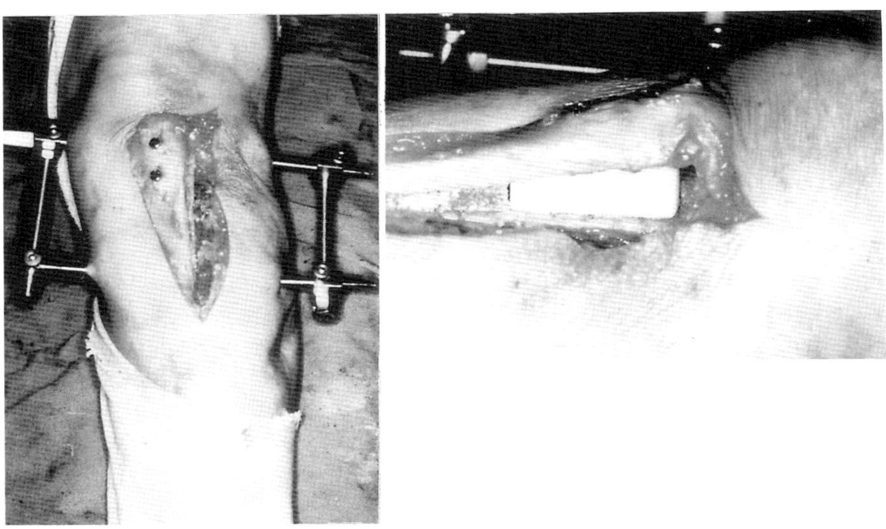

Fig. 2 Anterior displacement of tibial tubercle is performed concomitant with high tibial osteotomy.

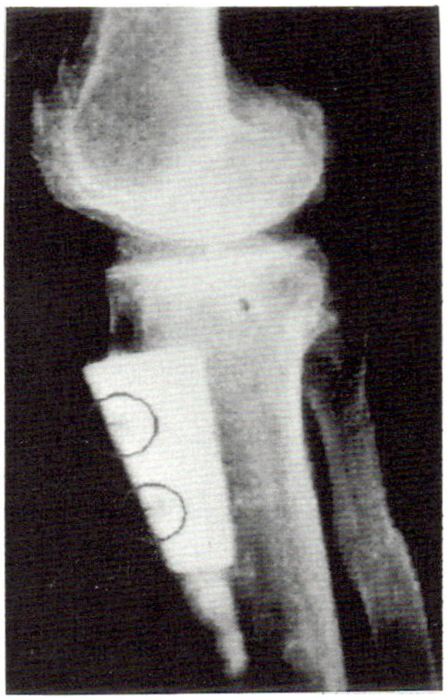

Fig. 3 X-ray film shows cracks at each of the screw holes of an HA spacer.

RESULTS

In all cases, patello-femoral pain was decreased and the ability to walk and climb up and down stairs improved. The average JOA score improved from 67.5 to 91.5 in the HA group and from 67.9 to 85.0 in the AW group. There was no obvious inflammatory reaction to these materials.

In 2 cases of the HA group, cracks developed in spacers during and after the operation. One was at the screw hole and the other was on the lateral side of the spacer (Fig. 3). However, these cracks caused no clinical symptoms.

Radiographic findings showed entire continuity of the HA spacer to the elevated tibial tubercle and the spacer to the tibia base in all cases from 6 to 9 months after operation. In the AW group, though radiographic continuity of the spacer to the tibia base occurred, some 6 areas between the spacer and elevated tubercle showed a persistent radiolucent line.

CASE PRESENTATIONS

Case I (HA group)

A seventy-two-year-old woman complained of right knee joint pain on the anterior and medial side. X-ray films showed osteoarthritic changes of the patello-femoral and medial femoro-tibial joints. A high tibial osteotomy of 16 degrees valgus correction and the elevation of the tibial tubercle with an HA spacer were performed at the same time. Radiographic findings 3 months post-operatively showed callus formation around the spacer. One year later, firm bonding of the spacer to the elevated tubercle and tibia base was confirmed. Her clinical symptoms have decreased and the JOA score improved from 85 to 95 points (Fig. 4).

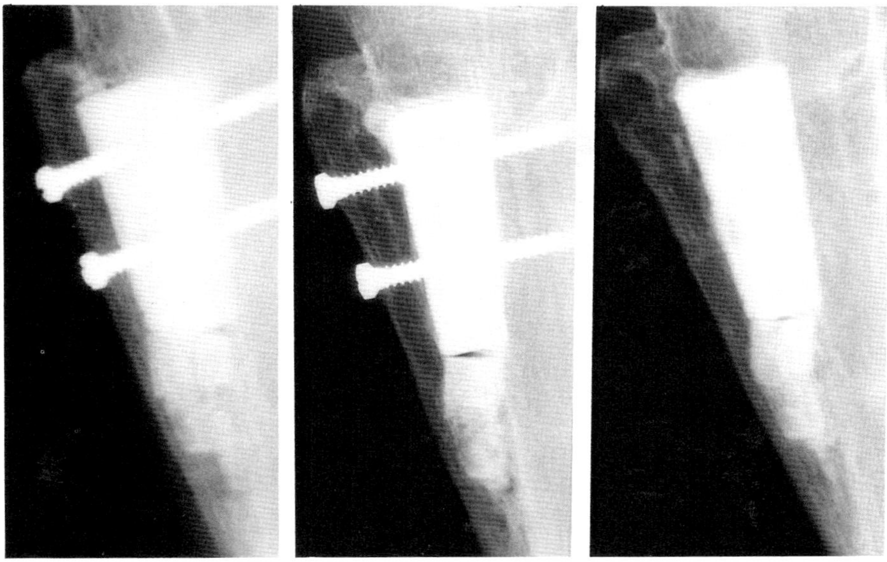

a b c

Fig. 4 X-ray films of case 1 (HA Group) a) 3 months after operation b) I year after operation c) after removal of 2 screws

Case 2 (AW group)

A sixty-year-old man complained of right knee pain especially when climbing up and downstairs. X-ray films showed osteoarthritic changes of the patello-femoral joint, but the femoro-tibial joint was not affected. The tibial tubercle was elevated with an AW spacer. Radiographic findings 3 months post-operatively showed a radiolucent line between the spacer and elevated tibial tubercle. On the X-ray film obtained 1 year after operation, although callus bridge formation was found between the proximal end of the elevated tubercle and anterior surface of the tibia, a radiolucent line between the spacer and elevated tubercle persisted. However, he was satisfied with this operation and even after the removal of 2 screws, there was no pain around the spacer. The JOA score improved from 80 to 90 points. (Fig. 5)

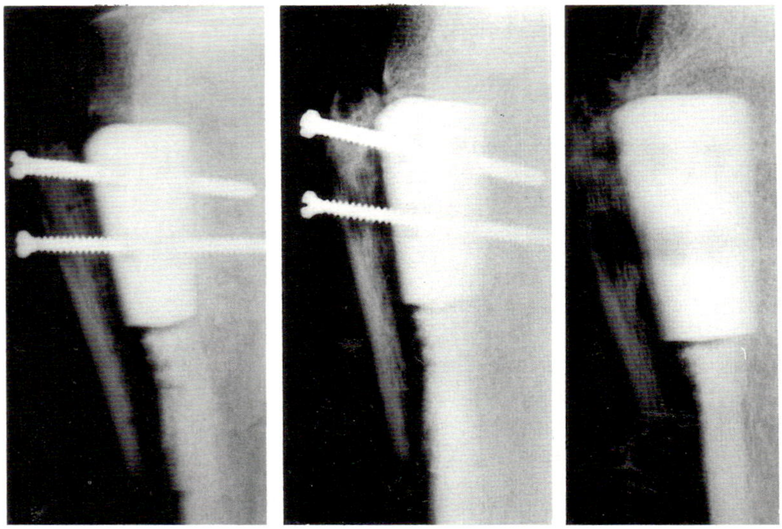

a b c

Fig. 5 X-ray films of case 2 (AW Group) a) 3 months after operation b) I year after operation c) after removal of 2 screws

DISCUSSION

We reported that hydroxyapatite ceramics show excellent osteoconductivity when used as a spacer in bony defects [7] or as a bone graft substitute in the treatment of bone tumor patients [8]. The HA ceramics also show firm bone bonding and the mechanism of the bonding occurs through the cascade of osteogenic differentiation on the ceramic surface [9]. Osteogenic differentiation also occurs on the bioactive glass ceramic surface [10]. Our results confirm the beneficial application of bioactive ceramics for bone reconstructive surgery. Although hydroxyapatite can show good osteoconduction the poor mechanical properties are a problem in this kind of application. In fact, two of our cases showed cracks of the HA spacer.

The strength of the AW spacer is sufficient for use as a spacer between the elevated tibial tubercle and base bone in this operation. No cracking was seen during or after operation. As for the bonding capacity, Yamamuro reported in his experimental animal study that when a sheep's lumbar vertebra is replaced by an A-W glass ceramic prosthesis, it takes at least I year for the bonding to be complete. He also suggested the possibility of much earlier bone bonding if more rigid fixation of the prosthesis is provided [11]. In our clinical study, radiographic findings showed a regional radiolucent line between the spacer and the elevated tubercle even more than I year after operation. Though the radiolucent line was restricted to an isolated area insufficient osteogenic cell source in the elevated tubercle. To overcome this problem, we recently applied an osteo-periosteal flap from the antero-medial surface of the tibia to cover the lateral side of the spacer and elevated tubercle. In all cases operated by this technique, 6 month postoperative X-ray films showed good bonding of the spacer to the elevated tubercle and tibia base.

CONCLUSION

I. Anterior displacement of the tibial tubercle for patello-femoral osteoarthritis was performed with either Hydroxyapatite spacers or A-W glass-ceramic spacers.
2. All cases showed satisfactory clinical results in both HA and A-W groups.
3. HA spacer showed more abundant bone formation around the spacer than AW spacer, but its low mechanical strength is a problem for this kind of operation.

REFERENCE

1. Maquet, P. *Rev Rhum Mal Osteoartic* 1963, 30, 779-785.
2. Maquet, P. *Second Edition. Berlin, Springer Verlag* 1984, 144-146.
3. Schmid, F. *Clin Orthop* 1993, 294, 254-258.
4. Kokubo, T. *Bull Inst Chem Res Kyoto Univ* 1982, 60, 260-268.
5. Kitsugi, T. *Orthopaedics (SICOT)* 1989, 13, 199-206.
6. Fujisawa, Y. *Operation [Jpn]* 1979, 33, 787-293.
7. Ohgushi, H., *et al., Acta Orhtop. Scand.* 1989, 60, 334-339.
8. Ohgushi, H., *et al., In Bioceramics* Volume 3, Rose-Hulman Institute of Technology 1992, 279-286.
9. Ohgushi, H., *et al., J. Biomed. Mat. Res.* 1993, 27, 1401-1407.
10. Okumura, M., *et al., Bioceramics* Volume 6, Butterworth-Heinemann, Oxford 1994, 337-340.
11. Yamamuro, T. *J. Bone Joint Surg. [Br]* 1990, 72, 889-893.

FOLLOW-UP STUDY OF CEMENTLESS THA WITH HYDROXYAPATITE COATED IMPLANTS

M.Inomoto, S. Miyakawa, H. Okada, H. Mishima, M. Sakane, J. Yasumoto, T. Ishii, Y. Miyanaga, K. Hayashi

Department of Orthopaedic Surgery, Institute of Clinical Medicine, University of Tsukuba, 1-1-1 Tennodai, Tsukuba-city, Ibaraki pref. 305 Japan

ABSTRACT

This is a report of 26 cases of total hip arthroplasties, using HA coating (3M,England), which were for osteoarthrosis. The average prospective follow-up period was fifteen months. Titanium femoral components had a proximal HA coating, usually with an HA-coated hemispherical cup with the rim-bearing flange. On clinical examination the incidence of pain was low immediately post-operatively. On radiographic examination, there was a rapid bony integration of implants. Compared with non-coated implants, HA-coated implants produced a rapid bony fixation and better clinical results. Implant fixation using HA coatings is a reliable procedure for good bony fixation and clinical results.

INTRODUCTION

The major problem concerning any cementless total hip arthroplasty has been how to stabilize the prosthesis in the skeleton reliably and reproducibly. Various factors influence this, material and design of the implant, levels of patient's activity and the method of fixation. Recent efforts to improve the interface between implant and bone have involved the use of bioactive materials. Hydroxyapatite(HA) has the ability to bind chemically to bone [1]. Studies of implant fixation have shown that plasma-spray coating with HA on titanium prostheses provides early and strong fixation to the bone [2,3]. This is a report of 26 cases of total hip arthroplasties, using HA coated implants (3M, England).

MATERIALS AND METHODS

HA-coated total hip prostheses were implanted from December 1992 to December 1993 in 38 consecutive cases. There were no specific exclusions for the use of an HA-coated device. Preoperative diagnosis of patients were osteoarthrosis, avascular necrosis, and rheumatoid arthritis. Rheumatoid arthritis cases are not included in this study. This study represents a total of 26 cases and 24 patients mainly for osteoarthrosis. The total hip prostheses used in all cases were Ultrapore MTS Straight Stem and Shearer Cup (3M,England). The stem component was made of titanium alloy and had "Ultrapore Porous Surface", proximally placed on the anterior and posterior surface. The straight stem was coated with HA around 60% of the proximal stem length.

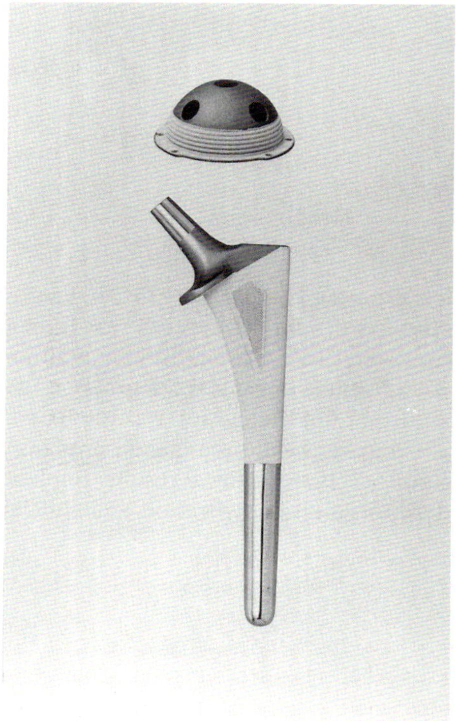

Figure 1. 3M HA-coated titanium cup and femoral stem.

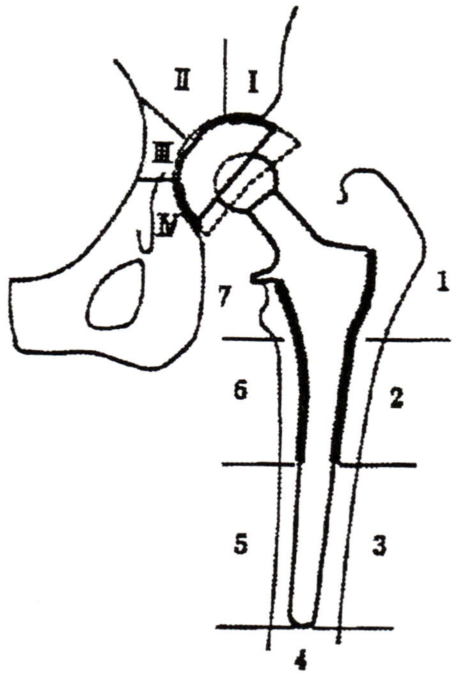

Figure 2. The zones of the acetabulum and the femur in the anteroposterior radiograph. The femoral zones 1,2,6,7 and the acetabular zones 1,4 were the HA- coated part.

The acetabular cup component was the titanium hemispherical cup with the rim bearing flange. The HA-coating was placed on the outside spherical surface and flange. The central dome of the acetabular component was not coated (Figure 1). The thickness of the plasma sprayed HA coating was 50 μm. All patients were included in a prospective follow up study. The average prospective follow-up period was fifteen months. There were 26 cases with an average age of 58.1 years (range 36-72 years). All patients entered were for primary arthroplasty, there were no revisions. Two patients had bilateral arthroplasty. Routine postoperative management included antibiotic prophylaxis (cephalosporin). Partial weight bearing was allowed after four weeks and full weight bearing was allowed after six weeks. Before surgery, each patient was evaluated using the Japan Orthopaedic Association hip score (JOA score). At follow-up intervals of 3, 6, 12, 18 months, all patients were evaluated using the same hip-scoring system. Emphasis was placed on evaluation of pain, especially thigh pain. No patients were lost to follow-up. During each follow-up visit, anteroposterior radiographs were taken of the lower pelvis. Radiographs of the stem and cup were evaluated using the zones shown in Figure 2. Signs of endosteal bone formation, reactive line formation around HA-coated and noncoated parts of the femoral stem, pedestal formation around the distal stem tip, calcar atrophy, bone resorption, subsidence and interface deterioration were evaluated. In interpreting the results, the distal termination of the HA coating separated the femoral zones 2 from 3 and 5 from 6. For this reason, the femoral zones 1, 2, 6 and 7 were upper HA-coated parts and

Table 1. JOA hip score and JOA hip ratings.

	Points (full mark)	Pre	Post-operatively 3	6	12 months
Pain	40	14.2	29.6	33.5	36.9
Walking ability	20	8.1	14.4	15.8	17.1
ROM	20	13.9	16.2	17.1	18.6
ADL	20	10.8	13.5	14.6	15.7
TOTAL	100	47.0	73.8	81.0	88.3

the femoral zones 3, 4 and 5 were distal, noncoated parts. In the acetabular area, the HA coated parts were in zones 1 and 4.

RESULTS

Clinical results

Clinical results for pain, limp, and overall JOA hip score are shown in Table 1. The results indicate a low incidence of pain immediately after surgery. One year postoperatively, none of cases had remaining pain of clinical significance.

Radiographic findings (stem side)

The development of areas with endosteal bone formation (cancellous condensation or spotwelds) is shown in Table 2. The typical pattern was endosteal bone formation in zones 2 and 6 (Figure 3). The endosteal bone formation first appeared at three months and was present in all cases at 18 months. Pedestal formation around the distal stem tip appeared in 11.5% at 18 months. Due to stress shielding effects on endosteal bone formation, bone atrophy in the proximal femur (zones l, 7) appeared in 42% at one year. Reactive line formation was regularly seen around the distal, noncoated part of the stem (zones 3, 4, 5) and in the upper part of zone 1 near the shoulder of the

Table 2 Endosteal bone formation per HA-coated femoral zone (% cases)

	Post-operatively 3	6	12 months
Zones		%	
1	0	0	0
2	3.8	53.8	80.8
3	0	0	0
4	0	0	0
5	0	0	0
6	7.7	65.4	80.8
7	0	0	0

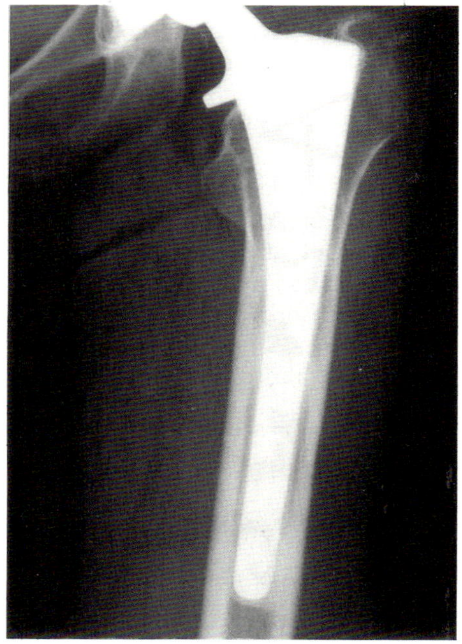

Figure 3. Early formation of spot-welds in the femoral zones 2 and 6.

Table 3 Reactive line formation per HA-coated femoral zone (% cases)

	Post-operatively 3	6	12 months
Zones		%	
1	11.5	30.8	34.6
2	0	0	0
3	0	23.1	23.1
4	0	53.8	88.5
5	0	42.3	57.7
6	0	0	0
7	0	0	0

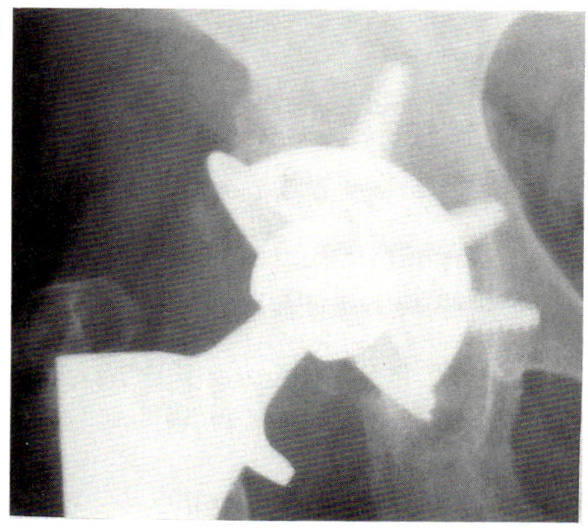

Figure 4. Radiograph of the acetabular side. There was no radiographic change.

stem, where the HA-coating begins, between 3 and 12 months (Table 3). With time this line in zone 1 extended more distally. Calcar remodeling was slow to appear. There were no signs of severe calcar resorption, radiolucent lines, subsidence or loosening of the femoral stem.

Radiographic findings (acetabular side)

Radiographic changes around acetabular components were much slower to appear than around the femoral stem. In only two cases (7.7%), reactive line formation was visible. Radiolucent lines, bone atrophy and the signs of loosening were completely absent (Figure 4).

DISCUSSION

This discussion concentrates on the evaluation of HA coated implants in comparison with their non-coated counterparts. Non-HA-coated total hip prostheses of identical design were implanted from 1991 in 40 patients (40 hips). For both groups total hip arthroplasties were performed by the same surgeon. The demographics of the two groups are listed in Table 4.

Table 4. Comparison of HA group vs. non-HA group.

	HA group	non-HA group
Age	58.1 (range .36-72)	57.7 (range .40-75)
Sex	2 Male (2 Hips) 22 Female (23 Hips)	4 Male (4 Hips) 36 Female (42 Hips)
Diagnosis	Osteoarthrosis	Osteoarthrosis

Clinical results

The JOA scores of the two groups are presented in Figure 5. The HA group showed significantly higher average JOA scores at all follow-up intervals. At one-year follow-up, the average JOA scores were 88.3 points for the HA group and 81.5 points for the control group. When the thigh pain was analyzed separately, the HA group was significantly better than the control group. At six-month follow-up, the percentage of the incidence of thigh pain was 3.8% in the HA group and 43.5% in the control group. Only one case in the HA group had thigh pain at six month follow-up. By the one-year follow-up, the thigh pain had disappeared.

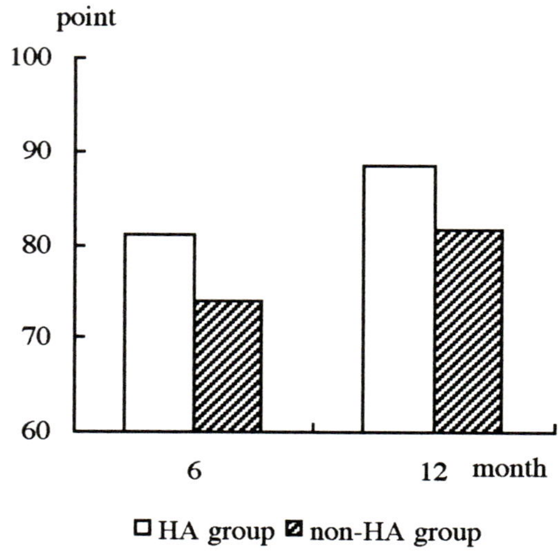

Figure 5. Comparison of JOA score between HA group vs. non-HA group. HA group showed significantly higher average JOA scores at all follow-up intervals. ($p<0.01$)

Radiographic findings (stem side)

Figure 6 compares the radiographic data for the stems. Endosteal bone formation at six months was found in zones 2 and 6 in 65.4% of the HA-coated group and 2.2% of the control group. At one year, endosteal bone formation was observed in 88.5% of the HA-coated group and 47.8% of the control group. The HA-coated group showed significantly earlier evidence of endosteal bone formation. For both groups, endosteal bone formation was observed in the same places (zones 2, 6).

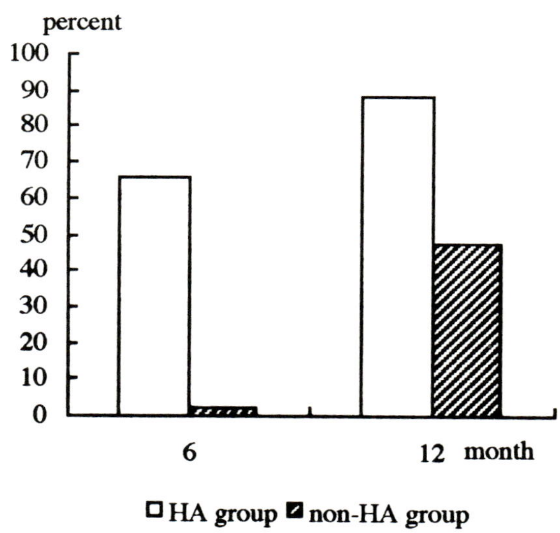

Figure 6. Comparison of endosteal bone formation for femur between HA group and non HA group. HA group showed significantly earlier evidence of endosteal bone formation($p< 0.01$).

Reactive line formation was observed most often around the uncoated distal tip in zones 3, 4 and 5, and the coated shoulder area of the stem in zone 1 for both groups. The incidence of reactive line at six months was in 61.5% of the HA-coated group and 43.5% of the control group. At one year, it was 84.6% of the HA coated group and 89.1% of the control group.

These distal reactive lines became visible after the sixth months, a small delay (approximately three months) in comparison with the signs of proximal endosteal bone formation. These distal reactive lines were probably the result of some micromotion between the stiff distal stem and the more elastic bone, caused by their relative differences in modulus of elasticity [4]. This phenomenon was enhanced because of the strong proximal fixation of the HA-coating. For this reason, the HA-coated group showed earlier evidence of reactive line formation. There was no cortical hypertrophy, subsidence and radiolucent line for both groups before 18 months postoperatively. The HA-coated parts of the stem were in zones 1, 2, 6, and 7, but endosteal bone formation was observed only in zones 2 and 6. HA coating did not alter the zones where the femoral endosteal bone formation occurred. The HA-coated group showed earlier evidence of endosteal bone formation, and the percentage of femoral stems exhibiting endosteal bone formation was significantly greater at all follow-up intervals. With time the incidence of endosteal bone formation in the same zones increased in the control group.

Radiographic findings (acetabular side)

At one year postoperatively, reactive line formation was observed in 50% of the control group and 7.7% of the HA coated group. For the HA-coated group, reactive line formation was observed in neither in the HA-coated parts of the cup (zones 1, 4) nor in the uncoated parts (zones 2, 3). This is understandable, as it is known that titanium can achieve spontaneous osseointegration provided that micro-motion between bone and implant is very low [5]. The uncoated parts fixed early and strongly to bone. This could not be achieved without the initial fixation and immobilization by the HA coating on the outside surface of the cup [6].

CONCLUSION

HA-coated total hip prostheses (3M,England) were implanted in 24 patients (26 hips) for osteoarthrosis. HA-coated implants appeared to achieve a more rapid bony fixation and better clinical results than non-coated implants.

REFERENCES

1. Geesink RGT, deGroot K, Klein CPAT, *Clin. Orthop.* 1987,225,147.
2. Geesink RGT, *Clin. Orthop.* 1990, 261,39-58.
3. Shyunpei Miyakawa, *et al., Bioceramics* Volume 6, Butterworth-Heinemann, Oxford 1993, 425430.
4. James A. D' Antonio, *et al.,* In: *Hydroxylapatite Coatings in Orthopaedic Surgery* Raven Press, New York 1993, 209-226.
5. Albrektsson T, Albrektsson B, *Acta Ortho. Scandinavica* 1987, 58,567-577.
6. Aspenberg P, *et al., Acta Ortho. Scandinavica* 1992, 63,141- 145.

THE NECK LENGTH CONTROL SYSTEM BY ALUMINA-BALL (28mm) IN Y-U TOTAL HIP ARTHROPLASTY-EXPERIMENTAL AND SHORT TERM CLINICAL STUDIES

H. Ida[1], M. Hamasakl[2], M. Takagi[1]

[1]Department of Orthopaedic Surgery, Yamagata University School of Medicine, 2-2-2 Iida-Nishi, Yamagata 990-23, JAPAN
[2]Department of Orthopaedic Surgery, Yamagata Saisei Hospital, 2-3-1 Kojirakawa, Yamagata 990, JAPAN

ABSTRACT

We have been using the system of ultra high molecular weight polyethylene and alumina-ball in total hip arthroplasty (THA) since 1988. Three types of femoral head, 28mm in diameter, have been available for controlling the neck length since 1991. We have performed two experimental studies. The static destructive load revealed 4900-9100 kgf in average and shock destructive energy 48.0-117.6 J in average. The experimental studies of Y-U neck length control system showed excellent mechanical properties and its short term clinical study revealed no mechanical failure in 320 THAs with this system, which have been followed from 1 year to 4 years. This system was useful for labor-saving in surgery.

INTRODUCTION

We have performed total hip arthroplasties since 1974 to 1988 and used metal head, 28mm in diameter femoral components. The materials were stainless steel or cobalt-chromium alloy. Recently, polyethylene-metal wear has become one of the factors of prosthetic loosening and the wear particles of high density polymer (HDP) have been considered important in the loosening of interface between bone and implants. According to clinical reports and experiences, we have been using the system of ultra high molecular weight polyethylene and alumina-ball since 1988. Alumina-ball has been shown to provide low friction and low wear in total hip arthroplasty. The usage of a 28mm diameter head was aimed at obtaining a larger range of motion for the Japanese life style. During ten year follow up, the ratios of the HDP socket wear of 28mm head was nearly same as that of 22mm heads [7]. At the beginning of this series, four types of stem size (extra-small, small, medium and large) and three neck lengths totaling 12 types of stem configuration were prepared according to the variation of femoral canal and limb lengths. The neck length control with alumina-ball was possible to reduce the numbers of the implants and to be useful for labor-saving in surgery. We have used this neck control system with the alumina-ball, namely Y-U neck length control system, since 1991.

MATERIAL AND METHODS

The alumina-ball used was 28mm in diameter. Three types of neck length (+4mm, ± 0mm, -4mm) were available for each size of Y-U stems. The +0mm ball was used as conventional type and +4mm and -4mm were applied when the neck length was short and long, respectively. We have performed two experimental studies of the static destructive load test (n=5) and shock destructive load test (n=5).

1) The static destructive load test: The test of cone cavity contact was performed by using the instrument, inserted ring bound in copper between metal cone cavity and alumina-ball combined taper-cone (Figure 1A). The cross-head speed was 0.5mm/min. This static load test was compression load and its load was gradually delivered until the alumina-ball was broken. The destructive load was monitored as kgf.

2) The shock destructive load test: The shock load test was performed by an instrument like Figure 2A. We dropped the weight from one meter height. The weight ranged from 2kg to 12kg. If the alumina-ball was not broken, the weight was increased gradually. When the specimen was broken, we evaluated the energy (J), calculated by the weight and height of fall.

3) Clinical evaluation: We have used this neck control system with the alumina-ball since 1991. The ball size was 28 mm in diameter. The numbers of THA's with the alumina-ball system included 609 cases from 1988 to 1994. These cases, included the neck control systems in 425 arthroplasties. Follow-up was from 1 month to 4 years. 320 cases which were followed over one year were evaluated in this study. We investigated age and gender at surgery, classification of disease and X-rays for the clinical evaluation.

RESULTS

1) The static destructive load test: The static load test revealed 9100 kgf average load for the -4mm ball, 6800 kgf for the ± 0mm and 4900 kgf for the +4mm ball. All of these alumina balls were broken (Figure 1B).

2) The shock destructive load test: The results of shock load tests revealed 117.6 J average for the -4mm ball, 88.2 J for the +0mmand 48.0 J for the +4mm ball. All -4mm balls were not broken. The other alumina-balls were broken in the experiment (Figure 2B).

3) Clinical evaluation: The cases followed included 21 male and 299 females. The classification of disease was 269 cases of osteoarthritis, 20 cases of rheumatoid arthritis and 31 cases of revision of THA. The age ranged from 35 to 89 years and the average was 63.6 years. The follow-up term was from one year to 4 years. 61 cases of -4mm ball, 152 cases of ±0mm ball and 107 cases of +4mm ball were studied. Cases of mechanical failures were not observed in the alumina-ball system. Two cases that were removed due to infection were revised.

DISCUSSION

Several systems of THA have been used to decrease socket-head wear. Boutin *et al.*, [1] reported the usage of combined system of alumina head and alumina socket in 1971, and reported long-term clinical results for ten years. But there were several reports of fracture of alumina head and socket, (this type of combination was problem due to more

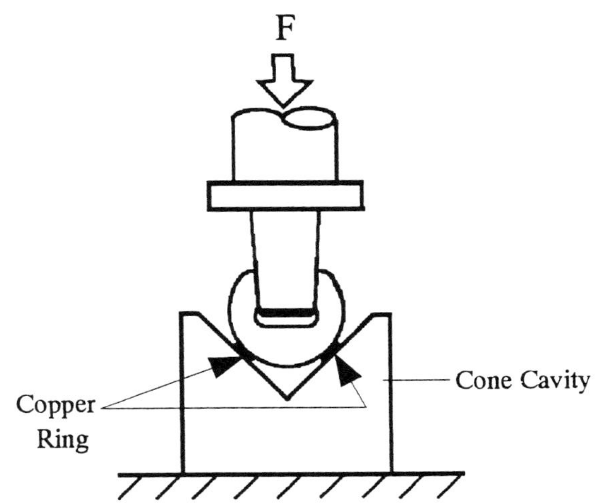

1A

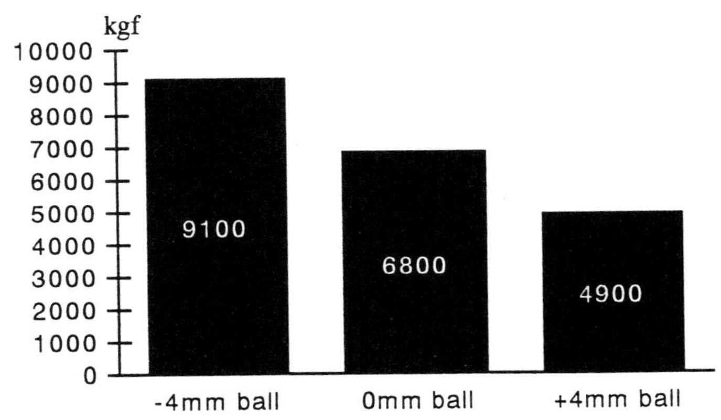

1B

Figure 1A and 1B. Instrumentation of static load test. Illustration showing the static destructive load in average and five balls being used each of three types. The shock destructive test by Kyocera Co. Ltd.

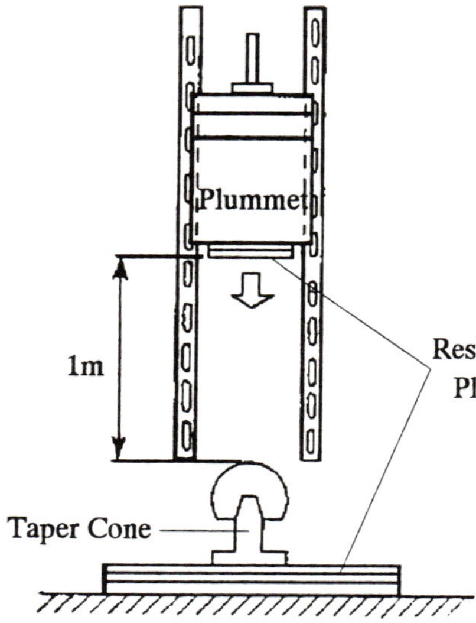

2A

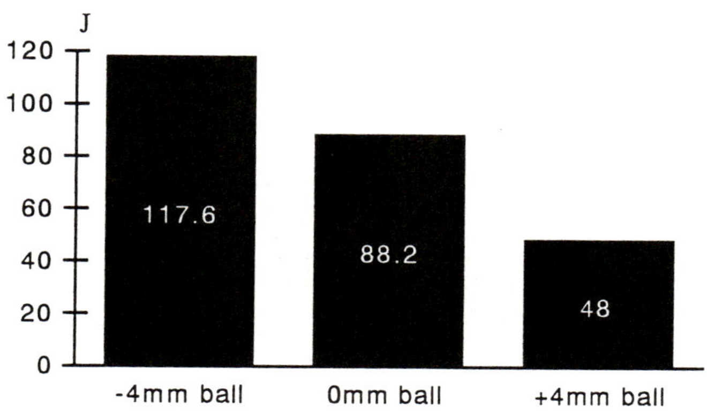

2B

Figure 2A and 2B. Instrumentation of shock load test. Illustration showing the shock destructive energy in average and five balls being used each of three types. The shock destructive test by Kyocera Co. Ltd.

hardness than metallic materials). Therefore Semlitsch *et al.,* [9], Dorlot *et al.,* [4] and Ziehner *et al.,* [11] have reported on the combination of HDP socket and alumina head in Europe. They reported that HDP socket and alumina head produced less wear debris than metal HDP system. In Japan, Oonishi and Shikita reported on the combination of the HDP socket and alumina head in 1978 with good results of both experimental and clinical studies [8]. Several cases of ball fractures were reported in these systems. Burckhardt *et al.,* [2] reported 3 cases of fracture within 3 months after surgery and Holmer [5] reported 5 cases of fracture after 1-2 years following primary hip arthroplasty. However, the mechanism of these failures has not clarified.

Mechanical failure were not observed in our usual alumina-ball system from 1988 to 1990. With the neck length control and alumina-ball, it was possible to reduce the numbers of the implants and to be useful for labor-saving in surgery. We have used this neck control system with the alumina-ball, namely Y-U neck length control system since 1991. The problem was ball strength in this neck control system. We have performed experimental studies of two strength tests. A ±0mm ball was on the current model, and ball strength was no problem. In addition, we compared -4mm ball and +4mm ball with ±0mm ball. The static destructive load test revealed 9100 kgf in average load in -4mm ball, 6800 kgf in ±0mm and 4900 kgf in +4mm ball. As load on the hip joint has been reported to be 1300-2000 kgf in an average 60kg human (3,6,10), this neck control system was adequate for clinical application. The results of shock load tests revealed 117.6 J in average energy in -4mm ball, 88.2 J in ±0mm and 48.0 J in +4mm ball, although -4mm ball was not broken. These results also support suitability of the system, because the energy by the shock load tests of fracture of the femoral neck bone of cadavers was reported to be 40 J or less (8). Thus, 48.0 J in +4mm ball should be sufficient for a usual life. Based on these experimental studies, we have used 3 types of alumina-ball. Mechanical failure cases were not observed in the alumina-ball system in the follow-up term over one year. We considered the neck control system in this THA was good and labor-saving system.

REFERENCE

1. Boutin, P. and Blanquaert, D., *Rev. Chir. Orthop. Reparatrice Appar.* Mot.(France) 1981, 67(3), 279-287.
2. Burckhardt, A. and Berberat, C., *Arch Orthop. Trauma Surg.* 1993, 112(5), 215-219.
3. Denham, R.A., *J. Bone Joint Surg.* 1959, 41-B, 550
4. Dorlot, J. M., Christel, P. and Meunier, A., *J. Biomed. Mater. Res.* 1989, 23, 2993I0.
5. Holmer, P. and Nielsen, P. T., *J. Arthroplasty* (United States) 1993, 8(6), 567-571.
6. Muller, M. E., *Die Huftnahen Femurosteotomien.* G. Thieme, Stuttgart 1971.
7. Togashi, K., Ida, H. and Watanabe, Y., *J. of Joint Surg.*(Japan) 1993, 12(6), 191-198.
8. Oonishi, H. and Shikita, T., *Orthop. Surgery* (Japan) 1983, 3, 264-279.
9. Semlitsch, M., Lehmann, M., Weber H., Dorre E., Willert, H.G., *J. Biomed. Mater. Res.* 1977, 11(4), 537-552.
10. Williams, M. and Lissner, H., In: *Biomechanics of Human Motion,* 1967, W.B. Saunder, Philadelphia
11. Zichner, L.P. and Willert, H.G., *Clin. Orthop.* 1992, 282, 86-94

COMPARATIVE STUDY ON POTENTIAL OF NATURAL CORAL AND TRICALCIUM PHOSPHATE CYLINDERS IN HEALING A SEGMENTAL DIAPHYSEAL DEFECT IN SHEEP

T.J. Gao, T.S. Lindholm, B. Kommonen*, P. Ragni**, A. Paronzini**, T.C. Lindholm and K.J.J. Pajamäki

Bone Transplantation Research Group, Medical School, University of Tampere, P. O. Box 607, FIN-33101,Tampere, Finland.
*Department of Surgery, College of Veterinary Medicine, Hämeentie 57, FIN-00580, Helsinki, Finland.
** II Orthopaedic Clinic, University of Milan, Milan, Italy.

ABSTRACT

The osteocompatibility, ossointegration and mechanical strength of natural coral and tricalcium phosphate cylinders implanted in a sheep tibial defect were established to evaluate the potential of two bioceramics in healing a segmental diaphyseal defect. A distinguishable increment of area and integrated intensity of callus in coral-implanted tibial was defined using a computerized image analyser at 3 weeks. Significantly increased maximal torque capacity, the maximal angle of deformation and absorption of energy were obtained in coral-implanted tibae at 16 weeks compared with TCP-implanted tibiae. Natural coral seems to be clinically superior to TCP in the repair of segmental diaphyseal defects.

INTRODUCTION

Screening biomaterials for an ideal bone substitute still challenges investigators in materials research and orthopaedic surgeons in clinical practice. An appropriate bone substitute must be characterized by its biocompatibility, mechanical performance, biodegradability and clinical accessibility. Tricalcium phosphate, which possesses inorganic components similar to those of bone, has been commonly used as an implantable material [1]. Natural coral, a bioceramic processed from the mineral skeleton of scleractinian coral, has been used in neurosurgery, orthopaedic and periodontal surgery since 1970 [2, 3, 4, 5]. Using tricalcium phosphate (TCP) and natural coral (NC) cylinders, the potential of healing segmental tibial defects in sheep was investigated. The purpose of this study was to compare the osteoconduction, ossointegration and mechanical strength obtained by the two different implants in an osteotomized diaphyseal defect model.

MATERIALS AND METHODS

Tricalcium phosphate (B247, DePuy, Warsaw, IN, USA) and natural coral cylinders (Biocoral©, Inoteb, LeGuernol, Saint-Gonnery, France) were used as trial bone substitutes. All cylinders were shaped to identical dimensions, 15 mm in diameter and 16 mm in length, with a plug of 3 mm in each end. A central longitudinal hole 4 mm in diameter was drilled to reproduce a medullary canal. Segmental osteotomy 16 mm in length was performed subperiosteally with a Gigli saw on the midshaft of the right tibia in 12 adult sheep under general anaesthesia. Six defects were replaced with TCP and six with NC cylinders. The osteotomized tibia was firmly immobilized by two overlapped AO plates. The muscles and skin were closed in layers. The experiment was terminated at 16 weeks. Sequential X-ray views of the osteotomized tibiae were taken at 3, 6, 12 and 16 weeks after surgery. All radiographs from 3 to 12 weeks were scanned by a computerized optical density scanner in the Bio Image System (6 XRS, Millipore, Corporation, USA) to follow quantitatively the changes in area and integrated intensity of callus formation around the implants. After removal of soft tissue and the plates, the bone ends of the osteotomized tibiae were embedded into a symmetrical circular aluminium moulds using polyester resin. A torsion test was carried out by loading at an angular velocity of 6.5 degrees per second with a modified torsional test machine until failure point [6]. The maximal torque capacity (MTC), the maximal angle of deformation (MA), the absorption of energy (AE) and the bone stiffness (BS) were calculated and compared between TCP- and NC-implanted tibia. The sites of the fracture lines were recorded and compared between the two groups. After mechanical tests undemineralized histological sections 12-20 μm were prepared using a cutting and grinding method (Exakt-Apparatebau, Hamburg, Germany), stained with Van Gieson and evaluated by light microscopy. Student's t test was used for statistical comparison.

RESULTS

Eleven sheep were available for evaluation. The appearance of subperiosteal callus began at 3 weeks after the operation. The external callus bridged the defects completely at 6 weeks and consolidated at 12 weeks (Figure. 1). Clinical healing was reached at that time. Quantitative analysis of the area and integrated intensity of callus formation in radiographs showed that a larger area and more highly integrated intensity of callus were obtained in NC- than TCP-implanted tibiae at 3 weeks ($p<0.05$). No difference was noticed at 6 and 12 weeks (Figure. 2).

Better osseointegration between newly-formed bone and materials was found in NC than in TCP cylinders. There was no sharp demarcation between new bone and coral at 12 and 16 weeks. An advanced remodelling bone was seen microscopically grown into macropores and connected channels of the porous materials. No interposed fibrous tissue was seen between ingrown bone and trabeculae of NC or TCP cylinders. A greater proportion of mature Harversian units were demonstrated in remodelled bone inside and around NC compared to TCP cylinders (Figure. 3.). The difference between the resorption rates of NC and TCP was apparent radiographically and histologically. More resorption took place in NC than TCP.

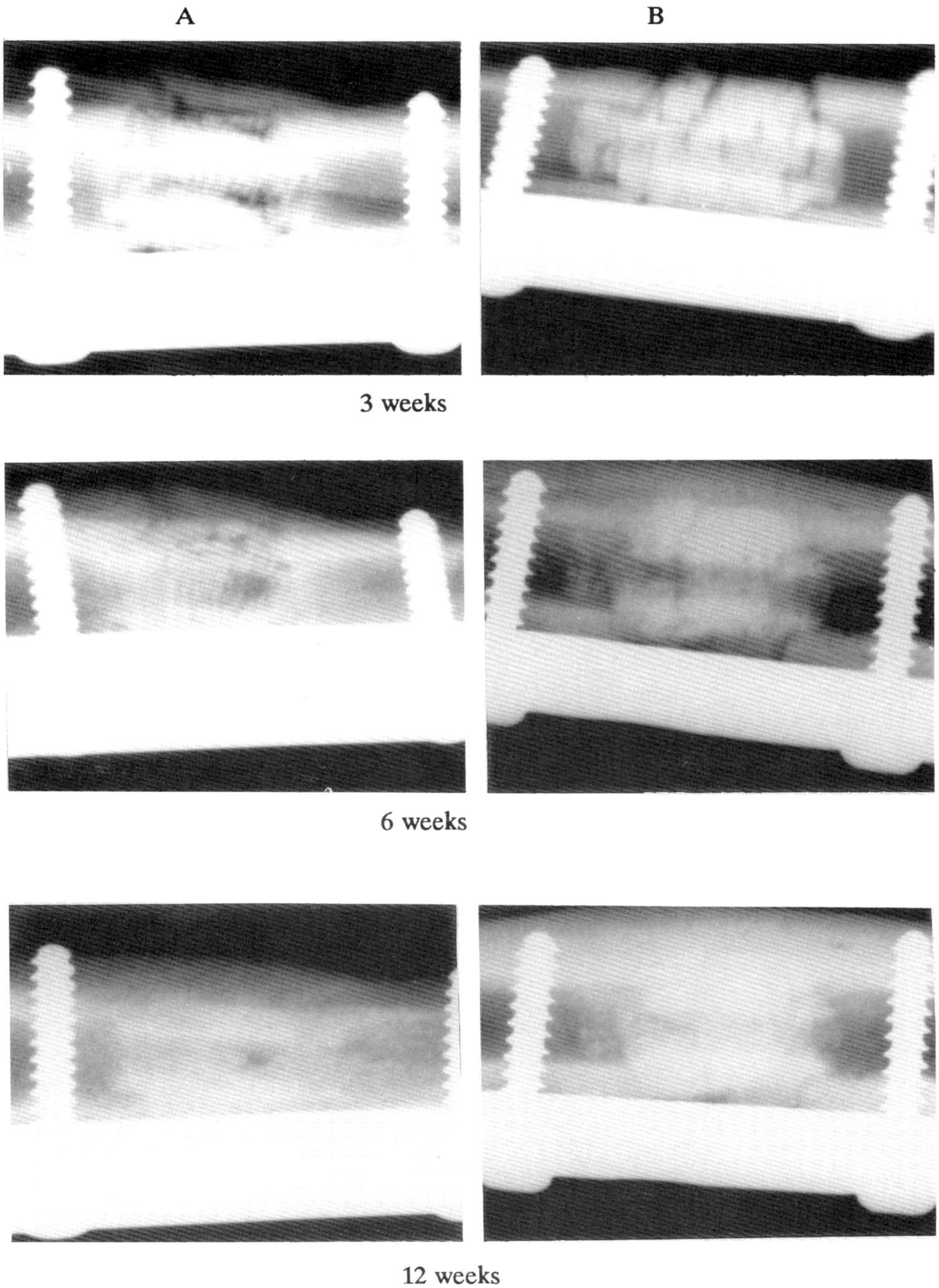

Figure 1. A-P views of radiograph of natural coral-(1a) and TCP-(1b) implanted tibiae. Visible periosteal callus formed at 3 weeks (3w), bridged defect at 6 weeks (6w) and consolidated at 12 weeks (12w).

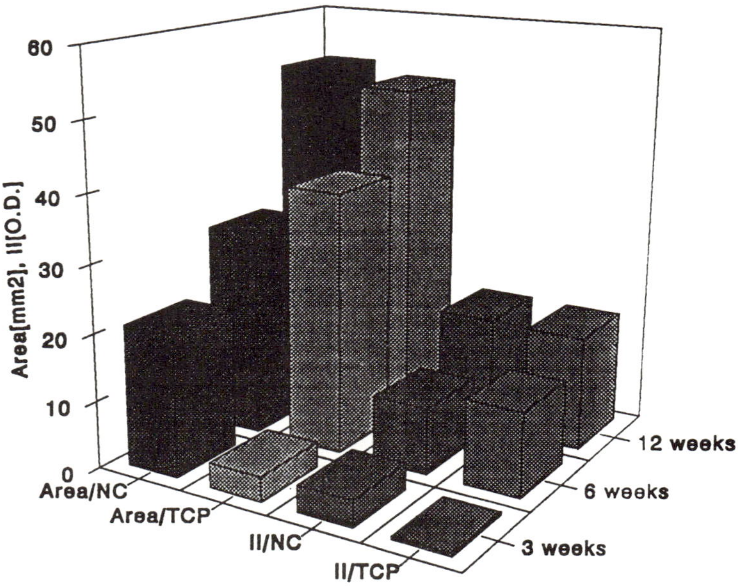

Figure 2. Three-dimensional column graph demonstrates variances of area (Area, mm^2) and integrated intensity (II, Optical Density) in coral-(NC) and TCP-(TCP) implanted tibiae at 3, 6 and 12 weeks.

In comparison with TCP-implanted tibiae, a significant enhancement of maximal torque capacity, maximal angular deformation and absorption of energy in NC-implanted tibiae was noted except for bone stiffness in the torsion test at 16 weeks after implantation (Table. 1). The fracture line through the conjunction of implant with sheep tibiae stump occurred in 1/5 (20%) of NC but in 3/6 (50%) of TCP implanted tibiae.

Table 1. Mechanical Parameters in Natural Coral- or TCP-Implanted Sheep Tibia at 16 Weeks

Parameters	Natural Coral	TCP	p Value
MTC (Nm)	40.40 11.35	23.08 4.70	0.018 *
MA (Degree)	18.55 4.28	13.59 2.29	0.05 *
MAE (Nm.degree)	337.6 126.4	159.3 44.4	0.014 *
BS (Nm/degree)	2.85 0.87	2.11 0.49	0.14

* Statistical significance at $p < 0.05$, Students' t test.

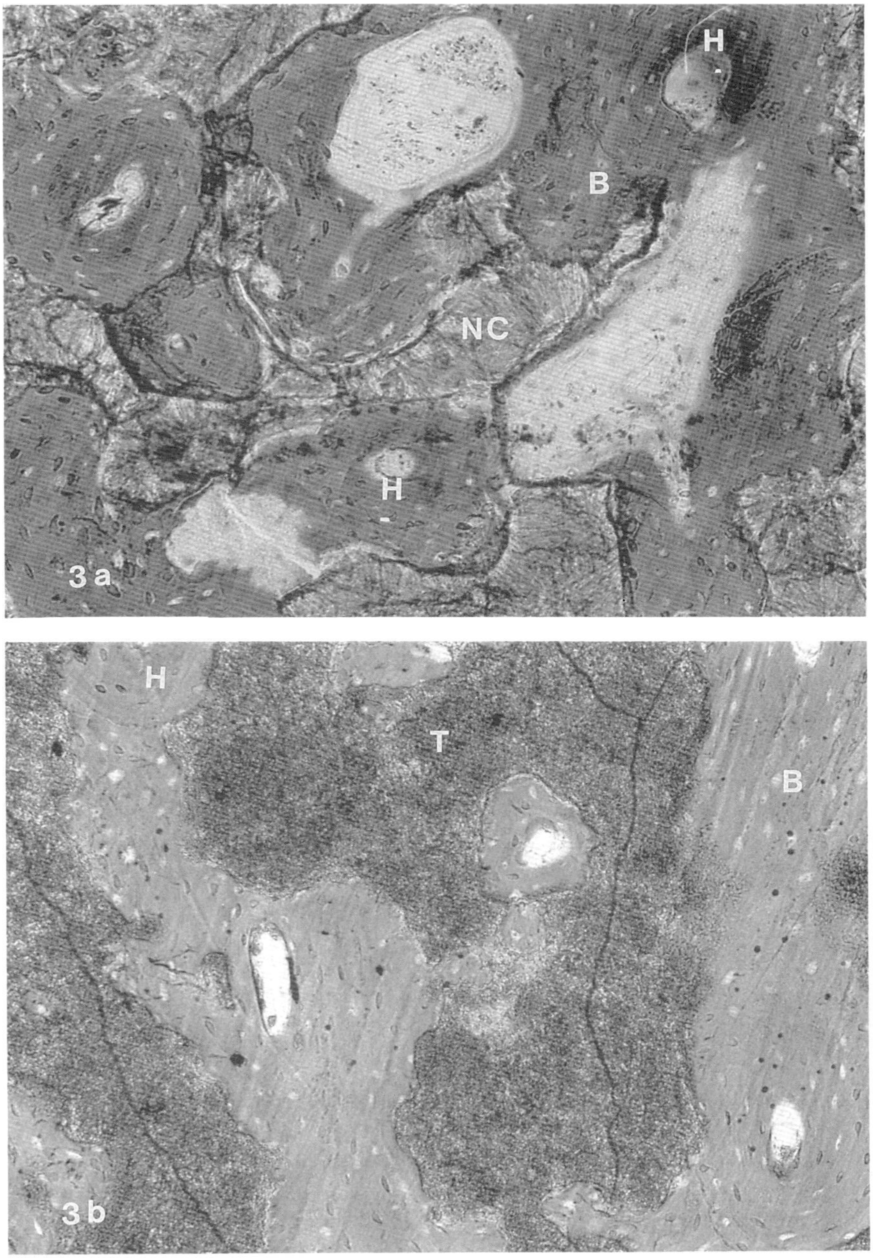

Figure 3. Photomicrograph(x100) of natural coral-(a) and TCP-(b)cylinders implanted in sheep tibiae defect for 16 weeks. New bone(B) ingrown into the pore of the ceramics. There was no interposed tissue between new bone and coral(NC) or TCP(T) material. More mature Harversian units(H) were observed in coral-implanted tibiae than in TCP.

DISCUSSION AND CONCLUSION

In this study, an early significant increment of area and integrated intensity of callus formation was induced by the NC cylinder in comparison with the TCP cylinder under identical conditions. The cellular and tissue events involved have also been cited by Hott in a rat cortical bone model [7]. Woven bone was found to be formed directly along the coral fragments by osteoblasts as early as 8 days after implantation. Perigranular calcification has been observed 2 weeks earlier in an NC-implanted mandible defect than in TCP [8]. This was attributed to the osteoinductive effect of the coral [7]. However, the osteoinductivity of the coral was not confirmed. A more conceivable explanation of this phenomenon is that the carbonate-dominated components of coral play a critical role in initiation and increment of bone apposition, as well as in biointegration with new bone [9]. Formation of a Ca-P rich layer on the surface of the material was considerably quicker in coral than TCP. The augmentation of early bone formation showed better osteocompatibility for coral than for TCP [8].

The better mechanical performance in NC- than in TCP-implanted tibiae was attributed to a good osseointegration of natural coral with host bone and mechanical integrity of the raw material. A rigid mixed bone-coral structure persisted with time and reinforced the implanted limb [7]. The fracture line passing through the implant-bone interface in 20% of NC as against 50% of TCP provides further evidence of intimate osseointegration between coral and newly-formed bone. The dimension and size of pore and interconnecting channels in natural-origin coral might be more suitable for new bone ingrowth. Compared with the TCP cylinder, superior degradation of the NC cylinder took place. This was considered to be a combined effect of cell-mediated resorption and enzyme hydrolysis with physiochemical dissolution on the surface of the material [8, 9]. The process resulted in an advanced remodelling of newly-formed bone and formation of mature callus.

With osteocompatiblity, mechanical integrity, biodegradation and clinical handling superiority, the results confirm that natural coral has advantages over TCP as a desirable bone substitute in the repair of experimental and clinical segmental diaphyseal defects.

REFERENCE:

1. Hoffmann,A.A., Bachus, K.N., Bloebaum, R.D.. *J Arthroplasty* 1993, 8, 157-166.
2. Yukna R.A. *J Periodontal* 1994, 65,177-85.
3. Roux F.X., *et al., J Neurosurg* 1988, 69, 510-13.
4. Patat J.L., *et al., Actualites En Biomateriaux* Romillat, 1990, 167-175.
5. Kehr P.H. *et al., Orthop Traumatol* 1993, 3, 287-93.
6. Lepola V, Väänanen H.K., Jalovaara P. *Clin Orthop* 1993, 297, 55-61.
7. Hott, M., Marie, P.J., Guillemin,G., Patat, J.L. In: *Ceramics in Substitutive and Reconstructive Surgery*. Elsevier Science Publishers B.V., 1991, 345-352.
8. Ouhayoun, J.P., Shabana, A.H.M., Issahakian, S., Patat, J.L., Guillemin, G., Sawaf, M.H., Forest, N. *J Mater Med* 1992, 3, 222-228.
9. Damien. C.J., Ricci, J.L., Christel, P., Alexander,H., Patat, J.L. *Calcif Tissue Int* 1994, 55, 151-158.

OXIDE CERAMICS FOR ARTICULATING COMPONENTS OF THPs - CERAMIC\POLYETHYLENE CERAMIC/CERAMIC

Gerd Willmann

Cerasiv GmbH, Medical Products Division, Fabrikstr. 23 - 29, D - 73207 Plochingen, Germany

ABSTRACT

Alumina ceramics were introduced 20 years ago as a material for bearing surfaces in total hip replacements to minimize the wear rate. More than 2 million alumina femoral heads have been used. The combination offering a low wear rate is alumina/polyethylene. The combination guaranteeing the lowest wear rate is alumina/alumina.

Due to their attractive mechanical properties zirconia heads have been introduced more recently.

The state-of-the-art is reviewed, e.g. basic properties, results of tribological testing, improvement of material properties, and safety.

INTRODUCTION

Currently the main problem in total hip replacement (THR) is the wear debris that causes osteolysis. Alumina according to ISO 6474, proved to be a material offering the required properties listed in Table 1 [1].

The most successful system in THR has been the combination of an alumina femoral ball head articulating against an acetabular cup made of polyethylene (UHMWPE) because this combination offered a wear rate that was up 10 times lower than the standard combination head of metal articulation against a PE-cup. Since 1974 more than 2 million alumina heads have been used. The most widely used alumina head is Biolox® developed by Feldmühle. The lowest wear rate can be guaranteed when an alumina head is articulating against an alumina cup. Typical wear is between 1 and 5 μm/year if there was no loosening [2,3].

Table 1. Important properties of ceramic heads.

Property	Dimension	alumina ISO 6474	zirconia Y-TZP
grain size	μm	<2	<0.5
strength	MPa	up to 580	up to 1.000
fracture toughness	MPa $m^{1/2}$	4	up to 10
hardness	HV 0.1	2.200	1.200

Due to the attractive mechanical properties of high purity zirconia, zirconia femoral heads have been introduced. The Y-TZP heads may be combined with PE-cups. They show similar wear rates to alumina heads. So far about 200.000 Y-TZP heads have been used. Zirconia is not suitable for acetabular cups.

SAFETY

In orthopedics the most important objective is product reliability. It must have an extremely low failure rate. According to statistics [4] the failure rate *in vivo* of Biolox® heads is 0.01 % (= 1:10,000). A low failure rate can only be achieved if the processing and the manufacturing is organized according to the rules of Good Manufacturing Practice and ISO 9001.

It is always possible to practice a 100 % quality control to check dimensions and to detect flaws by using dye penetrants. Unfortunately all known non-destructive methods are unsuitable for ceramics. For a 100 % control of the mechanical strength, a proof test improves safety.

Table 2. Typical wear rates.

Combination head/cup	Wear rate μm/year	References
alumina/PE	20	[1]
alumina/alumina	< 5	[2]
zirconia/PE	controversial reports	
zirconia/zirconia	not recommended	
metal/PE	up to 560	[6]
metal/metal	disastrous in the past	[3]
others	still R & D	[3]

Table 3. Improvements to medical-grade alumina.

Property	Dimension	ISO 6474	Biolox®	Biolox® forte
density	g/cm^3	3.94	3.96	3.98
bending strength	MPa	400	500	580
grain size	μm	〈4.5	〈3	〈1.8

The objectives to achieve high reliability have always been and still are: high purity ceramics, maximize the density, minimize the grain size in the microstructure, maximize the strength and fracture load according to ISO 7206-5, and minimize the flaw population. Bioceramics can achieve these objectives by using purified raw materials and clean room processing [5].

Strength and fracture load of a ceramic head are strongly correlated with density and grain size. The density has to be maximized and the grain size of a microstructure has to be minimized. If the ceramic heads are sintered and then additionally hipped, the material properties and the fracture load can easily be optimized, see Table 2.

All ceramic heads have to be marked with an identification number. It was found out that laser etching causes fewer critical flaws than green engraving and therefore improves the strength and reduces the failure rate.

The fracture load depends on the flaws in the bulk and on the surface which was ground and polished. If critical flaws exist in the bulk of the material they cannot be detected. Using a proof test, components with a critical flaw will be detected and the component will fracture during the test, so they are rejected and destroyed. This proof test improves the reliability of ceramic heads far above the already achieved failure rate [4].

CONCLUSION

Alumina and zirconia ceramic heads have proved to reduce the wear particle problem which causes osteolysis, which should lead to a renaissance for the combination of alumina/alumina. Reliability can be improved by hipping, laser etching, and proof testing.

REFERENCES

1. Clarke, I.C. and Willmann, G. In: *Bone Implant Interfaces,* Mosby, St. Louis 1994, 203-52.

2. Henssge, E.J., Bos, I. Willmann, G. *J.Mat.Sci.Mat. in Medicine,* 1994, 5, 657-61.

3. Buchhorn, G.H., Willert, H.G. (eds). *Proc. 6th Biomaterials Symposium,* Hogrefe & Huber Publ., Seattle 1995 (in print).

4. Semlitsch, M., Dawihl, W. In: *Technical Principles, Design and Safety of Joint Implants,* Hogrefe & Huber Publ., Seattle 1994, 99-101.

5. Nagel, A., Jaschinski, W., Richter, H.G., Willmann, G. Keram. Z., 1994, 46, 618-23.

ACTIVE BRAZING FOR BIOMEDICAL APPLICATIONS

E. Lugscheider*, A. Nyland*, M. Knepper**, R. Sicking*

*Materials Science Institute, Aachen University of Technology, 52056 Aachen, Germany
** Graduate School of Biomedical Engineering, University of New South Wales, Sydney, NSW 2052, Australia

ABSTRACT

The fabrication of structural components made of high performance technical ceramics as well as the fabrication of medical implants made of biocompatible ceramics with a complicated geometry is limited due to the ceramics brittleness. Active Brazing is a modern and successful joining technique to enable the fabrication of ceramic-ceramic/metal joints and has thus the ability to overcome this problem and to open new perspectives in the field of load-bearing implants. This paper shows the current state of the art in this technology and addresses its application for joining bioceramics.

INTRODUCTION

Increasing demands on technical components and, therefore, on the materials employed, lead to a great industrial interest on ceramic materials due to their specific mechanical and/or electrical properties. Nevertheless the wide range of ceramic-applications in different industries is limited by their high brittleness and the related difficulty of producing monolithic components of complex geometry. This limitation occurs as well in the field of bioceramics, especially for alumina and zirconia, being employed for load-bearing orthopedic implants. A possible way of solving this problem is the use of a close fitting joining technique with which ceramic-ceramic and ceramic-metal joints of sufficient strength and biocompatibility can be manufactured.

Initial movements in the direction of strength as well as heat and chemical resistance have already been researched in the thirties when Siemens [1] developed the well known Tungsten or Molybdenum-Manganese process as a metallization process for joining alumina. Unfortunately the use of Ni or Cu as a metallic interlayer excludes this technology for biomedical applications. Recently, a new technology that offers promising features in ceramic joining has been developed. The so-called active brazing process is a one-step process where a specially designed filler metal is placed between the two base materials and then heated under vacuum or shielding gas conditions to wet the ceramic [2].

MATERIALS AND METHODS

From a metallurgical viewpoint, the wetting of a ceramic material by a liquid brazing metal represents an extremely complex problem due to the combination of two material groups with fundamentally different atomic structures. In order to wet a ceramic material with a liquid metal, which is distinguished by metallic bonds, it is necessary that chemical interactions take place at the interface, so that the filler metal adheres sufficiently to the ceramic for technical use. For this reason, active brazes contain small amounts of transition metals (e.g. Ti, Zr, Hf, Nb, Ta, etc.) which are able to cause a dissociation on the ceramic surface through chemical reactions (formation of new phases, dissolution reactions) [3,4]. Figure 1 shows the effect towards the wetting behavior of doped active brazes in contrast to conventional brazes.

Most of the commercially available active brazes are based on Ag, Cu or the Ag-Cu eutectic (Table 1) and are employed at brazing temperatures between 800°C and 1100°C owing to thermodynamic activation of the ceramic. Titanium is used almost exclusively as the reactive agent with a content between 1 to 4 wt.-%. To reduce the risk of preoxidation during the vacuum brazing process, the reactive component is homogeneously embedded in the metallic matrix system. The most convenient and flexible way to apply active brazes is as foil of 50-200 μm in thickness. Besides the employed materials, the actual brazing parameters like heating rate, brazing temperature and dwell time are of decisive interest for the mechanical properties of the joint.

RESULTS AND DISCUSSION

High performance ceramics that are of importance in technical structures are silicon-nitride, silicon-carbide, aluminum-carbide as well as the biocompatible ceramics alumina and zirconia. Most of those ceramics have been investigated regarding active brazing, and the active brazing process has proved to be successful or showed at least very promising results [5, 6]. Figure 2 shows some bending strength values for different Al_2O_3-Al_2O_3/FeNiCo joints. In Figure 3 the microstructure of an Al_2O_3-Steel joint is presented. In contrast to the direct metal-metal brazing, the phase formation in the ceramic-metal interface is essential for the joints strength. Different thermal expansion coefficients might lead to residual stresses in the ceramic while cooling down from brazing temperature.

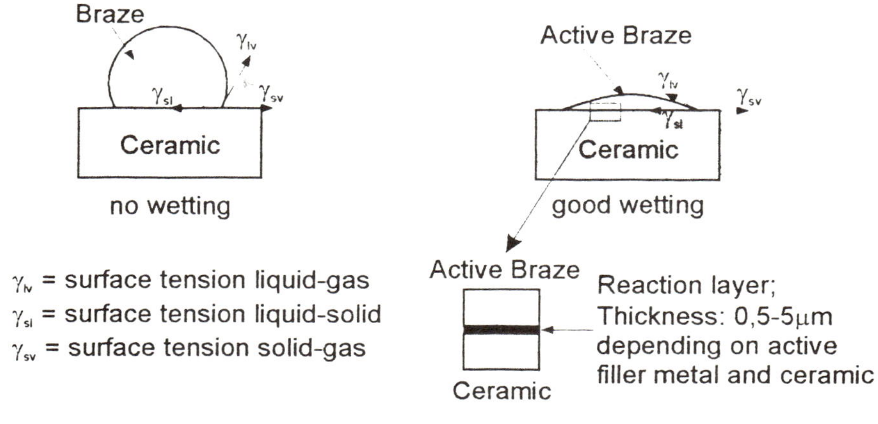

Figure 1. Wetting of a ceramic material with a liquid braze.

Table 1. Schedule of commercially available active brazes.

Filler Metal Composition in Weight-Percent								
Ag	Cu	In	Ni	Al	Ti	Others	T_{sol}	T_{liq}
72,5	19,5	5,0	--	--	**3,0**	--	730	760
96,0	--	--	--	--	**4,0**	--	970	970
70,5	26,5	--	--	--	**3,0**	--	780	805
64,0	34,5	--	--	--	**1,5**	--	770	810
98,0	--	1,0	--	--	**1,0**	--	950	960
10,0	--	--	--	--	**4,0**	86,0 Sn	221	300
--	--	4,0	--	--	**4,0**	92,0 Pb	320	325
--	--	--	33,0	--	**67,0**	--	942	980
--	15,0	--	15,0	--	**70,0**	--	910	970
68,8	26,7	--	--	--	**4,5**	--	830	850
--	--	--	3,0	--	**0,6**	96,4 Au	1003	1030
--	92,75	--	--	2,0	**2,25**	3,0 Si	958	1024
92,75	5,0	--	--	1,0	**1,25**	--	860	912
63,0	35,25	--	--	--	**1,75**	--	780	815
63,0	34,25	--	--	--	**1,75**	1,0 Sn	775	806
59,0	27,25	12,5	--	--	**1,25**	--	605	715
--	--	--	15,5	--	**1,75 V**	AuMo 0,75	940	960

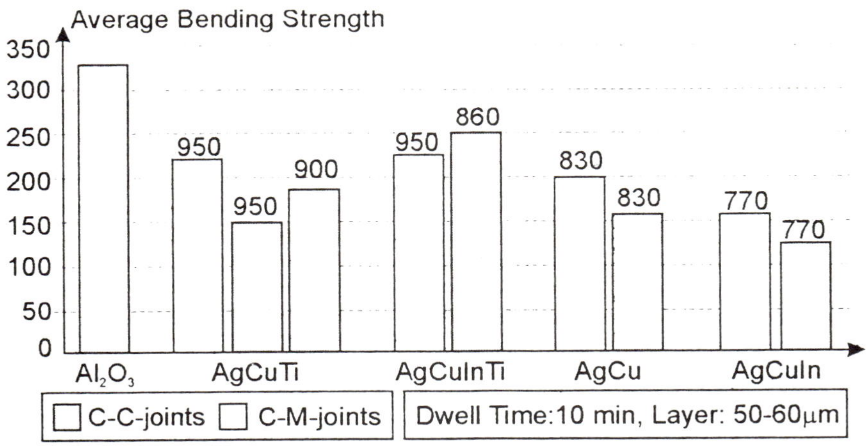

Figure 2. Four point bending strength of different Al_2O_3-Al_2O_3/FeNiCo joints [7].

Hence, an optimized design as well as a sufficient thickness and ductility of the filler metal is required above all with joining ceramics to metals. Figure 4 shows a successful example of combining the advantages of metal and ceramic. The stressed surface of a rocker arm for the automobile industry (carbon steel) can be protected against wear by brazing an armour plate (Si_3N_4) onto this surface, employing an active braze (AgTi). Other current applications in mechanical engineering like ceramic turbo-chargers, heat exchangers or electrical sensors use either the outstanding wear-protective and high-temperature properties or the electrical properties of both, oxide and nonoxide ceramics in combination with metals [8].

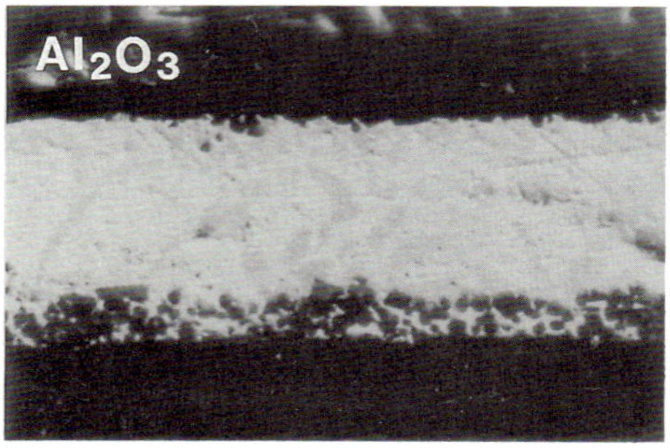

Figure 3. Micrograph of Al_2O_3-Cr Ni Steel joint; filler metal; AgCuTi.

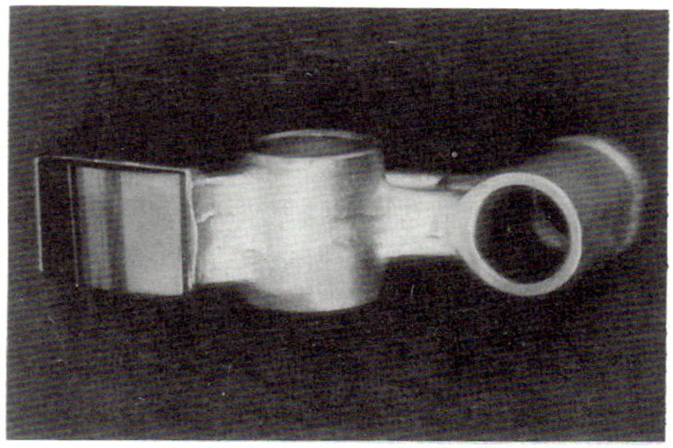

Figure 4. Rocker arm with ceramic armour plate.

To date the active brazes themselves have not been a subject of biomedical research, although there are comparable problems and limitations concerning the use of biocompatible ceramics as bulk materials, especially in orthopedic surgery. Similar to the rocker arm (Fig. 4), the utilization of a composite femoral component, whose sliding surface is made with an oxide ceramic and whose structural part, in contact with the bone, is made with a biocompatible metal alloy, could lower the harmful UHMWPE wear for hip or knee prostheses.

CONCLUSIONS

Active Brazing has proved its ability to produce reliable ceramic-ceramic/metaljoints for engineering applications. The facility of joining ceramics to themselves or to metals results in promising perspectives in the field of load-bearing implants. Therefore new filler metals on the base of biocompatible alloying elements have to be developed.

REFERENCES

1. Meyer, A., Berichte der DKG, Vol. 42, No. 11, 1965, 405.
2. Loehman, R.E., Ceramic Bulletin, Vol. 68, No. 4, 1989, 891.
3. Klomp, J.T., Ceramic Microstructures ´86, Plenum Press, New York, 1986, 307.
4. Naka, M. and Okamoto, I., Transactions of IWRI, Vol. 14, No. 1, 1985, 29.
5. Lugscheider, E. and Boretius, M., AIF-report 7310, Aachen 1990.
6. Nicholas, M.G., Mortimer, D.A., Jones, L.M. and Chrispin, R.M., Journal of Materials Science, Vol. 25, 1990, 2679.
7. Lugscheider, E., Boretius, M. and Tillmann, W., Schweißen und Schneiden, Vol. 43, No. 7, 1991, 392.
8. Boretius, M., Lugscheider, E. and Tillmann, W., ISBN 3-18-401272-7, 1995, 195-219.

BIOACTIVITY OF BIOACTIVE FILLER-RESIN CEMENT

T Kokubo, Y. Morita, F. Miyaji, K. Nakanishi, N. Soga and T. Nakamura,*

Division of Material Chemistry, Faculty of Engineering, Kyoto University, Sakyo-ku, Kyoto 606-01 Japan,
*Department of Orthopedic Surgery, Faculty of Medicine, Kyoto University, Sakyo-ku, Kyoto 606-01 Japan

ABSTRACT

Much attention has been paid to bioactive filler-resin composite cements, since they can solidify in a few minutes to give high mechanical strengths and bond to living bone. Their surface structural changes due to exposure to a simulated body fluid (SBF), which govern their bioactivity and mechanical properties, were investigated in terms of the kind of fillers and resins. PMMA shows no apatite formation on its composite, whereas Bis-GMA/TEGDMA does. Composites of a $CaO\text{-}SiO_2\text{-}P_2O_5\text{-}CaF_2$ glass, glass-ceramic A-W and sintered hydroxyapatite with Bis-GMA/TEGDMA all gave apatite formation on their surfaces, but with different surface structures. The first one formed a dense and uniform apatite layer, but accompanied by an underlying, less dense layer. The second one formed a dense and uniform apatite layer without forming the less dense layer. The third one formed the apatite only on the individual sintered hydroxyapatite grains, discontinuously.

INTRODUCTION

Polymethyl methacrylate has been mainly used as a cement for fixing metallic and polymeric implants to the surrounding bones and for filling bone defects. However, it does not bond to living bone, and hence its fixation is liable to degrade over a long period. Although some attempts have been made to prepare bioactive cements by mixing calcium phosphate crystalline powders [1] or $CaO\text{-}SiO_2$-based glass powders [2] with some aqueous solutions, the resultant cements had poor mechanical strengths. Much attention has recently focused on composite cements of bioactive inorganic fillers with organic resins [3-4]. These can exhibit fairly high mechanical strengths as well as high bioactivity. These properties are, however, largely influenced by their surface structural changes when exposed to body fluid. In this study, surface structural changes of composite cements exposed to simulated body fluid were investigated.

EXPERIMENTAL

Powders 3 μm average size of a CaO, 46.7, SiO_2 35.6, P_20_5 17.0 and CaF_2 0.7 wt% glass (CSG), which was prepared by a conventional melting technique [2], 5 μm average size of which AW-CC [5], supplied by Nippon Electric Glass Co. and HAp powders 5 μm average size sintered at 1200°C, supplied by Mitsubishi Material Co., were used as fillers. These fillers were treated with a silane coupling agent of 3-methacryloxy-propyltrimethoxysilane.

Methyl methacrylate (MMA) and a 50:50 mixture by weight of bisphenol-a-glicidyl methacrylate (Bis-GMA) with triethylene glycol dimethacrylate (TEGDMA) were used as monomers for forming resins.

For PMMA-based composites, the fillers were mixed with PMMA powder and dibenzoyl peroxide was added as a polymerization initiator in 100:15:2 weight ratio. Liquid MMA was added with N,N-dimethyl-p-toluidine as a polymerization promotor in a 100:2.5 volume ratio. The powders were mixed with the liquid in 115:28 weight ratio, to give filler to resin ratio of 70:30 by weight. For Bis-GMA/TEGDMA-based composites, the fillers were mixed with dibenzoyl peroxide in 100:0.4 weight ratio. Liquid Bis-GMA/TEGDMA was mixed with N,N dimethyl-p-toluidine in 100:0.2 volume ratio. The powders were mixed with the liquid in 100:43 weight ratio, to give a filler to resin ratio of 70:30 in weight. These mixed pastes, which solidify in 5 min, were cast into a Teflon mold 6 mm in diameter and 6 mm in length. At 3 min after mixing, the mold containing the composite was soaked in a simulated body fluid (SBF) with ion concentrations Na^+ 142.0, K^+ 5.0, Mg^{2+} 1.5, Ca^{2+} 2.5, Cl^- 147.8, HCO_3^- 4.2, HPO_4^{2-} - 1.0 and SO_4^{2-} 0.5 mm did pH 7.25 at 36.5°C [6].

After various periods, the mixtures were removed from SBF. Their flat surfaces were analyzed by thin-film X-ray diffraction (TF-XRD) and scanning electron microscopy (SEM). Concentrations of ions and organic components of SBF were analyzed by an inductively coupled plasma emission spectroscopy (ICP) and gel permeation chromatography (GPC), respectively.

RESULTS AND DISCUSSION

TF-XRD gave no peak on the surface of CSG-PMMA composite even after soaking in SBF for 2 weeks, whereas it gave apatite peaks on that of CSG-Bis-GMA/TEGDMA (abbreviated as CSG-Bis-GMA hereafter) composite within 8 h. This indicates that the former is not bioactive, whereas the latter is [7]. SEM showed no change in surface structure of the former composite where the resin completely covered the glass particles even after soaking in SBF for 4 weeks. (Figure 1 (a)). On the other hand, it showed dissolution of the resin from the surface of the CSG-Bis GMA composite within 1 h and precipitation of fine particles on the glass grains within 8 h, (Figure 1 (b)). GPC showed that the organic substance dissolved from the composite is mainly TEGDMA monomer. Therefore, apatite formation on the surface of the latter composite is attributed to the dissolution of TEGDMA from its surface, to expose the glass grains to SBF. ICP showed that the apatite precipitation on the surface of the glass grains was performed by consuming theCa^{2+} and PO_4^{3-} ions from SBF.

TF-XRD, SEM, GPC and ICP showed that A-W- and HAp-Bis-GMA composites also release TEGDMA from their surfaces into SBF and form the apatite on their fillers by consuming the Ca^{2+} and PO_4^{3-} ions from the surrounding SBF, (Fig.1 c,d).

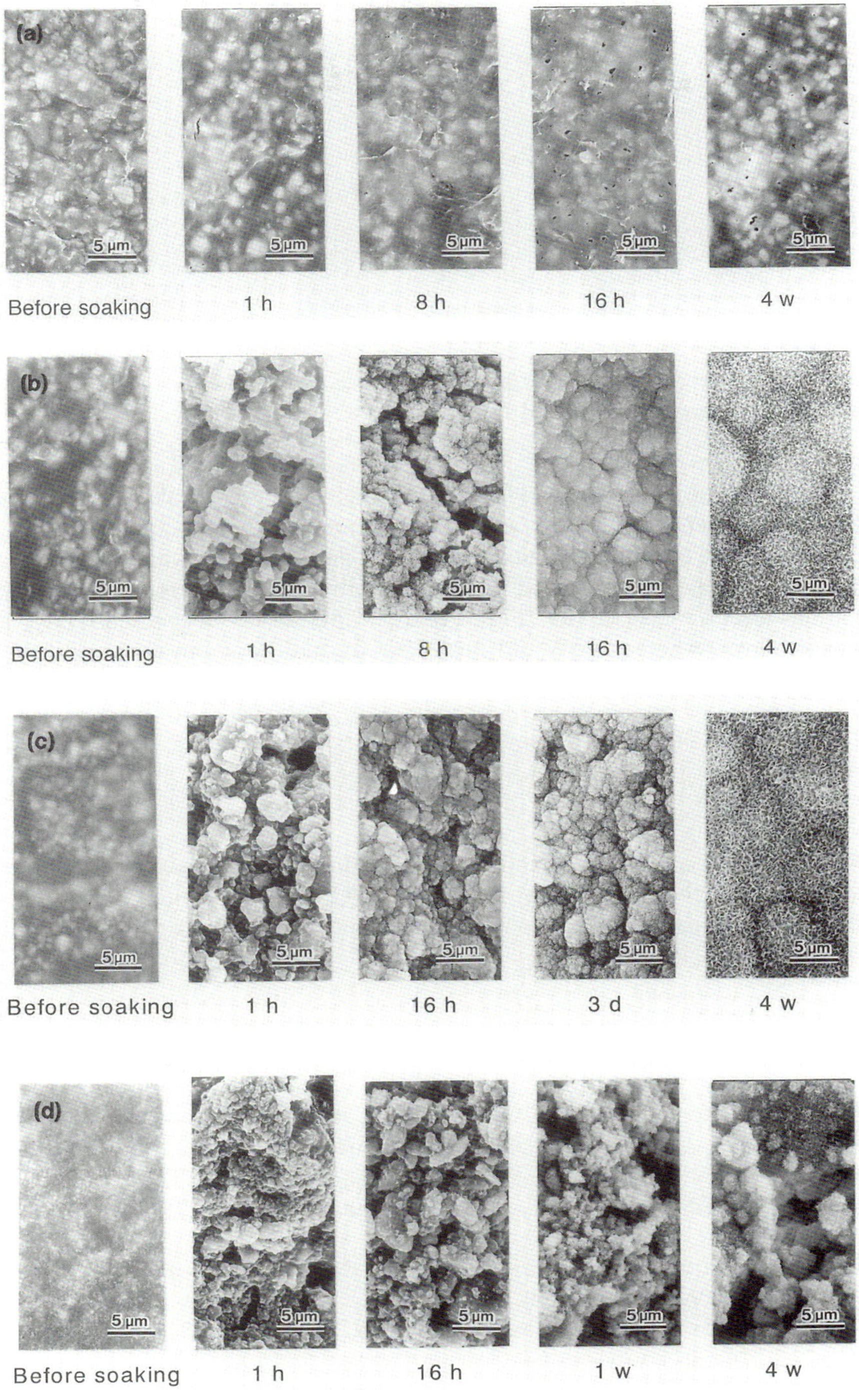

Figure 1. SEM photographs of surfaces of CSG-PMMA (a), CSG- (b), AW- (c) and HAp-Bis-GMA (d) composites soaked in SBF for various periods.

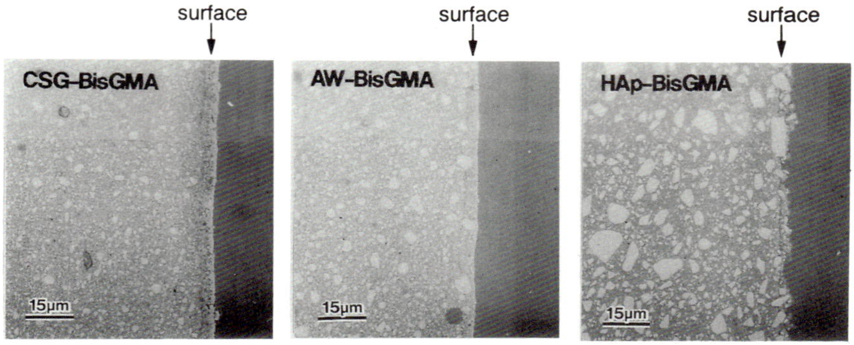

Figure 2. Back-scattering electron images of cross sections of CSG-, AW- and HApBis-GMA composites soaked in SBF for 4 weeks.

The rate of apatite formation varied with the kind of fillers. It takes 8 h, 16 h and 1 week, respectively for CSG, A-W and HAp to start to precipitate apatite. Both CSG and A-W formed a dense and uniform apatite layer on the whole surface of the composites, whereas HAp formed the apatite only on the surfaces of the individual filler grains after 4 weeks in SBF (Figs. 1 and 2). CSG formed a less dense layer under the apatite layer, whereas A-W did not. The formation of the dense and uniform apatite layer for CSG and A W was attributed to the catalytic effect of silicate ions dissolved from CSG and A-W and adsorbed on the composites for apatite nucleation [8]. The formation of the less dense layer for CSG was attributed to the fast dissolution of the glass grains into SBF.

CONCLUSION

PMMA-based composite cement does not form apatite on its surface in SBF and hence is not bioactive. CSG, A-W and HAp-Bis-GMA composite cements all form apatite and are bioactive. Only A-W filler cement forms only a dense and uniform apatite layer.

REFERENCE

1. Chow, H. C., *J. Ceram. Soc.* Japan, 1991, 99, 954-954.
2. Kokubo, T., Yoshihara, S., Nishimura, N., Yamamuro, T. and Nakamura, T., *J. Am. Ceram. Soc. ,1991,* 74, 739-1741.
3. Kawanabe, K., Tamura, J., Yamamuro, T., Nakamura, T., Kokubo, T. and Yoshihara, *S., J. Appl. Biomater.* 1992, 4, 135-141.
4. Saito, M., Maruoka, A., Mori, T. Sugano, N. and Hino, J., *Biomaterials.* 1994, 15, 156 160.
5. Kokubo, T., Ito, S. Sakka, S. and Yamamuro, T., *J. Mater. Sci.* 1986, 21, 536-540.
6. Kokubo, T., Kushitani, M., Sakka, S. Kitsugi, T. and Yamamuro, T., J. *Biomed. Mater. Res.,* 1990, 24,721-734.

7. Kokubo, T. *:Bone-bonding biomaterals,* Reed Healthcare Communications, the Netherlands. 1992, 31-46.
8. Abe, Y., Kokubo, T. and Yamamuro, T., J. *Mater. Sci. Mater in Medicine* 1990, 1, 233 238.

BONE-BONDING BEHAVIOR OF THREE TYPES OF BIOACTIVE BONE CEMENT CONTAINING BIOACTIVE GLASS OR GLASS-CERAMIC POWDER

J. Tamura[1], T. Kitsugi[1], H. Fujita[1], T. Nakamura[1], T. Kokubo[2], S. Yoshihara[3], and T. Shibuya[3]

[1]Department of Orthopaedic Surgery, Faculty of Medicine, Kyoto University, Kawahara-cho 54, Shogoin, Sakyo-ku, Kyoto 606, Japan, [2]Division of Material Chemistry, Faculty of Engineering, Kyoto University, Kyoto, Japan, [3]Nippon Electric Glass Co. Ltd., Otsu, Japan

ABSTRACT

Three types of bioactive bone cement (Types A, B, and C) were made from bioactive glass or glass-ceramic powder and BIS-GMA resin, and their bonding strengths to bone were evaluated. Rectangular plates (2 x 10 x 15 mm) of Type A (containing MgO-CaO-SiO_2-P_2O_5-CaF_2 glass powder), B (MgO-CaO-SiO_2-P_2O_5-CaF_2 glass-ceramic powder) and C (CaO-SiO_2-P_2O_5-CaF_2 glass powder) bioactive cements, PMMA cement, and A-W-glass-ceramic were implanted into the metaphysis of the tibia of male rabbits and the failure load was measured by a detaching test 10 weeks later. The failure loads of Types A, B and C bioactive cements, PMMA cement and A-W-glass-ceramic at 10 weeks were 3.01, 4.23, 2.88, 0.03, and 8.23 kg, respectively. Observation of the cement-bone interface revealed direct bone formation around all the bioactive bone cements.

INTRODUCTION

We have reported new bioactive bone cements consisting of bioactive glass or glass-ceramic powder and bisphenol-*a*-glycidyl methacrylate (BIS-GMA) resin [1, 2, 3]. These cements show direct contact with living bone and have high mechanical strength. In the present study, the bonding strengths of these bioactive bone cements were evaluated by a detaching test, and the cement-bone interface was observed.

MATERIALS AND METHODS

Cement Preparation

Glass with the composition of CaO 44.7, MgO 4.6, SiO_2 34.0, P_2O_5 16.2, and CaF_2 0.5 by weight ratio was melted in a SiC furnace at 1500°C for 4 h. The melt was quenched between water-cooled steel rollers to form ribbons, and then pulverized in an alumina ball mill to produce the glass powder for Type A cement [3]. Glass-ceramic with the same composition as the glass for Type A cement (A-W-glass-ceramic) was synthesized by the method reported previously [4]. The glass-ceramic plate was pulverized in an alumina ball mill to produce the glass-ceramic powder for Type B cement. Glass with a nominal composition of CaO 46.7, SiO_2 35.6, P_2O_5 17.0, and CaF_2 0.7 by weight ratio was prepared, melted and pulverized by the same procedure to produce the glass powder for Type C cement [5]. The average particle size of the glass and glass-ceramic powder was 5 μm. The powder was then treated with γ -methacryloxy propyl trimethoxy silane (Shinetsu Chemical Industry, Tokyo Japan) and benzoyl peroxide was added at a unit weight ratio of 0.4%. The BIS-GMA resin was prepared from equal weights of BIS-GMA and triethylene-glycol dimethacrylate (TEGDMA) (Shin-nakamura Chemical Industry, Wakayama, Japan) and N.N-dimethyl-p-toluidine at 0.2% per unit weight of resin, was dissolved in the mixture [1].

Each cement was prepared by mixing the powder (at a 70% weight ratio) into the BIS-GMA resin and stirring for 1 min. Polymerization occurred within 4 to 6 min.

Animal Experiments

Rectangular plates (10 x 15 x 2 mm) of Types A, B, and C bioactive cement, PMMA cement and A-W-glass-ceramic were abraded with #2000 alumina powder and sterilized in ethylene oxide. The plates of cement were made by solidifying the cement in molds.

The plates were implanted into the metaphyses of mature male rabbits weighing between 3.0 and 3.5 kg. A 16 x 2-mm hole was made from the medial cortex to the lateral cortex parallel to the longitudinal axis of the proximal metaphysis. The plates were implanted in a frontal direction perforating the tibiae and protruding from both the medial and lateral cortex. Each experimental group contained 5 animals (10 legs), which were sacrificed at 10 weeks after surgery (25 rabbits in total). A segment of the tibia containing the implant was excised and prepared for the detaching test using Nakamura's method [6]. The bone segment with the implant was placed horizontally and pulled in the opposite direction using an Instron-type machine at a cross-head speed of 3.5 cm/min.

Histological Examination

After the detaching test, the specimens were fixed in 10% phosphate-buffered formalin solution. The specimens were dehydrated in serial concentrations of ethanol and then embedded in polyester resin. Thin sections (500 μm thick) were cut perpendicular to the axis of the tibia with a band saw (EXAKT BS-3000, EXAKT Apparatebau, 2000 Norderstedt, Germany). The sections were polished with diamond paper for analysis of the interface between the implant and bone using a scanning electron microscope (Hitachi S-800, Tokyo, Japan) connected to an energy-dispersive X-ray microanalyzer (Horiba E-MAX5770, Tokyo, Japan). X-ray intensities for calcium, phosphorus, silicon, and magnesium were analyzed across the implant-bone interface.

RESULTS

Evaluation of Bone-Bonding Strength

Some implants of PMMA cement were detached from the bone before being detached by the Instron. Therefore, the failure load was defined as 0 kg. Macroscopically, every implant was detached at the implant-bone interface.

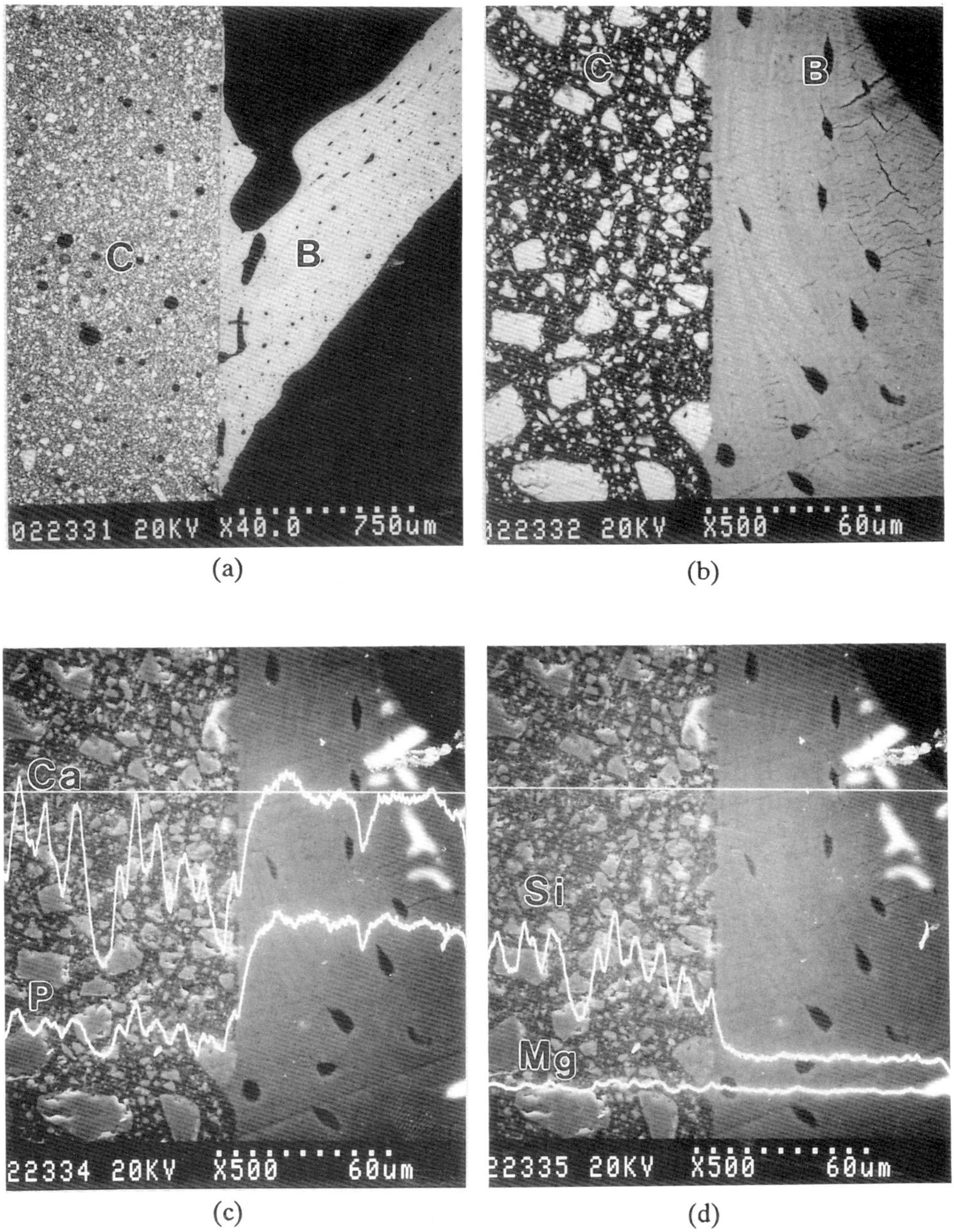

(a) (b) (c) (d)

Figure 1. Scanning electron micrograph and electron-probe microanalysis at the interface between Type B cement and bone 10 weeks after implantation in rabbit tibiae. (a,b) back-scattered electron image, (c) Ca and P, (d) Si and Mg. C: cement, B: bone.

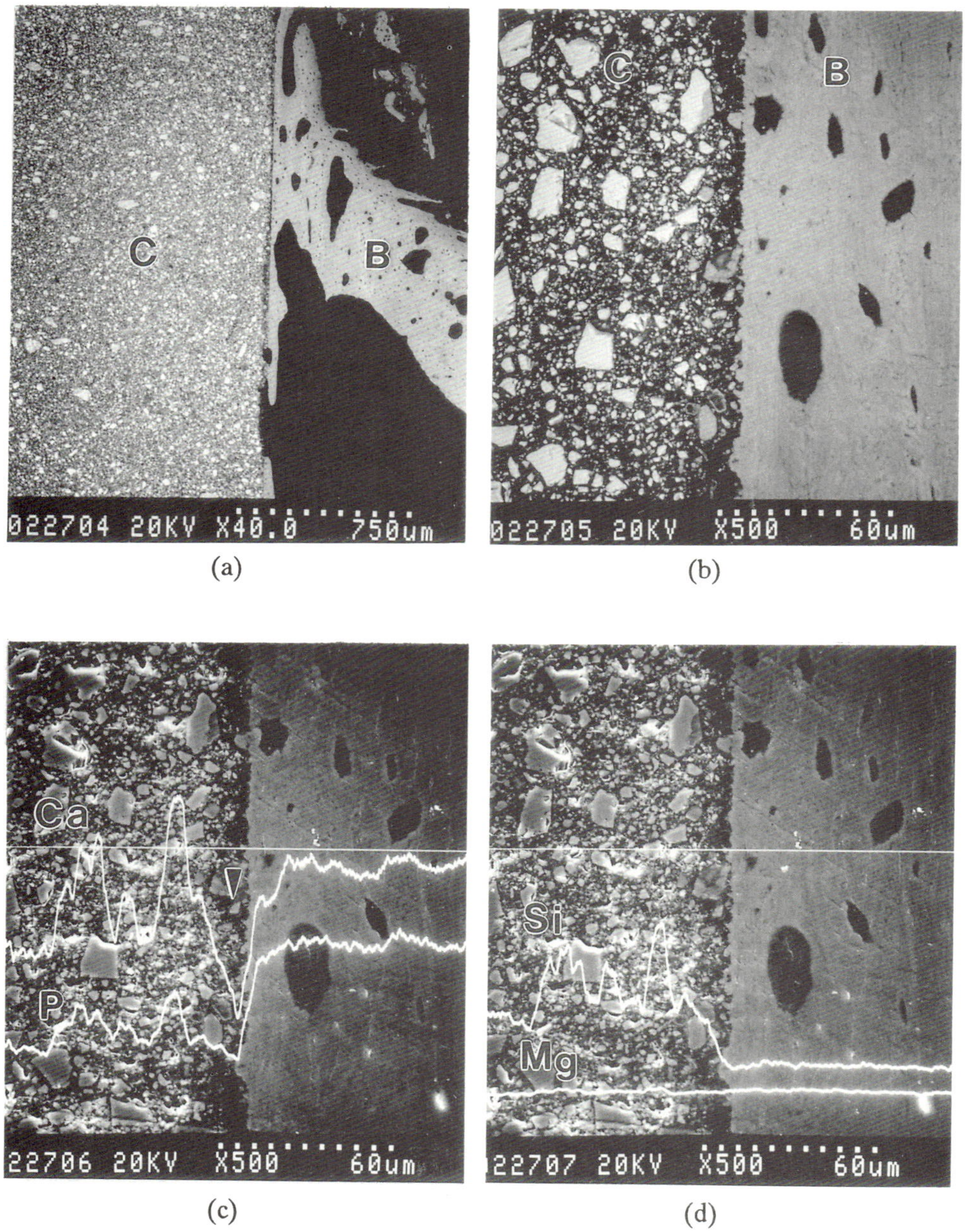

Figure 2. Scanning electron micrograph and electron-probe microanalysis at the interface between Type C cement and bone 10 weeks after implantation in rabbit tibiae. (a,b) back-scattered electron image. (c) Ca and P, (d) Si and Mg. A low calcium level layer is observed at the interface (arrowhead). C: cement, B: bone.

The failure loads of Types A, B, and C cement were 3.01, 4.23, and 2.88 kg, respectively, whereas those of PMMA cement and A-W-glass-ceramic were 0.03 and 8.23 kg (mean).

Evaluation of the Implant-Bone Interface

Scanning electron microscopy revealed direct bone bonding at the interface in the bioactive bone cements and A-W-glass-ceramic. Electron-probe microanalysis did not detect a Ca-P-rich layer at the interface in the bioactive bone cements, whereas one was observed in A-W-glass-ceramic. In specimens of Types A and C cement, a layer showing a low calcium level was seen at the interface (Figs. 1, 2).

DISCUSSION

We have been trying to make bioactive bone cements using bioactive glass powder or glass-ceramic powder combined with BIS-GMA resin [1, 2, 3]. These cements showed good bioactivity and high mechanical strength. The compressive strength of each type of bioactive bone cement (165-239 MPa) was more than twice that of PMMA cement (68 MPa), and bioactivity was high.

In the present experiment we attempted to evaluate the bone-bonding strength of the cements using solid cement plates. A detaching test showed that the failure loads of the bioactive cements were lower than that of A-W-glass-ceramic, but higher than that of PMMA cement. As bone cements are usually solidified *in situ* and mechanical interlocking reinforces this fixation to the bone, these values for bioactive cements should be sufficient. Among the bioactive bone cements, Type B (containing glass-ceramic powder) showed higher bonding strength than Types A and C (containing glass powder).

SEM-EPMA demonstrated a low-calcium layer at the interface, the calcium in the glass powder may have leached from this layer. In specimens with cement containing glass-ceramic powder (Type B), this layer was narrow or absent. These results confirm the higher degradability of glass powder compared with glass-ceramic powder of the same composition. The lower bonding strengths of Types A and C cement compared with Type B suggest a lower mechanical strength for this layer.

All the bioactive bone cements we tested have the ability to bind to bone, and also to function as a bioactive, low-modulus composite material.

This work was supported in part by a Grant-in-Aid for Scientific Research (No.05558112) from the Ministry of Education, Science and Culture, Japan.

REFERENCES

1. Kawanabe, K., et al ., *J. Appl. Biomater.*, 1993, 4, 135-141.
2. Tamura, J., et al., *J. Biomed. Mater. Res.*, in press.
3. Tamura, J., et al., *Bioceramics* Vol.7, Butterworth-Heinemann, Oxford 1994, 279-284.
4. Kokubo, T., et al., T., *J. Mater. Sci*, 1985, 20, 2001-2004.
5. Kokubo, T., et al., *J. Am. Ceram. Soc.*, 1991, 74, 1739-1741.
6. Nakamura, T., et al., *J. Biomed. Mater. Res.*, 1985, 19, 685-698.

HYDROXYAPATITE-TRICALCIUM PHOSPHATE FILLER FOR BONE DEFECTS ASSOCIATED WITH DISTAL RADIAL FRACTURE: COMPARISON WITH AUTOGENOUS ILIAC BONE GRAFTS

Katsuji Suzuki, Mitsuko Yamada, Kohsuke Yamamoto, and Kohichi Muramatsu.

Department of Orthopaedic Surgery, Fujita Health University School of Medicine. 1-98, Dengakugakubo, Kutsukake, Toyoake, Aichi, 470- 11, Japan.

ABSTRACT
The efficacy of a hydroxyapatite-tricalcium phosphate (HAP-TCP) filler for traumatic bone defects of the distal radius was studied by comparing 12 patients treated with HAP-TCP and 11 who received iliac autografts. The prevalence of osteoporosis was significantly higher in the HAP-TCP group (75%) than in the iliac autograft group (27%), but there was no significant difference in the range of motion (ROM) and grip power recovery times or in the volar and radial tilt angles. There was no significant difference in the radio-ulnar distance on the preoperative and immediate postoperative X-rays of the two groups, but at 1 year postoperatively the radio-ulnar distance was significantly greater in the HAP-TCP group than in the iliac autograft group.

INTRODUCTION
Filling of bone defects is necessary in patients with splintered or depressed distal radial fractures. Iliac autografts are often used, but problems arise due to the limited amount of bone which can be harvested and symptoms at the donor site. In the present study, we compared the effectiveness of repairing traumatic bone defects of the distal radius with a hydroxyapatite-tricalcium phosphate (HAP-TCP) filler or with iliac autografts.

SUBJECTS
Twenty-three patients who had distal radial fractures associated with defects which required filling were operated on in our department between January 1991 and July 1994.

Iliac autograft group: Iliac autografts were used in 11 patients from January 1991 to April 1992 (7 males and 4 females; mean age: 35.9 years; range: 16-76 years). Three of them had osteoporosis. Six patients were injured in motor cycle accidents, 3 were injured by falls, 1 had a bicycle accident, and 1 was injured in a fall from a height.

HAP-TCP group: HAP-TCP was used in 12 patients from May 1992 to July 1994 (7 males and 5 females; mean age: 54.0 years; range: 11-66 years). Nine of them had osteoporosis. Seven patients were injured by falls, 4 were injured in falls from a height, and 1 was involved in a traffic accident.

METHODS

In both groups, we investigated the prevalence of osteoporosis, ROM recovery time, grip power recovery time, and complications. The changes of the volar tilt angle, radial tilt angle, and radio-ulnar distance on X-ray films were also studied.

ROM recovery time: We determined the time required for wrist joint range of motion to recover to above 80% of that of the healthy side .

Grip power recovery time: We determined the time required until grip power recovered above 80% of that of the healthy side.

Volar tilt angle: We measured the volar tilt angle preoperatively, immediately postoperatively, and 1 year postoperatively on lateral radiographs (Figure 1-A).

Radial tilt angle: We measured the radial tilt angle preoperatively, immediately postoperatively, and 1 year postoperatively on anteroposterior radiographs (Figure 1-B).

Radio-ulnar distance: We measured the radio-ulnar distance preoperatively, immediately postoperatively, and 1 year postoperatively on anteroposterior radiographs (Figure 1-C).

RESULTS

Osteoporosis: The proportion of patients with osteoporosis was 75% in the HAP-TCP group and 27% in the iliac autograft group ($P<0.01$ x^2 test).

ROM recovery time: The ROM recovery time was 14.5+5.5 (M±SD) weeks in the HAP-TCP group and 15.1±7^2. weeks in the iliac autograft group (P=N.S.; Wilcoxon test).

Grip power recovery time: The grip power recovery time was 18.9±5.4 weeks in the HAP-TCP group and 20.1±8.1 weeks in the iliac autograft group (P=N. S.; Wilcoxon test).

Volar tilt angle: On preoperative X-rays, the volar tilt angle was -12.2± 10.2° in the HAP-TCP group and -2.9±16.8° in the iliac autograft group (P=N.S.; Wilcoxon test). On immediate postoperative X-rays, the volar tilt angle was 7.3±8.1° in the HAP-TCP group and 12.2±9.4° in the iliac autograft group (P=N.S.). At 1 year postoperatively, the volar tilt angle was 5.9±8.4° in the HAP-TCP group and 12.6±8.0° in the iliac autograft group (P=N.S.).

Radial tilt angle: Preoperatively, the radial tilt angle was 17.9±8.5° in the HAP-TCP group and 14.6±O.3° in the iliac autograft group (P=N.S.). In the immediate postoperative period, the radial tilt angle was 16.6±6.2° in the HAP-TCP group and 19.0±5.6° in the iliac autograft group (P=N.S.). At 1 year postoperatively, the radial tilt angle was 16.8±4.9° in the HAP-TCP group and 16.8±7.9° in the iliac autograft group (P=N.S.).

Radio-ulnar distance: Preoperatively, the radio-ulnar distance was 6.3±3.1 mm in the HAP-TCP group and 6.9±3.8 mm in the iliac autograft group (P=N.S.). In the immediate postoperative period, the radio-ulnar distance was 11.8±3.5 mm in the HAP-TCP group and 11.3±2.6 mm in the iliac autograft group (P=N.S.). At 1 year postoperatively, the radio-ulnar distance was 10.5±2.3 mm in the HAP-TCP group and 6.9±3.0 mm in the iliac autograft group (P<0.01; Wilcoxon test).

Complications: Postoperative infection did not occur in either group. Pain at the site of bone removal occurred in 3 patients from the iliac autograft group, while there were no complications in the HAP-TCP group.

CASE REPORTS

Case 1 was a 64-year-old woman from the iliac autograft group with an intra-articular comminuted fracture of the distal right radius due to a fall. The ROM

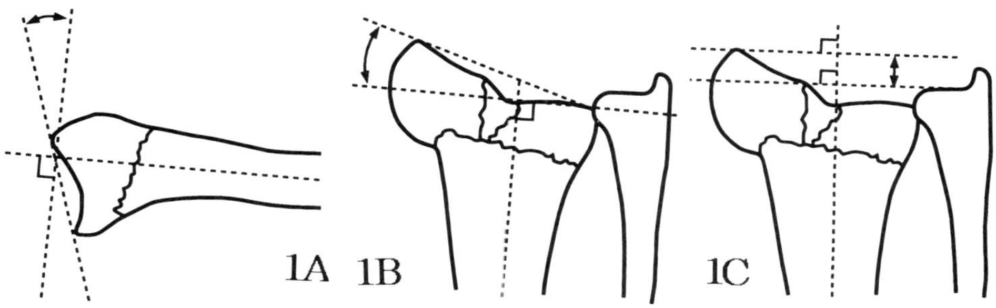

Figure 1. The measurements made on X-ray films. I-A:Volar tilt angle. The normal volar tilt angle was 11° (1 ° -21°). I-B:Radial tilt angle. The normal radial tilt angle was 23° (13° -30°). I-C:Radio-ulnar distance. The normal radio-ulnar distance was 12 mm.

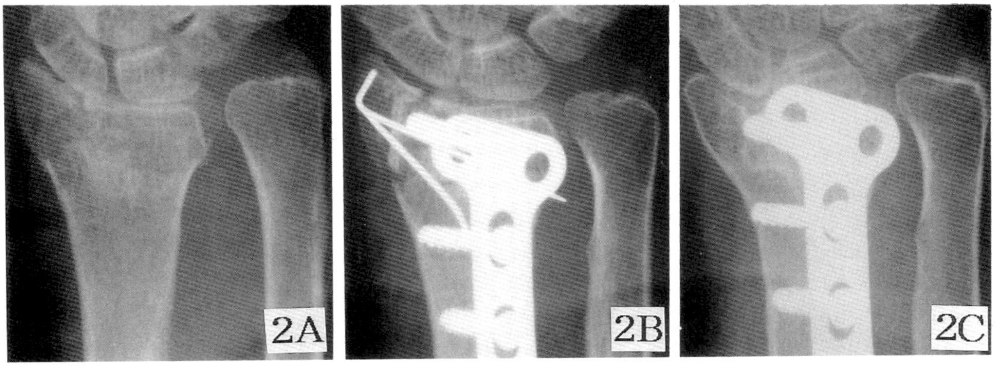

Figure 2. Case 1. A 64-year-old woman (iliac autograft group). 2-A:Intra-articular comminuted fracture of the distal right radius. 2-B:Immediately after surgery. 2-C:One year postoperatively.

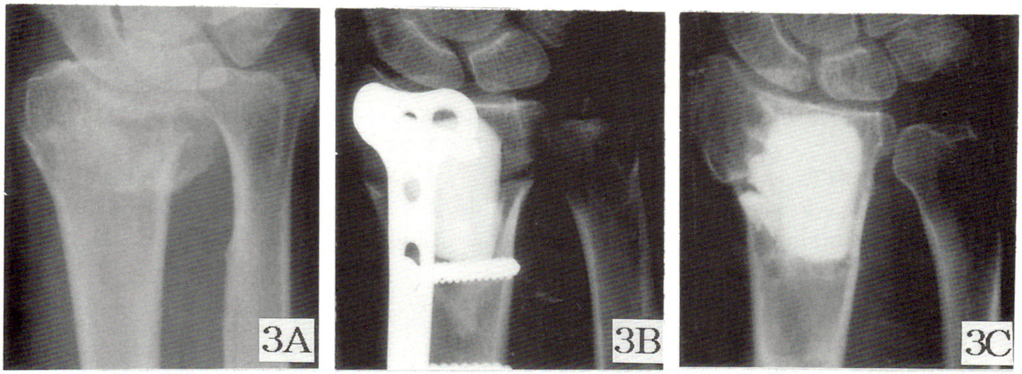

Figure 3. Case 2. A 61-year-old woman (HAP-TCP group). 3-A Intraarticular depressed fracture of the distal right radius. 3-B Immediately after surgery. 3-C One year postoperatively.

recovery time was 32 weeks and the grip power recovery time was 40 weeks. The volar tilt angle was -11° preoperatively, 14° in the immediate postoperative period, and 18° at 1 year postoperatively. The radial tilt angle was 18° preoperatively, 24° in the immediate postoperative period, and 8° at 1 year postoperatively. The radio-ulnar distance was 5 mm preoperatively, 9 mm immediately postoperatively, and 2 mm at 1 year postoperatively (Figures 2-A,B,C).

Case 2 was a 61-year-old woman in the HAP-TCP group who suffered an intra-articular depressed fracture of the distal right radius in a fall. The ROM recovery time was 10 weeks and the grip power recovery time was 12 weeks. The volar tilt angle was -25° preoperatively, 7° immediately postoperatively, and 120 at 1 year postoperatively. The radial tllt angle was 10° preoperatively, 12° immediately postoperatively, and 15° at 1 year postoperatively. The radio-ulnar distance was 2 mm preoperatively, 12 mm in the immediate postoperative period, and 10 mm at 1 year postoperatively (Figures 3-A,B,C).

DISCUSSION

Nakamura [1] inserted fresh autogenous bone grafts into rats and found that the compressive strength was reduced by 25%, 8 weeks after grafting. When autogenous bone was used as the filler, the graft was gradually replaced by new bone and its mechanical strength decreased during this process.

In experiments using rabbits, Hori *et al.,* [2] found that the compressive strength of HAP was only 11% of that of cancellous bone. However, the compressive strength of HAP increased to 71% of that of cancellous bone when it was packed into a bone defect and then removed after 4 weeks.

Suzuki *et al.,* [3] packed traumatic bone defects of the tibia with HAP-TCP filler and compared the efficacy of this filler with that of autogenous bone. The weight-bearing recovery time was significantly shorter in the HAP-TCP group than in the autogenous bone group. When HAP-TCP was used as the filler, it fused directly with the surrounding bone from an early stage. TCP also formed a strong union with the surrounding bone by gradual progressive substitution, and the HAP filler gradually increased in strength after grafting because of its excellent bone conductivity. Thus, the final strength of the filler approached that of normal cancellous bone.

In the present study, the radio-ulnar distance was normal immediately after surgery but decreased significantly by 1 year postoperatively when iliac autografts were used. In contrast, the radio-ulnar distance had not changed 1 year after surgery when HAP-TCP was used.

CONCLUSIONS

The prevalence of osteoporosis was significantly higher in the HAP-TCP group, but there was no significant difference in the ROM recovery time, grip power recovery time, volar tilt angle, and radial tilt angle. In addition, the 1 year postoperative radio-ulnar distance was significantly greater in the HAP-TCP group than in the iliac autograft group.

REFERENCES

1. Nakamura, S. *Kitazato lgaku* 1988, 18, 406-419
2. Hori , M., Munemiya, M., Takahashi, S., Sawai, K., Niwa, S.Tagai, H., Kobayashi, M., Ono, M. and Takeuchi, K *J.Chubu Orthop.Traumatol.*1984, 27, 2133-2135
3. Suzuki,K. and Kurabayashi, H. *Bioceramics,*Volume7, Butterworth-Heinemann, Oxford, 1994, 435-440

BIOMECHANICAL ANALYSIS OF THE FEMORAL STEM IN TOTAL HIP ARTHROPLASTY USING BIOACTIVE BONE CEMENT

M. Saito, A. Murakami*, N. Sugano**, T. Shibuya**, K. Yamaguchi, K. Hino***, and T. Ochi**

Department of Orthopaedic Surgery, Osaka Koseinenkin Hospital, 4-2-78 Fukushima, Fukushima-ku, Osaka 553, Japan, *Department of Chemical Engineering, Himeji Institute of Technology, 2167 Shosha, Himeji-shi, Hyogo 671-22, Japan, **Department of Orthopaedic Surgery, Osaka University Medical School, 2-2 Yamadaoka, Suita-shi, Osaka 565, Japan, ***R&D Department of Medical Products Division, Kuraray Co. Ltd., 1621 Sakazu, Kurashiki-shi, Okayama 710, Japan

ABSTRACT

We developed a hydroxyapatite composite resin (CAP) as a new type of bioactive bone cement. In this study, we examined the strength of the implant-CAP interface and performed finite element stress analysis of the femur after insertion of a total hip prostheses using CAP. The strength of metal-CAP bonds was greater than that of metal polymethylmethacrylate (PMMA) bonds. A marked decrease of bonding strength was found after distilled water immersion of the metal-PMMA specimens, while metal-CAP bonds showed less weakening. Finite element stress analysis showed that the high elastic modulus of CAP increased the stress acting on the cement compared with PMMA. However, this was not considered to be a significant problem because of the superior mechanical properties of CAP. In addition, the stress distribution in the bone was very similar for CAP and PMMA.

INTRODUCTION

We developed a hydroxyapatite composite resin (CAP) as a new type of bioactive bone cement [1,2]. CAP is composed of 80% w/w hydroxyapatite (HA) granules and a bis-phenol-A glycidyl methacrylate (BIS-GMA)-based resin. Although PMMA cement provides secure initial fixation of implants for patients, component loosening remains a major concern in long-term follow-up studies of total hip arthroplasty, especially in younger individuals. Development of a fibrous tissue membrane at the cement-bone interface and thermal damage to the surrounding bone during polymerization are causes of component loosening. These problems can be avoided by using CAP instead of PMMA, because CAP can bond directly with bone and the peak curing temperature is only 46°C [1]. Thus, CAP can provide a tight link with bone, but the strength of bond between the implant and CAP has not been determined. Recently, some authors have suggested that debonding at the implant-cement interface might initiate the process of component loosening [3]. The first objective of the present study was to examine the strength of the metal-CAP interface compared with the metal-PMMA interface. The second was to perform a theoretical analysis of the stresses acting throughout the stem, the cement (CAP), and the proximal femur, when a femoral stem was implanted using CAP. It has previously been reported that CAP has better mechanical strength and fatigue properties then PMMA cement [1,4]. However, the high elastic modulus of CAP is likely to alter the stress distribution in cement and bone compared with that obtained using PMMA [5]. Accordingly, the finite element analysis (FEM) method was applied to evaluate stresses in the human femur when CAP was used for total hip arthroplasty.

MATERIALS AND METHODS

Composition of CAP

CAP is a composite of HA granules (80% W/W) with a mean particle size of 2 μm and acrylic monomers plus a self-curing catalyst system. The HA granules are first sintered at 1200°C and treated with a silane coupling agent. The acrylic monomers used are BIS-GMA, 2,2'-bis-(4-methacryloylethoxyphenyl) propane (BIS-MEPP) and triethyleneglycol dimethacrylate (TEG-DMA). Polymerization is started by mixing approximately equal volumes of the two materials, mixtures of monomers and HA.

Strength of the metal-CAP interface

The strength of the bond between metal and CAP was determined by performing push-out tests on cylindrical specimens and was compared with values for metal and PMMA. The three metals used in this study were SUS316L, Ti_6Al_4 V, and CoCr alloys. Specimens were prepared by the method of Raab et al. [6] using cylindrical metal rods 6.4 mm in diameter and 25.6 mm long. The surfaces of the test rods were grit blasted and passivated in HNO_3 (30% V/V) for 30 min at room temperature followed by a thorough rinse in distilled water before autoclaving. The prepared rods were placed into Teflon molds and 4 ml of CAP in the dough phase (3 min after the start of mixing) was poured into each mold. Then the mold stopper was placed over the rod and pressed firmly against the mold surface. On completion of cement curing, the specimens were removed and stored at room temperature for 24 hours or immersed in distilled water at 37°C for 30 and 90 days to simulate the physiological environment. PMMA cement (Zimmer LYC, Zimmer, Warsaw, IN) was used as the control and metal-PMMA specimens were prepared by the same procedure.

Push-out tests were performed on an Instron, mechanical testing machine at a crosshead speed of 1 mm/min, and the bonding strength between metal and cement was determined from the maximum load at failure divided by the interface area. For each set of conditions, six specimens were tested. Differences in bonding strength between CAP and PMMA were assessed by the Student's t-test.

Stress analysis

A typical longitudinal section of a femur with a cemented prostheses was used as the analytical model. The thickness of the cement mantle along the stem was assumed to be 3 mm The elastic modulus was set at 20 GPa for cortical bone and 4.0 GPa for cancellous bone, while Poisson's ratio was 0.28 and 0.32, respectively. The elastic modulus and Poisson's ratio of the femoral stem were set at 200 GPa and 0.27, respectively, values characteristic of SUS316L or CoCr alloy implants. To model an object for stress analysis by the two-dimensional finite element method, it was divided into 230 elements. FEM V Post Data software was used. A 200-N load was applied to the head of the femoral component at an inclination of 16 degrees from the vertical.

Models employing CAP or PMMA to fix the femoral stem were examined and the predicted stresses within the stem, cement, and bone were compared. The elastic modulus of CAP was 15 GPa, a value relatively close to that of cortical bone and 5 times greater than that of PMMA (3 GPa). Poisson's ratio was 0.28 for CAP and 0.35 for PMMA. In addition, variations in the material properties of femoral stem were imparted to the basic model, and the changes of stress distribution were examined. The elastic modulus of the femoral stem was assumed to be 100 GPa (corresponding to that of Ti_6Al_4V implants) and 400 GPa (some ceramic materials).

RESULTS AND DISCUSSION

Strength of the metal-CAP interface

The strength of the SUS316L-PMMA bond was 14.6 MPa and that of the SUS316L-CAP bond was 13.3 MPa, with no significant difference between the two. However, the strength of the Ti_6Al_4V-CAP and CoCr-CAP bonds was greater than that of the Ti_6Al_4V-PMMA and CoCr-PMMA bonds, respectively. Ti_6Al_4V-PMMA bonds had a strength of 11.0 MPa and Ti_6Al_4V-CAP bonds had a strength of 17.6 MPa, the values were respectively 9.0 MPa and 11.4 MPa for CoCr-PMMA and CoCr-CAP bonds (Fig. 1).

Reduction of bond strength with water immersion was significant for all interfaces, except for SUS316L-CAP (Fig. 2). The strength of SUS316L-PMMA bonds decreased by more than 50% after water immersion. On the other hand, that of the SUS316L-CAP was 13.7 MPa after 90 days of water immersion and there was no significant decline. For both Ti_6Al_4V-PMMA and Ti_6Al_4V-CAP, the decline in bond strength occurred during the first 30 days of immersion, and the bond strength of Ti_6Al_4V-CAP (13.2 MPa) was significantly greater than that of Ti_6Al_4V-PMMA (6.1 MPa) after 90 days. With CoCr specimens, a decline in bond strength also occurred, but the CAP interfaces (9.3 MPa) remained stronger than the PMMA interfaces (5.7 MPa) after 90 days of immersion. Thus,

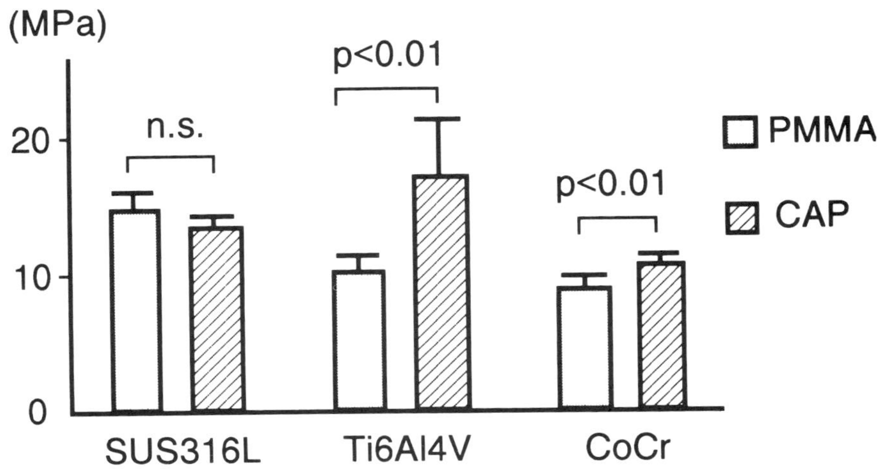

Figure 1. The strength of the bond between metal and cement.

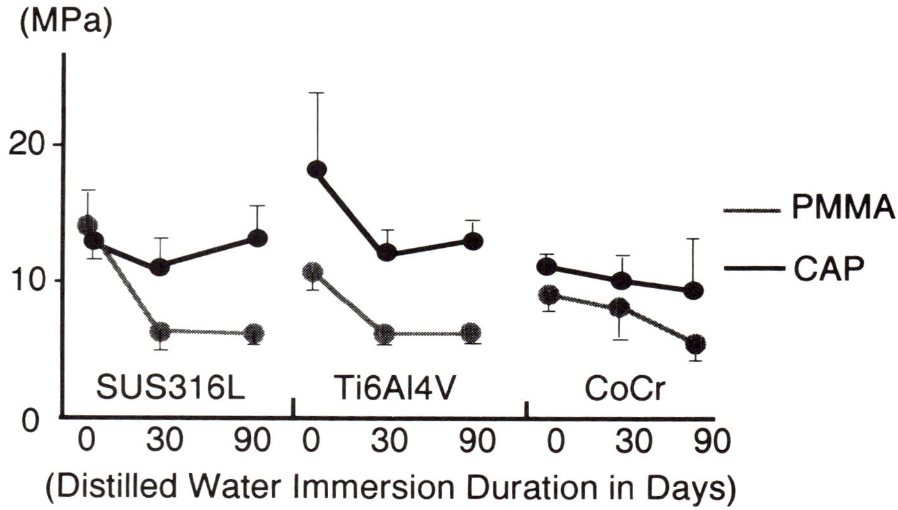

Figure 2. The effect of water immersion on the metal-cement bond.

CAP maintained stronger metal-cement interfaces than PMMA when stored in distilled water, and consequently might improve the *in vivo* durability of prostheses.

Stress analysis

Increasing the modulus of the cement from 3 GPa (PMMA) to 15 GPa (CAP) caused a 2.4-fold increase in the predicted value of the maximum compressive stress acting on the cement and a 1.3-fold increase in the maximum tensile stress. However, this was not considered to be a significant problem because of the superior mechanical properties of CAP. The compressive strength of CAP was about 3 times greater and the tensile strength has previously been expected to be about 1.4 times greater than that of PMMA [1]. Furthermore, the fatigue properties of CAP were also superior to those of PMMA [4]. The pattern of stress distribution in the cement differed between

CAP and PMMA. In the case of PMMA, the highest stress and strain within the cement was observed near the tip of the stem, while CAP cement showed a more uniform stress distribution (Fig. 3). On the other hand, the stress distribution in the bone was very similar for CAP and PMMA. Variations in the material of the femoral stem influenced the predicted stresses acting on both the stem and the cement. A decrease of the modulus of the stem increased the stress on the cement. Therefore, in order to reduce the stress on the cement, SUS316L or CoCr alloy stems, with a high elastic modulus, were preferable to the Ti_6Al_4V stem.

CONCLUSIONS

The strength of the metal-CAP bond was greater than that of the metal-PMMA bond, especially after storage in distilled water. Thus, CAP can provide a tight link not only with bone but also with the implant. The stress analysis study showed that the high elastic

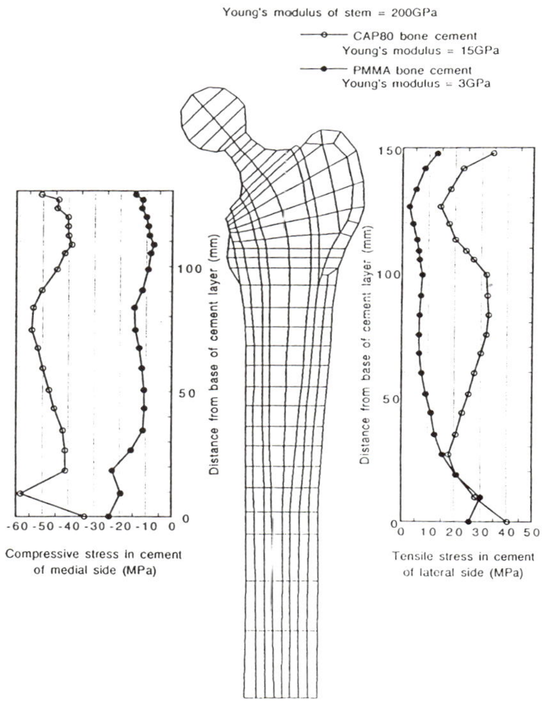

Figure 3. Predicted stresses acting on the cement.

modulus of CAP increased the compressive and tensile stresses within the cement when compared to PMMA. However, this should be compensated by the superior mechanical strength of CAP and the tight link provided with both bone and implant.

REFERENCES

1. Saito, M., Maruoka, A., Mori, T., Sugano, N. and Hino, K. *Biomaterials* 1994, 15, 156-160.
2. Maruoka, A., Saito, M., Sakai, H., Sugano, N. and Hino, K. Jn: *Bioceramics* Volume 7, Butterworth-Heinemann, Oxford 1994, 285-290.
3. Jasty, M., Maloney, WJ., Bragdon, C.R., Haire, T. and Harris, WH. *J. Bone Joint Surg. 1990,* 72-A, 1220-1229.
4. Saito, M., Maruoka, A., Mori, T., Kawakami, H. and Sugano, N. *Transactions of the 40th Annual Ueeting of the Orthopaedic Research Society* 1994, 19, 601.
5. Crowninshield, R.D., Brand, R.A., Johnston, R.C. and Milroy, J.C. *J. Bone Joint Surg.* 1980, 62-A, 68-78.
6. Raab, S., Ahmed, A.M. and Provan, J.W. J. *Biomed. Mater. Res.* 1981, 15, 159-182.

ENT AND MAXILLOFACIAL

BIOGLASS® MIDDLE EAR DEVICES: TEN YEAR CLINICAL RESULTS

June Wilson,[1] Ellis Douek[2] and Kevin Rust[3]

Bioglass® Research Center,[1] Division of Otolaryngology,[1,3] University of Florida, Gainesville, Florida, USA and Department of Otolaryngology, Guys Hospital, University of London, London, U.K.[2]

ABSTRACT

The clinical performance of middle ear devices made from 45S5 Bioglass® has been studied in two clinical trials. Long term, follow-up data of more than 10 years shows that extrusion has been eliminated and that hearing gains persist. A small incidence of late fracture *in situ* has been overcome by a modification of the original design. The modified MED has been in use since 1992 with no problems.

HISTORY

In the 1950's Wullstein was the first surgeon to recognize that plastic materials could be used to form a columella in cases with a destroyed stapes superstructure. Wullstein and Zollner presented their results in 1956 [1] and after that this new treatment concept spread world-wide. John Shea in 1957 began to use polyethylene; steel and tantalum wires were also used. Plester in his introduction to the proceedings of the Biomaterials in Otology meeting held in Leiden in 1983 [2], reviews this early work and states that *"The short-term results with all the alloplastic materials were usually excellent but the implants tended to extrude with time when they were in contact with the eardrum."* At the time of that meeting many materials were being tested to treat conductive hearing loss. They included Plastipore®, Proplast®, Ceravital®, hydroxyapatite, and aluminum oxide. In every case extrusion was frequent while in contact with the tympanic membrane and could only be postponed by the intrusion of cartilage or bone pâté between tympanic membrane and implant.

Preclinical research in the development of Bioglass® for middle ear devices was presented to the 1983 meeting [3,4] and Prof. Wullstein, who was present, was interested in the peculiar properties of this new material and how they might be used to improve middle ear devices. His advice, *"You have a very promising new material here, but you must be careful not to allow anyone to play with it."*, is sound advice which has, as far as possible, been followed. The property of bonding to the soft tissue of the tympanic membrane is the one which has reduced extrusion of devices made from Bioglass® to virtually zero, a decade and more after the discussions in Leiden.

INTRODUCTION

Conductive hearing loss is the consequence of a wide variety of pathological states and treatment depends on restoration of the ossicular chain between the tympanic membrane and the oval window. The clinical success depends on a multitude of factors and may be measured variously as improvement in hearing, change in the speech reception threshold (SRT) the air-bone gaps (ABG) and the pure tone average. However the alleviation of the deafness for which the restoration was required may be compromised by factors unrelated to the device, such as the need for a graft to replace or repair the tympanic membrane and the persistence of pathology, such as poor Eustachian tube function. Because the underlying clinical need varies from patient to patient it is not sufficient to measure device success or failure solely by the improvement or otherwise in measures of hearing ability. The major cause of failure, extrusion through the tympanic membrane, must be addressed before any middle ear device can usefully treat conductive hearing loss.

In this chapter, clinical results will be presented in terms of retention of the devices and other factors which result from the material used as well as hearing improvement measured by SRT, and ABG changes.

CLINICAL TRIALS

There have been two clinical trials, one at the University of Florida directed by the late Dr. G.E. Merwin, MD and the second at Guy's Hospital of the University of London and in his private practice by Mr. Ellis Douek, FRCS.

The University of Florida Trial

Between April 1984 and November 1987 devices were placed in 37 patients who were informed volunteers. Patients were usually worst case patients for whom no autograft ossicle was available and in whom previous reconstructions had failed [5]. Twenty five patients had total replacement of the ossicular chain and twelve a partial. Three had suffered traumatic disruption of the ossicular chain. All of the others had various levels of chronic otomastoiditis with and without cholesteatoma. In all patients, except the trauma patients, Eustachian tube function was poor or very poor.

Five designs of the middle ear prostheses were available to the surgeon who chose the most suitable size and shape and who could modify the device if necessary. [6] Such modifications most usually involved shortening or faceting the strut or shaping the device to accommodate a protruding facial nerve. These shapes are shown in Figure 1. Those with a rectangular platform were used when the malleus handle was present and were grooved to fit. The disc-shaped platforms were used when there was no malleus. The most bulky "blank" device was used when displaced or eroded ossicles were to be spanned.

The implantations were done using standard otological techniques, placed by two surgeons and their associated residents. Care was taken to remove the mucosa of the remaining ossicles where they contacted the bioactive surface to facilitate bonding. Once in place devices were supported by a suitable resorbable material, such as

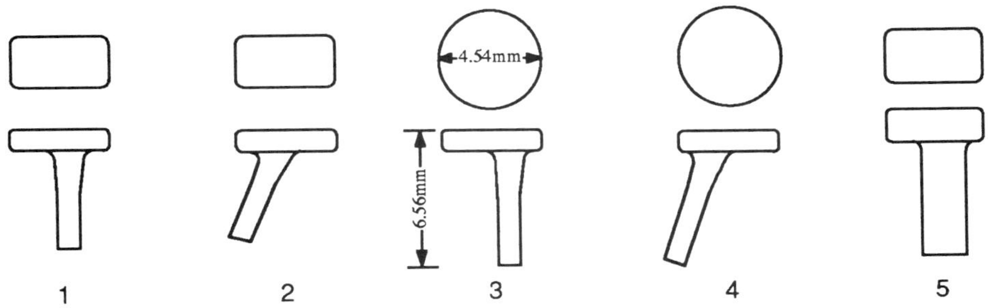

Figure 1. The five shapes available for the clinical trials.

Gelfoam® and the tympanic membrane, or fascial graft, where needed, replaced. No cartilage, bone pâté or any other material was placed between device and drum.

In 1994 all patients were contacted by mail and by telephone and asked to return for a follow-up examination. Of the 37, those who lived within a reasonable travelling distance of the University of Florida clinic returned for a complete otological examination conducted by K R. Others were examined elsewhere and the results were sent to the clinic. Failures were identified and the most recent follow-up times established for those patients who could not be traced. Those with follow-up times of more than 2 years have been included in the results.

RESULTS

Failures

Devices were removed intact from three patients with poor Eustachian tube function in whom the grafted eardrum failed. The graft functioned for three months in two cases and twelve months in the third. The devices were bonded to the ear drum when removed.

Device failures

No device failed by extrusion, but there were four fractures. These occurred after many years of successful function and were discovered at exploratory tympanotomy for worsening conductive loss after 38, 50, 84 and 126 months. In the first three cases the devices were removed and replaced. In the fourth case the fracture had gone unnoticed until the patient returned at the 10 year recall. In each case fragments of Bioglass® were found on the outer aspect of the tympanic membrane, held in place by squamous epithelium with no sign of inflammation. The eardrum was intact. In Figure 2 fragments seen after 84 months are shown. All of the fractured devices were those with disc-shaped platforms and right angle or obtuse angled stems, numbers 3 and 4 in Figure 1.

Device retention

Eleven patients were given a complete examination more than ten years after their original surgery. All were doing well, with the devices functioning as expected, although fragments were discovered on the outer aspect of the eardrum in one case, the patient had detected no adverse effect on her hearing.

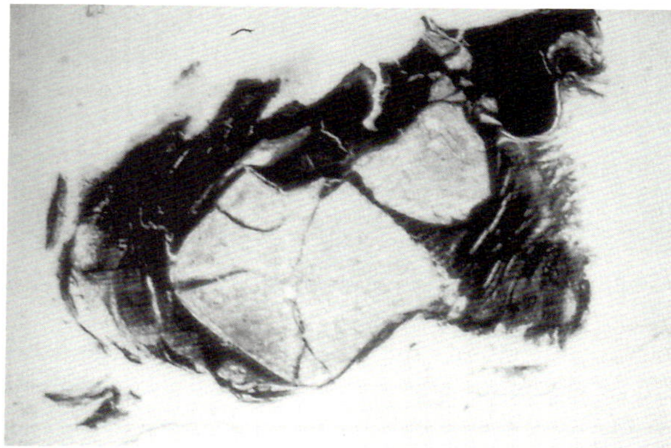

Figure 2. Small pieces of Bioglass® with associated squamous epithelium found on the outer aspect of the tympanic membrane.

In all, nineteen patients had follow-up data of more then 24 months, ranging from 24 to more than 120 months. The late fractures are included in this group. Fifteen more were lost to follow-up completely, although six of these had been functioning well at a 12 month follow-up visit.

In no case was there a failure of an intact device by extrusion. In the group followed for more than two years the mean SRT improved from 55 dB (range 30-95 dB) pre-operatively to 31 dB (range 5-75 dB) post-operatively and the pure tone average ABG from 46.5 dB (range 18-63 dB) pre-operatively to 24 dB (5-63 dB) post-operatively. The improvement in ABG was considered a success in 80% of the patients with partial replacement prostheses and 44% of those with total replacements. The hearing improvement has been maintained. The effect of the clinical condition and underlying pathology on these results, as well as more detail of the hearing data has been published elsewhere [7]. The distribution of patients in the UF trial is shown in Table 1.

Table 1

Follow-up of more than 12 months (includes one fracture)	11
Follow-up of 24 - 120 months (includes 3 fractures)	8
Lost to follow-up by 24 months	15
Unrelated failures	3
Total patients	37

The University of London Trial

In this study, which began early in 1985, twenty five patients were implanted between 1985 and 1986 under essentially the same conditions as those in Florida.

RESULTS

Failures

Devices were removed intact from five patients in whom postoperative hearing gain was minimal or non-existent. All had problems with poor Eustachian tube function and mobility of the footplate and the failure was not related to the device. In one patient with a failed, grafted eardrum, replacement graft and implant have functioned successfully for several years [8].

Device failures

Three devices in this study failed by fracturing, at approximately 48, 60 and 84 months. In two cases the devices were substantially drilled before implantation and were implanted with residual cracking. Post-retrieval histology on one showed fibrous tissue grown into and presumably widening the cracks. The third and latest device to fracture separated where the thin strut attached to the platform. All were successfully replaced with Bioglass® devices, of a different design.

Device retention

The remaining 16 patients have been followed to date. All are doing well and have maintained their hearing improvements for almost 10 years. The distribution of patients is shown in Table 2. Hearing data and clinical results will be published in the near future.

Table 2

Follow-up to approx. 120 months	16
Follow-up of 48-84 months (all fractured)	3
Unrelated failures	5
Total patients	24

Since the experiences in each trial were similar they have been combined to produce the overall distribution shown in Table 3.

Table 3.

Follow-up of 120 months	27
Follow-up 24 - 120 months	11
Lost to follow-up by 24 months	15
Unrelated failures	8
Total patients	61

DISCUSSION

The most important result to come from these trials is that no implant was lost by extrusion at any time.

There are already 27 which have survived for more than 10 years and a further 11 which are expected to do so. Of those lost to follow-up it is probable that many are functioning well even though they could not be traced for evaluation.

The patients in which the devices failed by fracture, had effective hearing treatment for at least four years and are thus included in the follow-up groups. This is longer than many other materials have functioned without extrusion. In some cases the design, or previous drilling on the device, was considered to be implicated in the failure. The discovery of fragments of glass on the outer aspect of the ear drum was decidedly unexpected, since the eardrums had no evidence of perforation. We can only suppose that these fragments had worked their way through the drum which had healed behind them. The time at which this had happened could only be guessed. However it can be assumed that the consequences of fracture may be considered benign.

Taking the fractures into account and the fact that experience had confirmed that devices made from Bioglass® could be easily contoured in the operating room by the surgeon, it was decided that the choice of shapes offered in 1984 was not essential and that a design which incorporated more bulk glass for contouring and a truncated cone shape which eliminated the vulnerable junction between platform and strut, might be more appropriate. Facets were added to facilitate handling in the operating theater and the new design seen in Figure 3 was produced in 1992 as the Douek-MED, it is a modification of the earlier devices seen in Figure 1. Twenty-two patients have been treated by E.D. with this new design since 1992. All are doing well with hearing improvement and no rejection or fractures.

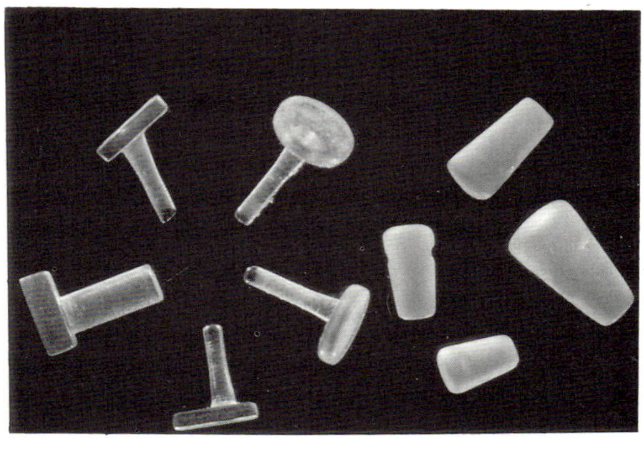

Figure 3. Middle ear devices in the original (LHS) and modified (RHS) designs.

CONCLUSION

Shea and Emmet, at the time of the 1984 conference believed that clinical success was dependant primarily on the underlying pathology and the skill of the surgeon and only secondarily on the properties of the implant material. [9] This is undoubtedly true and bourne out by the hearing results. However maximal support to the patient and surgeon is given by a material with properties which are optimal for this application, in this case soft and hard tissue bonding where needed and ease of shaping in the operating room, especially important where extrusion can be caused by too long a strut.

It is essential to understand both the importance of long term clinical data and the difficulty in acquiring it. Many materials, including porous and inert materials of many different compositions, have been studied in trials in which the data is given at 2 years, and which show relatively good results at that time with low incidences of extrusion. In many, if not most of these trials, the two year follow-up is the last one done since patients without problems tend not to return. Where published data for other materials exists it may be seen that the extrusion rate for polymeric materials can rise from an acceptable 5% at 2 years to an unacceptable 40% at five years [10]. Our results have used only the data collected after two years.

Finding and recalling those patients who had their implants more than ten years ago was frustrating, time consuming and expensive, but these results show as close to 100% success in avoiding extrusion as it is possible to achieve under the circumstances. No intact device has been extruded and the new design is expected to avoid the problem of late fracture associated with certain of the earlier shapes.

In a field in which failure by extrusion has been a major problem, devices made from Bioglass® do not extrude. Long term data of more than 10 years, presented here, make the results of these two trials unequalled in the field.

REFERENCES

1. Wullstein, H. (1956) *Laryngoscope* 66, 1076.
2. Plester, D. (1984) In: *Biomaterials in Otology* (J.J. Grote, Ed) Martinus Nijhoff, Boston, 1-5.
3. Hench, L.L., Wilson, J. and Merwin, G.E. (1984) *Ibid.* 62-69.
4. Merwin, G.E., Wilson, J. and Hench, L.L. (1984) *Ibid.* 220-229.
5. Merwin, G.E. (1986) *Ann. Otol. Rhinol. Laryngol.* 95, 78-82.
6. Wilson, J., Merwin, G.E. and Hench, L.L. (1985) *Sampe Journal,* 21-3, 6-8.
7. Rust, K.R., Singleton, G.T., Wilson, J. and Antonelli, P.J. (1995) In press, *Am. J. Otology.*
8. Wilson, J., Clark, A.E., douek, E., Kreiger, J. Smith, W. King and Zamet, J.S. (1994) In: *Bioceramics 7* (Andersson. Happonen and Yli-Urpo Eds.) Butterworth Heinemann, Oxford, 415-422.
9. Shea, J. and Emmett, J.R. (1984) In: *Biomaterials in Otology,* (J.J. Grote Ed) Martinus Nijhoff, Boston, 137-152.
10. Lobel , K.D. (1995) In: *Clinical Success of Skeletal Prostheses,* (L.L. Hench and J. Wilson, Eds.) Chapman and Hall, London 215-236.

DEVELOPMENT OF POROUS GLASS-CERAMICS IN AG-TITANIUM PHOSPHATES AND ITS ANTIBACTERIAL EFFECTS

Yoshihiro Abe,* Hideo Hosono,** Masayuki Nogami,* Toshihiro Kasuga* and Mitsuo Nagase***

* Department of Materials Science & Engineering, Nagoya Institute of Technology Gokiso-cho, Showa-ku, Nagoya 466, Japan; ** Research Laboratory of Engineering Materials, Tokyo Institute of Technology Nagatsuta, Midori-ku, Yokohama 227, Japan *** Department of Orthopaedic Surgery, Gunma University School of Medicine Showa, Maebashi, Gunma 371, Japan

ABSTRACT

New types of bioceramics for antibacterial or bacteriostatic application have been developed. In a previous paper [1] we prepared porous glass-ceramics with a skeleton of $CaTi_4(PO_4)_6$ crystal by controlled crystallization of glasses and subsequent leaching by HCl in the CaO-TiO_2-P_20_5 system. In this paper, the porous glass-ceramics with the surface crystalline phase of $AgTi_2(PO_4)_3$ and the interior phase of $LiTi_2(PO_4)_3$ are developed by ionic exchange of Ag^+ for Li^+. It is found that the resultant porous glass-ceramics show excellent bacteriostatic properties.

INTRODUCTION

Antibacterial or bacteriostatic materials such as zeolites and hydroxyapatite in which Ag^+ ions are adsorbed have been commercially used. We have developed a new type of bacteriostatic material of porous glass-ceramic whose surface consists of NASICON-type crystal of $AgTi_2(PO_4)_3$.

In our laboratory, calcium phosphate glass-ceramics containing no silica have been developed for biomedical uses such as bone implant materials and castable dental crowns. The glass-ceramic rods in CaO-P_20_5 prepared by unidirectional crystallization showed an unique fracture behavior of toughness similar to bone [1]. These were subjected to implantation in animal bone [2], but the mechanical strength decreased in a humid atmosphere. They are still in the improvement stage.

The durability of calcium phosphate glass-ceramics was improved drastically by the addition of alumina; these glass-ceramics (randomly crystallized) have received practical application since 1994 in Japan as castable dental crowns by using a lost-wax technique [3].

In 1989 porous glass-ceramics with a skeleton of $CaTi_4(PO_4)_6$ crystal [4] were prepared by a controlled crystallization of glasses in the CaO-TiO_2-P_2O_5 system and subsequent acid leaching of the resulting dense glass-ceramics composed of $CaTi_4(PO_4)_6$ and ß-$Ca_3(PO_4)_2$ phases which interlock with each other. The porous glass-ceramics in $CaTi_4(PO_4)_6$ have good immobilization properties of an enzyme of alkalophilic proteinase [5].

Since then, we have developed a series of porous glass-ceramics in $RTi_2(PO_4)_3$ (R = Li, Na, 1/2Ca) and found that Li^+ of $LiTi_2(PO_4)_3$ is easily exchanged for Ag^+. The resultant Ag^+-substituted porous glass-ceramics are found to exhibit bacteriostatic properties.

PREPARATION OF POROUS GLASS-CERAMICS OF $LiTi_2(PO_4)_3$

Neither chemical composition of NASICON-type crystal nor zirconium phosphate-type crystal can be prepared in a glassy state by the conventional quenching technique [6]. We found that there is a glass formation range in the pseudo-binary system at around equimolar compositions of $RTi_2(PO_4)_3$ and $Ca_3(PO_4)_2$.

The flow-chart of preparation process of the glass-ceramics (R = Li) is shown in Figure 1. Materials corresponding to equimolar composition of $LiTi_2(PO_4)_3$ (LTP) and $Ca_3(PO_4)_2$ (TCP) were melteld by using raw materials indicated in Figure 1, and quenched to form glass (1). After heating a dense glass-ceramic (1) without pores was obtained in which the crystalline phases consist of LTP and TCP; the former crystal is non-soluble and the latter is soluble in acid. Leaching of the dense glass-ceramic (1) with HCl resulted in the formation of porous glass-ceramic (2) with a skeleton of $LiTi_2(PO_4)_3$ (LTP).

POROUS $AgTi_2(PO_4)_3$ WITH INTERIOR SKELETON OF $LiTi_2(PO_4)_3$

Since the mobility of Li^+ ions in grain bulk of LTP ceramics is very high [7], it is expected that the materials will have excellent ion exchange properties. Recently we showed that porous LTP glass-ceramics have excellent ion exchanging properties and that the Li^+ ions in the LTP are exchanged with Ag^+ ions to form chemically stable $AgTi_2(PO_4)_3$ (AgTP) [8].

When the crystal compositions of the skeleton of porous glass-ceramics are changed from LTP to $Li_{1.4}Ti_{1.6}Al_{0.4}(PO_4)_3$ (LTAP), cation exchange rate is significantly enhanced, and the pore size is increased by a factor of 3 [9]. Table 1 shows the physical properties of these porous ceramics.

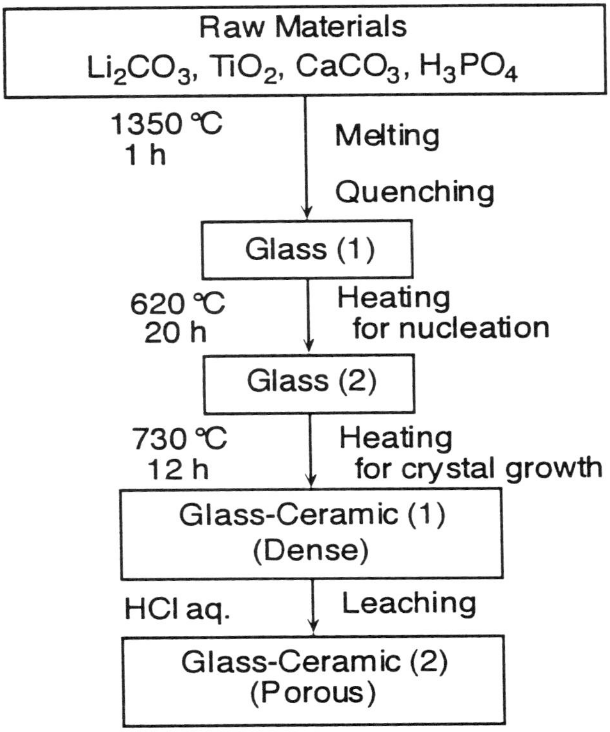

Figure 1. Preparation process of dense and porous glass-ceramics in Li_20-TiO_2-P_20_5 system.

Table 1. Physical and pore properties of porous $LiTi_2(PO_4)_3$ (LTP) and $Li_{1.4}Ti_{1.6}Al_{0.4}(PO_4)_3$ (LTAP) glass-ceramics.

	$LiTi_2(PO_4)_3$	$Li_{1.4}Ti_{1.6}Al_{0.4}(PO_4)_3$
Surface area (m^2/g)	30	8
Pore Volume (cm^3/g)	0.30	0.32
Porosity (%)	45	48
Apparent density (g/cm^3)	1.5	1.5
Bulk density (g/cm^3)	2.8	2.8

BACTERIOSTATIC PROPERTIES

The porous glass-ceramics (Ag-LTAP) with the surface crystalline phase of AgTP and with the interior phase of LTAP show excellent bacteriostatic properties.

Figure 2 shows the evaluation procedure of the bacteriostatic activity of Ag-LTAP porous glass-ceramics. In this test, alumina powders were used as a negative control material. Bacterial cell suspension was prepared by adding the bacteria (Escherichia coli: IFO 3301) at 10^4 cells/ml into the phosphate buffer solution. The granular samples, 30 to 300 μm in size, were sterilized by autoclaving at 120°C under a pressure of 100 kPa. A 2.5 mg of the glass-ceramic sample was added to 5ml of the suspension in a flask, and shaken well for 20 h at 25°C. The suspension was diluted with the phosphate buffer solution to bacterial concentrations of 10 - 10^3 cell/ml, and the resultant suspensions were added to soybean-casein-digest (SCD) culture medium. After the suspensions were incubated for 24 h at 36°C, the number of living bacterial cells were counted. Results are shown in Table 2.

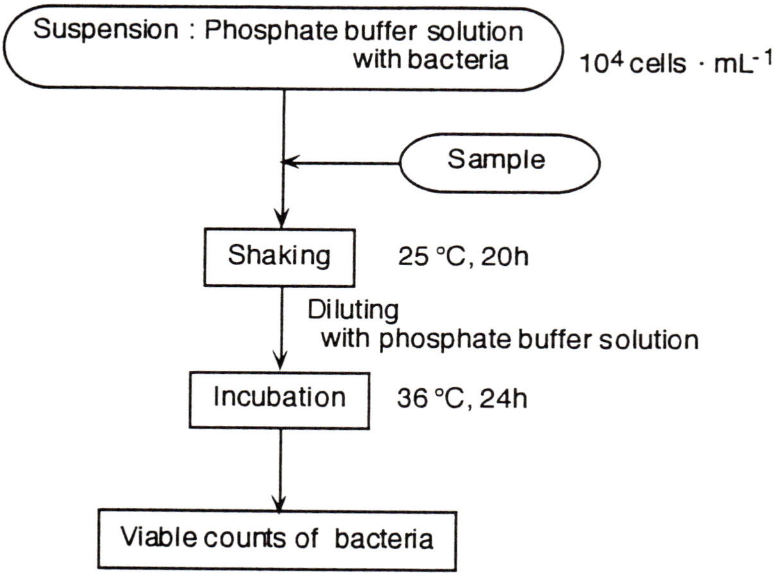

Figure 2. Evaluation procedure of antibacterial activity of the glass-ceramic obtained in this work.

Table 2. Result of bacteriostatic activity test using Escherichia coli.

Sample	**Viable Counts of Bacteria**
Alumina	2 x 10^5
Ag-LTAP	$<$ 1

CONCLUSIONS

Ag-LTAP porous glass-ceramics show excellent antibacterial or bacteriostatic effects (Table 2). Effectiveness against various other bacteria such as Staphylococcus aureus, Pseudomonas, and Streptococcus mutans has also been shown and the excellent bacteriostatic activities of the glass-ceramics confirmed [10].

REFERENCES

1. Abe,Y., Kasuga, T., Hosono, H. and de Groot, K *J. Am. Ceram. Soc.* 1984, 67, C142-144.

2. Klein, C.P.A.T., Abe,Y., Hosono, H. and de Groot, *Biomaterials* 1987, 8, 234-236.

3. (a) Kihara, S., Watanabe, A., and Abe, Y. *J. Am. Ceram. Soc.* 1984, 67, C142-44. (b) Abe, Y., Hosono, H., and Hosoe, M. *Phosphorus & Sulfur* 1987, 30, 337-340. (c) Watanabe, A., Mitsudou, M., Khara, S. and Abe, Y. *J. Am. Ceram. Soc.* 1989, 72 C1499-500.

4. Hosono, H., Zhang, Z., and Abe, Y. *J. Am. Ceram. Soc.* 1989, 72,1587.

5. Suzuki, T., Toriyama, M., Hosono, H., and Abe, Y. J. *Ferment Bioeng.* 1991, 72, 384-391.

6. Kishioka, A. *Bull. Chem. Soc. Jpn.* 1978, 51, 2559.

7. Aono, H., Sugimoto, E., Sadaoka, Y., Imanaka, N and Adachi, G. *J. Electrochem Soc.* 1989, 136, 590-591.

8. Hosono, H., Tsuchitani, F., Imai, K, and Abe, Y. *J. Mater. Res.* 1994, 9, 755-761.

9. Hosono, H. and Abe, Y., *Am Ceram. Soc.* 1992, 75, 2862-2864.

10. Hosono, H. and Abe, Y. *Mater. Res. Bull.* 1994, 29, 1157-1162.

INTERACTIONS BETWEEN THE FRONTAL SINUSITIS-ASSOCIATED PATHOGEN *HAEMOPHILUS INFLUENZAE* AND THE BIOACTIVE GLASS S53P4

P. Stoor*, E. Soderling*, O.H. Andersson** and A. Yli-Urpo*

*Institute of Dentistry, University of Turku, Turku, Finland
**Department of Chemical Engineering, Abo Akademi University, Turku, Finland

ABSTRACT
The bioactive glass S53P4 has been used as a filling material in treatment of sinusitis. The aim of this study was to find out if the sinusitis-associated pathogen, *H. influenzae* could colonize the glass and stay adhered to it during the formation of a Si-rich layer. Polished glass discs were first incubated with the bacterial suspension and then transferred to a simulated body fluid and incubated for 8 h at 37°C. The discs were examined with a scanning electron microscope. *H. influenzae* adhered to the glass surface, but after the 8 h incubation no microbes were detected on the discs. *H. influenzae* had left empty grooves on the surface of the discs suggesting that it would be metabolically active after its initial colonization. The bioactive glass S53P4, seems to be a good filling material with regard to avoiding *H. influenzae-associated* infections.

INTRODUCTION
Bioactive glasses containing SiO_2, Na_20, CaO and P_20_5 act in a surface reactive manner leading to a chemical bond with bone. *In vivo,* the bonding is due to the formation of Si and Ca,P- rich layers, to which osteoblasts adhere [1]. Thus bioactive glasses have been tested for use in various bone augmentation and as filling materials in operative treatment of maxillar and frontal sinusitis [2]. Bioglass®, a bioactive glass developed by Hench [1], has been extensively studied for various clinical applications.

Specific pathogens, like *H. influenzae,* are connected with complications of the conventional treatment of frontal sinusitis [3]. When using bioactive glass as filling material in frontal sinusitis the glass may come in direct contact with the pathogens. Sodium, calcium, phosphate and silica dissolve from the bioactive glass and the pH in its vicinity changes, which could affect the growth properties of bacteria or even act bactericidally. The first step in the development of biomaterial-associated infections is the colonization of a material [4]. In earlier unpublished experiments we showed that sinusitis-related microbes adhered to various bioactive materials and that these materials had no growth inhibiting effect on the microbes. The aim of the present study was to examine: 1) adherence of *H. influenzae* to the bioactive glass S53P4 [5] and 2) interactions between the bioactive glass and the microbe during the formation of a Si-rich layer on the glass.

MATERIALS AND METHODS

The bioactive glass S53P4 [SiO_2,53; Na_20,23; CaO,20; and $P_20_5$4 weight %] was prepared from reagent grade Na_2CO_3, $CaHPO_4$ x $2H_2O$, $CaC0_3$ (Merck, Darmstadt, Germany) and Belgium sand. The glass batches were melted in platinum-gold-alloy crucibles for 3 h at 1360°C. After melting the glass was cast into a plate in a graphite mould. The plate was cooled from 520°C to 220°C by 1°C/min in an annealing oven. At 220°C the oven was turned off and air cooled to room temperature. Discs of 4.0 x 4.0 x 1.5 mm were cut from the glass plates with a diamond saw. The glass discs were polished in ethanol on 4000 grit SiC-paper.

The microorganism used was *Haemophilus influenzae* (NCTC K1157 type b). It was grown in air supplemented with 7% CO_2 at 37°C on chocolate agar plates.

For the incubation experiments the growth of *H. influenzae* was tested in three different liquid media: 1) BHI (Brain Heart Infusion, Unipath LTD, England; calf brain infusion solids 12.5 g/l, beef heart infusion solids 5.0 g/l, proteose peptone 10.0 g/l, glucose 2.0 g/l, NaCl 5.0 g/l and Na_2HPO_4 2.5 g/l). 2) Simulated body fluid (SBF; 142.0 mM Na^+, 5.0 mM K^+, 1.5 mM Mg^{2+}, 2.5 mM Ca^{2+}, 193.8 mM $C1^-$, 4.2 mM $HC0^{3-}$ and 1.0 mM HPo_4^{2-}, pH 7.3) supplemented with 10 mM glucose and 3) SBF supplemented with 0.1 % casamino acids, 0.5 % yeast-extract and 10 mM glucose. The cultivations were performed in air supplemented with 7% CO_2. At the beginning the optical density of the cultures were adjusted to ~0.1 (A_{700}). Samples were collected every second hour to monitor pH, turbidity (A_{700}) and colony forming units (CFU)/ml .

The attachment and incubation of *H. influenzae* in the presence of the bioactive glass was performed as follows. After 10-20 h growth on chocolate agar plates, *H. influenzae* was harvested, washed once in TBS (Tris-buffered saline containing 10 mM Tris and 150 M NaCl, pH 7.4) and adjusted to an optical density of -1.0 (A_{700}) To attach the microorganisms to the polished glass discs, the discs were incubated with the microbial suspension for 15 min at room temperature, the surface area to solution volume (SA/V) ratio being 0.1 cm^{-1}. After the initial attachment the glass discs were carefully washed in TBS and transferred to SBF containing 10 mM glucose, and incubated without agitation at 37°C for 8 h, the SA/V-ratio being 0.1 cm^{-1}. The pH of the SBF was monitored every second hour. The control discs were incubated without bacteria.

To determine the possible bacterial growth in SBF during incubation, 100 μl samples of the 8 h SBF were transferred to 500 μl of anaerobic transport medium, serially diluted and cultivated at 37°C on chocolate agar plates overnight to determine CFU/ml.

For the scanning electron microscopy examination the glass discs were fixed for 5 min in 0.25% glutaraldehyde/TBS and dried in an ascending ethanol series for 15 min, once in 50% and 70% and twice in 96% and 100% and finally covered with a layer of carbon.

RESULTS

Three different liquid media were tested to find the optimal incubation conditions for *H. influenzae.* The two SBF-based media were used since the surface changes of the bioactive glass S53P4 in SBF are known [5]. BHI was used as a positive control medium. BHI was a good growth medium for *H. influenzae* (Table 1). The microbe was also able to grow in SBF supplemented with casamino acids, yeast-extract and glucose (Table 1). In these two media the pH decreased from 7.28 to 6.57 (BHI) and from 7.20 to 6.45 (SBF) during the 8 h incubation. SBF supplemented with glucose only kept the microbe viable and the smallest change in pH was observed for this medium (Table 1). Since the pH of the medium will affect the surface reactions of the glass the SBF supplemented with glucose was used in the incubation experiments of the colonized glass discs.

H. influenzae colonized the glass discs during the initial 15 min attachment period in TBS (Fig. l). The microorganism showed adhesion-mediated adherence to the glass surface (Fig. l). However, after the 8 h incubation in glucose supplemented SBF no microbes were detected on the glass surface. Empty grooves resembling the shape of initially attached bacteria were seen (Fig. 2). The numbers of the grooves and the initially attached bacteria appeared to be similar. Samples of the SBF collected after 8 h incubation showed no microbial growth. Even though *H. influenzae* decreased the pH of the SBF supplemented with glucose in the above growth experiments, in the experiment with the glass discs the pH of the medium increased from 7.25 to 7.49 during the 8 h incubation.

DISCUSSION

Adherence of bacteria to mucosal surfaces is generally believed to be the first step in the pathogenesis of many infectious diseases. *H. influenzae* possesses fimbriae which promote its adherence to epithelial cells [6] through specific receptors on the eucaryotic cells [7]. *H. influenzae* expresses also other kinds of adhesions since non-fimbriated bacteria adhere to epithelial cells as well [8]. The expression of fimbriae in *H. influenzae* appears to be subject to phase variation [9]. The colonization of a biomaterial is believed to lead to biomaterial associated infections [4]. In our experiments *H. influenzae* colonized the surface of the bioactive glass S53P4. Depending on the experimental conditions the adhesion of *H. influenzae* to the glass involved (present results) or did not involve (unpublished results) adhesions.

Table 1. Changes in medium pH and viable counts (log CFU/ml) of *H. influenzae* incubated in BHI, SBF supplemented with casamino acids, yeast-extract and glucose (1) and SBF supplemented with glucose only (2).

Time	BHI		SBF(1)		SBF(2)	
	pH	CFU/ml	pH	CFU/ml	pH	CFU/ml
Start	7.28	6.64	7.20	6.82	7.37	6.38
2 h	6.90	6.93	6.68	6.79	7.02	6.65
4 h	6.72	7.06	6.62	6.92	6.92	6.65
6 h	6.59	7.15	6.63	6.89	6.80	6.45
8 h	6.57	7.05	6.45	7.00	6.80	6.41

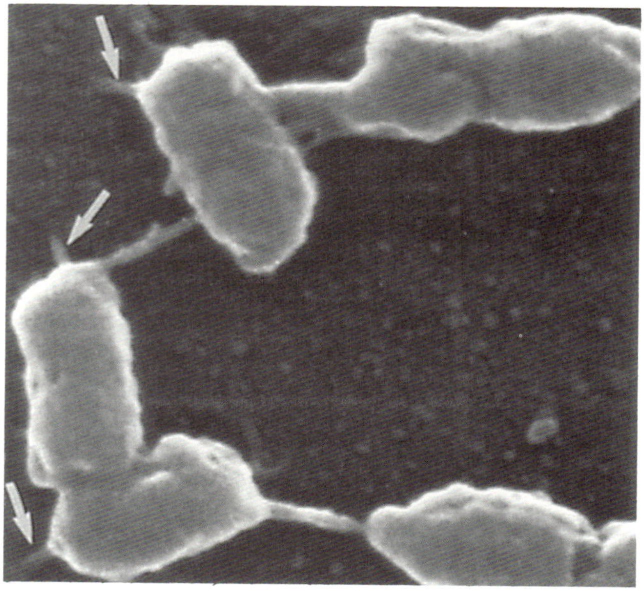

Figure 1. *H. influenzae* colonizing the surface of the bioactive glass S53P4 after the initial attachment. Adhesions indicated by arrows. The length of the figure is 2.5 μm.

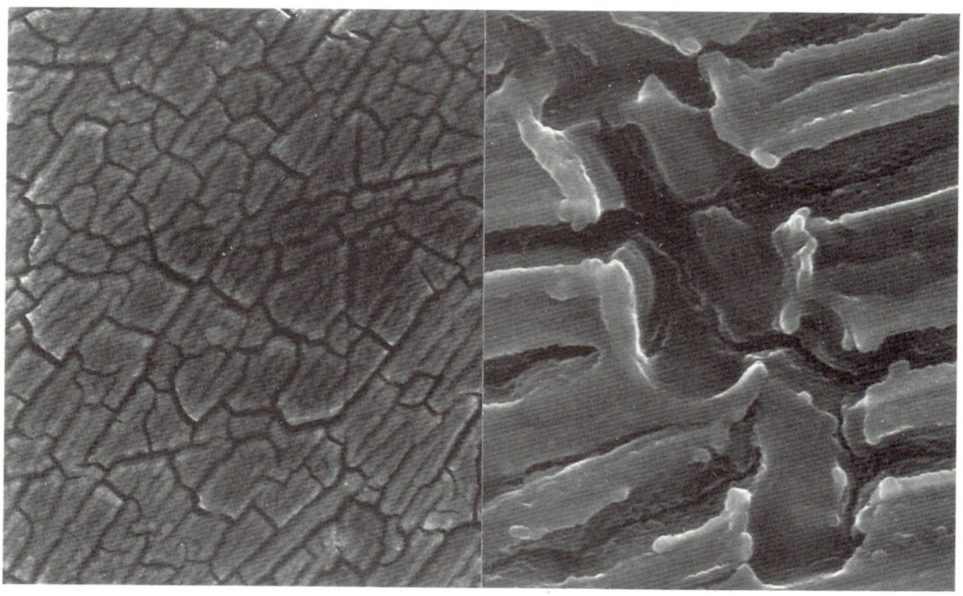

Figure 2. To the left; the Si-rich layer on the control disc after 8 h incubation, the length of the figure is 64 μm. To the right; close-up of two empty grooves on the *H. influenzae*-colonized glass surface after 8 h incubation, the length of the figure is 6.4 μm.

Since no proteins were involved in the present experimental design *H. influenzae* attached to the glass surface itself. The bond appeared strong since the bacteria could not be detached from the glass with mild sonication without loss of viability (unpublished results). Bioactive glasses have negative surface potentials in aqueous solutions above its isoelectric point, which is about pH 2 [10]. The surface attracts Ca^{2+} and Na^{+} ions as a result of the negative surface potential creating an electric double layer. At physiological pH, the *H. influenzae* cells have a negative net charge. Under these experimental conditions the initial binding between the bioactive glass and *H. influenzae* was most probably mediated by Ca^{2+}. This mechanism is commonly involved in adhesion between negatively charged bacteria and negatively charged surfaces or groups of proteins. According to Andersson [11] the accumulation of amorphous calcium phosphate at the surface of glass S53P4 at a SA/V ratio of 0.1 cm^{-1} in Tris-buffer, starts at about 1.2 h. It is expected that the same occurs in SBF. The formation of this Ca,P-rich layer will increase the ability of the glass surface to bind bacteria [12].

The detachment of the *H. influenzae* during the 8 h incubation was connected with the appearance of grooves in the glass surface. Several explanations for this phenomenon can be offered. Firstly, even though the pH changes in the experiments in which *H. influenzae* was attached to the glass were small during the 8 h incubation, local pH changes could be large. In fact, the pH of the SBF should have increased significantly due to dissolution of the bioactive glass if no microorganisms had been present. Kokubo reported that apatite did not form in SBF at pH 6 or pH 4 [13]. This suggests that also the accumulation of amorphous calcium phosphate, with a possible stabilizing effect on the Si-rich layer, might decrease with decreasing pH. Secondly, it has been reported that organic acids promote dissolution of glass by forming complexes with calcium and silicon in neutral solutions [14]. Bacteria, however, produce acids with low complex forming ability and thus, this explanation for the groove formation seems unlikely. Thirdly, the involvement of simple "physical" effects of *H. influenzae* on the groove formation in the glass surface cannot be excluded.

Since the grooves resembled the shape of the microbe it is possible that the detachment of the bacteria took place only at a late stage of the incubation. The detachment mechanism can only be hypothesized. It could involve the replacement of Ca^{+} mediating the cell bonding with protons produced by the bacteria. According to Rappaport et al. the detachment of mammalian cells from glasses occurs due to this phenomenon [15].

According to our earlier unpublished studies, the growth of *H. influenzae is* not inhibited by the presence of the bioactive glass S53P4. The present results show that *H. influenzae,* even though it can colonize the bioactive glass S53P4 and stay metabolically active when attached to the glass, was detached during the 8 h incubation period. Thus, to avoid *H.* influenzae-associated infections the bioactive glass S53P4 appears to be a good filling material. Our further studies with *H. influenzae* focus on the time dependency of the groove formation in different media as well as on the attachment mechanism in the presence of serum proteins.

REFERENCES

1. Hench, L.L. and Paschall, H.A. J. *Biomed. Mater. Res.* 1973, 3, 25-42.
2. Aitasalo, K., Peltola, M., Suonpää, J., Yli-Urpo, A., Andersson, O.H., Varpula, M. and Happonen, R-P. In: *Bioceramics* Volume 7, Andersson, O.H., Happonen, R-P.

and Yli-Urpo, A. Butterworth-Heinemann, Oxford 1994, 409-414.

3. Kilian, M. In: *Manual of Clinical Microbiology* 5th ed, Balows, A., Hausler, WJ., Herrmann, K.L., Isenberg, H.D. and Shadomy, HJ. American Society for Microbiology, Massachusetts, Washington DC 1991, 463-470.
4. Wadstrom, T., *J. Invest. Surg.* 1989, 2, 353-360.
5. Andersson, O.H., The Bioactivity of Silicate Glass, Thesis, Abo Akademi University, Finland 1990.
6. Guerina, N.G., Langermann, S., Clegg, H.W., Kessler, T.W., Goldmann, D.A. and Gilsdorf, JR. *J. Infect Dis.* 1982, 146, 564.
7. van Alphen, L., Geelen-van den Broek, L., Blaas, L., van Ham, M. and Dankert, J. *Infect. Immun.* 1991, 59, 4473-4477.
8. Read, R.C., Wilson, R., Rutman, A., Lund, V., Todd, H.C., Brain, A P., Jeffery, P.K. and Cloe, PJ. *J. Infect. Dis.* 1991,163, 549-558.
9. van Ham, S.M., van Alphen, L. and Mooi, F.R. *J. Inf.. Dis.* 1992, 165, 97-99.
10. Iler, R.K. *The Chemistry of Silica,* John Wiley & Sons, New York, 1979.
11. Andersson, (O.H. and Karlsson, K.H. In: *Bone-bonding biomaterials,* Ducheyne, P., Kokubo, T. and Van Blitterswijk C.A. Reed Healthcare Communications 1992,7984.
12. Stoor, P., Kirstilä, V., Soderling, E., Kangasniemi, I., Herbst, K. and Yli-Ürpo, A. Unpublished data.
13. Kokubo, T., Kushitani, H., Sakka, S., Kitsugi, T. and Yamamuro, T., *J. Biomed. Mater. Res.* 1990, 24, 721-734.
14. Bacon, F.R. and Raggon, F.C. *J. Amer. Cer. Soc.* 1959, 42, 199-205.
15. Rappaport, C., Poole, J.P. and Rappaport H P. *Exptl. Cell Research* 1960, 20, 465479.

AUGMENTATION OF THE MAXILLARY SINUS WALL USING BIOACTIVE GLASS AND AUTOLOGOUS BONE

T. Turunen[1], J. Peltola[1], I. Kangasniemi[2], J. Jussila[3], E. Uusipaikka[4], A. Yli-Urpo[2] and R-P. Happonen[1]

Departments of Oral and Maxillofacial Surgery[1], Prosthodontics[2], and Statistics[4], University of Turku and Faculty of Veterinary Science[3], University of Helsinki, Finland

ABSTRACT

Usefulness of bioactive glass (BG), autologous bone and BG (AB+BG), and autologous bone (AB) for augmentation of the maxillary sinus wall was studied in sheep. Space for augmentation was created by pressing the bone plate drilled on the lateral sinus wall into the sinus. Histomorphometrical analysis at 12 weeks showed that new bone occupied 5.9, 15.8, and 34.1 % of the augmentation area in BG, AB+BG, and AB groups, respectively. Bone and BG granules together comprised 47.2 % of the augmentation area in BG group and 44.4 % in AB+BG group. Mixture of BG granules and autologous bone chips may prove beneficial for sinus augmentation procedure.

INTRODUCTION

Various methods have been investigated to create sufficient amounts of bone for placement of endosseous implants in atrophic alveolar crests. Problems exist often in the posterior maxilla due to proximity of the maxillary sinus. Augmentation of the maxillary sinus floor with autologous bone graft is a widely used method to solve this problem [1]. However, harvesting of bone prolongs surgical procedure and results in increased postoperative morbidity [2]. For this reason, use of various bone substitute materials has been studied [3]. We have compared the use of bioactive glass (BG) granules and autologous bone (AB) chips for augmentation of the maxillary sinus wall.

MATERIALS AND METHODS

The chemical composition of BG used is SiO_2 53.0, Na_2O 23.0, CaO 20.0 and P_2O_5 4.0 in weight percentages [4]. Autologous bone was harvested from the mandibular angulus area through a submandibular incision. BG granules (800-1000 μm; BG group) and autologous bone chips (2-4 mm; AB group) were used for augmentation of 10 and 8 sinuses, respectively. A mixture of bone and BG granules (1:1) (AB+BG group) was used in 8 sinuses.

Adult sheep (weight 40-80 kg) were operated under general anesthesia and standard aseptic conditions. The lateral aspect of the maxillary sinus of each animal was exposed bilaterally through extraoral incisions. A bone window (10x15 mm) was drilled on the lateral wall. The space for augmentation was created by pressing the bone plate 8-10 mm into the sinus preserving the sinus mucosa intact (Fig. 1A). The animals were given benzylpenicillin procaine 30 mg/kg (Ilcocillin® 300 mg/ml, Lääkefarmos) and phenylbutazone 10 mg/kg (Reumuzol® 200 mg/ml, Lääkefarmos) i.v. at the operation and postoperatively for 2 days. The experiment periods were 8 and 12 weeks.

Resected bone blocks were fixed in 70 % ethanol and embedded in methylmethacrylate (Technovit 7200®, Kulzer GmbH). A cutting-grinding method [5]was used to prepare histological sections (20 μm) transversely through the sinus at

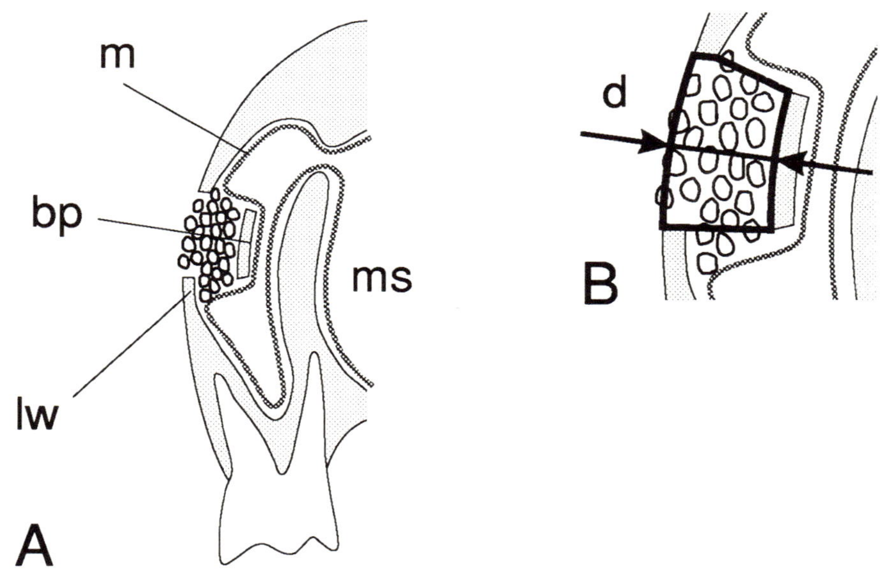

Figure 1. A. Space for augmentation was created by pressing the bone plate (bp) drilled on the lateral sinus wall (lw) into the maxillary sinus (ms). Attention was paid to avoid perforation of the mucosa (m).
B. Outlining indicates the augmentation area used in histomorphometrical analysis. Depth of the augmentation (d) was measured as the distance between the inner aspect the bone plate and the outer aspect of the sinus wall.

three levels. The sections were stained with toluidine blue and modified van Gieson method and analyzed by light microscopy. A computerized analysis system (Micro-Scale TC, Digithurst Ltd, Royston, England) was used for histomorphometrical evaluation. The amount of bone and BG was measured as percentages of the augmentation area (Fig. 1B). Furthermore, the depth of the augmentation was measured (Fig. 1B). The statistical computation was performed with SAS MIXED procedure [6].

RESULTS

In BG group, mostly dense connective tissue with foci of chronic inflammatory cells was seen between the BG granules (Figs. 2A-B). Bone formation was scanty at 8 weeks. Abundant bone formation was found by 12 weeks between BG granules in AB+BG group (Fig. 2C). Newly formed bone was in tight contact with BG granules (Fig. 2D). No giant cells or foreign body reaction was detected in either group. A considerable amount of bone was seen in AB group here shown at 8 weeks (Figs. 2E-F). Statistically significant differences were found in the amount of bone formation between BG and AB+BG groups (p=0.0003), BG and AB (p=0.0003) groups, as well as AB+BG and AB groups (p=0.0003) (Table 1). This difference was the same for both time periods. The mean depth of the augmentation was 5.0 mm. 4.9 mm, and 2.7 mm in BG, AB+BG, and AB groups respectively.

Table 1. Mean values (standard deviations) of bone and bone-bioactive glass (BG) area in the study groups given as percentages of the augmentation area.

	BG	AB+BG	AB*
8 WEEKS			
BONE	4.3 (1.5)	14.1 (8.8)	24.8 (6.6)
BONE+BG	47.5 (4.5)	43.5 (6.5)	-
12 WEEKS			
BONE	5.9 (1.2)	15.8 (4.5)	34.1 (16.4)
BONE+BG	47.2 (7.2)	44.4 (12.7)	-

*Considerable reduction of the augmentation due to resorption of the transplanted bone

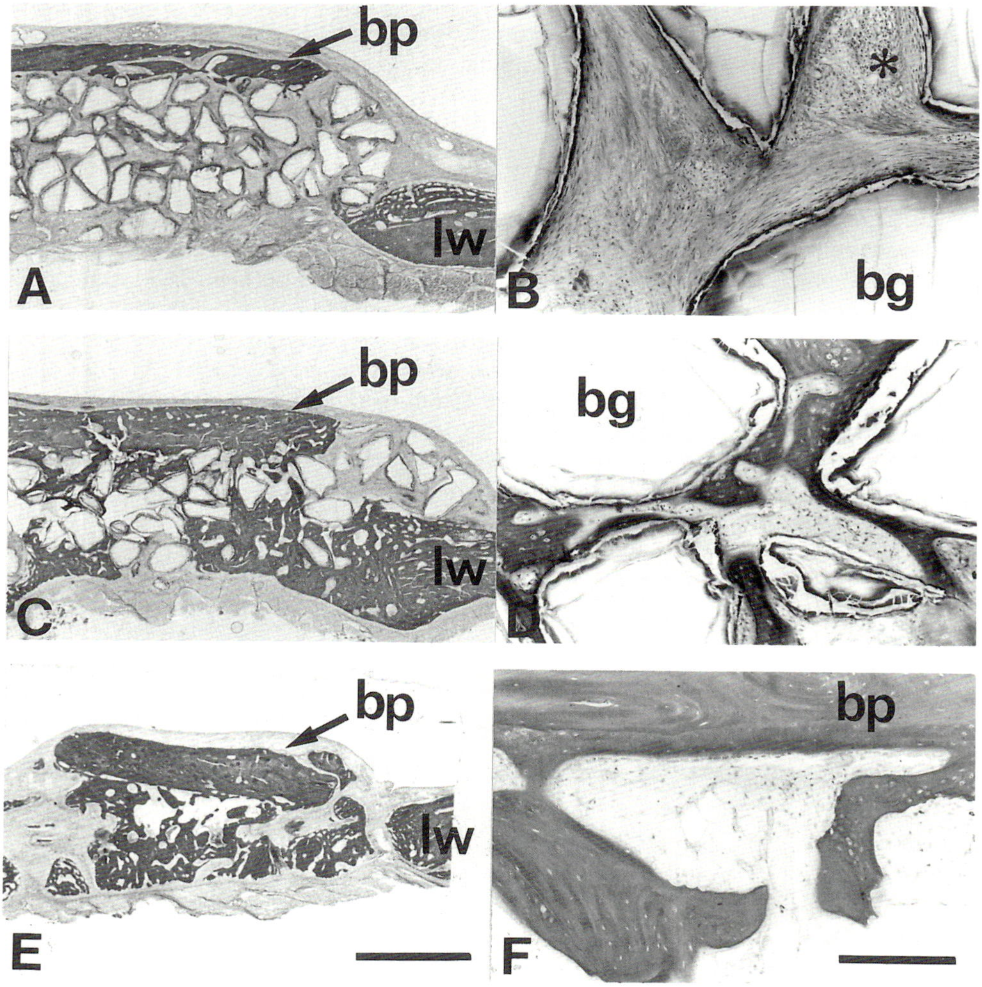

Figure 2. A. Micrograph of BG group shows dense connective tissue between the granules at 8 weeks. Bone formation is scanty. B. Note inflammatory cell focus in connective tissue (asterisk). C. Abundant new bone formation is seen between the granules in AB+BG group at 12 weeks. D. New bone is in tight contact with BG granules. E. Considerable amount of bone formation is seen in AB group at 8 weeks. Note that the depth of augmentation is smaller in this picture than in A and C. F. Higher magnification shows new bone formation in contact with the bone plate. Abbreviations: bp = bone plate pressed into the sinus; lw = lateral wall of the sinus; bg = bioactive glass. Bars: A, C, and E = 3 mm; B, D, and F = 250 μm.

DISCUSSION

Autologous bone grafts are widely used for augmentation of the maxillary sinus floor to increase support for dental implants in the posterior maxilla [1]. Hydroxylapatite and allogenic freeze-dried demineralized bone have been applied as alternative materials to avoid the problems related to the use of autologous bone [3,7,8]. The present study was prompted by the promising results obtained on repair of bone defects using BG granules [9-11].

BG, AB+BG and AB were used for augmentation of the lateral wall of the maxillary sinus in sheep. Growth factors and other proteins necessary for bone formation can be brought into the augmentation area by mixing BG granules with bone chips. The best augmentation was obtained in AB+BG group. It has been shown in earlier studies that newly formed bone bonds chemically with BG [4]. Consequently it is justified to consider the amount of bone-BG composite formed as the actual augmentation achieved in the AB + BG group. The use of BG granules in combination with bone chips reduces the amount of bone needed for augmentation.

The depth of the augmentation was smaller in AB than other study groups indicating that the augmentation area had diminished due to resorption of the bone grafted into the sinus. This is reflected in the histomorphometrical results as an increase of the figures for the bone area because results of the measurements are expressed in percentages of the augmentation area achieved. No significant reduction of the augmentation area occurred when BG granules were used.

Use of BG granules together with autologous bone chips seems to be a promising method for augmentation of the maxillary sinus wall. Incorporation of bone growth factors with BG granules would probably offer a more practical and efficient way to induce bone formation for this purpose. However, further experiments dealing especially with biomechanical properties of bone-BG composite are needed before any conclusions can be made on the clinical applicability of BG granules for the sinus floor augmentation procedure.

REFERENCES

1. Raghoebar, G.M., Brouwer, T.J., Reintsema, H. and Van Oort, R.P. *J. Oral Maxillofac. Surg.* 1993, 51, 1198-1203.

2. Keller, E. and Triplett, W. *J. Oral Maxillofac. Surg.* 1987, 45, 11-14.

3. Smiler, D.G., Johnson, P.W, Lozada, J.L., Misch, C., Rosenlicht, J.L. Tatum Jr., O.H. and Wagner, J.R. *Dent. Clin. North Am.* 1992, 36, 151-188.

4. Andersson, Ö.H., Liu, G., Karlsson, K.H., Niemi, L., Miettinen, J. and Juhanoja, J. *J. Mater. Sci. Mater. Med.* 1990, 1, 219-227.

5. Donath, K. and Breuner, G. *J. Oral Pathol.* 1982, 11, 318-326.

6. SAS/Technical Report P-229, SAS/STAT Software: Chances and Enchancements, Release 6.07, SAS Institute Inc., Cary, 1992, 289-366.

7. Small, S.A., Zinner, I.D., Panno, F.V., Shapiro, H.J. and Stein, J.I. *Int. J. Oral Maxillofac. Implants* 1993, 8, 523-528.

8. Tidwell, J.K., Blijdorp, P.A., Stoelinga, P.J., Brouns, J.B. and Hinderks, F. *Int. J. Oral Maxillofac. Surg.* 1992, 21, 204-209.

9. Turunen, T., Peltola, J., Yli-Urpo A. and Happonen, R.-P. *J. Mater. Sci. Mater. Med.*, 1994, submitted.

10. Turunen, T., Peltola, J., Helenius, H., Yli-Urpo, A. and Happonen, R.-P. *Clin. Oral Implants Res.* 1995, submitted.

11. Heikkilä, J.T., Aho, A.J., Yli-Urpo, A., Andersson, Ö.H., Aho, H.J. and Happonen, R.-P. *Acta Orthop. Scand.* 1993, 64, 678-682.

THE IMPORTANCE OF THE ADHESION THROUGH BIOLOGICAL GLASS TO THE ACOUSTIC MEMBRANE OF TOR PROTHESES

P. Laudadio[1], E. Cunsolo[1], L. Presutti[1], A. Krajewski[2], A. Ravaglioli[2], L.L. Hench[3]

[1]E.N.T. & H.N. Surgery Department of *Maggiore* Hospital - Bologna (Italy)
[2]Institute for Technological Research on Ceramics of C.N.R. - Faenza (Italy)
[3]Advanced Materials Research Center, University of Florida - Gainesville (FL, USA)

ABSTRACT

A solution of the problem concerning the instability of auricular TOR (Total Ossicle Replacement) protheses was successfully achieved by adopting inert ceramic coated with a biological glass at the extremities of the columnella, to encourage adhesion between tympanic membrane and the basal rim of the protheses. This study tries to identify the reason(s) for the good statistical results for Alumina TOR protheses with a layer of biological glass applied on the tympanic bearing at the base of the columnella.

INTRODUCTORY REMARKS, MATERIALS AND EXPERIENCES

Previous studies [1,2,3] developed ossicular ceramic prostheses for ossicular chain reconstruction. Such ceramic protheses proved to an improvement over those made of polymer. Their improved positive performances compensate for lesser surgical handiness and higher weight. These ceramic prostheses, are made up of hydroxyapatite, Al_2O_3 , were applied in patients requiring tympanoplasty at the E.N.T. & N.H. surgery department of the *Maggiore* Hospital of Bologna.

Today the problem relative to biomaterials for reconstruction of the ossicular chain remains unsolved. The impact of the intervention of ossiculoplasty revision surgery shows that up to now, the optimal biomaterial for use in such revision is still not known. Bioinert ceramics may tilt from the position surgically assigned although less frequently than polymeric prostheses. The fundamental problems remain: the extrusion at long term (particularly in the case of polymers); tilting from the tympanic membrane (particularly for the inert biomaterials); fixation with surrounding structures (specifically with bioactive materials).

A way to overcome these limits of the biomaterials now in use is to induce attachment between the tympanic membrane and TOR prostheses. Previous workers [4] altered the shape to allow for tympanic anchorage. We have designed a specific coupling between inert ceramic and biological glass, a composite prosthesis combining the good characteristics of the inert ceramic and the adhesion of soft tissue to bioactive material. To maximize anchorage, the side of the prostheses in contact with the membrane was covered with bioactive glass to improve adhesion with the tympanic membrane. The only problem was to control the tissue adhesion to avoid the risk of damaging the tympanic membrane. The material on which this coating was carried out until now is Al_2O_3 ceramic. A feasibility study to produce similar prostheses made with ZrO_2 is still in progress. Among all developed TOR (Total Ossicle Replacement) prostheses models, one of columnella type appeared suitable. The base of the columnella was covered with AP40 biological glass [5]. Grafts of these TOR prostheses in patients did not show any tilting from the position surgically allotted, which is reported to happen in 5-10% of cases, when other similar devices are used. Clinical test (otoendoscopy with Valsavae's method, High Resolution Computed Tomography, audiological tests; pure tone averages and speech reception threshold) showed clinical results suggested a linking between prostheses and tympanic membrane.

In the present work our first experiences with the clinical application of this type of prosthesis are reported. Table 1 shows the pathologies and the surgical methodologies adopted for the patients in this study. There are also a number of reinterventions in which the new prosthesis was substituted for failed (mainly polymeric) devices. Table 2 reports the distribution of follow-up. (Patient details appear in Table 4.)

In-vitro testing of the bioactive coating was also studied to detect chemical changes in the surface.

Table 1. Statistic data on the TOR surgical intervention with Alumina ceramic prostheses covered with AP40 in the plate in contact with tympanic membrane.

Patients	Whole number of patients: men: women:	33 13 20
Age (years)	minimum: maximum: mean:	12 70 42.1
Pathologies	cholesteomatosis chronic otitis: simple chronic otitis: oto-mucous anthritis: cholesterinic granuloma: tympanosclerosis: non-stabilized radical baudy operation:	21 5 1 1 3 2
Surgical procedures	intact canal wall tympanoplasty with ossiculoplasty: ossiculoplasty (with or without second look): reconstruction of bondy operation: ossiculoplasty revision surgery:	4 15 3 11
Follow-up (years)	mean value on all patients:	2.2

Table 2. Follow-up distribution.

Years	4	3.5	3	2	1	0.5
No. of patients	3	3	9	7	6	5

METHODS

Clinical audiometric tests were made on all patients in this TOR clinical study. The positioning of the applied prostheses was performed by HR-CT (High Resolution Computerized Tomography) of temporal bone. Statistical data are reported in the Table 1 and Table 4.

Bioactivity testing was done following those used to certify bioactivity for implants made under the US-FDA guidelines. A sample of 45S5 Bioglass® was used (U.S. Biomaterials Co.) for comparison. The samples were tested in both trisbuffer (TRB) and simulated body fluid (SBF #9) solution under static conditions at 37°C with a SA/V ratio of 0.1 $cm^{-2}ml^{-1}$ for time periods from one day to one week. After the samples were removed from solution, FTIR (Fourier Transform Infra Red) analysis was performed to determine the extent of HCA formation on their surfaces and solution analysis was performed for elemental concentrations of Ca, P, and Si ICP (Inductively Coupled Plasma) analysis.

RESULTS

The mean audiograms before and after surgical application of these TOR prostheses are reported in Figure 1. Mean values were obtained from audiometric results coming from all the patients. No prostheses has tilted up to now.

As concerns FTIR analysis, the spectrum from the "as produced" sample of the TOR device, exhibits peaks with maximum intensities at 589 cm^{-1} and 544 cm^{-1}. These peaks do not correlate to the P-O rocking vibrations at 604 cm^{-1}, and cannot be attributed to any crystalline calcium phosphate produced in these devices.

The 1 day spectrum of the samples reacted in trisbuffer exhibits peaks with maximum intensities at 603 cm^{-1} and 557 cm^{-1}. These peaks may be related to HCA as the spectra were collected at 2 cm^{-1} resolution which puts them in the range of the P-I rocking vibrations. A 7 days spectrum exhibits peaks with maximum intensities at 613 cm^{-1} and 562 cm^{-1}, which are still in the range of the P-O rocking vibration of HCA, but the relative intensities of these peaks change little as a function of reaction time, indicating that the chemical composition and thickness of the eventual reaction layer has not changed significantly with time. In practice there is no significant change from 1 day to 7 days treatment. The samples reacted in SBF #9 for 1 day and 7 days exhibit spectra in which peaks maximum intensities and locations change little with time, indicating in practice that there is relatively no change in chemical composition as a function of reaction time for these samples. There seems to be no indication of the presence of any HCA layer on these samples up to 7 days when treated with SBF #9. The 1 day spectra of the glass covered surface of these devices treated in trisbuffer and SBF #9 are reported in Figure 2 together with the spectrum of "as produced" devices and the spectrum of 45S5 Bioglass®, reacted in trisbuffer. The concentrations of Ca, P, Si and Al detected by ICP as a function of reaction time in trisbuffer are reported in Table 3. Although the amount of glass layer is very small also a development of surface (less than one fourth of the total surface of the prostheses), nevertheless the released amounts are very small. This indicates a low exchange of ions that reduces drastically bioactivity.

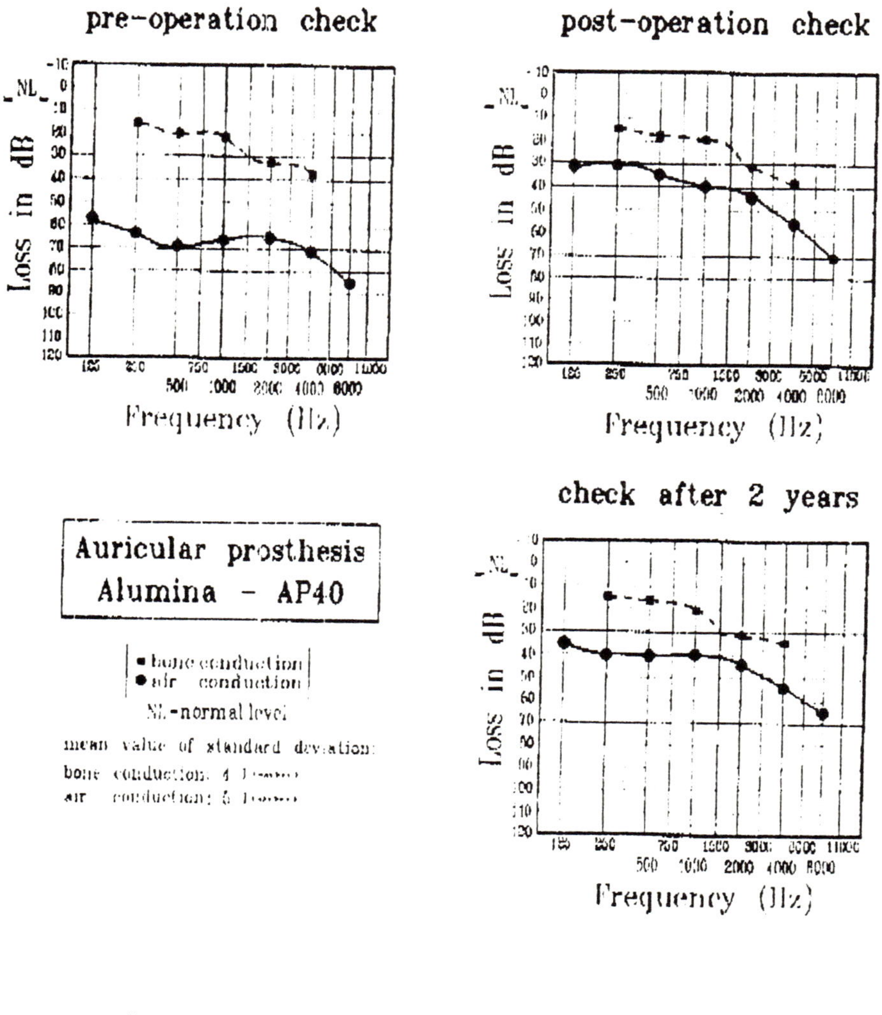

Figure 1. Audiograms reporting mean values coming from all patients subjected to ossiculoplasty with columnella like TOR prostheses covered by a layer of AP40 biological glass on the plate in contact with tympanic membrane. Comparisons between pre-operatory and post-operatory diagrams. Mean values expressed in dB.

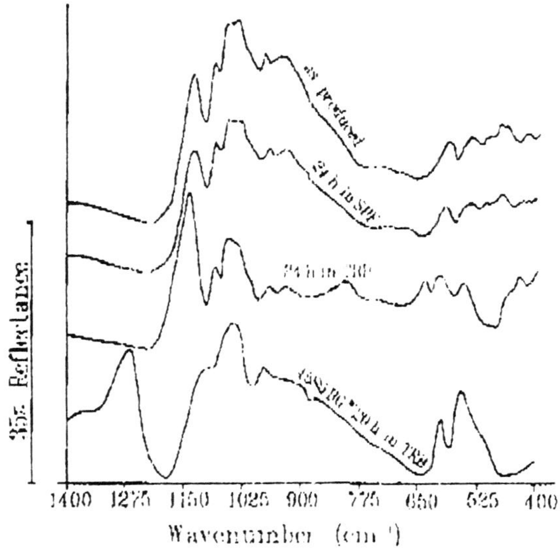

Figure 2. FTIR spectra of the glass covered surface after the indicated treatments, compared with a spectrum coming from 45S5 Bioglass® after treatment.

Table 3. ICP analysis on the reacted trisbuffer solution.

Reaction Time	Ion Concentration			
(days)	(ppm)			
-	Ca	P	Si	Al
1	nd	1.2	0.2	0.1
7	nd	1.5	0.6	-
14	nd	1.8	0.5	0.3

DISCUSSION

The very low bioactivity observed for the AP40 covering layer could derive from absorption of some Al^{+3} ions from the substrate by the biological glass deposited on it sufficient to destroy its bioactivity. Previously we found absorption of about 9.8 % [4]. As there is no bone growth involved, a first hypothesis can be advanced to interpret the observed joining between the covering glass layer and tympanic membrane. The scarce amount of ions released by the glass (Mg^{+2}, K^{+} and PO_4^{-3}) in contact with the tympanic membrane, although not sufficient to produce a HCA layer, can be enough to stimulate a small wished formation of fibrous connective between the

Table 4. List of the most significant cases with follow up more than 2 years.

Patient code	Sex	age	Ear pathology	Surgical procedure	ABG (*) (b.s.) (dB)	ABG(*) (a.s.) (dB)	ABG(*) (>2y) (dB)	Follow up (yrs)
NM	W	54	cholesteatomatosis chronic otitis	ossiculoplasty revision surgery	40/40/35	15/20/15	25/20/15	4
GD	M	12	cholesteatomatosis chronic otitis	ossiculoplasty	35/30/25	25/20/10	20/25/20	4
VC	W	33	cholesteatomatosis chronic otitis	ossiculoplasty	40/35/30	10/10/15	25/20/30	4
GS	M	19	cholesteatomatosis chronic otitis	ossiculoplasty	60/40/45	30/30/25	45/15/30	3.5
DF	M	42	cholesteatomatosis chronic otitis	ossiculoplasty	55/40/20	10/25/10	25/20/10	3.5
MS	M	50	cholesteatomatosis chronic otitis	ossiculoplasty	70/65/45	15/20/15	30/30/25	3.5
CI	W	68	cholesterinic granuloma	reconstruction of bondy operations	65/55/45	25/30/30	30/25/20	3
VA	W	14	cholesteatomatosis chronic otitis	ossiculoplasty	50/45/40	10/05/00	20/20/25	3
BL	M	36	cholesteatomatosis chronic otitis	tympanoplasty	40/45/40	15/20/10	20/25/15	3
SN	W	44	cholesteatomatosis chronic otitis	ossiculoplasty	45/40/20	15/15/15	15/20/15	3
ND	M	12	cholesteatomatosis chronic otitis	ossiculoplasty	65/45/40	30/25/20	35/30/25	3
SG	M	69	cholesteatomatosis chronic otitis	ossiculoplasty	50/75/55	20/20/15	25/25/30	3
BP	W	23	tympanosclerosis	ossiculoplasty	45/40/45	25/20/15	25/25/15	3
AN	W	29	cholesteatomatosis chronic otitis	ossiculoplasty	45/55/50	20/15/10	25/25/20	3
BC	M	37	chronic otitis	I.C.W.T.	55/60/50	25/30/20	35/25/20	3

anonymous list compiled under law permission
*: ABG at 500, 1000 and 2000 Hz respectively

rim of TOR prostheses and the auricular membrane. The release of such ions should be furthermore favored by weak acidic environment of the middle ear. Probably this not emphasized by bioactivity tests carried out *in vitro*, which operate in the weakly alkaline environment of the physiological solutions. Such adhesion does not take place in the remaining Al_2O_3 ceramic prostheses, simply since it is not able to release metabolic ions. According to this interpretation, assuming that the observed adhesion to the tympanic membrane is coming from the residual bioactivity of the applied biological glass, a fine regulation of its bioactivity could offer results of closer joining. A solution could be the increase of the thickness of the glass, by applying it through successive layers. Consequently the induction to the development of the connective layer should increase. With a covering process carried out in this manner, the greater is the number of layers and the smaller is the pollution of Al^{+3} suffered by the last layer.

Since however the *in vitro* tests did not give satisfactory and sharp answer to explain the observed adhesion to the membrane, a second hypothesis can be formulated that involves the physico-chemical nature of the resulting material. It could be possible that the adhesion is not induced by the supposed scarce residual bioactivity, but simply due to other reasons (e.g. formation of a surface gel, suitable Z potential, better wettability of important proteins including the cell membrane, etc.) that offer a higher affinity of the connectival cells towards the surface of the covering glass in respect to that towards Al_2O_3 ceramic.

CONCLUSIONS

The use of biological glass as covering the surface in contact with tympanic membrane was effective to improve the performance of the TOR prostheses, so that it may be clinically useful. The audiometric results are extremely reassuring and the post-operative ones very good. It was very difficult to interpret the reasons of the observed improved adhesion prostheses-membrane. The physico-chemical environment of the tympanic cavity is different to that of bone. The application of one layer of AP40 biological glass on the alumina surface has reduced the bioactivity of the glass. This reduction was due to an uncontrolled dissolution of Al^{+3}. We intend to adjust the bioactivity, if it is the cause of production of soft tissue linking. Results from histological tests from implantations on animals, will inform us about the kind of tissue formed, but probably will not answer in physico-chemical terms.

REFERENCES

1. P. Laudadio, L. Presutti, A. Ravaglioli and R. Martinetti, in Bioceramics and the Human Body, edited by Ravaglioli and Krajewski) Elsevier (London, 1992) 486-490.
2. A. Ravaglioli, A. Krajewski, P. Laudadio, L. Presutti, E. Cunsolo and R. Martinetti, Bioceramics Volume 5, edited by T. Yamamuro, T. Kokubo and T. Nakamura (Tokyo, 1992) 451-458.
3. P. Laudadio, L. Presutti, E. Cunsolo, A. Ravaglioli and R. Martinetti, Fourth World Biomaterials Congress, book of abstracts (Berlin, 1992) 344.
4. A. Ravaglioli, A. Krajewski, A. Piancastelli, G. Berger, K. Adam and R. Gildenhasr, Inter. Ceram. 41, (2) (1992) 69-74.
5. K. Jahnke, D. Plesser and G. Heimke, Biomaterials, 4, (1983) 137-138.

DENTAL APPLICATIONS

BIOCERAMICS IN DENTISTRY

K. de Groot and J.G.C. Wolke

Dept. of Biomaterials, Leiden University, School of Medicine, Rijnsburgerweg 10, 2333 AA Leiden, The Netherlands

ABSTRACT

Although bioceramics in dentistry covers a wide rage of materials, such as various dental cements (for restorations), in prosthodontics, in orthodontics, ceramic covers for dental crowns, and porcelain inlays, we limit ourselves in this article to bioactive ceramics, i.e. ceramics bonding to bone. Since in terms of clinical acceptance, hydroxyapatite (HA) coatings are -currently- the most relevant application, we further narrow our article to HA coatings.

This article shows that HA ceramics have their greatest advantage as a biocompatible coating on mechanically strong (i.e., metallic) substrates. The debate about crystallinity and required degradation rate has been intense; however, the current state of the art is that (1) high crystallinity does not improve compatibility, but rather slows down bioactivity compared with amorphous coatings; and (2) the required degradation rate is such that HA coatings do not need to stay for longer than one year.

INTRODUCTION

Although it has been recognized for decades that hydroxylapatite (HA) ceramics, have an excellent biocompatibility with bone, there exists still a controversy with respect to the usefulness of HA coatings on (titanium) dental implants. Incidentally, failures have been reported, although large scale evaluations show an improved bonding to alveolar bone [1] as compared with titanium implants. Animal experiments show the same difference. In this review optimal coating properties necessary to maintain bone bonding as discussed as well as clinical indications and contra-indications. After an overview of the coating process, animal studies will be presented, whereafter conclusions are drawn with respect to clinical uses.

The coating process

Currently, two coating processes are of interest. One of them, plasma spraying [2], is the only one commercially available, while the other, r.f. magnetron sputtering [3] may be the choice for the future.

Plasma spray coatings

Schematically the principle of plasma spraying is as follows. A DC electric arc is struck between two electrodes, while a stream of (mixed) gases passes through this arc. This results in an ionized gas of high temperature up to 30000°C, with a speed approaching the speed of sound due to the large expansion resulting from this temperature increase. Hydroxylapatite powder is suspended in the carrier gas stream which is fed into the plasma flame. It is well known that apatite is thermodynamically unstable at plasma spray temperatures, which means that the plasma spray process must be executed carefully. Ideally, only a thin outer layer of each powder particle gets into the molten plastic state which unavoidably undergoes some phase transitions. This plastic state however is necessary to ensure dense and adhesive coatings. By choosing an optimum relation between particle size, type of gas (the heat content of a plasma, and thus the ability to increase the temperature of a particle depends strongly on the gas used), speed of the plasma (the longer a particle resides in a plasma, the higher its temperature), and cooling process of the coated surface, one obtains coatings with the desired calcium phosphate(s) and crystallinity. Hydroxylapatite coatings are thus a compromise between being completely amorphous and being amorphous with a crystalline phase.

Different plasma gases influences the crystallinity of the coating. Argon mixed with hydrogen gives a higher degree of crystallinity but without hydrogen the powder particles cannot enter the gas. This is because the high velocity and viscosity of the argon gas cause the particles to bounce back from the flame, instead of entering it. Plasma gases also influence coating thickness: for example nitrogen as the plasma gas gives a thicker coating layer compared to argon. An important criterion is formation of calcium oxide; too much can react with water and destroy the coating layer.

Thus, plasma spray technology allows production of either amorphous or (partially) crystalline coatings of HA on dental (and other) implants. Most industrial companies prefer a thickness of about 50 microns, this being a compromise between (1) thinner coatings which are stronger than thicker ones, but (2) thinner coatings may resorb faster.

Magnetron sputter process

RF magnetron sputter-coating can be performed using a commercially available sputter unit (Edwards High Vacuum ESM100 system). The target material usually consists of a (110 mm diameter) copper disc, plasma-spray coated with a 1 mm thick HA layer. For the coating of the target commercially available HA powder can be used. The chemical composition and purity of the target-coating should be confirmed by X-ray diffraction (XRD) analysis.

Specimens are mounted on a rotating and water-cooled substrate holder. The target-to-substrate distance is about 80 mm. Before sputtering the metal specimens should be cleaned, for example by etching for 5 min. with argon ions. In our experiments, a liquid nitrogen cold trap was used for all sputtering runs and a base pressure of $< 10^{-5}$ mbar was obtained before the sputter process was started. Process pressure was 5×10^{-3} mbar using argon gas. The deposition rate of the ceramic on the substrate can be as high as 200-250nm/min of sputtering (power level 700W). The film thickness and rate of deposition were determined in our experiments using an Edwards FTM 5 quartz crystal film thickness monitor. Physicochemical analysis demonstrated that depending on sputter conditions amorphous or crystalline Ca/P coatings were deposited with an apatite structure.

It is concluded that RF magnetron sputtering is an excellent method for forming stable, dense, adherent, and homogenous Ca/P thin-films on metal substrates. The advantages of RF magnetron sputter-coating over other coating processes include the high adhesion of films, the excellent uniform layers and the ability to coat implants with difficult surface geometries. An important advantage, especially for dental implants, is that no grit blasting of the substrate surface is needed, contrary to plasma spraying. The thickness of such a coating should be around 10 microns: this is sufficient if one accepts the idea that HA coatings should stay for periods up to one year but not necessarily longer. As with coatings obtained by means of plasma spraying, RF magnetron sputter coatings can be obtained as either amorphous or (partly or completely) crystalline.

Biological considerations

We next address two important questions; 1) should the coatings be crystalline? and 2) should they be long lasting? i.e., should the coating stay?

In an earlier publication, [4] we have shown in animal tests that HA coated test specimens are rapidly bonded to bone, while non-coated Ti implants take much longer times (>6 months) to obtain a (not quite as) good bonding. Two important points were concluded: although the HA coating has degraded within 12 months, the strong bonding stays in existence, and titanium itself is (under unloaded conditions only) able to achieve a good bonding after longer times as well (although HA has -even in the long run- a consistently higher bond strength with bone).

This shows that the HA coating performs its most important function during healing and bone ingrowth. As soon as the bone reaches the HA surface, and a good bond is established, the coating may gradually disappear; i.e., even after disappearance of the HA coating, its effects are lasting. Therefore, the conclusion is that the coating does not need to stay, but may gradually resorb.

Should the coating be crystalline?

Crystalline coatings have the disadvantage that although resorption should theoretically be lower for crystalline materials than for amorphous ones, its resorption mode may be just a fragmentation process, leading to irritating particles between bone and implant, rather than a physiochemical dissolution process releasing only ions. The fragmentation process is unpredictable and may even lead to a relatively fast degradation of crystalline coatings. Therefore, the conclusion must be that HA coatings should be amorphous, or only partly crystalline, with the restriction that the crystalline areas are of nanometer size to avoid release of harmful particles.

CONCLUSION

Both plasma spraying and r.f. magnetron sputter-coating are capable of producing HA coatings that stay in place for periods of up to one year as required for optimal function of a dental implant. The positive effects are lasting even after complete resorption of the bioactive layer.

The required HA degradation rate can be controlled by crystallinity (high crystallinity, if crystallites in n.m. size are employed, reduces degradation rate) and thickness.

An interesting advantage of r.f. magnetron sputter-coatings, is that they can be made thinner than plasma sprayed coatings (lower limit < 1 micron versus > 30 micron respectively). Thus, r.f. sputter-coating changes the dimensions carefully machined dental implants less than plasma spray coatings. In addition, no sand blasting, as required for plasma spraying is required, hence again, there is no influence on dimensions of dental implants. Thus, in the future we foresee an increased interest in the use r.f. magnetron sputter-coated dental implants. Although we limited ourselves to HA materials, it should be emphasized that, generally, our conclusions hold for other bioactive ceramics as well. Due to their brittleness, they should be used as a coating and such coatings do not need to stay for longer periods than one year.

REFERENCES

1. Ochi, S., Morris, H.F., Gillette, W., Glasscock, W., Lambert, P., Laucillo, F., Stoffer, W., Weir, D. J. *Dent. Res.* 1994,73,219.
2. Groot, K. de. In: *Innovative Materials,* N.R.C. Italy 1993, 489-497.
3. Wolke, J.G.C., van Dijk, K., Schaeken, H.G., de Groot, K., Jansen, J.A. J. *Biomed. Mater. Res.* 1994, submitted for publication.
4. Wolke, J.G.C., de Blieck-Hogervorst, J.M.A., Dhert, W.J.A., Klein, C.P.A.T., de Groot, K. J. *Drermal Spray Technology* 1992, 1, 75-82.

BIOACTIVE GLASS IN PERIODONTAL BONE DEFECTS. INITIAL CLINICAL FINDINGS OF SOFT TISSUE AND OSSEUS REPAIR

E. Larmas*, L. Sewón*, T. Luostarinen**, I. Kangasniemi*** and A. Yli-Urpo***

The Departments of *Periodontology, **Radiology and ***Prosthetic Dentistry, Institute of Dentistry, University of Turku, Finland

ABSTRACT

A controlled study model was designed to study the healing and regeneration rate of periodontal bony defects with and without bioactive glass, S53P4 [1]. Patients with 2-3 wall vertical bony defects of the same depth on both sides of the mandible or maxilla were recruited. A modified Widman flap was performed on both sides of the jaw on the same day by the same clinician. The bony defects on the experimental side were filled with bioactive glass granules (size 630-800 μm). Initial findings revealed a good clinical and radiographic response to the treatment. Evidence of osteogenesis and osteointegration of the glass-granules could be seen in some radiographs.

INTRODUCTION

Improved probing attachment levels and bone-fill of intraosseus defects with minimal tissue loss is the goal of modern surgical methods in periodontal treatment. The methods vary from open curettage to the use of grafting materials and guided tissue regeneration [2,3,4,5,6,7,8,9,10]. According to our experience, the use of highly conservative surgical methods and meticulous professional removal of soft debris after surgery results in a surprisingly good and rapid osseous healing without any grafting or tissue guiding material [10,11]. On the other hand, the need for reconstructive and regenerative surgical methods in the treatment of periodontal bony defects is increasing at present. The use of nonresorbable grafting materials involves a risk of infection during the maintenance phase of the treatment. This leads to extra procedures to remove the infected tissue and the material.

Resorbable bioactive glass, S53P4, is potentially an ideal grafting material in periodontal treatment, because total resorption and replacement of the glass by osseus tissue are expected advantages. Using a highly controlled study model, we wanted to evaluate the possible advantages of bioactive glass, S53P4, when compared to the atraumatic periodontal surgery without grafting. In addition, we are aiming to further develop the presently used operative methods to gain optimal healing with the bioactive glass.

MATERIALS AND METHODS

Seven periodontal patients, 5 men and 2 women (age range 44-75 yrs) participated in the study. The subjects were selected based on radiographic findings from orthopantomograms (Fig 1). The following radiographic criteria were used to select the subjects: Patients with a 2-3 wall vertical bony defect of the same depth on controlateral sides of the mandible or maxilla were accepted. Subjects with systemic disease or medications were excluded. Control and experimental sites were randomly assigned. A modified Widman flap operation (MWF) according to Ramfjord [4] was performed on both sides of the jaw on the same day by the same clinician. The documentation of seven patients treated so far provided 14 individual evaluation sites. Half of these were debrided and root planed and grafted with bioactive glass, S53P4 (size 630-800 μm), while the other half was debrided and root planed only. The procedures were carried out under local anesthesia. The graft material prior to insertion was mixed with the patient's own blood obtained from the operation area. During the first 3 months after surgery, the patients had a minimum of 8 re-call visits including suture removal, exchange of surgical packages, oral hygiene control and professional removal of soft debris. Clinical recordings and radiographic examinations before the operation and 3, 6 and 12 months postoperatively are planned. Probing pocket depth (PPD) and probing attachment level (PAL) were recorded using a standardized, thin Michigan-O periodontal probe. Radiographic examination was planned before the operation, immediately after surgery as well as 3 and 6 months postoperatively. Bone loss i.e. the defect depths (DD) was determined according to Schei et al. [12] from the radiographs by measuring the distance between the alveolar bone margin and the cemento-enamel junction and by relating it to the total root length of the tooth. The measurements were carried out with computerized Digora system (Soredex/ Orion Corp., Helsinki, Finland). Wilcoxon's sign test was used in the statistical evaluation of the results.

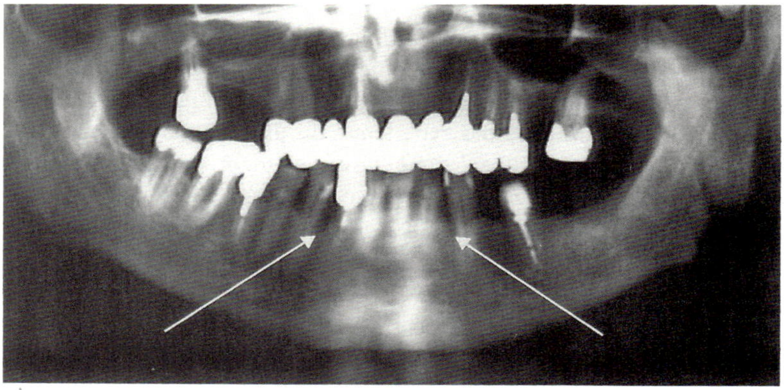

Figure 1. An example of the radiographic criteria used in patient selection. Note the identical bony defects on controlateral sites of the lower jaw (arrows).

RESULTS

Eight out of fourteen defects were from premolar sites, 4 from the area of second molars and 2 from canine region. Nine of the defects were located on the mesial and 5 on the distal sides of the teeth. Eight of the lesions were in the lower and 6 in the upper jaw. The available results from the five patients 3 months postoperatively are summarized in Table 1. Initial findings revealed a good clinical and radiographic response to treatment. The graft material was well tolerated by all patients.

There were no significant differences between the grafted and control sites with regard to either the soft tissue or the hard tissue measurements 3 months postoperatively. However, the controls revealed more positive mean value for soft tissue healing in terms of a more rapid reduction of probing pocket depth: the mean PPD reduction was 3.3 mm in the control group as opposed to 2.9 mm in the experimental group. The mean gain of probing attachment (PA) was 2 mm in the control and 1.5 mm in the experimental group. The measurements of the bony defects revealed the opposite: bone apposition was seen on the experimental side while bone reduction was seen on the control side 3 months postoperatively. In the experimental group a mean of 0.60 mm's *gain* of bone level and a mean of 0.30 mm's *bone loss* in the control group was measured. Tendency of osteointegration and osteogenesis could be observed in some radiographs (Fig 2c and d; Fig 3a and b). The radiographs on the control sites revealed an initial bone resorption, which after 6 months shifted to apposition (Fig 4).

TABLE 1. Clinical findings of soft tissue and osseous repair 3-months postoperatively.

No	SEX	AGE [yr]	AREA		GRAFTED		CONTROL		GRAFTED		CONTROL		GRAFTED		CONTROL	
			Graf	Cont	IPPD	PPPD	IPPD	PPPD	IPAL	PPAL	IPAL	PPAL	IDD	PDD	IDD	PDD
1	M	75	43^2	33^2	9	7	9	5	9	8	9	6	12	10.9	7.6	8.2
2	M	61	14^2	24^2	10	6	6	3	11	8	7	6	11.6	8.3	9	9.4
3	M	45	35^2	45^2	6	3	5	3.5	6	4	6	3.5	5.6	6.1	3.5	3.7
4	F	62	15^4	14^4	6	3.5	6	1.5	6	4	6	2.5	7.4	8.3	6.7	6.5
5	M	50	34^4	45^2	7	4	7	3.5	7	7.5	7	7	7.2	7.4	7.6	8.1
$\bar{x}$ ±SD					7.6 ±1.6	4.7 ±1.5	6.6 ±1.4	3.3 ±1.1	7.8 ±1.9	6.3 ±1.9	7.0 ±1.1	5.0 ±1.7	8.8 ±2.6	8.2 ±1.6	6.9 ±1.8	7.2 ±2.0
mean Change					2.9		3.3		1.5		2		-0.6		+0.3	

IPPD = Initial Probing Pocket Depth [mm]
PPPD = Postoperative Probing Pocket Depth [mm]
IPAL = Initial Probing Attachment Level [mm]
PPAL = Postoperative Probing Attachment Level [mm]
IDD = Initial Defect Depth [mm]
PDD = Postoperative Defect Depth [mm]

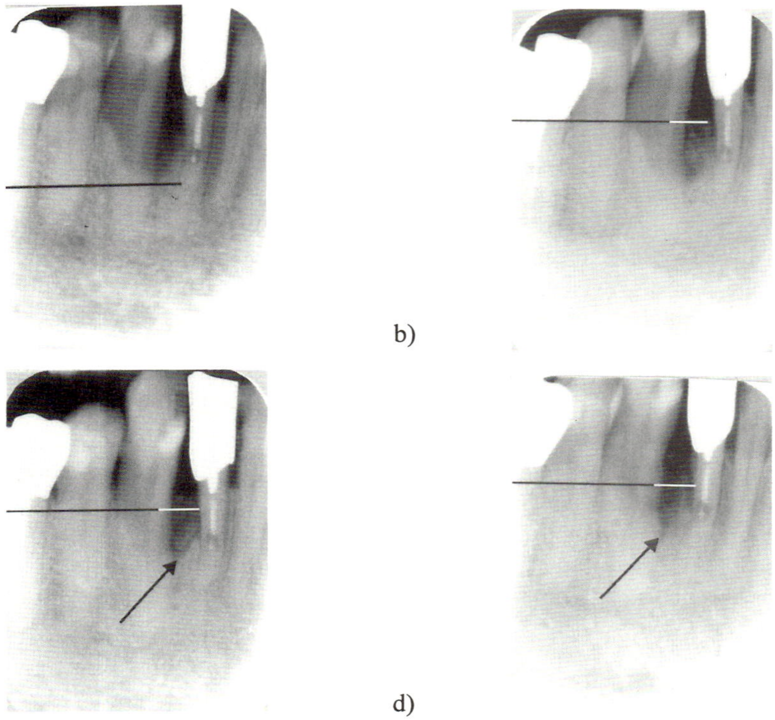

a) b) c) d)

Figure 2. A series of radiographs from the experimental side:
a.) Pre-operative condition. Note the bone margin. (line)
b) Post-operative radiograph immediately after grafting. Note the level of the defect fill. (line)
c.) 3 months post-operatively. Note the radiolucent zone between the graft material and the bone (arrow) as well as the level of the defect-fill.(line)
d.) 6 months post-operatively. Note the disappearance of the radiolucent zone (arrow) indicating osteointegration or osteogenesis.

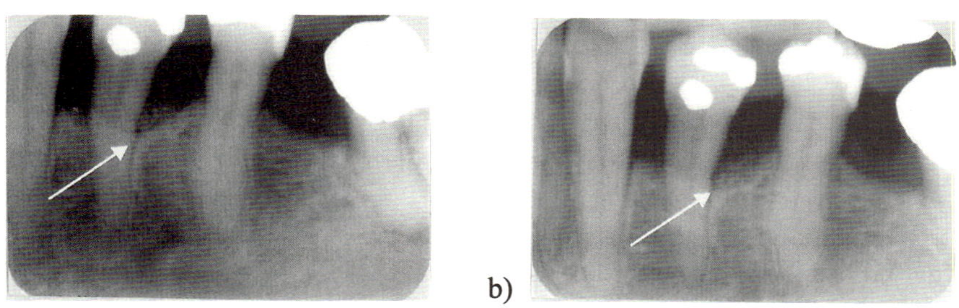

a) b)

Figure 3. A radiograph of patient # 3 from the experimental side:
a.) The vertical bone defect distally to 34 immediately after grafting. A strong sclerotic zone under the graft material can be seen (arrow) similar to the pre-operative radiograph.
b.) 3 months postoperatively the sclerotic zone seems to develop towards normal bone (arrow).

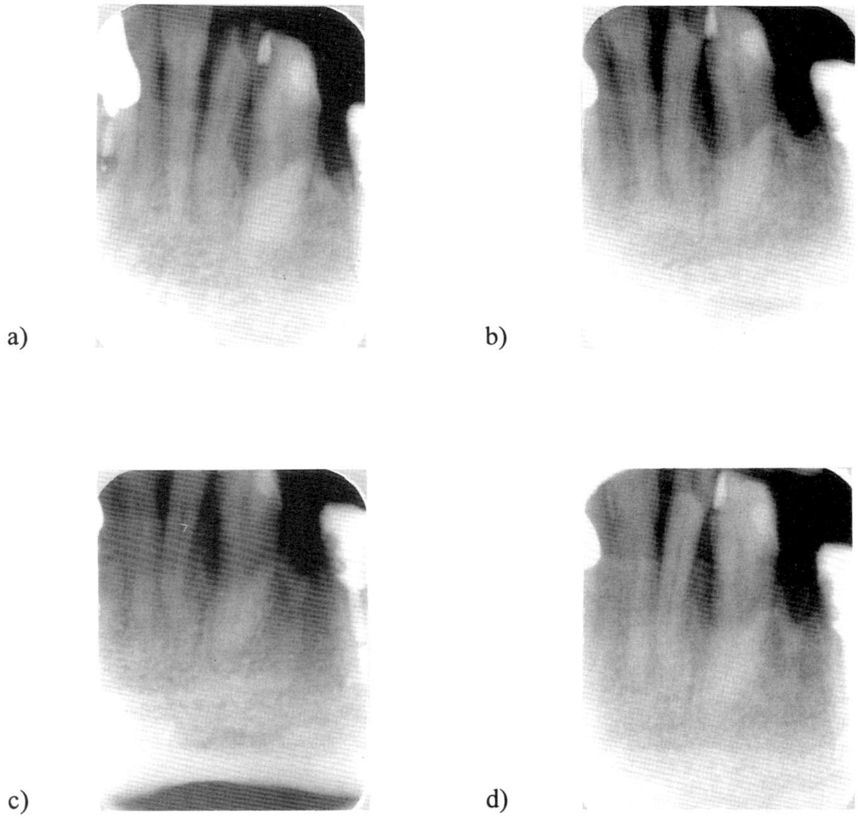

Figure 4. A radiograph from the control side prior to treatment (a) Note the initial resorption in the first (b) and second (c) postoperative radiographs. The last radiograph (d) reveals the initiation of bone apposition.

DISCUSSION

The present results give preliminary information on a bioactive glass, S53P4, as a grafting material in periodontal defects. The surgical procedures were carried out on both sides on the same day and by the same clinician. In this way, confounding factors related to host response, home-care and the operator's skill were well controlled .By using identical bony defects for both sides we wanted to minimize variation in radiographic diagnosis, and to exclude errors arising from local differences in healing depending on various bone and root anatomy and varying plaque accumulation rates.

The material is well tolerated resulting in a clinical healing as well as debridement only. More over the preliminary results suggest that osteointegration and osteogenesis start 3 months postoperatively. This starts with the resorption of the grafted material followed by the replacement with new bone. However, because traditional modified Widman flap with debridement only can also result in excellent bony healing, the determination of optimal selection of patients and area for grafting is one aim of further studies.

CONCLUSION

The present results suggest, that bioactive glass, S53P4, is a promising grafting material in periodontal bony defects which may lead to a faster hard tissue healing than without grafting.

ACKNOWLEDGEMENT

Financial support from Turku Finnish University Society is gratefully acknowledged.

REFERENCES

1. Andersson, Ö.H., The Bioactivity of Silicate Glass, Thesis, Åbo Akademi University, Finland, (1990)
2. Prichard, J.F., *J. Periodontol* 1957, 28, 202-216.
3. Rosling B., Nyman S., and Lindhe, J., *J. Clin. Periodontol* 1976, 3, 38-53.
4. Ramfjord, S.P., *J. Periodontol* 1977, 48, 558-565.
5. Polson A.M. and Heij, L., *J. Clin. Periodontol* 1978, 5, 13-23.
6. Mellonig, J.T., *Int. J. and Restor. Dent.* 1984, 4, 41-55.
7. Gottlow, J., Nyman, S., Lindhe, J., Karring, T., Wennström, J., *J. Clin. Periodontol* 1986, 13, 604-616.
8. Bowen, J.A., Mellonig, J.T., Gray, J.L., and Towle, H.T., *J. Periodontol* 1989, 60, 647-654.
9. Renvert, S., Nilveus, R., Dahlen, G., Slots, J., and Egelberg, J., *J. Clin. Periodont* 1990, 17, 356-363.
10. Sewón, L.A., *Scand. J. Dent. Res.* 1993, 101, 371-374.
11. Sewón, L.A. and Talonpoika, J., *Scand. J. Dent. Res.* 1992, 100, 159-163.
12. Schei, O., Waerhaug, J., Lövdal, A., and Arno, A., *J. Periodontol* 1959, 30, 7-16.

AN EVALUATION OF MATERIALS FOR ENDODONTIC SURGICAL APPLICATIONS USING THE RBC HEMOLYSIS ASSAY

Neville J. McDonald[1], Robert J. Sydiskis[2] and Leonard J. Litkowski[3]

Departments of Endodontics[1], Oral Craniofacial Biology[2] and Restorative Dentistry[3], Baltimore College of Dental Surgery, Dental School, The University of Maryland at Baltimore, Baltimore, Maryland, 21201-1586.

ABSTRACT
The purpose of this *in vitro* study was to determine the percent hemolysis, using changes in optical density as an indicator of toxicity, of red blood cells at 1, 10, and 30 days. Samples of Bioglass® (45S5, 54S and 77S all <90 μm in size), Super EBA, (Alumina reinforced Zinc Oxide Eugenol), with Zinc Oxide Eugenol (ZOE) and Amalgam as controls. The supernatants were placed in cuvettes and the O.D. read in duplicate and averaged. The percent hemolysis for each sample was calculated. These results show that there is no significant difference in hemolysis between the various preparations of 45S5 Bioglass®, and sol-gel preparations 54S or 77S at 1, 10 or 30 days.

INTRODUCTION
With the passage of the Medical Devices Amendments in 1976, the FDA received authority to evaluate the biological effects of all materials used in human beings [1,2]. Numerous devices and materials have been developed for use in the medical and dental professions. These come in intimate contact with bony and/or soft tissues in the body. Several *in vitro* methods have been used to assess potential cytotoxicity of these materials and leachates from solids, cements, sealants and enchants directly in contact with cells [3]. All of these assays detect overt morphologic changes and death of cells or hemolysis of RBCs. These tests have generally been used only as a screening mechanism before *in vivo* animal testing.

Bioglass® has been reported as a potential pulp capping agent for use when a mechanical exposure occurs during a dental procedure[4,5]. At this time the dental pulp is extremely susceptible to the toxic effects of any material which may be used to repair this exposure. Thus it is very important to be able to quantitate any potential cytotoxic effects of the materials used. Surgical endodontics often involves apical root resection and placement of a retrofilling material in order to achieve a fluid tight seal and prevent bacterial penetration. Bioglass® has the potential to provide a fluid tight seal in this type of application in addition to aiding the regeneration of bone and periodontal ligament.

Currently a material that possesses both of these properties is unavailable for use in endodontic surgery.

Bioglass® can be produced by several different manufacturing techniques. One of the techniques includes a sol-gel method in which the components are not heated to the same temperature as the traditional production methods [6,7]. A concern has been that the potential exists that some toxic elements would not be removed in the sol-gel production. An evaluation of this effect by a very sensitive system would be important prior to incorporating these materials into general clinical use. The material 54S and 77S used in this study were manufactured by the sol-gel process while the 45S5 samples were produced by heat and grinding. The size of the Bioglass® particles in all the groups was less than 90 μm.

The specific aim of this research was to evaluate the potential sensitivity and specificity of a red blood cell (RBC) Hemolysis Assay [7]. This assay detects potential cytotoxic components which may not affect the viability of cells in culture, but do affect the sensitive membranes of red blood cells. This results in the lysis of the RBC and release of hemoglobin which is easily detectable spectrophotometrically. The red blood cell hemolysis assay is used as a biocompatibility test for a variety of surgical, periodontal and restorative materials in dentistry [8,9].

MATERIALS AND METHODS

Fresh, whole defibrinated sheep blood (BBL, Cockeysville, MD) was diluted so that 0.2 ml, hemolyzed in 10.0 ml of distilled water, gave a spectrophotometric reading at 545 nm of 0.8 $\pm$ -0.5 O.D. The test materials, Zinc Oxide Eugenol (L.D. Caulk, Milford, DE), 45S5 Bioglass®, sol-gel 54S, 77S, (U.S. Biomaterials, Alachua Fl), (compositions of Bioglasses are shown in Table 1) Super EBA (Harry J. Bosworth, Skokie Ill),and Amalgam (L.D. Caulk, Milford, DE), were incubated for 1, 30, and 60 days at 37°C placed in tubes and 0.2 ml of the diluted blood was added to the samples and gently mixed and incubated in the water bath for 60 min.

A positive control of 100% cell lysis was made by adding and gently agitating 0.1 ml of the diluted blood to 5 ml of distilled water. The negative control, which is an estimate of spontaneous lysis in medium, was made by mixing 0.1 ml of the diluted blood with 5 ml of RPMI medium and incubated for 1, 30, and 60 days at 37°C. Positive and negative controls were also incubated for 60 min in the 37°C water bath. After the 60 min of incubation, all the tubes were centrifuged for 5 min at 2,000 RPM to pellet the blood cells and debris. The absorbance of hemoglobin in the supernatant was measured at 545 ñm in the spectrophotometer.

The percent hemolysis was calculated according to the following formula:

$$\%\ hemolysis = \frac{(O.D.\ test\ samples) - (O.D.\ negative\ control)}{(O.D.\ positive\ control) - (O.D.\ negative\ control)} \tag{1}$$

RESULTS

At day 1, there was no significant difference between the lysis of the experimental materials, Particulate Bioglass® 45S5, 54S, 77S. Amalgam showed significantly less and ZOE and Super EBA significantly greater lysis ($p < 0.05$). At day 10 the experimental materials showed the same trends as at day 1. At day 30 there was no difference between the lysis of the three particulate Bioglass® samples and Super EBA.

Table 1. Compositions of Bioactive Glass Powders (in mol %).

Sample ID	SiO_2	P_2O_5	CaO	Na_2O
45S5 (melt)	46.1	2.6	26.9	24.4
54S (sol-gel)	55.0	4.0	41.0	--
77S (sol-gel)	80.0	4.0	16.0	--

ZOE showed significantly greater and Amalgam significantly less lysis ($P<0.05$). This data is presented in Table 2.

DISCUSSION

These results indicate that particulate Bioglass® has a low percent hemolysis at 1 and 10 days but showed an increase at 30 days. This was not significant when related to manufacturing methods. All of the Bioglass® groups had a particle size of <90 μm, however the 45S5 group was produced by heating the glass, while the 54S and 77S were produced by the sol-gel process. This finding indicates that sol-gel produced Bioglass® does not retain any additional toxic components suring the production process.

It is reasonable to suggest that the increase in lysis at 30 days may be due to leaching of soluble products from the glass over time. This effect is most likely related to the change in the available surface area available for chemical interaction. The supernatant was not analyzed in this study to identify any soluble products that may have entered the supernatant at any of the time intervals (1, 10, or 30 days). The hemolysis recorded at these observation periods could have resulted either as a direct result of a soluble agent(s) leaching from the glass or as the result from an interaction between any of the individual chemicals that became soluble in the supernatant.

The pH of the supernatant has been shown to have dual effects on hemolysis assays. [10]. The pH of the supernatant can directly cause the red blood cell membrane torupture thus causing a positive reading to be recorded. The second effect related to pH is one of a change in the osmolality which could lead to either complete rupture of the

Table 2. Percent Hemolysis of Red Blood Cells of Samples Incubated for 1, 10, and 30 days at 37°C.

Material	DAY		
	1	10	30
ZOE	8.4	82	74
Bioglass® 45S5	3.2	2.4	5.5
Bioglass® 54S	2.6	2.2	4.7
Bioglass® 77S	2.9	2.8	5.4
Super EBA	3.9	4.6	5.1
Amalgam	0.9	1.6	1.4

RBC or leakage; both events would lead to a positive reading. It has been reported [10] that Bioglass® with a higher surface area to volume ratio shows a quicker increase in pH and a higher final pH. Similarly, phosphorous has been shown to undergo a drop in concentration, at least up to a 20 hour observation period [10]. This concentration change could be a factor in the hemolysis figures recorded at the day 1 (24 hour period) in this study. These findings suggest that additional insight into the mechanism of action of the red blood cell hemolysis should be done at closer time periods over the first 24 hours. Additionally, concurrent with an RBC hemolysis assay an ICP analysis for elemental phosphorous may provide information at an ion level as to the agents responsible for the red blood cell hemolysis.

Super EBA contains fused alumina particles and acetate, a component to accelerate the set of the material. This however, can affect the solubility of the final product and both the acetate and the free eugenol probably contributes to the hemolysis readings recorded in this investigation.

The hemolysis obtained from the ZOE and Super EBA can be potentially explained by the presence of free eugenol, a known lysant. Thus eugenal is free in the supernatant, due to it not being incorporated into the setting reaction of the two materials agents.

Amalgam, has been shown to be toxic in red blood hemolysis and agarose overlay tests. The lysant in this study is probably free mercury, which has not been incorporated into the gamma 1 phase of the material. Its levels are related to mercury controlled diffusion and the aging of the specimens [11].

A significant conclusion to be drawn from this study is the lack of toxicity of the Bioglass® materials. In addition there is no difference between the various formulations of the glass, an important finding, as the manufacturing processes for the samples used in this study wee both heat and sol-gel. Bio-compatibility and lack of toxicity of Bioglass® has also been reported by other investigators [12]. The <90 samples are very small particulate Bioglass® with a significantly higher surface to volume ratio than the other materials. It could be expected that the increase in surface area would result in an increase in surface area would result in an increase in the toxicity if the material was releasing toxic components. This was not seen. In addition, there was no difference between the sol-gel derived Bioglass® (54S and 77S) compared to the traditional preparation 45S5. These results demonstrate that sol-gel produced Bioglass® does not retain any additional toxic components during the production process.

REFERENCES

1. Federal Register, Vol. 43(247), Dec 22, 1978, Part II 59986-60025.
2. Federal Register, Vol. 43(93), May 12, 1978, 20726-20757.
3. Autian, J., *J Cri. Rev Toxicol* 1973, 2(1), 1-40.
4. Litkowski, L.J. & Niehaus-Rohde, C. *J Dent Res* 1994, 74:84.
5. Oguntebi, B., Clark, A., Wilson, J., *J Dent Res* 1993, 72:484-489.
6. Pereira, M., Clark, A.E., Hench, L.L. *J Dent Res* 1994, 28:693-698.
7. Wennberg, A., Hentsen-Pettersen, A. *J Biomed Mat Res* 1981, 15, 433-435.
8. ADA, ANSI/ADA document 41, *J Am Dent Ass* 1979, 99: 697-698.
9. ISO *International Organisation of Standardization* 1984, Technical report 7405.
10. Greenspan, D.C., *Bioceramics* 1994, 7:55-60.
11. Brune, D. *Int Endodon J* 1988, 21:135-142.
12. Wilson, J., Pigott, G.H., Hench, L.L. *J Biomed Mat Res* 1981, 15:805-817.

COMPARISON OF PULPAL INFLAMMATORY RESPONSE USING CALCIUM HYDROXIDE VERSUS PARTICULATE BIOGLASS® IN HUMAN TEETH

Leonard J. Litkowski and Carol Niehaus-Rohde*

Department of Restorative Dentistry, *Department of Endodontics, Dental School, University of Maryland at Baltimore, 666 W. Baltimore Street, Baltimore, MD 21201 USA

ABSTRACT

The purpose of this study was to compare the use of a particulate bioactive ceramic (Bioglass®) with calcium hydroxide as a pulp-capping agent in vital, human teeth. Pulps of vital, asymptomatic teeth were mechanically exposed in deep Class V or Class I cavity preparations and capped with Bioglass® or calcium hydroxide. Teeth were extracted at two intervals, 3 or 30 days post exposure and microscopically evaluated for inflammation and presence of bacterial invasion. Results showed a significant reduction in the amount of inflammation when using Bioglass® as a pulp capping agent.

INTRODUCTION

Direct pulp capping involves the application of a dressing to the exposed pulp in an attempt to preserve its vitality. Some believe that previously reported failures in pulp capping procedures were due to restorative microleakage and subsequent pulp infection rather than to the capping procedure or repair material utilized in these studies [1]. Various materials, medicaments, antiseptics, antinflammatory agents and antibiotics have been utilized as pulp capping agents. Calcium hydroxide, however, is generally accepted as the material of choice for pulp capping [2,3,4].

Stanley [5] histologically confirmed complete dentinal bridging with healthy radicular pulp under calcium hydroxide dressings. Pulp capping is indicated mainly for mechanical exposures in young teeth with incompletely formed root ends in which the vascular supply is greatest. With advancing age, the chances for successful pulp capping diminishes. Pulps in the teeth of older patients become fibrotic and reduced in volume and have increased calcific deposits [2,5,6] thereby limiting the vascular supply needed to maintain a vital pulp. Other factors to consider when doing a direct pulp capping procedure include the size of the exposure, contamination of the exposure site and poor coronal restorations with marginal leakage, all of which may produce unfavorable results.

The objective of pulp-capping is to facilitate pulpal healing. The efficacy of calcium hydroxide has been proven through years of clinical use as the treatment of choice.

However, the use of calcium hydroxide for treating pulp exposures in mature permanent teeth has been questioned. Some investigators have demonstrated degenerative changes such as tissue necrosis and a persistent inflammation of the pulp tissue [7,8].

The mechanism of action of calcium hydroxide revolves around the basic pH of the agent. This pH will kill bacteria and cause an inflammation of the pulp. Inflammation is beneficial to the pulp because it stimulates the formation of reparative dentin. However, persistent or severe inflammation over the exposure site can also lead to significant changes in the viability of the pulp tissue [3]. When calcium hydroxide is applied directly to pulp tissue, there is necrosis of the adjacent pulp tissue and inflammation of the contiguous tissue. Dentin bridge formation occurs at the junction of the necrotic tissue and the vital inflamed tissue. Beneath the region of necrosis, cells of the underlying pulp tissue differentiate into odontoblasts and elaborate dentin matrix. Occasionally, in spite of successful bridge formation, the pulp remains chronically inflamed or becomes necrotic. Therefore, a material which will enhance the formation of reparative dentin without causing severe pulpal inflammation would be a significant treatment modality.

In order to ensure predictable dentin bridge formation, the possible use of bioactive materials for pulp capping procedures may enhance the dentin formation with a reduction in inflammation. Bioglass®, a bioactive ceramic with an ability to bond to bone has recently been studied for pulp capping procedures in miniature swine with apparent success [9]. This study reported a layer of reparative dentin covering the whole exposure site in all pulp specimens capped with Bioglass®. The dentin bridge formed immediately below the Bioglass® layer without an intervening area of tissue necrosis. Bioglass® appears to be able to predictably produce a dentinal bridge with a minimal amount of inflammation in otherwise healthy mechanically exposed teeth.

Bioactive ceramics have been created by systematic examination of different tissue responses to a diverse range of inorganic-nonmetallic implant materials [10]. Since the discovery of Bioglass® by Hench, various kinds of bioceramics have been found to bond chemically to vital bone [11]. Calcium phosphate ceramics and glass ceramics have received much attention as potential bone implant materials because they can form a direct bond with bone tissue [12]. Bioactive ceramics release elements such as calcium, magnesium, phosphorous and silicon which form an apatite layer on their surface [13] and may have potential to induce dentinal bridging without the inflammatory response of calcium hydroxide. However, the use of Bioglass® as a potential agent for capping exposed, vital, human pulp tissue has never been studied. The purpose of this study was to compare the use of a bioactive ceramic (Bioglass®) with calcium hydroxide as a pulp capping agent in vital, human teeth.

METHOD/MATERIALS

The material used was 45S5 Bioglass® particulate in the size range of 90 - 710 μm (Perioglas®). This pilot study consisted of twelve human permanent teeth fromvolunteer patients. All of the teeth were free of caries and restorations, vital (as determined by a cold test) and asymptomatic. Of the 12 teeth, two were maxillary first premolars slated for extraction for orthodontic treatment. The other 10 teeth were fully erupted third molars treatment planned for extraction. Subjects who had taken antibiotics and/or anti-inflammatory medication within 2 weeks prior to treatment were not entered into the study.

Bioglass® was compared with calcium hydroxide as a pulp-capping agent. The calcium hydroxide product, Dycal, was used because of its proven efficacy as a pulp-capping agent (Cvek, 1978). Following review of medical history, local anesthetic (Lidocaine with Epinephrine 1:100,000) was given and the teeth isolated with a rubber dam. A 4-mm diameter buccal Class V or Class I cavity preparation 3-4mm deep was made with a new sterile #557 fissured bur in a high-speed handpiece with adequate water spray. A pulp exposure 2mm in diameter was made in the center of the preparation. The choice of which tooth to receive the experimental or control pulp-capping material was decided by random selection prior to the cavity preparation and pulp exposure. The pulp-capping agent randomly selected was placed directly over the exposure, a sterile 3 mm diameter Goretex® membrane was placed over the pulp-capping agent to separate the pulp capping material from the restorative material. The cavity prep was restored with IRM cement. Patients were asked to monitor any changes in the tooth (i.e. pain, cold sensitivity) and record them. The teeth were extracted in pairs at randomly selected intervals of either 3 days or 30 days with 6 teeth per interval.

The roots of the extracted teeth were cut off and the coronal portion fixed in 10% buffered formalin for 72 hrs. Following fixation, the teeth were sectioned and divided into two groups. One group was demineralized and serial sections prepared. The other group was prepared for staining by use of the Exakt® system for evaluation of non decalcified samples. The amount of pulpal inflammation was determined by histologic examination.

Microscopic examination

The H&E stained serial histological sections made through the exposure site in each specimen were examined under a Nikon Labophot microscope, and the pathological changes in the dental pulp was graded according to the following criteria.

None (0) - no disruption of the odontoblast layer and no inflammatory cells;

Mild(1) - disruption of the odontoblast layer, absence of inflammatory cells adjacent to the dentin bridge and fewer than 10/mm inflammatory cells in the central pulp.

Moderate (2) - disruption to or absence of the odontoblast layer, local accumulation of inflammatory cells below the dentin bridge, with no inflammatory cells in the central pulp and absence of foci of tissue necrosis.

Severe (3) - absence of odontoblast layer, accumulation of inflammatory cells below the dentin bridge and involving 1/3 or more of the coronal pulp, and presence of areas of local tissue necrosis.

Alternate sections stained according to Brown and Brenn were examined for the presence or absence of bacteria on the cavity margins and the underlying pulp. Results were evaluated based on the above criteria. Statistical analysis for the comparison of the $Ca(OH)_2$ to the Bioglass® were performed on the inflammatory response data using an ANOVA with a Scheffe F-test to compare the values within groups and a Mann-Whitney U test to compare the Bioglass® group to the $Ca(OH)_2$

RESULTS

The results of the inflammation scores after histologic preparation are shown in Table 1. There was no presence of bacteria on any sample for both the Bioglass® and $Ca(OH)_2$ groups. Two subjects complained of pain which lasted for about an hour in the experimental tooth capped with Bioglass® at approximately 24 hours after the procedure.

Table 1. Inflammation score of each sample at day 3 and day 30.

	3 Day	30 Day
Bioglass®	1,1,0	0,0,0
$Ca(OH)_2$	2,1,2	2,1,2

However, both subjects denied the need to take any analgesic medication. None of the subjects complained of pain in the control teeth.

An ANOVA was performed on the data which showed a significant difference ($p<.05$) among the groups. A Scheffe's F-test was performed to determine if there was a difference between the individual groups. It was found that there was no difference between the 3 and 30 day Bioglass® group and no difference between the 3 and 30 day $Ca(OH)_2$ group. Therefore the two groups were combined and evaluated for statistical significance using a Mann-Whitney U test. There was a significant difference between the Bioglass® and the $Ca(OH)_2$ groups at the $p<.05$ level.

DISCUSSION

The main goal of pulp capping is to facilitate pulpal healing following mechanical exposure. The ability of the pulp to form reparative dentin as a result of injury is a fundamental defense mechanism. Since reparative dentin forms after the pulp is subjected to inflammation from injury, the presence of mild inflammation may desirable for healing to occur.

The efficacy of calcium hydroxide has been proven over the years as the treatment of choice. The theory of the mechanism of calcium hydroxide is due to the basic pH and antibacterial properties of the material. Calcium hydroxide also induces inflammation which stimulates odontoblasts to produce dentin. However, persistent or severe inflammation over the exposure site sometimes causes necrosis and subsequent changes in the viability of the pulp. The necrosis is apparently initiated by damage to the blood vessels in the pulp. Therefore, a material which induces only minimal inflammation without damage to blood vessels may be clinically useful in mechanically exposed pulps of the older patient population. It should be remembered that the ultimate protection for dentin and the underlying pulp depends on a leak-proof coronal restoration.

In the present study two patients reported a transient pain in the tooth containing Bioglass®. The pain was described as mild and no analgesic was necessary and it diminished completely within one hour. Although the source of this discomfort is not known, there are possibly two mechanisms to attempt to explain these findings. Bioglass® has a rapid release of sodium from the surface of the particle. This leads to a rapid change in the pH of the local environment. This change in pH could be implicated in the pain or the osmotic changes that could be induced by the high level of sodium present leading to a transient swelling of the pulp with the resultant rise in pressure. In addition the presence of sodium ions in the pulp could be stimulating the release of cytokines to begin the repair process which have also been implicated in the pain.

Although it was not possible to quantitate the reparative dentin bridge formation it was noted on all the samples of both Bioglass® and $Ca(OH)_2$. This finding is significant in showing that the repair mechanism is established. The repair of an exposure as large as 2 mm in this study could have significant value in clinical practice. It will be necessary to expand this group and evaluate patients in various stages of carious exposures with bacterial contamination present.

REFERENCES

1. Cox, C.F. and Bergenholtz, G., Fitzgerlad, M., *J. Oral Pathol.* 1982, 11, 327-339.
2. Vernick, S. and Nedelman, C., *J. Endo.* 1975, 3, 88.
3. Cox, C.F. and Bergenholtz G., Heys, S.R., *J. Oral Pathol.* 1985, 14, 156.
4. Cvek, M., *J. Endo.* 1978, 4, 232-237.
5. Stanley, H.R. and Lundy, T., *Oral. Surg.* 1972, 34, 818.
6. Stanley, H.R. and Ranney, R.R., *Oral. Surg.* 1962, 15, 1396.
7. Masterson, J.B., *Br. Dent. J.* 1965, 118, 241-249.
8. Patterson, SS., *Int. Dent. J.* 1967, 17, 490-505.
9. Oguntebi, B., Clark, A., and Wilson, J., *J. Dent. Res.* 1993, 72 (2), 484-489.
10. Hench, L.L. and Paschall, H.A., *J. Biomed. Mater. Res.* 1974, 5, 49-64.
11. Kokubo, T., *Biomater.* 1991, 12(2), 155-63.
12. Hyakuna, O., Yamamuro, T., Kotoura, Y., Oka, M., Nakamura, T., Kitsugi, T., Kokubo, T., and Kushitani, H.J., *Biomed. Mater. Res.* 1990, 24, 471-88.
13. Cheol, K.Y., Clark, A.E., and Hench, L.L., *J. Non-cryst. Solids* 1989, 113, 195-202.

EFFECT OF CHONDROITIN-SULFATE CONCENTRATION OF A ROOT CANAL SEALER CEMENT MADE WITH CALCIUM PHOSPHATES

M. Yoshikawa*, T. Toda*, H. Oonishi**, Y. Mandai*** and F. Sugihara***

*Department of Endodontics, Osaka Dental University, 5-31, Otemae 1-chome, Chuoku, Osaka 540, Japan **Department of Orthopedic Surgery, Artificial Joint Section and Biomaterial Research Laboratory, Osaka-Minami National Hospital, 677-2, Kido-cho, Kawachinagano-shi, Osaka 586, Japan ***Department of Research and Development, Nitta Gelatin Inc., 2-22, Futamata, Yao-shi, Osaka 581, Japan

ABSTRACT
Solubility and disintegration, and histocompatibility of two newly developed root canal sealer cements (sealer) composed of tetracalcium phosphate, dicalcium phosphate dihydrate and 1% or 2% of chondroitin-sulfate (CS) were estimated. The sealers were implanted into the dorsal subcutaneous tissue, and also placed in prepared mandibular first molar canals of rats. The new sealers showed less than 2% solubility and disintegration. In the subcutaneous tissue, it was found that both of them had excellent histocompatibility. In the periapical region, it was considered that they promoted wound healing. These results indicate that the newly developed sealers are endodontically useful.

INTRODUCTION
At the 7th International Symposium on Ceramics in Medicine, we reported on the excellent biocompatibility of cement prepared by kneading an equimolar mixture of tetracalcium phosphate (TeCP) and dicalcium phosphate dihydrate (DCPD) with a modified McIlvain's buffer solution containing cellulose [1]. The cement was superior to conventional sealers in biocompatibility, but inferior to them in respect to viscosity for handling. We, therefore, tried to develop a new sealer containing CS to improve the viscosity and promote wound healing. The effect of the concentration of CS (1%:CS-l, 2%:CS-2) on solubility and disintegration of the sealers was studied. The histocompatibility and wound healing ability of CS were also estimated using rats *in vivo*.

MATERIALS AND METHODS
The components of CS-1 and CS-2 are shown in Table 1. TeCP was prepared by heating the stoichiometric mixture of calcium phosphate dihydrate and calcium carbonate at 1400°C. The particles obtained from the manipulation ranged from 0.6 μm to 44.0 μm

Table 1 Components of newly developed sealers (%: P/L=1.5)

		CS-1	CS-2
Powder phase	TeCP	68.0	68.0
	DCPD	32.0	32.0
Liquid phase	Citric acid	2.1	2.1
	Dibasic sodium phosphate	7.2	7.2
	CS	2.5	5.0
	Distilled water	88.2	85.7

(mean 12-13 μm) in size. DCPD was purchased from Wako Pure Chemical Inc. (Japan). The solubility and disintegration of the sealers were examined according to the methods in the International Standard ISO 6876 [2]. Both sealers were implanted into the dorsal subcutaneous tissue of 6 week old, male, Sprague Dawley rats. The tissue was trimmed out *en bloc* including the implant at 1, 2, 3 and 4 weeks after implantation. The sealers were also placed into the rat mandibular first molar canals after opening of the chamber. The root canals had been prepared to the file size #25 before the placement of sealers. At the same experimental periods, the mandibles were resected. All specimens were fixed and immersed in ethylenediaminetetra-acetic acid. Then 6 μm thick serial sections were made and stained with hematoxylin and eosin (H. & E. stain).

RESULTS AND DISCUSSION

Solubility and disintegration of CS-1 and CS-2 were 1.18+0.05% and 1.92±0.04% respectively. Both sealers satisfied the ISO standard that solubility shall not exceed 3% by mass nor shall the specimen show evidence of disintegration [2].

No inflammatory response around the implanted sealers was observed. However, multinucleated giant cells (MGC) were present around both implants at early experimental periods. The number of MGC increased with the CS-concentration. As mentioned by Chow, the reaction rate of the sealers might be decreased by using a liquid phase containing water-miscible non-aqueous liquids [3]. MGC are commonly seen in tissue associated with intracellular digestion-resistible particulate matter [4]. Many fibroblasts, collagen fibers and small blood vessels infiltrated the implants 4 weeks after implantation, especially in the case of CS-2 (Figs. 1, 2). In this study, no inflammatory response was found in the periapical region after placement of each cement into the root canal. At 2 or 3 weeks after placement of each sealer, many polarized osteoblast-like cells were arranged along the margin of alveolar bone. It has been reported that CS is able to promote or maintain the polarized state of the odontoblasts [5]. The periapical wound caused by mechanical root canal preparation had repaired after 4 weeks in the CS-1 group (Fig. 3). At 4 weeks after placement of CS-2 into the canal, deposition of osteocementum-like hard tissue was found around the apical foramen (Fig. 4). Judging from the results, a combination with CS is preferable for the histocompatibility of the calcium phosphate-based sealer.

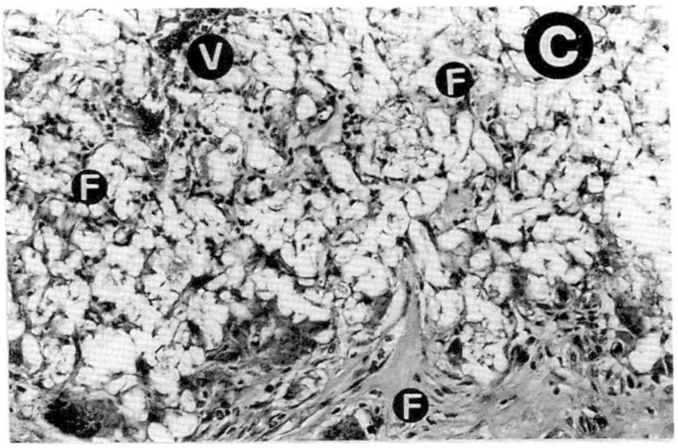

Fig. 1. 4 weeks after implantation of CS-1 F:collagen fiber, V:small vessel C:sealer (H. E. stain X50)

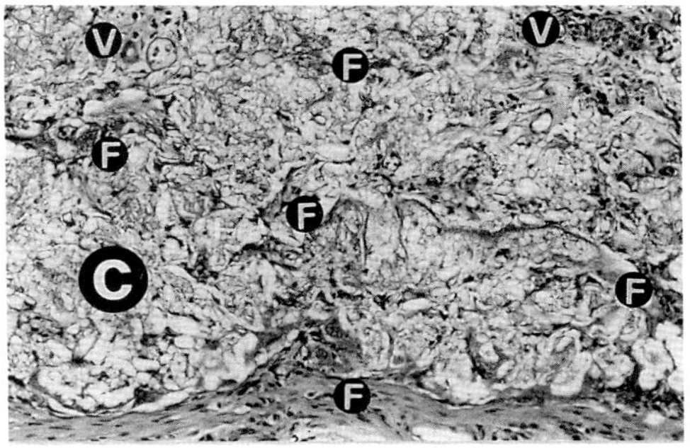

Fig. 2. 4 weeks after implantation of CS-2, F:collagen fiber, V:small vessel, C:sealer (H. E. stain X33)

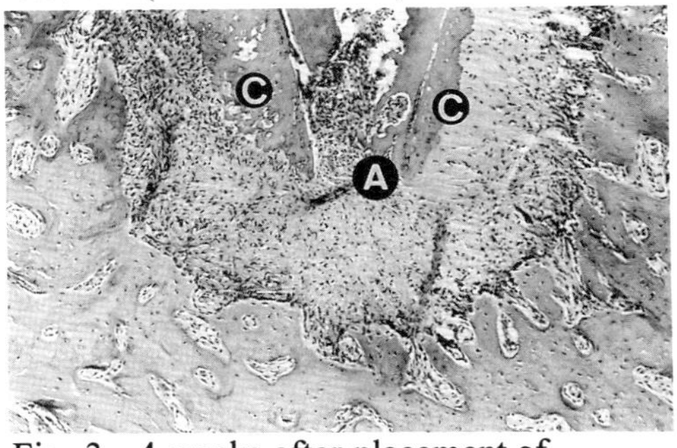

Fig. 3. 4 weeks after placement of CS-1 into a root canal A:apex, C:cementum (H. E. stain X20)

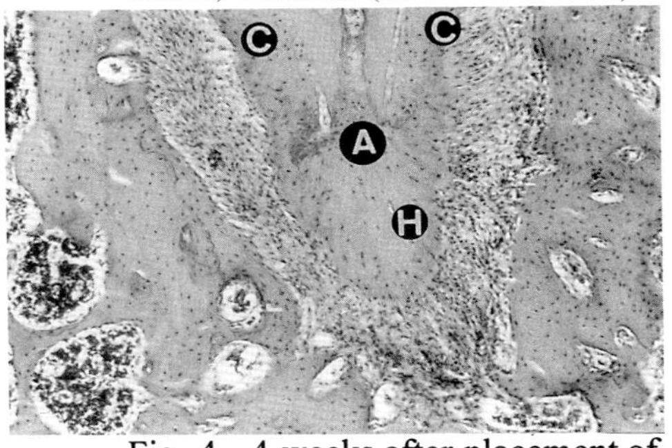

Fig. 4. 4 weeks after placement of CS-2 into a root canal A:apex, C:cementum, H:hard tissue (H. E. stain X20)

CONCLUSIONS

The results of this study indicate that the use of CS in a calcium phosphate-based sealer is valuable because it promotes wound healing in the periapical tissue and can induce osteocementum-like hard tissue around the apex.

REFERENCES

1. Yoshikawa, M., Toda, T., Oonishi, H., Kushitani, S., Yasukawa, E., Hayami, S., Mandai, Y. and Sugihara, F.: *Bioceramics* Volume 7, Butterworth Heinemann, Oxford 1994, 187-192.
2. *ISO Standard,* 6876, 1986.
3. Chow, L.C. *Adv. Dent. Res.* 1988, 2, 181184.
4. Glowacki, J., Jast, M. and Goldring, S. *J. Bone Mineral Res.* 1986, 1, 327-331.
5. Tziafas, D., Amar, S., Staubli, A., Meyer, J.M. and Ruch, J.V. *Archs oral Biol.* 1988, 33, 735-740.

GLASS-CERAMICS FOR DENTAL RESTORATIONS

W. Höland, V. Rheinberger, M. Frank, M. Schweiger

Ivoclar Company Limited, FL - 9494 Schaan, Principality of Liechtenstein

ABSTRACT

The aim of this paper was the development of glass-ceramics for dental restorations. It was possible to develop glass-ceramics in two systems. Glass-ceramics of the SiO_2-Al_2O_3-K_2O system were processed by viscous flow and combined with a new opal glass-ceramic. If fluorine, CaO and P_2O_5 were added, the base glass-ceramic contained needle-like apatite and leucite. Dental glass-ceramics of the SiO_2-Li_2O-ZrO_2-P_2O_5 system possessed basic strength of approx. 280 MPa.

INTRODUCTION

High requirements with regard to the combination of properties are placed on bioceramics used as dental restorative materials. Thus bioceramic crowns and inlays must demonstrate a translucent optical quality, high strength, biocompatibility and favourable processing properties. To achieve these special properties, two material systems were analyzed with regard to their crystallization behaviour and their properties.

LEUCITE-APATITE GLASS-CERAMICS

In the SiO_2-Al_2O_3-K_2O ceramic system with added components such as Na_2O, B_2O_3, CeO_2, CaO, BaO and TiO_2, controlled leucite crystallization was shown [1]. From these examinations it becames apparent that a special mechanism, controlled surface crystallization of leucite, K $(AlSi_2O_6)$, could be used. The resulting glass-ceramic possesses basic strength of 120 MPa, which could be increased to 170 MPa (bending strength) by sinter-fusing additional ceramic layers. The dental crown is translucent and following a special procedure involving a viscous flow process, the material also acquires the processing properties desired by dental technicians.

Based on these investigations, it was possible to develop a dental opal glass with the composition of 48-66 wt.-% SiO_2, 5-20 Al_2O_3, 3-15 K_2O and the addition of 3-12 Me(II)O, with Me(II): Ca, Mg, Sr, Ba, 0.5-5 P_2O_5 and 3-12 Na_2O under the simultaneous influence of up to 6 wt.-% additives, such as Li_2O, ZrO_2, TiO_2, La_2O_3. Phase separation

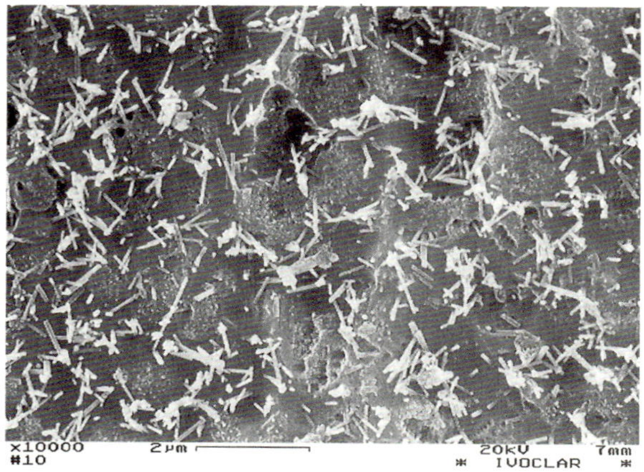

(a)

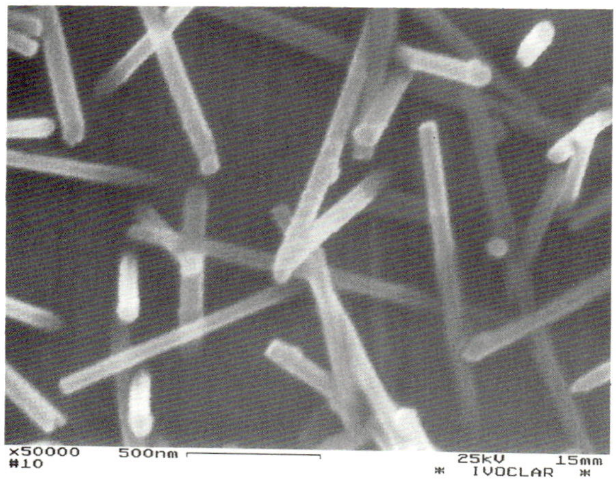

(b)

Fig. 1. Microstructures of leucite-apatite glass-ceramics for dental restorations (SEM). (a) Leucite-apatite crystals after heat treatment at 1050°C. (b) Needle-like apatite after heat treatment at 1150°C.

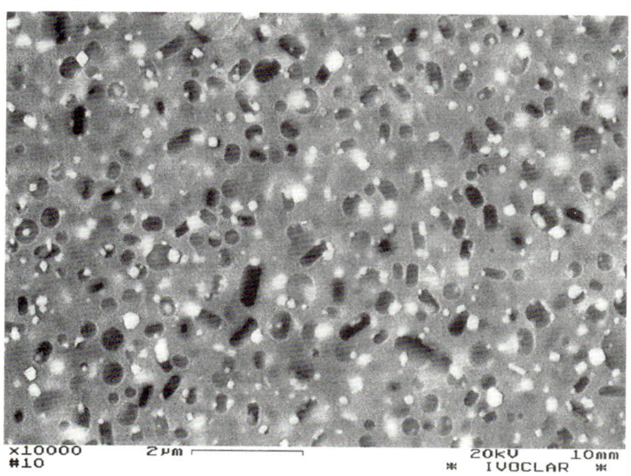

Fig. 2 Microstructure of zirconia based glass-ceramic after HF-etching (SEM).

processes took place in the microstructure and the glass showed opalescence. In parallel to phase separation processes, surface nucleation at grain bounderies resulted in a very high linear thermal expansion coefficient of approx. 120-190 x $10^{-7}K^{-1}$. Therefore, it was possible to combine this dental opal glass with the leucite glass-ceramic to form special dental restorations, dental crowns in particular.

If fluorine was added to the SiO_2-Al_2O_3-K_2O-CaO-P_2O_5 opal glass system, a new phenomenon was observed. Two different mechanisms took place: surface crystallization of leucite and bulk crystallization of needle-like apatite. The composition of this new glass-ceramic is characterizedby 49-58 wt.-% SiO_2, 11-19 wt.-% Al_2O_3, 9-23 wt.-% K_2O, 2-12 wt.-% CaO, 0.5-6 wt.-% P_2O_5, 0.2-2.5 wt.-% F and up to 9 wt.-% additives of $Me(I)_2O$, Me(II)O, $Me(III)_2O_3$ and $Me(IV)O_2$. The microstructure is seen in Fig. 1a and b. Leucite is the main crystal phase but phosphate phases as secondary crystals were determined by X-ray diffraction. Apatite or rather fluorine apatite, in a mixed phase of fluorine/hydroxylapatite could also be determined. The crystallization of needle-shaped apatite is new and had previously been reported in apatite formation by hydrothermal synthesis [2]. The low contents of CaO, P_2O_5 and F are interesting to note in this context.

ZIRCONIA BASED GLASS-CERAMICS

ZrO_2 glass-ceramics having high fllexural strength were developed [3,4,5]. Our aim was to develop a high strength and at the same time partially translucent glass-ceramic that would exhibit viscous flow at temperatures below 1200°C.

This was possible by developing a glass-ceramic in the 42-59 wt.-% SiO_2, 7-15 Li_2O, 15-28 ZrO_2 and 4-14 P_2O_5 system when up to 14 wt.-% additives, such as $Me(I)_2O$, Me(II)O, $Me(III)_2O_3$, $Me(IV)O_2$ and F were used. The final dental glass-ceramic was produced after melting a glass, processing of a raw glass-ceramic, pressing and viscous flow of the raw glass-ceramic at about 1000°C. The characteristic micro-structure of the final glass-ceramic is shown in Figure 2. Lithium phosphate (Li_3PO_4), ZrO_2 (tetragonal and baddeleyite) and $ZrSiO_4$ are the main crystal phases. The glass-ceramic exhibits a flexural strength of 280 MPa, K_{IC} of 1.9 MPa $m^{1/2}$, and translucency at a thickness of approx. 0.5 mm.

In addition, pigmentation of the glass-ceramic microstructure was successfully tested, used as abutments in dental applications.

REFERENCES

1. Höland, W., Frank, M. and Rheinberger, V., *J. Non-Cryst. Solids* 1995, 180, 292-307.
2. Newesely, H., *Mechanism and action of trace elements in the mineralization of dental hard tissues,* Zyma SA 1972.
3. Echeverria, L.M. and Beall, G.H., *Ceram. Trans.* 1991, 20, 235-244.
4. Budd, M.I., *J. Mat. Sci.* 1993, 28, 1007-1014.
5. Uno, T., Kasuga, T., Nakayama, S. and Ikushima, A.J., *Bol. Soc. Esp. Ceram VID* 1992, 31-C, 5, 73-78.

ENDODONTIC IMPLANTATION USING HYDROXYAPATITE-COATED TITANIUM STICKS

H. Oguchi, Y. Karube, K. Mizoue, M. Kinoshita, K. Seto

The First Department of Oral and Maxillofacial Surgery, Tsurumi Unversity, School of Dental Medicine, 2-1-3 Tsurumi Tsurumi-ku Yokohama, 230 JAPAN

ABSTRACT

In 1988, titanium sticks (Ti-6Al-4V) coated with hydroxyapatite (HA) using a high-velocity flame-spraying technique (HVFST) were developed for endodontic implants. Fifty-four patients involving 79 anchored teeth were treated between April 1989 and November 1994. Their clinical diagnoses were radicular cysts (30 patients, 48 teeth), tooth luxation (12 patients, 17 teeth), marginal periodontitis (6 patients, 8 teeth), root fracture (6 patients, 6 teeth). The complications were infection, tooth luxation during operation and root fracture. As a result, seventy-three were saved by applying this method, making the preservation rate 94%. Our results indicate that this implant is effective in preserving teeth which heretofore would have had to be extracted.

INTRODUCTION

The recent development of novel biomaterials has been remarkable, offering many new possibilities in dentistry. However, biomaterials are more fragile than living bone. To solve stress-related problems and improve strength, many investigators have applied HA [1] onto the titanium alloys using a plasma-spraying technique. In 1988, a titanium alloy (Ti-6Al-4V) sprayed with HA by a high-velocity flame-spraying technique(HVFST) was jointly developed by ASAHI Optical Co., Ltd. and our department [2]. Furthermore, HVFST was used to apply HA onto the titanium alloy of endodontic-endosseous implants (PTH stick; Asahi Optical Co., Ltd.). By using a porous-type surface structure, the adhesion strength has been significantly improved between the implant and bone, sprayed-HA and substrate. We also investigated the biocompatibility of the interface between bone and HVFS-HA using tibias of adult male rabbits. Both light and electron microscopic examination of histological sections showed that inflammatory responses of tissues at the implantation site were completely resolved and the interface between the bone and the implant was filled with newly formed bony substrate. Based on these results, the clinical application of PTH sticks was started in April 1989 [3].

This report describes the clinical results obtained over the past 6 years with our endodontic implantation procedure using titanium coated with HVFS-HA.

MATERIALS

Figure 1 shows the HA-sprayed titanium sticks (PTH sticks) prepared by HVFST for use as endodontic implants. The implants were 31 or 34 mm long, made of titanium alloy (Ti-6Al-4V), and sprayed with HA (thickness about 50) from the apex to the mid-point at 20 mm. The diameters of these implants were 1.8 mm and 2.0 mm, in line with the dental root width. The sprayed part was indented every 1.8 mm or 0.7 mm reciprocally until 20 mm from the apex to increase surface area contact with the bone and to determine the length inserted into the bone. The apex of the implant was bullet-shaped to facilitate insertion into the bone and to decrease apex stress. The surface of the non-sprayed portion of the PTH stick was modified by adding a transverse channel (width 0.2 mm) and sand blasting it to prevent rotation and to increase the supporting strength of the crown part. Figure 2 shows the microsurface structure of HVFS-HA. The surface is irregular owing to diverse sizes and shapes of particles and pores, resulting in a pattern similar to that of a coral reef. Regarding the other chemical and physical propertities, see reference 2.

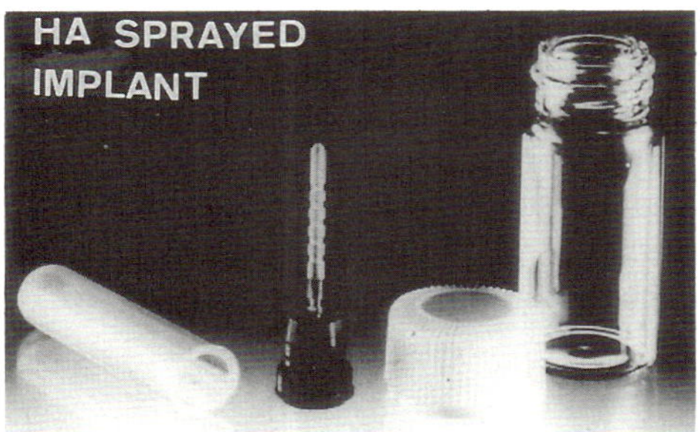

Figure 1: HA sprayed implant

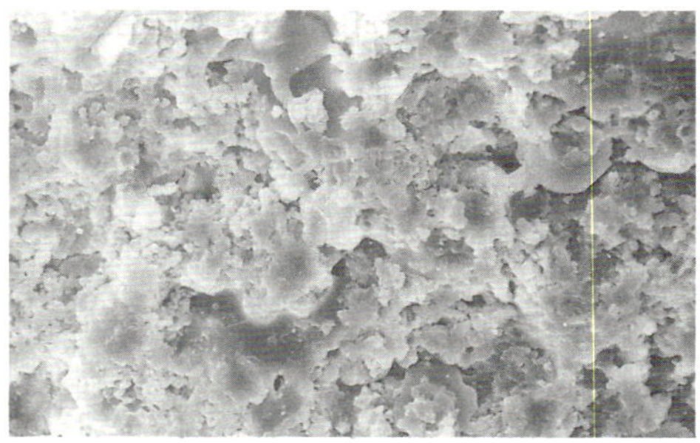

Figure 2: Microsurface structure

The following indications are recommended for these implants:

1) Apical lesions such as radicular cysts and radicular granulomas where the dental root is extensively resected by apicoectomy and marked tooth mobility is observed.

2) Dental root fractures perpendicular to the dental root due to trauma; if the fractured piece is moved from the apical area, cases where it is difficult to preserve the tooth because the remaining dental root is too short.

3) Internal and external absorption, extending for more than half of the length of the dental root, which is associated with high tooth mobility.

4) Significant absorption of the alveolar bone where it is impossible to preserve the bone because of tooth mobility.

5) Teeth highly loaded with abutments for fixed bridges, or retainers for partial dentures, which must be reinforced.

RESULTS

Fifty-four patients involving 79 anchored teeth were treated between April 1989 and November 1994. The age of the patients ranged from 8 to 58 years. The age distribution was: 10 years old or younger - 5 patients, 11 to 20 years old - 14 patients, 21 to 30 years old - 13 patients, 31 to 40 years old - 6 patients, 41 to 50 years old - 13 patients, 51 years or older - 3 patients. Their clinical diagnoses were radicular cysts (30 patients, 48 teeth), tooth luxation (12 patients, 17 teeth), marginal periodontitis (6 patients, 8 teeth), and root fracture (6 patients, 6 teeth).The implants were applied in the following regions: upper median incisor, 37 teeth, upper lateral incisor, 26 teeth, upper canine, 1 tooth, lower median incisor, 4 teeth, lower lateral incisor, 3 teeth, lower canine, 2 teeth, lower first premolar, 3 teeth, and lower second premolar, 3 teeth.

Consequently, 73 teeth were saved by this method over the past 6 years. The preservation rate was 94%. The main complication was infection (10 cases, 12 teeth), treated by antibiotics and iodine-application. However,3 implants were removed in 2 cases. Other complications were tooth luxation during operation (1 tooth, treated by refixing the tooth), root fracture while enlarging the dental root (1 tooth) and retrauma (3 teeth, 3 cases).

Figure 3 is a postoperative radiograph taken 6 years after implantation for a radicular cyst. The tooth was firmly fixed and there have been no complications thus far. Figures 4 and 5 show the microsurface structure of a case in which the implant was removed (retrauma). In this case, it was very difficult to remove the PTH stick from the bone. Therefore, we removed the implant with the surrounding bone. The HA-sprayed portion showed bone-like tissue and the interface between the bone and

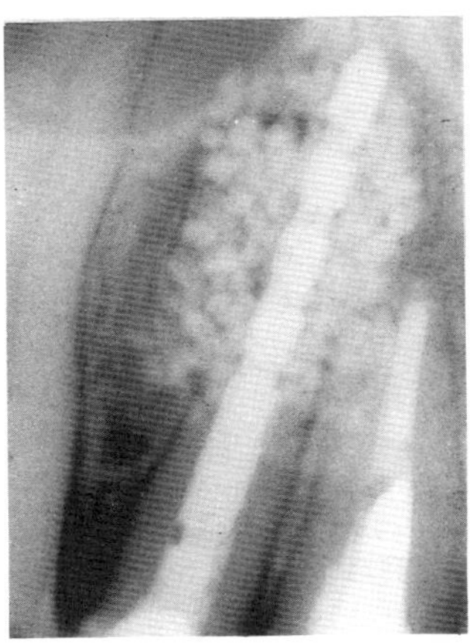

Figure 3

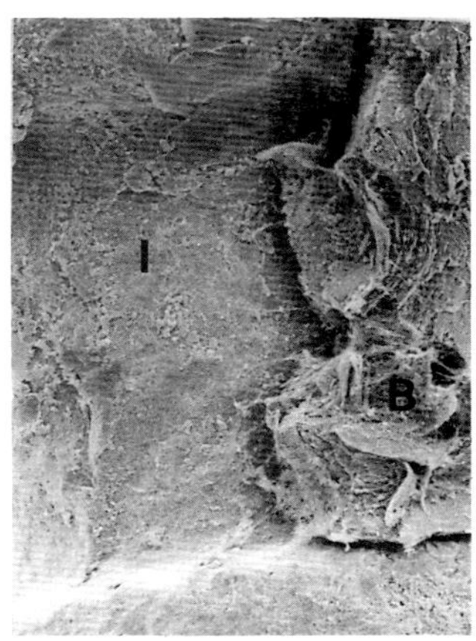

Figure 4: Removal case (SEM)
B: Bone I: Implant

HA in close contact. Figure 6 is a light micrograph of the interface between bone, sprayed-HA and HA granules which filled in the bone defect. The new bone was mature and directly adhered to the implant. Furthermore, resorption of sprayed HA was not clearly evident.

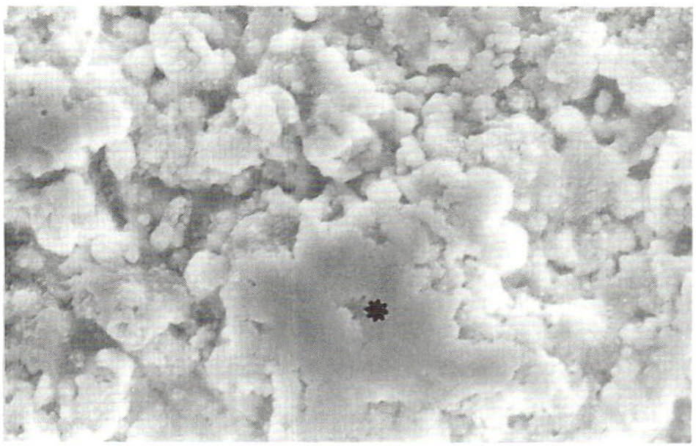

Figure 5: Surface Microstructure(SEM)
* Bone like tissue

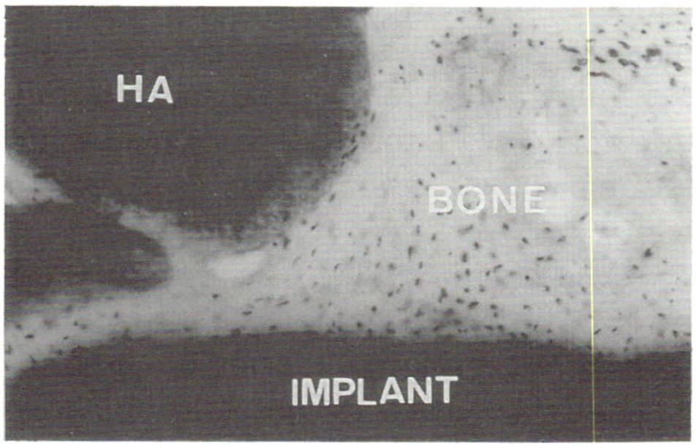

Figure 6: Toluidine blue stain (~100)
HG: HA granule

CONCLUSION

In 1943, Strock [4] first reported the endodontic implantation of a tooth using Vitallium. Orlay [5] and other investigators subsequently established operative methods. Our implant system relies on these techniques. Materials which have been previously used include Vitallium®, single sapphire, titanium, and oxide-coated alloy. Unlike these previous reports, we used a HA-coated stabilizer, and consequently obtained a success rate comparable with previous reports. In particular, firm fixation was demonstrated between coated HA and bone in a case from which the implant was removed. Based on these results, we concluded that the tooth preservation properties of this material are clinically superior to many other biomaterials. At present, the main clinical benefit of HA-coating is good initial fixation to bone, because of the theory that the HA-coating is resorbed. If the HA is not resorbed or if resorption proceeds very slowly, HA-coated materials may have excellent long-term properties in addition to good initial fixation. Jansen *et al.,* [6] have reported that progressive dissolution was observed for all coatings, and in some areas the HA coating totally disappeared, 12 weeks after implantation in the tibia of rabbits. Wang [7] and Maxian [8] have also reported cellular or body fluid resorption of Plasma-HA *invivo* and *in vitro*. Histopathological examination of coated HA materials removed from one patient after three years did not reveal any clear-cut signs of resorption. At the 7th Conference of Ceramics in Medicine, we reported the evaluation of HA sprayed by different coating methods [9]. Although the reasons for resorption of HA are still not completely understood, the density of coated HA seems to be the most important factor.

REERENCES

1. DeGroot K., Geesink, R.G.T., Klein, C.P.A.T. and Serekian.P. *J. Biomed. Mater.Res.* 1987, 21, 1375-1381.
2. H. Oguchi., K.Ishikawa., S. Ojima., Y. Hirayama., K.Seto and G. Eguchi. *Biomaterials.* 1992, 13, 471-477.
3. H. Oguchi., K. Seto., K. Ishikawa and G.Eguchi. *Bioceramics 4* (Bonfield, Hasting & Tanner Eds), Butterworth Heinemann, Oxford, 1991, 363-369.
4. Strock AE., Strock MS. *J. Oral. Surg.* 1943, 1, 252-255.
5. Orlay HG. *J. British Dental.* 1959, 2, 118-121.
6. J.A. Jansen. *J. Biomed.Mater.Res.* 1993, 27, 603-610
7. B.C. Wang. *J. Biomed.Mater.Res.* 1993, 27, 1315-1327
8. S. H. Maxian. *J. Biomed.Mater.Res.* 1993, 27, 111-117
9. H.Oguchi., G.W. Hastings. *Bioceramics. 7* (Andersson, Happonan and Yli-Urpo Eds.) 1994, Butterworth Heinemann, Oxford, 1994, 215-221.

CALCIUM PHOSPHATE COATINGS

STRUCTURAL CHANGES INDUCED DURING THERMAL SPRAYING OF HYDROXYAPATITE. A COMPARISON OF THREE DIFFERENT SPRAYING METHODS.

J.C. Knowles,[1] K. Gross,[2] C.C. Berndt[2] and W. Bonfield[1]

[1]IRC in Biomedical Materials, Queen Mary and Westfield College, Mile End Road, London, E1 4NS. UK.
[2]Thermal Spray Laboratory, Department of Materials Science and Engineering, State University of New York at Stony Brook, New York 1 1794-2275, USA.

ABSTRACT

HA is commonly applied to orthopaedic implants by thermal spraying. The thermal spraying methods used induce differences, not only in the macroscopic and microscopic properties of the coating, but also at the atomic level, which may compromise the long term stability of the coating. Three different thermal spray methods were investigated to determine the effect each would have on the final coating produced at the atomic level. The methods investigated were flame spraying, plasma spraying and high velocity oxy-fuel spraying. All three methods induced a distortion into the hydroxyapatite structure. The high velocity method was expected to produce the highest distortion, but this was not seen due to an annealing effect. Changes were also seen on the chemical level and carbonate found in the precursor powders was removed as determined by both X-ray diffraction (XRD) and Fourier Transform Infra Red spectroscopy (FTIR). Furthermore, hydroxyl groups were removed during spraying, to form oxyapatite.

INTRODUCTION.

Hydroxyapatite (HA) has been established as a material for use in surgery [1,2] and is commonly processed by thermal treatment. However, thermal processing has been shown to induce changes in the structure of HA [3]. Thermal spraying is currently a commonly used method for coating prostheses to produce cementless fixation. The thermal spraying methods utilise high temperatures and velocities, to give the desired coating, but these vigorous conditions can induce significant changes in the HA. Microstructural analysis has shown that the thermal processing methods considerably alter the morphology of the powder and XRD also has detected changes in the HA to an amorphous state, to give a semi-crystalline coating. However, XRD can detect more subtle changes in the coatings, down to the atomic level, by Rietveld analysis. These effects have previously been shown to be significant [3]. The changes detected may be used, not only to assess the chemical quality of the coating, but also as a means of optimising the coating process.

MATERIALS AND METHODS.

HA was sprayed by three different techniques: flame spraying (FS), plasma spraying (APS) and high velocity oxy fuel (HVOF) spraying. The powders and variables used are detailed in Table 1.

Table 1. Conditions used for producing coatings.

	FS	APS	HVOF
Gases	Acetylene/ oxygen	Argon/ nitrogen	Propylene/ oxygen
Stand off distance (cm)	10	10	10
Power level (kW)		18	
Torch type	Terodyne	Metco 3MB	Jet Kote II
Powder particle size (μm)	10-40	30-80	10-40
Spraying velocity (ms^{-1})	50-80	150-180	280-320
Spraying temperature (°C)	1800	2900	1700

Following coating, the HA was carefully removed from the substrate and analysed by X-ray diffraction (XRD). A data set was collected between 5 and 110°2θ, using a step size of 0.02° and a sample time of 12 seconds. CuKα radiation was used. The data set was analysed using General Structure Analysis Software. Samples were also analysed using a Nicolet 800 FTIR spectrometer.

RESULTS

When spraying a powder by thermal methods, there are two main variables in the spraying, namely the temperature and the velocity. The three different methods used in this study were chosen to have markedly different temperatures and velocities, to highlight differences that the techniques may introduce. The first variable examined was the velocity, which was measured indirectly by calculation of any physical distortion in the HA from the distortion of the PO_4 tetrahedra, as shown in Figure 1. The precursor powders show a relatively low distortion index of around 2. Following spraying, irrespective of method, this index increases. Consideration of the source of the distortion leads to the conclusion that velocity is the major influencing factor. However, the HVOF method, while having a significantly higher spraying velocity, does not introduce the highest distortion. This result may be accounted for by the annealing effect in the HVOF method. The HVOF method has a large heat zone, which extends as far as the substrate. The substrate is heated and thus distortion is annealed out. The APS method however, has a localised heat zone and no annealing occurs, giving the high distortion index.

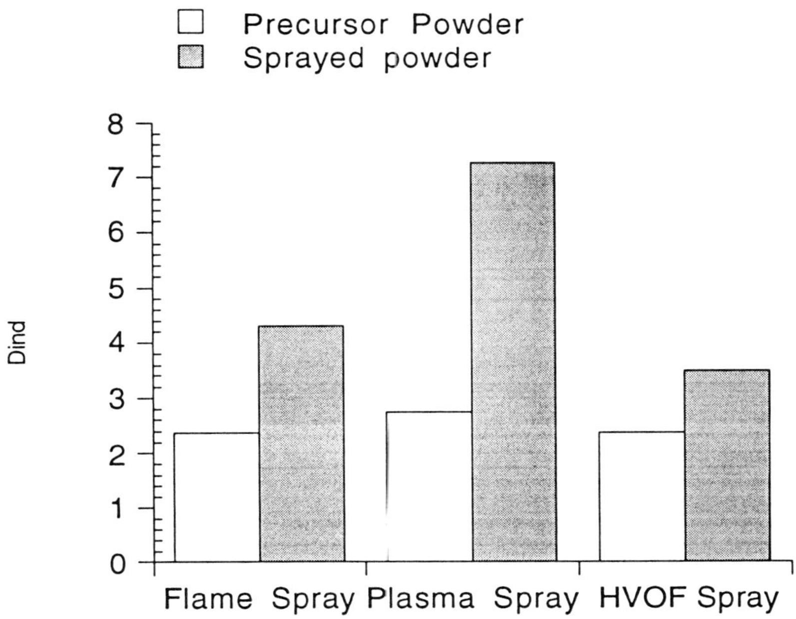

Figure 1. Change in distortion index using different thermal spray methods.

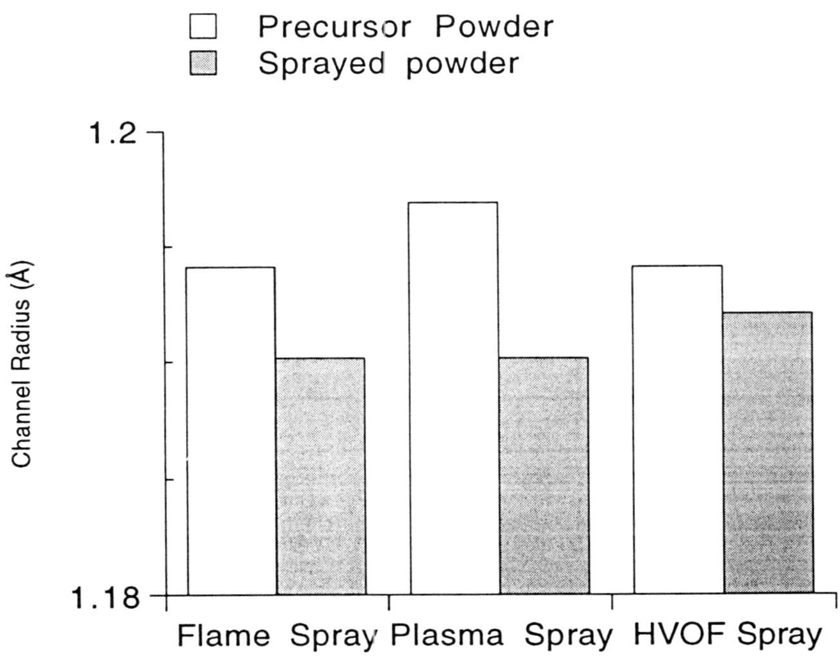

Figure 2. Effect of spraying methods on the hydroxyl channel radius.

Situated within the apatite structure, channels running parallel to the 'c' axis are seen and the radius of these channels may be measured, as shown in Figure 2. As expected, a comparison of before and after spraying shows that the channels shrink. In order to determine why the channels are shrinking, further analysis was performed for specific bonds associated with the hydroxyl channels (so designated, because the hydroxyl groups reside within these channels). Measurement of the $Ca(OH)_2$ bond length reveals significant changes following thermal spraying. The precursor powders both show bond lengths of approximately 2.4 Å Following spraying, these bond lengths all drop to values of between 2.355 and 2.365 Å, a significant reduction in bond length. Determination of the hydroxyl oxygen occupancy (not detailed here) show a reduction in occupancy from above 0.5 to values below 0.5. A value of 0.5 is expected when hydroxyl groups occupy this site. If carbonate groups are located on this site, the occupancy rises to a value above 0.5. However, if only oxygen is associated with the site, the occupancy drops to below 0.5. From the results obtained, it may be inferred that carbonate is present in the precursor powder and is lost on thermal spraying. Furthermore, the rigorous conditions have also formed oxyapatite. In order to confirm this conclusion, FTIR analysis was carried out on both the precursor powders and the sprayed surfaces.

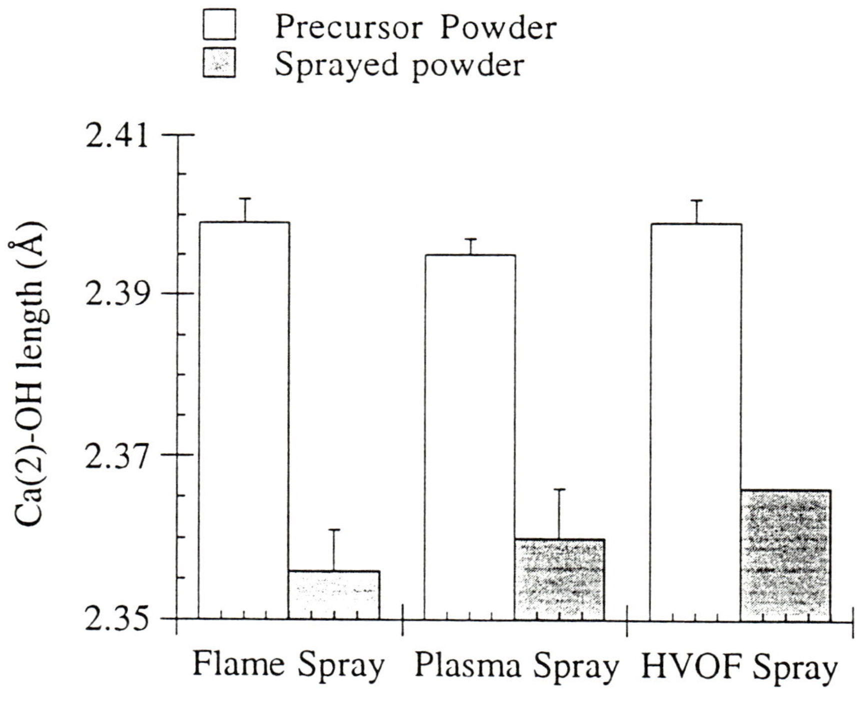

Figure 3. Effect of different thermal spray methods on the $Ca(OH)_2$ bond length.

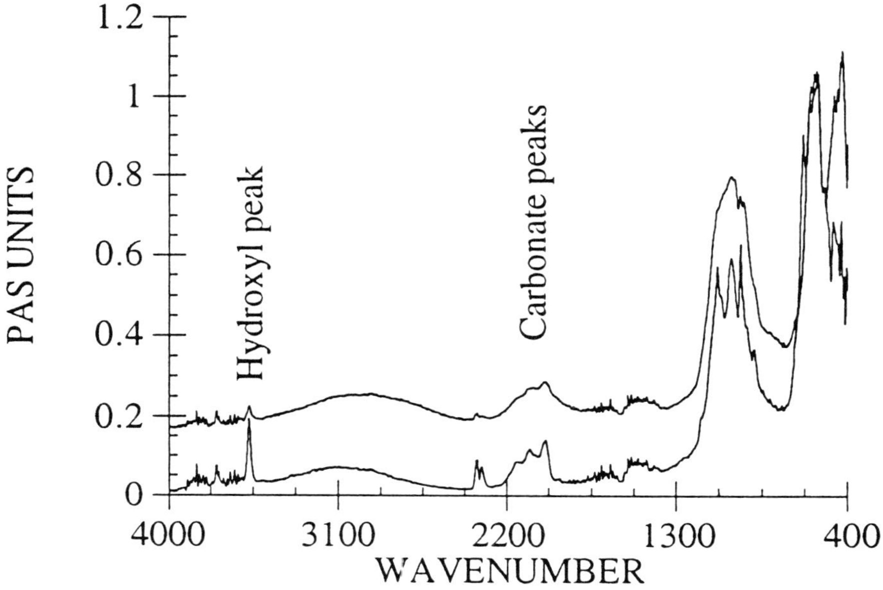

Figure 4. Infra red spectra for HA, before (lower) and after (upper) flame spraying.

Labelled in Figure 4 are the peaks of interest, the hydroxyl peaks and the carbonate peaks. It can be seen that the starting powder contains significant amounts of carbonate in the structure. The hydroxyl peaks are also present in the starting powder as expected. Following spraying, the carbonate peaks show a reduction in intensity, indicating loss from the structure and furthermore, the hydroxyl peaks also show a reduction in intensity. Figure 5, shows an FTIR analysis of the precursor powder before and after plasma spraying. This again shows a disappearance of both the hydroxyl peaks and also loss of the carbonate groups. Thus the FTIR results confirm the conclusions drawn from the data calculated from Rietveld analysis.

CONCLUSIONS.

The thermal spraying induces considerable changes in the structure of HA, detected by XRD in conjunction with FTIR. XRD analysis is able to detect subtle changes in the structure of the sprayed HA, with distortion induced by the extremely high particle velocities used. Small chemical changes were also detected and confirmed by the use of FTIR analysis.

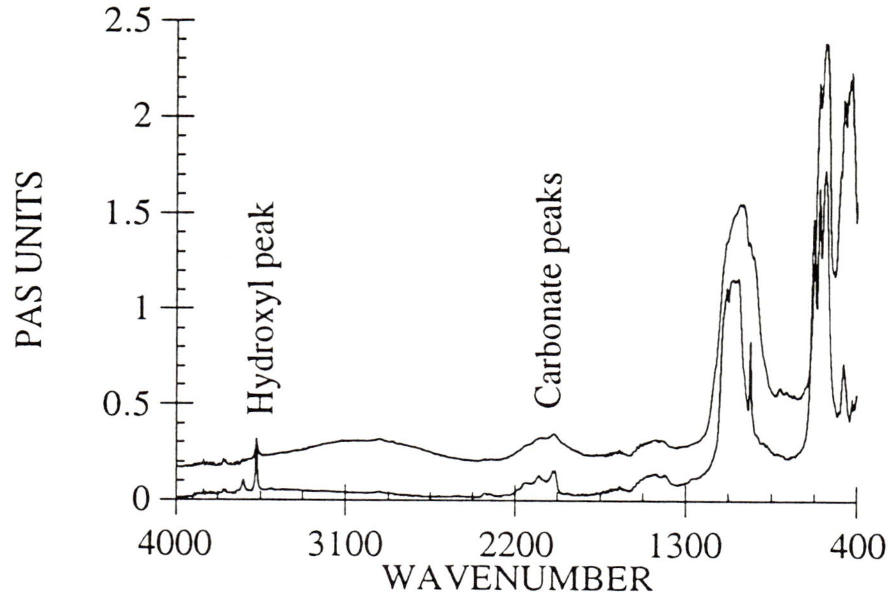

Figure 5. Infra red spectra for HA, before (lower) and after (upper) plasma spraying.

ACKNOWLEDGEMENTS .

The continued support of the EPSRC for the IRC programme grant in Biomedical Materials is gratefully acknowledged. The authors also thank Dr. I. Rehman for his help with the FTIR analysis.

REFERENCES.

1. Wolke, J.C.G., Klein, C.P.A.T., de Blieck-Hogervorst, J.M.A. and de Groot, K., In: *Proceedings of the 1993 National Thermal Spray Conference,* Ed. by Berndt, C.C. and Bernecki, T.F. ASM International, 619-628.
2. Almby, B. and Hierton, T. *Acta Orthop. Scand.,* (1982) 53, 398-406.
3. Abrahams, I. and Knowles, J.C. *J.Mat.Chem.,* (1994), 4(2), pl85-188.

PLASMA SPRAYED COATINGS OF CALCIUM TITANIUM PHOSPHATE: A NEW GENERATION OF BIOACTIVE COATINGS.

E. Lugscheider[1], G. Berger[2], M. Knepper[3], R. Sicking[1], A. Nyland[1]

[1]Materials Science Institute, Aachen University of Technology, 52056 Aachen, Germany,
[2]Federal Institute for Materials Research and Testing, Laboratory for Biomaterials, 12200 Berlin, Germany,
[3]Graduate School of Biomedical Engineering, University of New South Wales, Sydney, NSW 2052, Australia

ABSTRACT

Plasma spraying is one of the most modern techniques for processing powders to make functional coatings. However, depending on the physical properties of the materials they may undergo chemical and structural changes during this energetic process. This paper presents and dicusses the production of plasma sprayed CaTiP coatings which were evaluated with regards to the phase composition and purity and the mechanical stability, including tensile strengths. Investigations of the surface microstructure and porosity were also conducted. The most important results are presented and compared to plasma sprayed hydroxyapatite coatings.

INTRODUCTION

Plasma sprayed coatings of bioactive materials have been introduced in the early eighties. The most important coating material is hydroxyapatite (HAp) [1,2], the main calcium-phosphate phase of natural bone. The advantage of employing calcium-phosphate coatings on orthopaedic and dental implants is their surface bioactivity. This leads to a strong chemical bond between bone and implant, strengthening the bond in the bone/implant interface in comparison with uncoated implants.

In the early nineties, calcium-metal-phosphate (CaMP (M=Ti, Zr)) coatings were reported. For example, material with the chemical composition $CaTi_4(PO_4)_6$ (CaTiP) as bulk material has been shown to exhibit good biocompatibility with respect to biological stability [3]. Dissolution rates lower than those of HAp could be observed. However, plasma sprayed coatings of CaMP have not yet been processed. This paper describes the formation of bioactive coatings on implants by using atmospherical plasma spraying.

MATERIALS AND METHODS

During plasma spraying the plasma gas jet is created by an electric arc burning between a finger-type tungsten cathode and a nozzle-type copper anode inside the burner. Plasma gases used are noble gases (argon, helium) or mixtures with diatomic gases (nitrogen, hydrogen). The powder is fed by a powder gas jet into this high energy plasma. The injected powder particles enter the molten state and the material is deposited onto the roughened substrate surface. Depending on the plasma gas composition the velocity of the molten powder particles during spraying is in the range of 300 to 600 ms^{-1}. Figure 1 shows the plasma burner in a cross section of an atmospheric plasma spray system [6].

In this project atmospheric plasma spraying was carried out by applying argon and hydrogen as plasma gases and argon as the powder carrier gas. To keep substrate material at low temperatures cooling was performed by means of compressed air. The powders were sprayed on samples made of surgical grade of titanium alloys (TiAl6V4). Previous investigations led to optimized spray conditions which are listed below:

Plasma power:	40 kW	
Plasma gas composition:	Ar	50 SLPM
	H_2	10 SLPM
Spray distance:	90 cm	
Passes:	5	

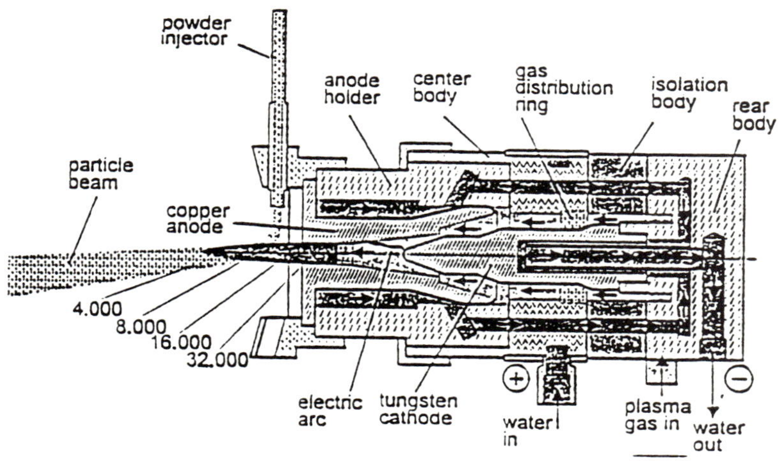

Figure. 1: Principle of a plasma burner.

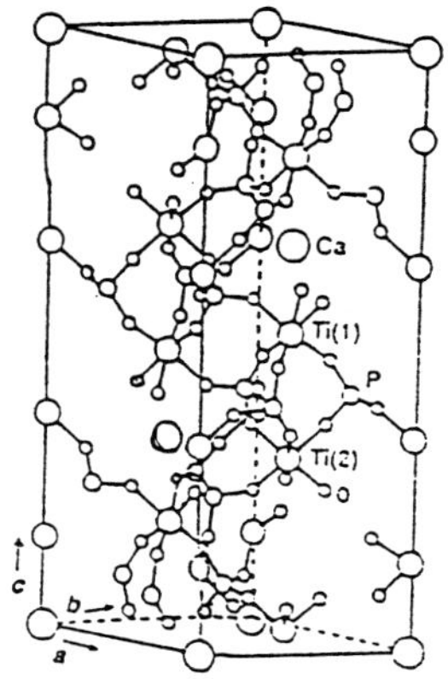

Ionradius (10^{-10} m)	1,00
a (10^{-10} m) (0.01)	8,38
c (10^{-10} m) (0.02)	22,03
Volume of the unit (10^{-10} m)^3	1139,00

Figure 2. Crystallite structure and properties of an elemental unit. [4,5]

In addition to hydroxyapatite, calcium-titanium-phosphate ($CaTi_4(PO_4)_6$) is an other suitable example of a bioactive material. The bioactive nature and the permanence as a bulk material has been well documented [3]. Figure 2 show the crystallite structure and the properties of an elemental unit.

First step in the coating production is the manufacturing of suitable particle sizes of powders. In this project different paricle sizes were used:

- 45 - 200 μm
- 90 - 200 μm
- 45 - 90 μm
- less than 45 μm

Aim of the powder variation was to optimize the quality of the coatings, especially the tensile bond strength, the degree of crystallinity and the homogenity of microstructure.

RESULTS AND DISCUSSION

Optical and Scanning Electron Microscopy

To illustrate the microstructure of a calcium-titanium-phosphate coating, optical and scanning electron microscopy investigations was done. Figures 3 to 6 show the different coating qualities, depending on particle size, taken by optical microscopy.

All coatings show the typical lamellar structure of plasma-sprayed coatings, the density and the degree of homogenity are also obvious. The variation of the powder size leads to great differences in the deposition rate. The minimum deposition rate was achieved by using powder size of 45 - 200 μm. The plasma power is too low for melting large particles. The best results were achieved with the smallest powder size distribution (⟨45 μm). The photo shows a homogeneous microstructure with low porosity and good bonding between substrate and coating simular to HAp-coatings.

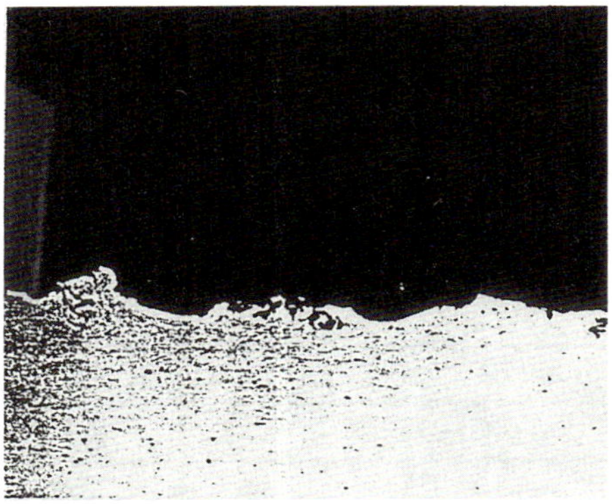

Figure 3. Microstructure (45-200 μm)

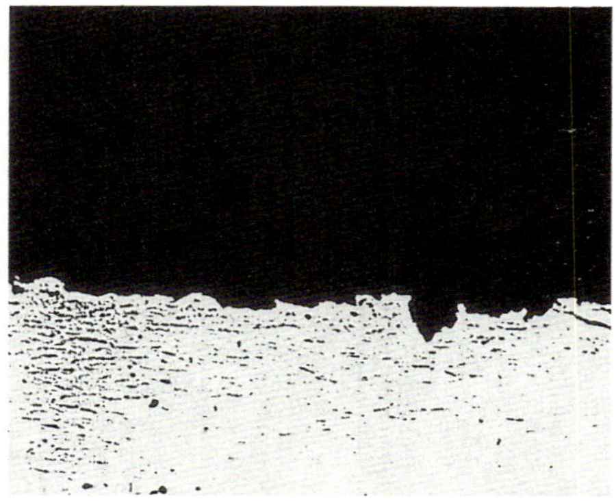

Figure 4. Microstructure (90-200 μ m)

Figure 5. Microstructure (45-90 μm)

Figure 6. Microstructure (⟨45 μm)

The determination of phase composition was investigated using EDX-analysis (energy dispersive x-ray spectral analysis). Three different phases were analyzed (Figure. 7). The light color phase 1 contains high amounts of titanium, but nearly no phosphorus. Therefore it can be concluded that there exists a calcium-titanium phase,

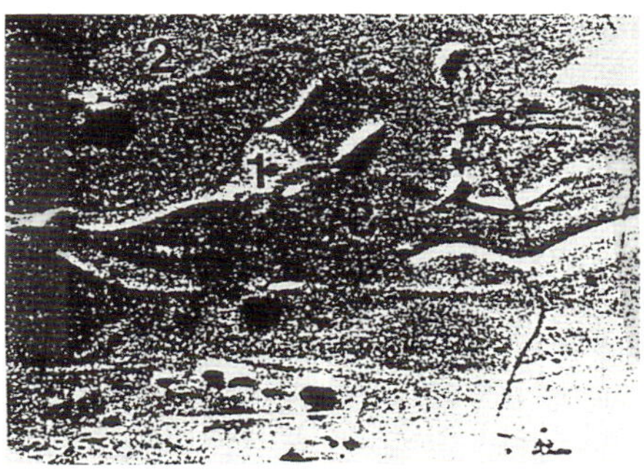

Figure 7. Phase composition of $CaTi_4(PO_4)_6$.

e.g. Ca_2TiO_4. Due to the unknown bioactive behaviour of this oxidation phase, phase 1 should be avoided. Just as the middle dark phase 2, the dark phase 3 shows more phosphorus, but less titanium. Probably both phases are different modifications of calcium-titanium-phosphates.

X-ray diffraction

Investigations by X-ray diffraction starting powder and resultant coatings were conducted to compare compositions of coatings with the powders used. Previous investigations showed that the influence of the spray powder on the coating is significant [4]. It was noticed that, during spraying, a decomposition process takes place. Compared to the initial powder (Fig. 8) the degree of crystallinity of all coatings decreased.

The content of amorphous phase is maximum when using the smallest particle distribution of ⟨45 μm (Fig. 8). The results illustrate that with decreasing particle size the degree of crystallinity also decreases. However, there is still a potential for increasing the calcium-titanium-phosphate phase in air-plasma-sprayed coatings.

Measurement of mechanical strength

Investigations of tensile strength according to European standard EN 582 [7] were performed. In case of Ca_2TiO_4 the influence of particle size distribution on tensile strength was of special interest. Coatings for this test were made on stainless steel samples. Results show that with increasing particle size distribution the tensile strength decreases. Hence the sample with the most homogeneous microstructure shows the highest value of tensile strength.

45 - 200 μm	90 - 200 μm	45-90 μm	⟨45 μm
26,8 MPa	33,4 MPa	39,6 MPa	52,3 MPa

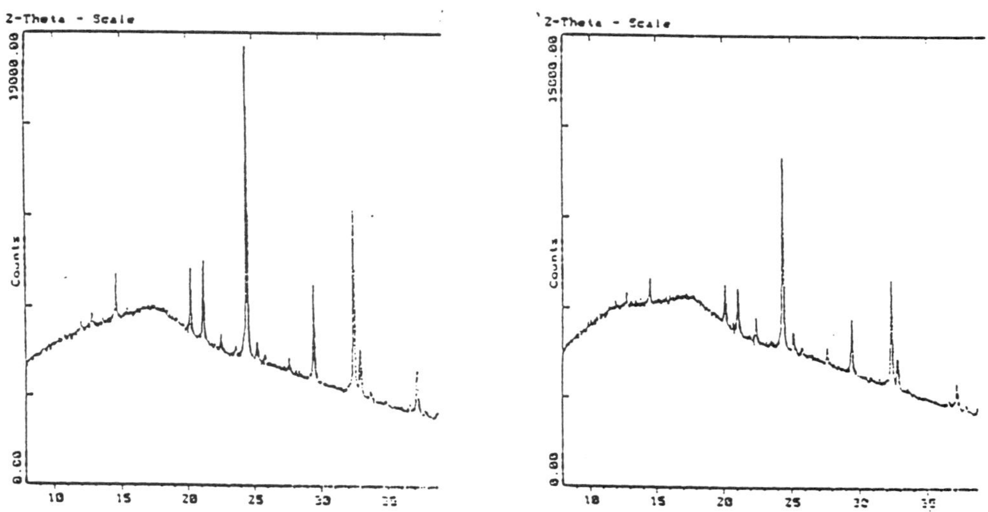

Figure 8. X-ray analysis of initial powder (left) and coating (right).

CONCLUSION

The results so far suggest that functional coatings of CaTiP can be produced, but the crystallinity of the coatings decreases during the spray process. A two step process (plasma spraying - thermal post treatment of the surface) is expected to improve the coating crystallinity. The mechanical stability is higher than that of HAp, but the brittleness has still to be evaluated.

From the results of particle sizes variation the following conclusions can be drawn:

- the most homogenious microstructure could be achieved by using the particle size distribution of $\langle 45\ \mu m$.
- during plasma spraying different phases occur.
- the degree of crystallinity increases with increasing particle sizes.
- with increasing particle size distribution the tensile strength decreases.

This joint project is supported by the German Research Foundation (DFG), Bonn.

REFERENCES

1. Lugscheider, E., Weber, T., Knepper, M., Vizethum, F. Production of Biocompatible Coatings by Atmospherical Plasma Spraying. Materials Science and Engineering 1991, A139, 45-48.

2. Knepper, M. Entwicklung plasmagespritzter Calciumphosphat-Schichten für den Einsatz in der Medizintechnik Dissertation, RWTH Aachen, 1993

3. Szmukler-Moncler, S., Daculsi, G., Deudon, C., Passuti, N. *9th European Conference on Biomaterials,* Chester, UK, 9th-11th Sept. 1991

4. Senbhagaraman, S., Guru Row, T.N., Umarji, A.M. *Journal Mater. Chem.,*1993, 3 [3] 309-314.

5. Senbhagaraman, S., Umariji, A.M. *J. Solid State Chemistry,* 1990 85, 169-172.

6. Lugscheider, E., Nyland, A., Sicking, R. *VIIIth Colloquium on Biomaterials,* February 16-17th, 1995, Abstract

7. EN 582, Ermittlung der Haftzugfestigkeit

BIOACTIVE TITANIUM ALLOYS PREPARED BY CHEMICAL SURFACE MODIFICATION

F. Miyaji, H.M. Kim, T. Kokubo, T. Kitsugi* and T. Nakamura*

Division of Material Chemistry, Faculty of Engineering, Kyoto University, Sakyo-ku, Kyoto 606-01, Japan
*Department of Orthopedic Surgery, Faculty of Medicine, Kyoto University, Sakyo-ku, Kyoto 606-01, Japan

ABSTRACT
The validity of a novel chemical method for inducing bioactivity was examined for titanium based alloys as well as other metallic biomaterials. Ti-6Al4V, Ti-6Al-2Nb-Ta and Ti-15Mo-5Zr-3Al alloys, SUS316L and Vitallium® were soaked in 10 M-NaOH aqueous solution at 60°C for 24 h and then heated up to 600°C at a rate of 5°C/min. All the Ti alloys examined formed an amorphous alkali titanate layer on their surfaces by these treatments and formed a dense and uniform bone-like apatite layer after subsequent soaking in simulated body fluid with ion concentrations nearly equal to those of human blood plasma. SUS316L and Vitallium® did not form them. The apatite layer tightly bonded to the titanium alloy substrates because of the compositional gradient from the outer apatite layer to the inner metal. The present chemical surface modification provides bioactive Ti and its alloys, useful as artificial bones under load-bearing conditions.

INTRODUCTION
Some metallic materials such as Ti, Ti-6Al-4V, SUS316L and Vitallium® have been widely used as orthopedic implants. None of these metallic materials, however, directly bonds to living bone. Thus, various surface modifications have been attempted for providing these metals with bone-bonding ability. Ti metal and its alloys, coated with hydroxyapatite (HA) by the plasma spray method, are currently widely used as bone substitutes under load-bearing conditions [1]. Plasma spraying is usually performed at extremely high temperature, about 10,000°C. This gives rise to various problems in controlling composition, crystallinity and structure of HA owing to its thermally unstable character. As a result, degradation of the HA coating layer is inevitable. In addition, the HA coating is only bonded mechanically to the substrate, and the HA layer is liable to peel off. We have shown [2] that pure Ti metal which is soaked in a NaOH or KOH aqueous solution (alkali treatment) and subsequently subjected to a heat treatment forms a bone-like apatite layer on its surface in simulated body fluid with ion concentrations nearly equal to those of human blood plasma [3]. This indicates

that Ti metal thus treated will be able to form a biologically active apatite layer in the body. In the present study, the validity of such treatment for inducing bioactivity is examined for Ti based alloys as well as other metallic biomaterials.

MATERIALS AND METHODS

Table 1 shows the chemical compositions of the metallic substrates used in this work. The dimensions of the substrates were 10x10x1 mm^3. They were polished with #400 diamond paste and washed with pure acetone and distilled water in an ultrasonic cleaner. Alkali treatment was performed by soaking these substrates in 5 ml of 10M NaOH aqueous solution at 60°C for 24 hr. After alkali treatment, the substrates were carefully washed with distilled water, and dried at 40°C for 24 hr in air. The alkali-treated substrates were placed on an alumina boat, heated to 600°C at a rate of 5°C min^{-1} in an electrical furnace, kept at that temperature for 1 h, and cooled to room temperature in the furnace.

The bioactivity of the alkali- and heat-treated specimens was evaluated by examining apatite formation on their surfaces in an acellular simulated body fluid, (SBF) [3]. Each specimen was soaked in 24 ml of SBF for 1-4 weeks. After the soaking, the specimens were removed from the fluid, washed gently with pure acetone, and dried.

After alkali and heat treatments and subsequent soaking in SBF, surface structural and morphological variations of the specimens were characterized by a thin-film X-ray diffractometer (TF-XRD; thin-film attachment CN2651A1, Rigaku-Denki Co.,Tokyo, Japan), and a scanning electron microscope (SEM; S-2500CX, Hitachi Co., Tokyo, Japan) with an energy dispersive electron probe X-ray analyzer (EDX; EMAX-3700, Horiba Co., Kyoto, Japan). The variations in elemental concentrations of SBF due to immersion of the specimens were characterized by an inductively coupled plasma (ICP) emission spectroscope (Model SPS-1500 VR, Seiko Instruments Inc., Tokyo, Japan). The changes in pH were also measured by a pH meter (Model D- 14, Horiba Co., Kyoto, Japan).

RESULTS AND DISCUSSION

Figure 1 shows the TF-XRD patterns of the surfaces of the alloys after alkali and heat treatments. The broad halo is due to the amorphous phase and appears at about 23 to 30° and 47-49° in 2θ for all the Ti alloys after alkali treatment. This is attributed

Table 1. Chemical compositions of substrates used in this work (Wt%)

Alloy	Ti	Fe	Co	Mn	Cr	Ni	Mo	Al	V	Nb	Ta	Zr
Ti-6Al-4V	Bal.	0.18	-	-	-	-	-	6.45	4.16	-	-	-
Ti-15Mo-5Zr-3Al	Bal.	0.03	-	-	-	-	15.17	3.5	-	-	-	5.13
Ti-6Al-2Nb-Ta	Bal.	0.20	-	-	-	-	0.72	6.25	-	1.93	1.00	-
SUS316L	-	Bal.	-	1.23	17.5	12.15	2.12	-	-	-	-	-
Vitallium	-	0.48	Bal.	0.71	28.5	0.18	6.04	-	-	-	-	-

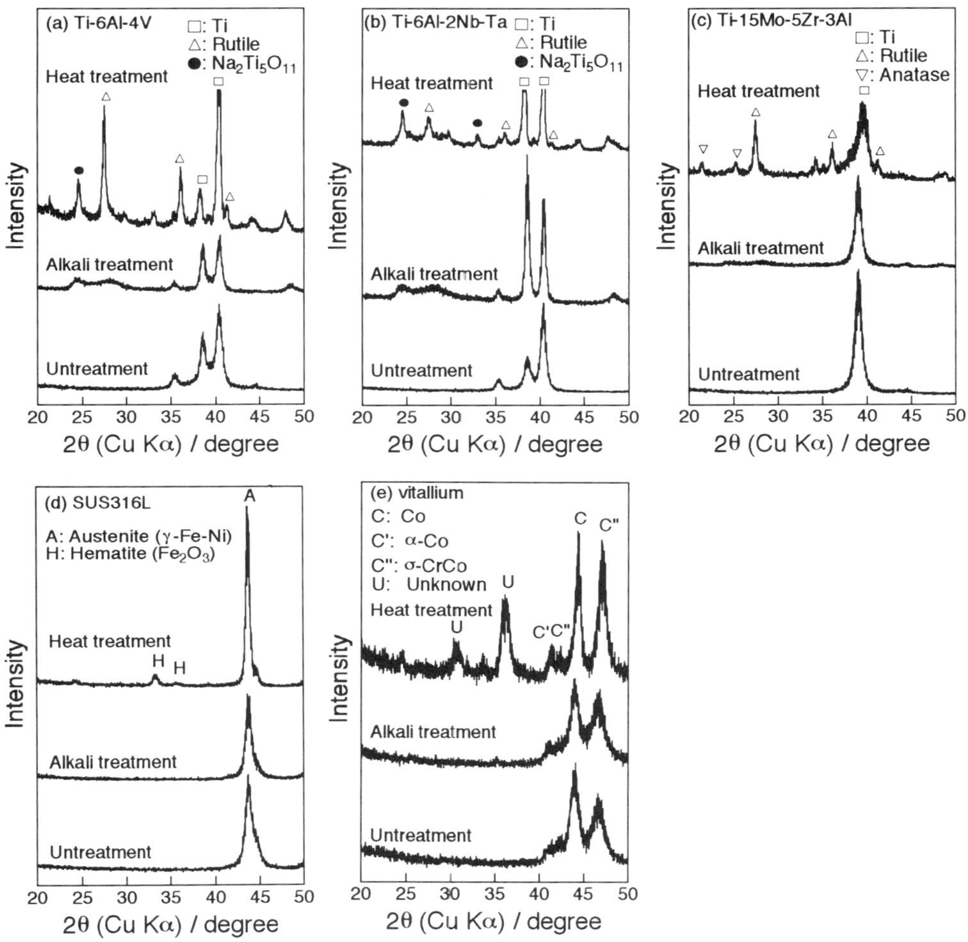

Figure 1. TF-XRD pattems of the surfaces of (a) Ti-6AI 4V, (b) Ti-6AI2Nb Ta, (c) Ti-lSMo-SZr3AI, (d) SUS316L and (e) Vitallium® subjected to alkali and heat treatments.

to the formation of the alkali-containing TiO_2 hydrogel layer on their surfaces similar to the case of pure Ti [2]. Ti-6Al-4V and Ti-6Al-2Nb-Ta alloys precipitate rutile and $Na_2Ti_5O_{11}$ after the heat treatment at 600°C, and Ti-l5Mo-SZr-3Al alloy precipitates rutile and anatase. The halo based patterns are, however, still noticable after the heat treatment for all the Ti alloys similar to the case of pure Ti [2]. This might be attributed to formation of a dehydrated amorphous alkali titanate layer. On the other hand, SUS316L and Vitallium® show almost no change after alkali treatment. SUS316L precipitates hematite (Fe_20_3) after the heat treatment, while Vitallium® precipitates appreciable amounts of an unknown phase, which we speculate to be a certain complex

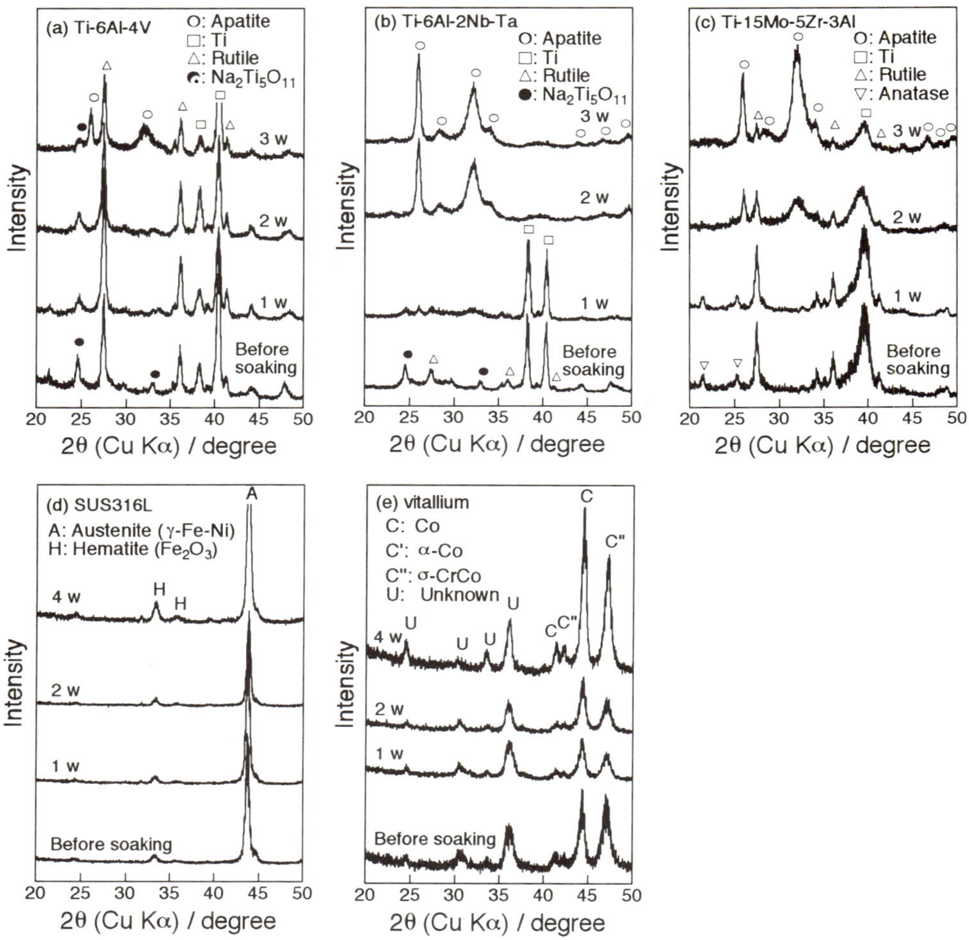

Figure 2. TF-XRD pattems of the surfaces of (a) Ti-6A14V, (b) Ti 6AI2Nb-Ta, (c) Ti l5MoSZr-3AI, (d) SUS316L and (e) Vitallium® subjected to alkali and heat treatments and the subsequent soaking in SBF for various periods.

oxide. Neither SUS3 16L nor Vitallium® formed an amorphous layer on their surfaces after the alkali and heat treatments.

Figure 2 shows the TF-XRD pattems of the surfaces of the Ti alloys treated with 10M NaOH, heated at 600°C and then soaked in SBF for various periods. It is found tbat all the Ti alloys forms an apatite layer on their surfaces in SBF within 3 weeks The soaking periods required for apatite fommation are 1, 2 and 3 weeks for Ti-6Al-2Nb-Ta, Ti15Mo5 SZr-3Al and Ti-6AI-4V, respectively. On the contrary, no apatite was formed on the surfaces of SUS316L and Vitallium® even after soaking in SBF for 4 weeks.

Figure 3 shows the SEM micrographs of the (a) surface and (b) cross-section of

Ti 6Al-2Nb-Ta alloy subjected to alkali and heat treatment and the subsequent soaking in SBF for 4 weeks. It is found that a uniform and dense apatite layer, which was confirmed by EDX analyses, is formed on the alloy. When a tensile stress was applied normaly to the substrate, the fracture occurred not at the apatite-substrate interface but in the glue or the apatite layer. This indicates that the formed apatite layer bonded tightly to the substrate.

Figure 4 shows the variations in elemental concentrations and pH of SBF with soaking of Ti-6Al-4V and Ti-6Al-2Nb-Ta alloys subjected to alkali and subsequent heat treatment. It is observed that the sodium concentration and the pH steeply increase at the initial soaking period up to 1-3 d. Tbis indicates that the alkali ions first release from the amorphous alkali titanate layer via ion exchange with H_30+ species in SBF. Ti and other main metal elements are not found to release into SBF in ppm level, excepting Al release below 0.002 mM. Thus, the amorphous alkali titanate layer formed on the Ti alloys is essentially unresorbable. The apparent decrease in Ca- and P-concentrations as well as pH after 3 days' soaking of each substrate is due to the apatite formation and the growth which proceeds via consumption of these species from SBF.

The previous and present results indicate that chemical surface modification using an alkaline solution is a quite simple as well as effective method for inducing bioactivity on pure Ti metal and its alloys. The process of apatite formation on Ti alloys is considered as follows. When the Ti alloys are soaked in alkaline solution, the hydrated TiO_2 gel layer, containing alkali ions is formed on their surfaces. Previous results have suggested that the Ti and alkali concentrations respectively gradually increase and decrease from the outer surface to the interior, for pure Ti metal [2]. This may be also the case for the present Ti alloys. As expected, this gel layer contains a considerable amount of water or hydrated ions. It is densified to form an amorphous

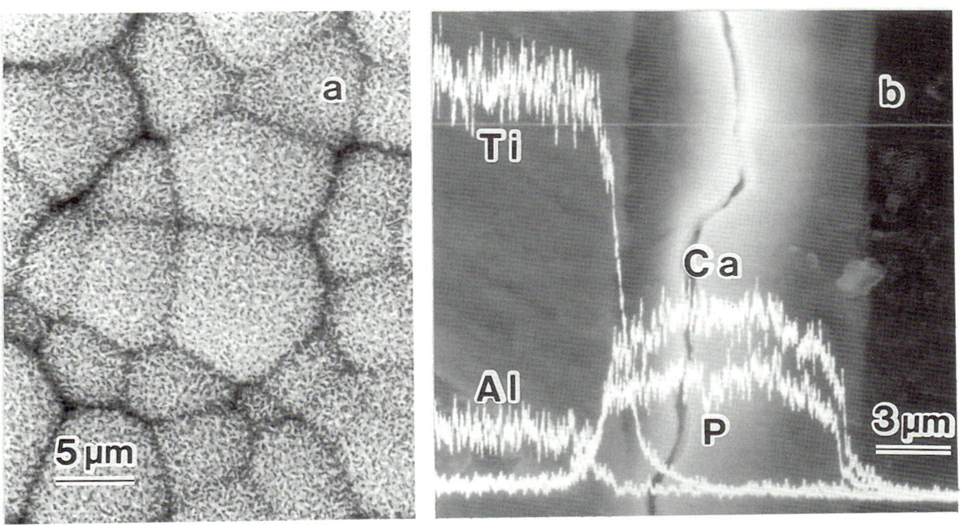

Figure 3. SEM micrographs of the (a) surface and (b) cross-section of Ti-6AI-2Nb-Ta

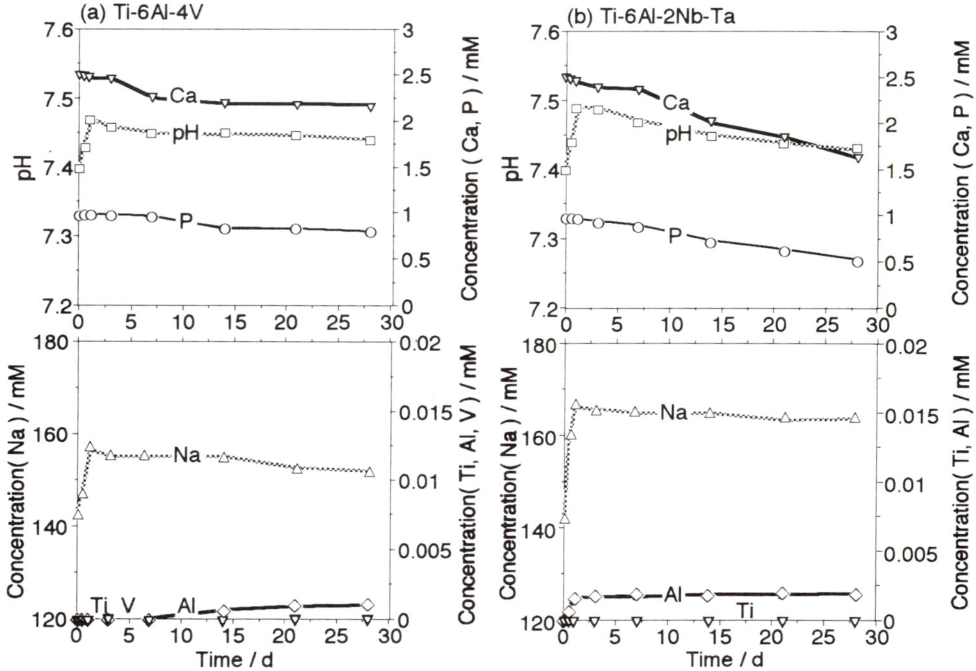

Figure 4. Variations in element concentrations and pH of SBF with soaking of (a) Ti-6AI-4V and (b) Ti-6AI-2Nb-Ta subjected to alkali and heat treatments .

alkali titanate layer and tightly bonded to the substrate by heat treatment although a part of the gel layer precipitates crystalline TiO_2 and/or alkali titanate phases. Simultaneously, the concentration gradient of Ti and alkali may be stabilized by the heat treatment. When alkali- and heat-treated Ti alloys are exposed to SBF, the alkali ions are dissolved from the amorphous titanate layer and H_30+ ions enter into the surface layer, resulting in the formation of TiO_2 hydrogel layer. The dissolved alkali ions increase the degree of supersaturation with respect to apatite by increasing pH, and the TiO_2 hydrogel induces apatite nucleation on its surface [4]. Once the apatite nuclei are formed, they spontaneously grow by incorporating the Ca^{2+} and PO_4^{3-} ions from the surrounding nuid which is already supersaturated with respect to apatite.

The SBF-soaking period required for apatite formation was different for the various Ti alloys. The intrinsic characteristics of each alloy, such as the degree of surface hydration by alkali treatment and the crystallization behavior by heat treatment, might affect the ultimate apatite-forming ability. SUS316L and Vitallium® did not form the apatite layer on their surfaces with this chemical surface modification. This is attributed to the lack of the amorphous alkali titanate layer which is responsible for the apatite formation.

The apatite layer formed on the Ti and its alloys shows the compositional gradients from the outer apatite layer to the inner metals [2]. It is therefore expected that not only the surface apatite layer bonds strongly to the substrates but also a uniform gradient of stress transfer from bone to implant effectively occurs *in vivo*. Moreover, the Ti metal and its alloys, treated by the present chemical method, can form a bone-like apatite layer even in the body. It is expected that the apatite layer thus formed *in vivo* can exhibit high bioactivity as well as strong bonding to substrates.

REFERENCES

1. Pilliar, R. M. and Filaggi, M.J. *Bioceramics* Volume 6, Butterworth-Heinemann,Oxford 1993, 165-171.
2. Miyaji, F. Zhang, X. Yao, T. Kokubo, T. Ohtsuki, C. Kitsugi, T. Yamamuro, T.and Nakamura, T. *Bioceramics* Volume 7, Butterworth-Heinemann, Oxford,1994, 119-124.
3. Kokubo, T. Kushitani, H. Sakka, S. Kitsugi,T. and Yamamuro, T. *J. Biomed. Mater. Res.* 1990, 24, 721-734.
4. Li, P.; Ohtsuki, C.; Kokubo, T.; Nakanishi, K.; Soga, N.; Yamamuro, T.; Nakamura, T. *J. Biomed. Mater. Res.* 7, 1994, 2S30.

CHARACTERISATION OF HYDROXYAPATITE PRECIPITATED FROM DIFFERENT REACTANTS

N. Asaoka, S. Best, J. C. Knowles and W. Bonfield

IRC in Biomedical Materials, Queen Mary and Westfield College
Mile End Road, London E1 4NS, UK

ABSTRACT

Hydroxyapatite suspensions were prepared at temperatures of 90, 25 and 2°C, with final HA concentrations of 1, 2.5 and 5% using two different reactions. The two reactions consist of (i) orthophosphoric acid and calcium hydroxide and (ii) diammonium hydrogen phosphate and calcium nitrate. The properties of the crystallites obtained were compared by using XRD, TEM and particle size analysis. The crystallinity and morphology of the crystallites were more affected by the precipitation temperature than the reactant concentration. Of the two routes, the reaction between orthophosphoric acid and calcium hydroxide was found to produce a more crystalline precipitate.

INTRODUCTION

Hydroxyapatite (HA) is one of the most interesting materials for biomedical application because of its similarity with the composition of bone mineral and there are now many HA products clinically in use. There are a number of techniques by which HA may be prepared including precipitation [1,2], solid state synthesis [3], hydrolysis [4], hydrothermal synthesis [5] and sol-gel method [6], although in terms of industrial processing the precipitation process appears to be most regularly used. Of the range of precipitation routes available, the two most popular are: (i) orthophosphoric acid (H_3PO_4) and calcium hydroxide ($Ca(OH)_2$) [1], and (ii) diammonium hydrogen phosphate ($(NH_4)_2HPO_4$) and calcium nitrate ($Ca(NO_3)_2$) [2]. The effect of reaction temperature during precipitation on the morphology of hydroxyapatite crystallites has been reported previously [7]. However, there has been no systematic investigation of the influence of reaction temperature and concentration for contrasting reaction systems. In this investigation, HA suspensions were prepared using the two aqueous precipitation reactions above and a comparison was made of the properties of crystallites produced.

MATERIALS AND METHODS

HA suspensions were prepared through the following two different reaction routes.

(1) $10Ca(OH)_2 + 6H_3PO_4 \rightarrow Ca_{10}(PO_4)_6(OH)_2 + 18H_2O$

(2) $10Ca(NO_3)_2 + 6(NH_4)_2HPO_4 + 2H_2O \rightarrow Ca_{10}(PO_4)_6(OH)_2 + 12NH_4NO_3 + 8HNO_3$

The syntheses were performed at temperatures of 2, 25 and 90°C, with final HA concentrations of 1.0, 2.5 and 5.0 wt%. In each case, the reactants were carefully weighed so that the Ca/P molar ratio in the system was maintained at the stoichiometric value for HA (1.67). Samples from reaction (1) were prepared as follows: H_3PO_4 aqueous solutions (0.12 to 0.60 mol/dm^3) and $Ca(OH)_2$ suspensions (0.20 to 1.00 mol/dm^3) were prepared from reagent grade chemicals and distilled water. Then, the H_3PO_4 solution was slowly added to the beaker, which contained equivalent volume of the $Ca(OH)_2$ suspension. The suspension was stirred for one day.

Samples from reaction (2) were also prepared in a similar manner, but the pH of the $Ca(NO_3)_2$ and $(NH_4)_2HPO_4$ solutions (0.12 to 0.60 mol/dm^3 and 0.20 to 1.00 mol/dm^3, respectively) were adjusted to 11 with ammonium hydroxide before they were mixed.

The precipitates were washed with distilled water, and approximately 1g of each batch was collected and dried at room temperature. The precipitates were characterised using an X-ray diffractometer (XRD; Siemens D5000), a laser diffraction particle analyser (Master Sizer X; Malvern Instruments) and a transmission electron microscope (TEM; JEOL JEM-100CX).

RESULTS

Preparation temperature

XRD analysis showed that all the precipitates were crystallographically pure HA, although crystallinity was found to vary according to preparation conditions. Figure. 1 shows the diffraction patterns obtained for the precipitates prepared at 2, 25 and 90°C. The pattern for reaction (1) at 90°C had very sharp and well defined peaks, which indicated that the precipitates were crystalline, while (211) and (112) peaks were merged in the pattern for a sample prepared at 25°C. For the reaction performed at 2°C, the peak was further broadened by the inclusion of the (300) reflection. However, the patterns for reaction (2) performed at 25 and 2°C were similar and exhibited broad peaks, and the pattern for the material produced at 90°C showed that the precipitates were highly crystalline.

The change in morphology of the precipitates with temperature is shown in Fig. 2. In both reactions, the particles prepared at 90°C were markedly different. The particles from reaction (1) were spherical (30 to 60 nm; Fig. 2a), while the precipitates prepared at 25 and 2°C were of elongated particles which were interlaced, with little difference in size between them (100-200 X 20-30 nm; Fig. 2b and c). However, the precipitates from reaction (2) were columnar in shape (100-300 x 20-80 nm; Figure. 2d).

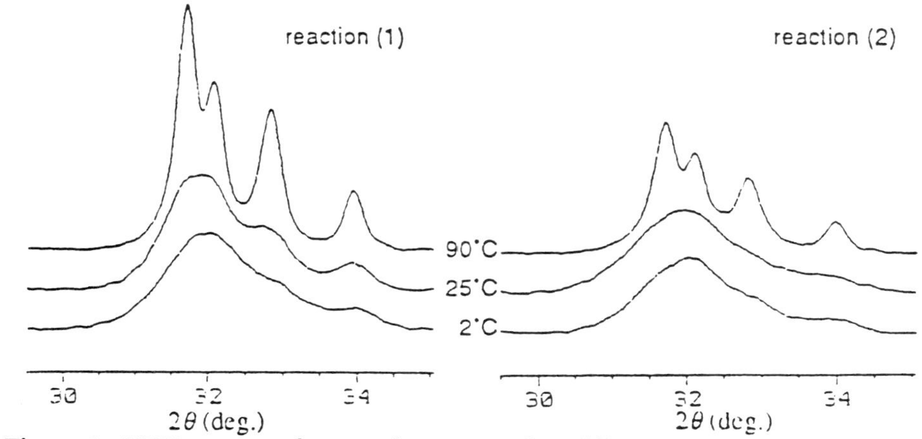

Figure 1. XRD patterns for samples prepared at different temperature.

As well as the precipitates from reaction (1), those prepared at 25 and 2°C also consisted of interlaced, elongated particles, whose sizes were similar (50-100 x 10 nm; Fig. 2e and f). However, observation at higher magnification revealed that each elongated particle was a chain of fine primary crystallites (about 10 nm in diameter; Fig. 3).

Concentration of the suspension

A reaction temperature of 25°C was selected for this series of experiments. From the XRD results, the crystallinity seemed to increase slightly with an increase in concentration from 1 to 5 wt% (Fig. 4). However, there was no clear difference in particle morphology between them (Fig. 5). Particle size analysis indicated that

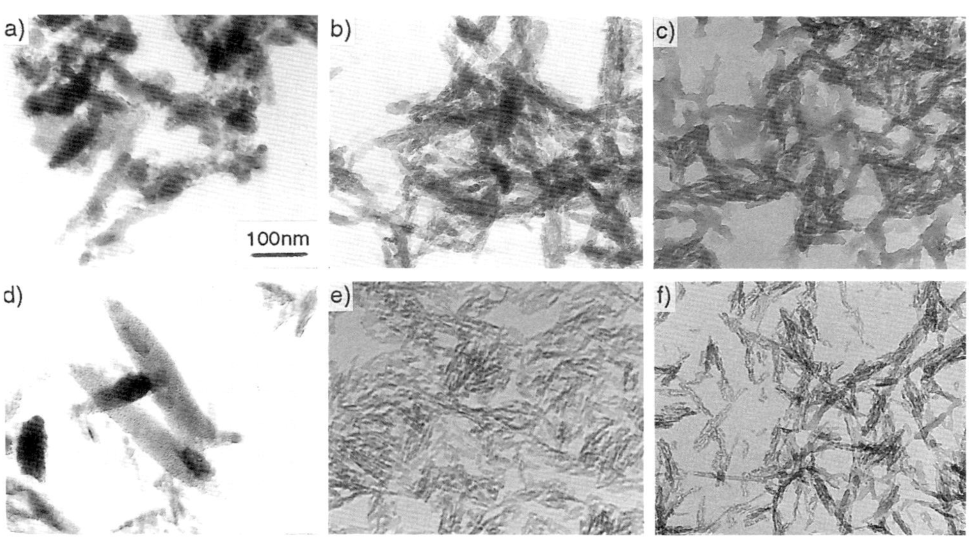

Figure 2. Precipitates at different reaction temperatures from reaction (1) (a - c) and (2) (d-f). (left; 90°C, middle; 25°C, right; 2°C)

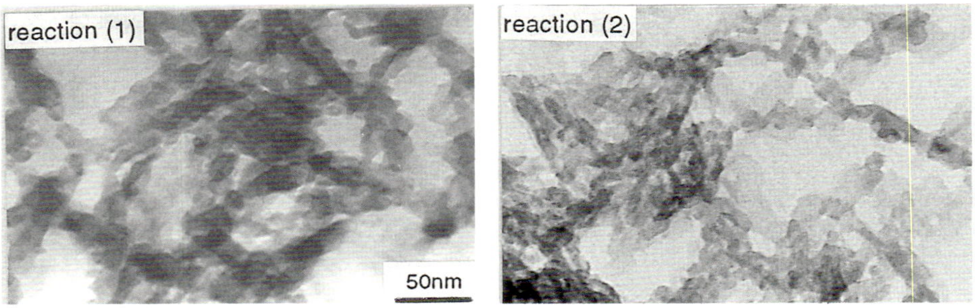

Fig. 3 Precipitates from reaction (1) (left) and (2) (right).

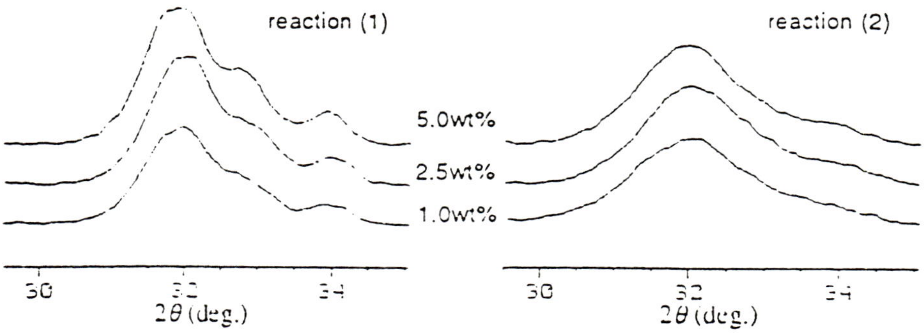

Fig. 4 XRD patterns for HAs prepared at different reactant concentrations.

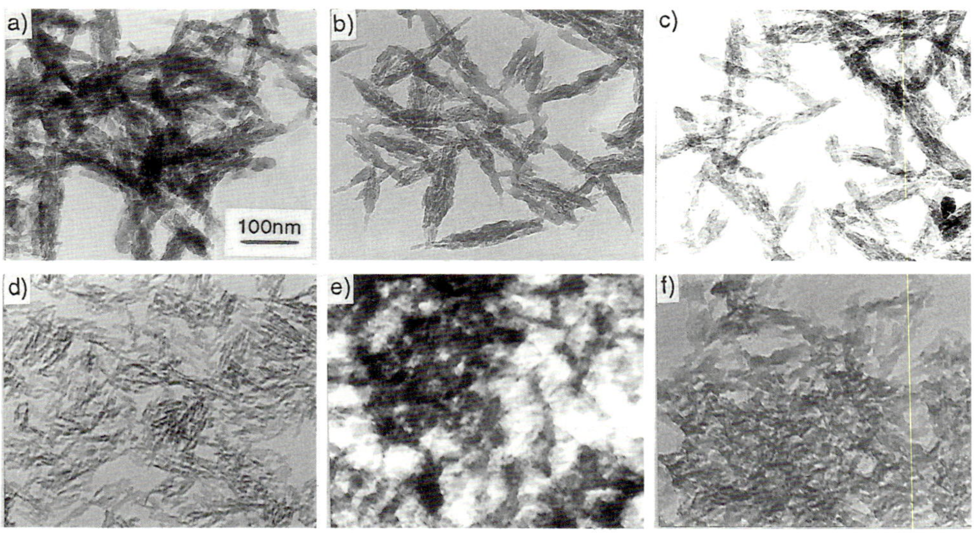

Figure. 5 Precipitates at different reactant concentrations from reactions (1) (a-c) and (2) (d-f). (left; 5.0 wt%, middle; 2.5 wt%, right; 1.0 wt%)

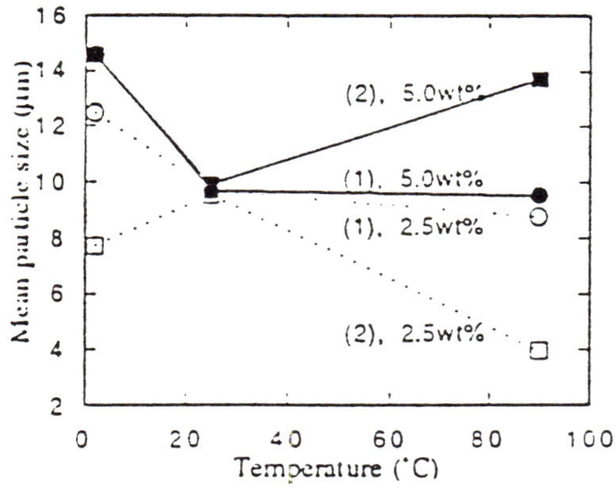

Fig. 6 Variation of HA mean particle sizes with preparation conditions.

the particles were extensively agglomerated in the suspension, since the mean particle size obtained using this technique was about 10 μm, while their size observed with TEM was sub-micron. The degree of agglomeration seemed to increase with increasing concentration (Fig. 6).

Reactants

The effect of the reactants themselves on the HA products was studied at given reaction temperatures and concentrations. Fig. 7 shows a comparison of the XRD patterns obtained for the samples. The precipitates from reaction (1) had higher crystallinity than those from reaction (2) at all synthesis temperatures. The difference was most significant at 90°C where the intensity of each peak in the XRD pattern for reaction (1) was twice that of the products from reaction (2) (Fig. 7a). At 25°C, the difference in the intensities was less marked (Fig. 7b). However, the peaks of the (102) and (210) planes were clearly discernible in the pattern for reaction (1), while they were not in the pattern of reaction (2). At 2°C, the peaks in the pattern from reaction (1) were of slightly higher intensity, although the diffraction patterns for products from both reactions appeared to be similar (Fig. 7c).

TEM observation also revealed some differences between the products of the two reactions, as mentioned above. The difference in morphology was most obvious at 90°C (Fig. 2a and d). As mentioned above, the particles from reaction (1) were spheroidal in shape, while those from reaction (2) were columnar. As for the specimens prepared at 25 and 2°C, the size of the chained particles from reaction (1) were larger than those from reaction (2).

DISCUSSION

When all the samples were compared within each reaction group, there appeared to be a stronger influence from the reaction temperature than the reactant concentration. The particles prepared at 90°C were larger and more crystalline in comparison with those produced at lower temperatures. It is known that crystallite size can also affect X-ray diffraction results [8], but differences observed seem to have been related, not only to crystallite size but to the degree of distortion in the lattice of the HA crystals.

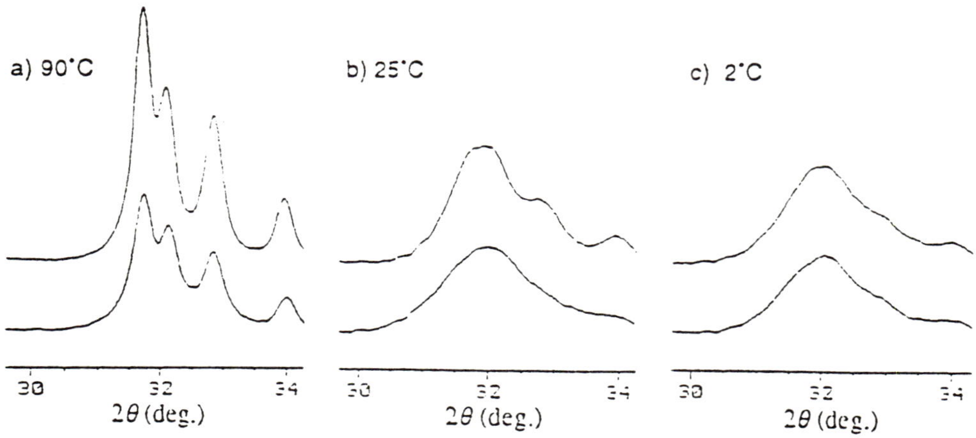

Figure. 7 Comparison of XRD patterns for HA precipitates from reaction (1) (upper) and (2) (lower).

Therefore a comparison of the two reaction routes revealed that reaction (1) resulted in more crystalline precipitates than reaction (2), under the identical temperature and concentration conditions. In addition, there were differences in the morphology of the resultant crystallites. At 90°C, the products from reaction (1) were spherical in shape, while those from (2) were columnar. At 25 and 2°C, a particle from (1) was larger in size than that from (2), although they were similar in shape. When chemical species are considered in reaction (2), ammonium and nitrate ions are found in addition to the calcium and phosphate ions, which are exclusively present in reaction (1). Some of the ions might be incorporated within or on the surface of the particles, so that the nucleation and growth characteristics of the system would be altered. Further investigation is in progress to consider these effects.

As for the particle size analysis, the results seem to be predominantly affected by the concentration of the suspension, rather than other factors. The mean particle size became larger with increasing concentration. The relation between particle size and the pH of the suspension was also examined, because agglomeration is dependent on zeta-potential. However, in the present study there appeared to be no clear relation between them.

CONCLUSION

a. During the precipitation of HA, crystallinity and morphology of the particles were more affected by synthesis temperature than by reactant concentration.
b. Products obtained from the reaction of $Ca(OH)_2$ and H_3PO_4 were more crystalline than those prepared from $Ca(NO_3)_2$ and $(NH_4)_2HPO_4$.
c. For a given reactant concentration at 25 and 2°C, the products obtained from $Ca(OH)_2$ and H_3PO_4 were larger in size than those from $Ca(NO_3)_2$ and $(NH_4)_2HPO_4$, although all of them consisted of chains of fine crystallites. At 90°C, however, the products of the former reaction were spheroidal, while those of the latter were columnar.

ACKNOWLEDGEMENTS

The support of EPSRC for the IRC in Biomedical materials and of Mitsubishi Materials Corporation for one of the authors (N. A.) are gratefully acknowledged.

REFERENCES

1. Avinmelech, Y., Moreno, and Brown, W. E., *J. Res. Nat. Bur. Stand.*, 1973, 77A, 149-155
2. Jarcho, M., Bolen, C. H., Thomas, M. B., Bobick, J., Kay, J. and Doremus, R. H., *J. Mater. Sci.*, 1976, 11, 2027-2035
3. Rootare, H. M., Powers, J. M. and Craig, R.G., *J. Dent. Res.* 1978, 57, 777-783
4. Perloff, A. and Posner, A. F., *Inorg. Synthesis,* 1960, 6, 16-18
5. Young, R. A. and Holcomb, D. W., *Calcified Tissue Int.*, 1982, 34, S17-S32
6. Deptula, A., Lada, W., Olczak, T., Borello, A., Alvani, C. and di Bartolomeo, A., *J. Non-Cryst. Solids.,* 1992, 147&148, 537-541
7. Barralet, J., Best, S. and Bonfield, W., *Bioceramics* Volume 6, Butter-worth, Oxford 1993, 179-184
8. Cullity, B. D., *Elements of X-ray Diffraction 2nd ed.*, Addison-Wesley, Massachusetts, 1978, 281-295

ENVIRONMENTALLY INDUCED CRACKS AND DETACHMENT OF PLASMA-SPRAYED HYDROXYAPATITE COATINGS UNDER ULTRASONIC TREATMENT

J. Weng[1,2], J.G.C. Wolke[1], X. Zhang[2], K. de Groot[1]

[1]Biomaterials Research Group, University of Leiden, The Netherlands;
[2]Institute of Materials Science and Technology, Sichuan Union University, Chengdu 610064, P. R. China

ABSTRACT

Since ultrasonic cleaning is not only a widely accepted pretreatment of coatings but also a dynamic process rather than static immersion, the present study focuses on induced cracks and detachment of laminas in plasma-sprayed hydroxyapatite coatings with different properties under ultrasonic treatment in different solutions. The results show that the performance of the hydroxyapatite coatings is solution-sensitive under ultrasonic treatment. In aqueous solutions, microcracks nucleate quickly around the irregular pores and unmelted particles, even after the coating is treated for only 1 min. Prolonged treatment causes detachment of weakly bonded particles and results in the pit-erosion-like morphology of coatings with a large quantity of cross cracks. On the contrary, ultrasonic treatment of the coatings in acetone for as long as 20 hr initiates no additional microcracks in coatings and induces no evident changes on their morphology. It is suggested that the more homogeneous coatings without unmelted particles are more suitable in clinical applications, and that acetone, rather than aqueous solutions should be used when ultrasonic cleaning is considered.

INTRODUCTION

Hydroxyapatite (HA) coatings by plasma-spraying are now used clinically for cementless fixation of surgical prostheses to bone. Animal studies [1,2,3] have shown that HA coatings on metallic substrates promote bone formation around implants and enhance the bonding strength of implants to bone. Recently, Geesink [4] reported in a five year HA-coated total hip replacement study that *"current clinical results of HA-coated implants are excellent and are among the best available with any hip system"*. But concerns have been raised about this retention of coatings in body environments.

Accumulated evidence has shown that the integrity of the plasma-sprayed coating is not quite maintained in physiological environments. [1,5,6] This is mainly ascribed to the induced amorphous HA and other less stable calcium phosphates which are more both *in vitro* and *in vivo*.[1,6] *In vivo* experimental results [5,7,8] also reveal that soluble coating thickness may decrease with the implantation time and that coatings might disintegrate into a mass of loose particles. Coating remnants were sometimes seen in surrounding bone tissue. The observed disintegration and disappearance of coatings may imply that their microstructure also plays an important part in their performance in physiological environments.

The immersion of the HA coatings in solutions is a widely adopted *in vitro* method to evaluate their solubility. [7,9] This static process does not represent the *in vivo* solubility of the HA coatings in a dynamic system. Ultrasonic treatment is a dynamic process and widely accepted in pretreatment of coatings. Therefore, the present study focuses on the environmentally induced cracks and detachment in the plasma-sprayed HA coatings under ultrasonic treatment. It is also intended to reflect how the microstructure of the coatings influences their performance in different solutions during ultrasonic treatment.

MATERIALS AND METHODS

Titanium alloy Ti6A14V plates ($20x20x8mm^3$) were used as substrates. They were sandblasted with $Al_2 0_3$ powder to produce a surface roughness of 3.5-4.0 μm. HA powder was obtained from Merck (Germany) with particle size less than 45 μm. A Metco MN system (USA) was used to plasma spray HA powder onto titanium alloy plates. The variation in the coating crystallinity was obtained by varying the spraying conditions. For example, coatings with a 60% crystalline component were obtained in the present study by lowering the arc current in order for the partially melted particles to impinge onto the substrates. This results in coating with a special microstructure. [10]

Ultrasonic treatment was carried out in a Bransonic® (USA) ultrasonic cleaner with HF-output power 30W and working frequency 47kHz. During ultrasonic treatment, the coatings were immersed in three solutions: pure acetone, deionized water and simulated body fluid (SBF). [11] After different periods of time in the ultrasonic treatment, the coatings were taken out, dried and sputter-coated with gold for scanning electron microscopy (SEM).

RESULTS

The 50 μm coating kept its original morphology with the weakly adhesive particles on the surface being shaken off after ultrasonic treatment in pure acetone for 20 hr (Figure 1a). Upon treatment in SBF for 30 min, the as-received morphology was extensively destroyed as shown in Figure 1b. Some unmelted particles or cores were detached to form erosion-like pits and a large quantity of microcracks existed in the pancake-like particles.

Figure 2 shows the morphologies of the HA coatings (50 μm) ultrasonically treated in deionized water for different periods of time. In the 1 min treatment, the weakly adhesive particles were detached and microcracks appeared (Figure 2a). After 5 minutes; the morphology of the coating was approximately the same as with the 1 minute treatment but there appear erosion-like pits in the early stage (Figure 2b). After 30 minute's treatment, the erosion-like pits became deeper and the detachment of laminas occurred (Figure 2c). The original smooth morphology of pancake-like particles became microscopically rough with a large quantity of cross microcracks. After 60 minutes the erosion-like pits enlarged and the integrity of the coating was significantly compromised (Figure 2d).

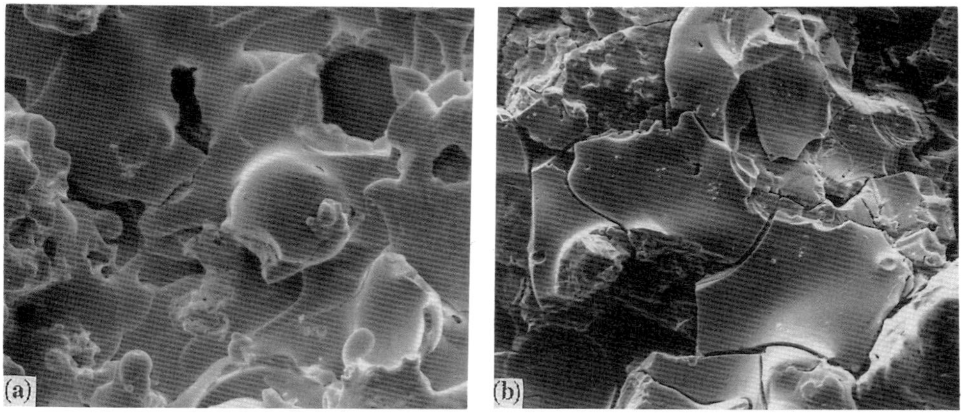

Figure 1 SEM morphologies of the HA coatings (5O>m) ultrasonically treated (a) in pure acetone for 20 hr and (b) in SBF for 30 min. (Magnification 820X), lb) (c) (¢

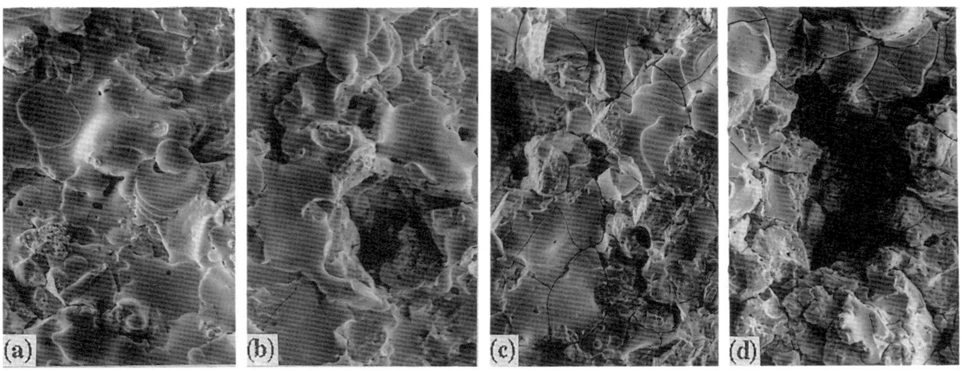

Figure 2 SEM morphologies of the HA coatings (5O μm) ultrasonically treated in deionized watér for (a) 1 min; (b) 5 min; (c) 30 min and (d) 60 min respectively. (Magnification 320X)

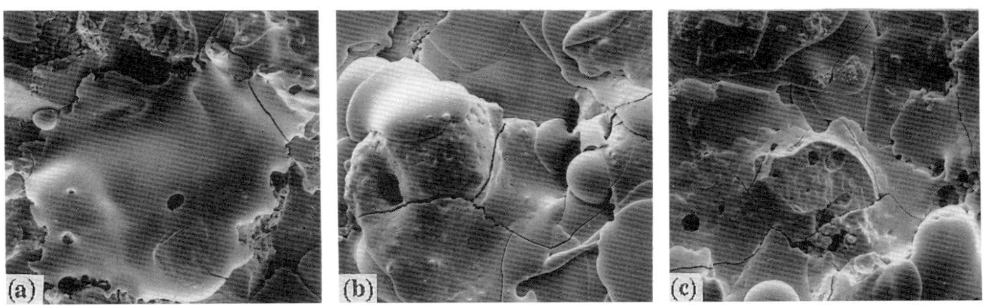

Figure 3 SEM morphologies of different coatings ultrasonically treated in deionized water for different periods. (a) separated pancake-like particle for 3 min; (b) 10 μm coating for 3 min and (c) 50 μm coating for 1 min. (Magnification 620X)

The performance of the coatings with different thicknesses in the ultrasonic treatment was examined in deionized water. The nucleation of microcracks began at the irregular pores in the separated pancake-like particles deposited upon the metallic surface (Figure 3a). In the 10 μm coating, the microcracks initiated more easily in the unmelted area than in the pancake-like particles (Figure 3b). In the 50 μm coating, the microcracks quickly initiated around the unmelted particles or cores (Figure 3c). The thicker the coating, the more easily the microcracks nucleated.

DISCUSSION

The performance of the plasma-sprayed HA coatings in the ultrasonic treatment is environmentally or solution-sensitive. If the coated prostheses are immersed in a water-free solution such as pure acetone or ethanol, ultrasonic cleaning is effective and nondestructive. In Figure la, the coating shows the same morphology as that of the as-received coating even after the 20 hr ultrasonic treatment. There is no evidence that additional microcracks have initiated in the coating.

Water is critical to the performances of the coatings during ultrasonic treatment in an aqueous solution. Although SBF is supersaturated for apatite, in which the dissolution of the HA coating is supposed to be retarded, the morphology of the coating was still destroyed extensively after the 30 min ultrasonic treatment. This means that the nucleation of microcracks and detachment of laminas are governed mainly in a water controlled way rather than the pure dissolution of the calcium phosphates during the ultrasonic treatment. The water environment was also reported to reduce the bending strength of polycrystalline alumina ceramics after they were exposed to a saturated stream or aged in deionized water [12,13].

The immersion of the plasma-sprayed HA coatings in different fluids used to fix tissue resulted in a variety of surface morphologies. [14] Coatings fixed in ethanol showed no recognizable alterations in morphology while microcracks were prominent in the coating after the 7 day immersion in water. Residual stresses were reported to exist in the plasma-sprayed HA coatings and to increase with coating thickness [15]. The stress release, which initiates microcracks in the coatings, is water-sensitive. In an inert environment, the ultrasonic treatment of the as-received coatings even for a long time resulted in no nucleation of additional microcracks (Figure la), and therefore little stress release. In the short time treatment in deionized water, the microcracks initiated at the irregular pores and near the unmelted particles or cores (Figure 3). This means that the residual stresses concentrate at the irregular pores and near the unmelted particles or cores, resulting in stress concentration which allows microcracks to form more easily, especially in thicker coatings (Figure 3).

Water molecules may debond the interface between the HA ceramic grains. In an *in vivo* experiment, the interface degradation at the sintered necks between the HA grains was observed after the HA ceramics were implanted for weeks [16]. In the present study, the timed treatment was too short to degrade the interface between the HA grains. But the interface area, concentrated with defects such as dislocation and imperfect contact etc, is the weak link in the coatings especially with the existence of residual stresses. The ultrasonic treatment enhances water molecules penetrating the strained interface areas. Water molecules may promote the debonding between the HA grains through a kind of water-enhanced stress corrosion process, and thus nucleation of microcracks may occur in the high stress areas such as at irregular pores and near unmelted particles.

The formation of erosion like pits during ultrasonic treatment reflects the inhomogeneity of cohesive bonding between laminas in the plasma-sprayed HA coatings. The plasma-sprayed HA coatings consist of unmelted particles or cores, completely melted parts of pancake-like particles and splashed droplets [10]. As the deposition of the coating occurs layer by layer by plasma spraying, the weakly bonded particles, which were shaken off, as shown in Figure la, are embedded within the coating. McPherson and Shafer [17] observed directly by transmission electron microscope the imperfect contact between laminas within the plasma sprayed $Al_2 0_3$ coatings. At the early stage of the treatment, the microcracks are quickly initiated around the unmelted cores or imperfectly bonded particles with the release of the residual stresses. The further treatment makes them detach from the outer layer of the coating to form the erosion like pits with the enhancement of water.

In an *in-vivo* physiological environment, the release of the residual stresses may also initiate microcracks around the unmelted crystalline particles or cores. Further attack of the body fluid through the microcracks and pores could make the particles detach with the mediation of cells such as osteoclasts and macrophages. This could finally result in the disintegration of the coatings into a mass of loose particles, with coating remnants in the surrounding bone. [5,8]

CONCLUSION

The nucleation of microcracks and detachment of laminas in plasma-sprayed HA coatings are environment or solution-sensitive under ultrasonic treatment. These processes are related to the microstructure and the residual stresses of the HA coatings. Ultrasonic cleaning of the coatings is suggested as unsuitable in an aqueous solution, such as deionized water, even for a few minutes before surgical operation.

ACKNOWLEDGEMENTS

The authors thank Mr. Jurren Koerts for the preparation of titanium alloy substrates and Mr. Joost v. 't Noordende for his assistance with SEM observation.

REFERENCES

1. Geesink,G.R.T., de Groot,K., Klein,C.P.A.T., *J Bone Joint Surg* 1989, 70, 17-23
2. Soballe, K., B-Rasmussen, H., Hansen, E.S., Bunger, C., *Acta Orthop Scan* 1992, 63, 128-140
3. Cook, S.D., Thomas,K.A., Kay,J.F., Jarcho,M., *Clin Orthop* 1988, 232, 225-243
4. Geesink,G.R.T., In: *Hydroxylapatite Coatings in Orthopaedic Surgery*, Raven Press, New York 1993, 171-208
5. Klein, C.P.A.T., Patka,P., Wolke, J.G.C., de Blieck-Hogervorst,J.M.A., de Groot,K., *Biomaterials* 1994, 15, 146-150
6. Thomas,K.A., Cook,S.D., Haddad,R.J., Kay,J.F., Jarcho,M., *J Arthroplasty* 1989, 4, 43-53
7. Jansen, J A., van der Waerden, JP.C M., Wolke, J.G.C., *J Biomed Mater Res* 1993, 27, 603610
8. Dhert, W.J.A., Klein, CP.A.T., Jansen, J.A., van der Velde, E.A., Vriesde, R.C., Rozing, P.M., de Groot, K., *ibid.* 1993, 27, 127-138

9. Klein, C.P.A.T., Wolke, J.G.C., de Blieck-Hogervorst, J M.A., de Groot,K.,*ibid.*1994, 28, 961-967
10. Chen,J., Wolke,J.G.C., de Groot,K., *Biomaterials* 1994, 15, 396-399
11. Kokubo,T., Kushitani,H., Ohtsuki,C., Sakka,S., Yamamuro,T., *J Mater Sci: Mater in Med* 1992, 3 79-83
12. Day,D.E., *Am Ceram Soc Bull* 1982, 62, 624-626
13. Frakes,J.F., Brown,S.D., KeMer,G.H., *ibid.* 1974, 53, 183-187
14. Kieswetter,K., Bauer,T.W., Brown,S.A., Van Lente,F., Merritt,K ., *J Biomed Mater Res* 1994, 28, 281-287
15. Brown,S.R., Tumer,I.G., Heiter,H., *J Mater Sci: Mater in Med* 1994, 5, 756-759
16. Lin,H., Xu,H., de Groot,K., *J Biomed Mater Res* 1992, 26, 7-18
17. McPherson,R., Shafer,B.V., *Thin Solid Film* 1982, 97, 201-204

IMPROVEMENT OF THE INTERFACE STRENGTH AND OSTEOINTEGRATION OF EXTERNAL FIXATION PINS COATED WITH HYDROXYAPATITE

A. Moroni, L. Orienti, S. Stea, M. Visentin, and C. Maltarello

Rizzoli Orthopaedic Institute, via Pupilli,1 40136 BOLOGNA, ITALY

ABSTRACT

The present study was designed to compare the bone pin interface in two groups of external fixation pins; uncoated and coated with hydroxyapatite. Twenty pins made of stainless steel were utilized. Half of the pins were plasma-sprayed with hydroxyapatite and the other half remained uncoated. Two adult sheep were selected. Each sheep tibia was implanted with five pins. Sheep were killed four months after surgery. Extraction torque was higher in the hydroxyapatite coated pins compared to the uncoated ones ($p \leq 0.0005$). An extensive bony coverage of the hydroxyapatite coated pins without any hydroxyapatite coating resorption and delamination from the metallic substrate was observed. Fibrous tissue encapsulation was found in the uncoated pins.

INTRODUCTION

It is generally accepted that pin loosening is related to improper pin insertion [1]. In spite of this, pin loosening and infection can be observed with apparent proper pin insertion technique [1]. Aro *et al.*, [2], and Pettine *et al.*, [1], in recent experimental studies, demonstrated that a severe progressive reduction of pin extraction torque occurs with time independently of the pin position. Bone damage during pin insertion, fibrous tissue encapsulation of the pin, and pin loading could be all responsible for this deterioration of the bone pin interface strength.

Unfortunately, the effect of these factors on pin loosening and infection are still not established. Furthermore, very little information is available in the literature on the behavior of the bone pin interface under unloaded conditions.

On the other hand, synthetic hydroxyapatite has shown the ability to bind chemically to bone [3,4,5,6]. The high biocompatibility and the low degradation of this bioceramic material have also been demonstrated [3,4,5]. For these reasons, we proposed hydroxyapatite as a suitable coating material to improve the bone pin interface [7,8].

In a very recent *in vivo* experimental study under loaded conditions we demonstrated a significant enhancement of the interface strength in hydroxyapatite coated external fixation pins compared to uncoated ones [7,8].

However, data on unloaded conditions were not provided. For these reasons, the present study was designed to evaluate the bone pin interface in an unloaded experimental model in two groups of pins; uncoated and coated with hydroxyapatite. This study compares the biomechanical, histological and histomorphometric results in two groups of pins, uncoated and hydroxyapatite coated implanted into sheep tibiae free of external fixation and thus not subject to either the static or dynamic compression forces.

MATERIALS AND METHOD

Implant characteristics

Twenty bicylindrical external fixation pins made of stainless steel were utilized (Superfixation pins, Citieffe, Lippo di Calderara di Reno, Bo, 40100, Italy). The outer threaded pin diameters were 4 and 5 mm respectively.

Half of the pins were plasma-sprayed in air with hydroxyapatite and the other half remained uncoated (Biocoatings, Flametal, Fornovo Taro, Pr, 43045, Italy). The hydroxyapatite coating thickness ranged from 30 to 60 μm. The crystallinity ratio of hydroxyapatite, calculated after X ray spectroscopy, was more than 70%, and purity by mass spectroscopy, more than 97%. The Ca/P ratio was 1.67+0.01. The hydroxyapatite powder contained small traces of heavy elements below the limits of the ASTM standard F1185-88 (As < 2ppm; Cd < 1ppm; Hg < 1ppm; Pb < 1ppm; total heavy elements < 30 ppm; Cu < 1 ppm; Mn < 100 ppm; Fe < 100 ppm).

Surgical procedures

Two adult female sheep of similar size and weight (45 ± 5 kg mean body weight) were selected for this study. Maturity was determined by radiographic examination of the physes of the proximal tibiae and distal femora to confirm closure. The surgical procedures were performed under assisted general anaesthesia following a standardized protocol: premedication with intramuscular Ketamine (10 mg/Kg), Xylazine (0.2 mg/Kg) and Atropine sulphate (0.0125 mg/Kg), induction with intravenous Thiopenthone sodium (8 mg/Kg) and maintenance with oxygen, nitrous oxide and Halothane (1-2.5%) under assisted ventilation. Perioperative antibiotics (Cefazolin 22 mg/kg) were given starting the day before surgery, for five days.

The hind limbs were clipped, and right and left tibiae aseptically prepared for surgery. The hydroxyapatite coated and uncoated pins were implanted bilaterally in the sheep's tibial diaphyseal bone in an alternate manner. Each sheep received five hydroxyapatite coated and five uncoated pins. The pins were numbered proximal to distal and from one to five, with the most proximal pin being number one. In each sheep the first pin implanted into the right tibia was a hydroxyapatite coated pin and the first pin implanted into the left tibia an uncoated pin. Small (6 mm) incisions were made in the skin and a trochar-centered drill guide passed through the fascia and muscle to the tibia. The pins were placed on the anterior-lateral surface of the tibia 2.5 cm apart each other. A 3.5 mm drill was used to drill a hole in the tibial cortices, then the holes were tapped with individual tapers for either the hydroxyapatite coated and uncoated pins, and finally pins were manually inserted.

Following surgery, the sheep were placed in recovery rooms in heated cages and closely monitored over twenty-four hours. Unrestricted weight-bearing was allowed immediately after the operation. Ketoprofen (500 mg/day) was given for pain relief for two days. Twenty-four hours after recovery the sheep were returned to regular housing facilities where they were monitored twice a day and allowed normal activity. The sheep were killed four months after surgery.

Biomechanical analysis

Software for measuring and recording the pin torque resistance was developed (Moon System, Bo, 40100, Italy). An adaptor was manufactured to connect the pins to the torque measuring machine (BLM, Cusano Milanino, Mi, 2095, Italy) connected to a computer. After a pin had been inserted into the bone to its desired depth, torque was applied through the torque measuring machine in the direction of tightening the pin and final insertion torque was measured. After sheep were killed, extraction torque was measured on four pins (pins 1 to 4) from each tibia with the same system. Thus, a total of sixteen pins, half uncoated and half hydroxyapatite coated, was used for the measurement of pin extraction torque.

Histological analysis

Two pins from each animal (the hydroxyapatite coated pin in position 5 in the right tibia, and the uncoated pin in position 5 in the left tibia) were processed for morphological analyses. The retrieved bone pin blocks were embedded in methylmethacrylate and processed without decalcification. Samples were cut perpendicularly to the tibial longitudinal axis with a diamond saw (Exakt system, Kulzer System, Germany). After grinding to 30 μm thickness, sections were stained with acid fuchsin and light green to distinguish the mineralized bone (green) from the osteoid tissue (red). These sections were utilized for morphological qualitative analyses of the bone pin interfaces.

RESULTS

All the animals recovered from surgery and were walking normally and no major complications occurred.

Biomechanical Results

Biomechanical results are reported in Table 1. No significant differences of insertion torque between the hydroxyapatite coated and uncoated pins were found. Mean extraction torque was significantly higher in the hydroxyapatite coated pins compared to the uncoated ones, ($p \leq 0.0005$). Furthermore, in the hydroxyapatite coated pins a significant improvement with time of the interface strength was found. In fact, in these pins mean extraction torque was higher compared to the corresponding mean insertion torque ($p \leq 0.0005$). On the contrary, in the uncoated pins, mean extraction torque was slightly but not significantly lower compared to the corresponding mean insertion torque ($p \leq 0.375$).

Table 1: Biomechanical results for the pins implanted in the sheep killed 4 months after implantation (Mean ± SD values; N = 8)

Measurement	Uncoated	Hydroxyapatite coated	P
Insertion torque	769±450	1079±125	0.1
Extraction torque	552±535	6116±2096	0.0005

Histological Results

The histological patterns observed in the sheep were very similar. An extensive bony coverage of the hydroxyapatite coated pins with direct contact between bone and the Bioceramic coating was observed (Figure 1). No hydroxyapatite coating delamination from the metallic substrate or resorption were seen. On the contrary, fibrous tissue encapsulation with an average thickness of 10 μm was observed on the uncoated pins (Figure 2).

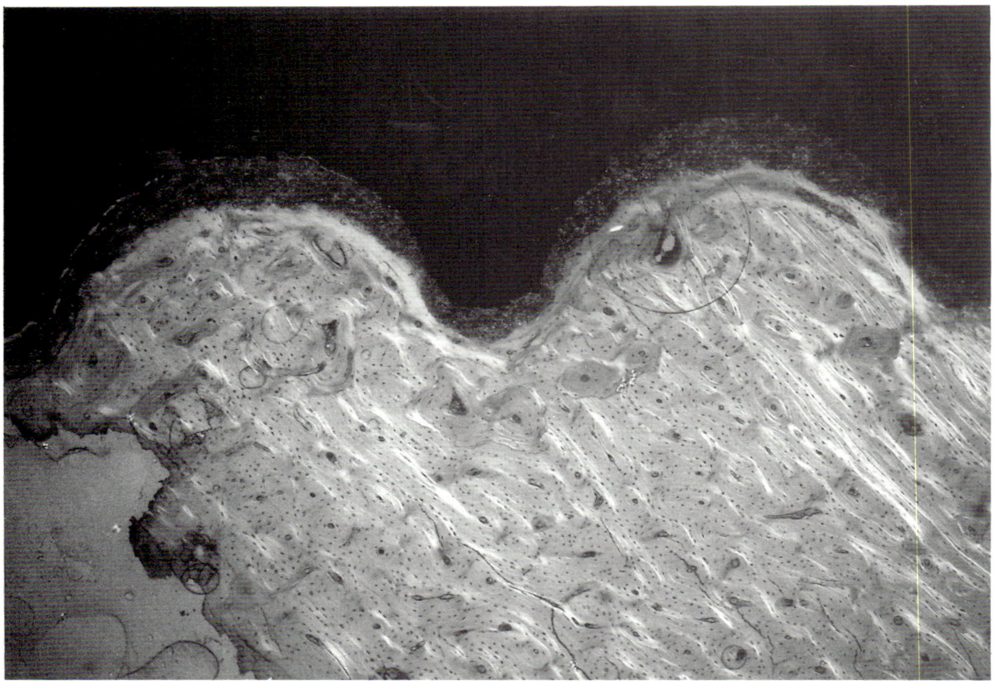

Figure 1: Histological cross section of a hydroxyapatite coated pin. Extensive direct contact between bone and the hydroxyapatite coating can be seen. No coating delamination or degradation is visible.

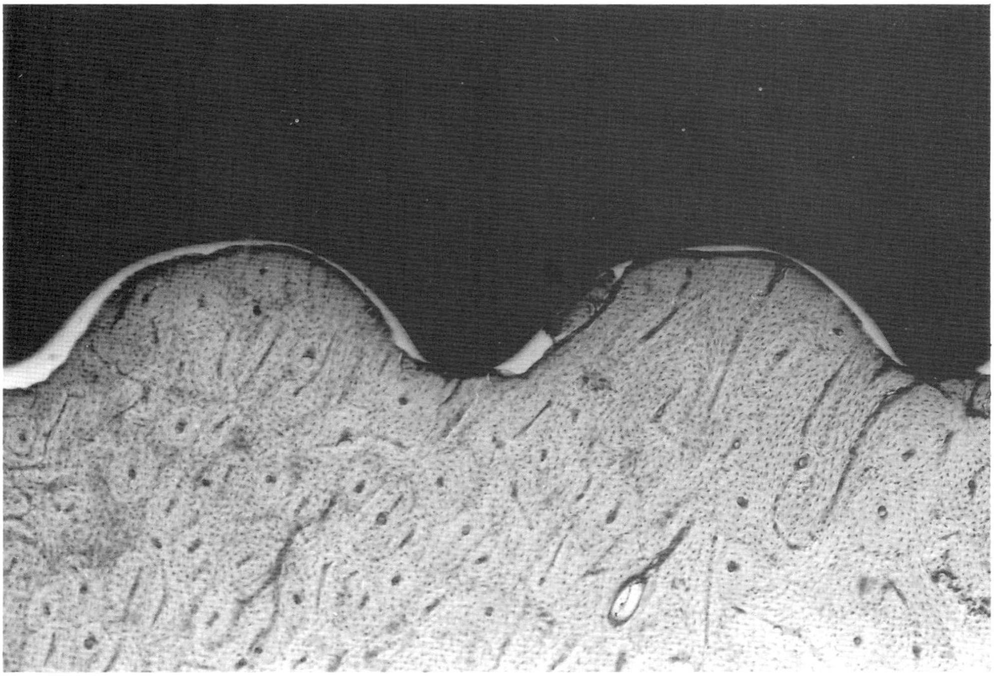

Figure 2: Histological cross section of an uncoated pin. A continuous severe gap at the bone pin interface is seen.

No histological sign of infection was observed in any pin. No mineralization changes occurred in the bone surrounding both the hydroxyapatite coated and uncoated pins.

DISCUSSION

In the uncoated pins extraction torque was slightly but not significantly lower than to the corresponding insertion torque. This result stresses the importance of the load as cause of deterioration of the bone pin interface. In fact Aro *et al.,* [2], and Pettine *et al.,* [1], in experimental studies on external fixation pins with load applied on the bone pin interface, demonstrated that a severe progressive reduction of pin extraction torque occurs with time.

On the other hand, in the hydroxyapatite coated pins a significant improvement of the bone pin interface strength was observed. In these pins extraction torque was approximately six times greater than the corresponding insertion torque. We have already reported similar results in a previous loaded study in which hydroxyapatite coated and uncoated pins of the same type had been implanted in sheep tibiae [7,8]. In that study, at six weeks after implantation the bone hydroxyapatite coated pin extraction torque was approximately twice the corresponding insertion torque, but no long term results had been given [7,8]. No direct comparison is possible between the results of these studies because of the different loading mode, but it is interesting to observe that in the previous study, mean hydroxyapatite coated pin extraction torque

was 1485±1308 N/mm [7,8]. This value is four times lower than to the mean extraction torque observed in the present study 4 months after implantation in the same pin type. This difference could to be due to both the effect of the load and the different animal survival period.

The improvement of the bone pin interface strength observed for the hydroxyapatite coated pins was explained by the morphological observations which showed an extensive, close, direct contact between the bone and the hydroxyapatite coating.

In the uncoated pins soft tissue encapsulation around the pin threads was observed. The osteoconductivity of the hydroxyapatite coating has facilitated bone remodelling and direct bony coverage of the pin surface and mechanically improved the interface strength.

It should also be noted that no deterioration or degradation of this bioceramic coating was found. This result is important because of concern about hydroxyapatite coating durability. This experimental model was unloaded, but absence of any visible deterioration of this coating is a very positive sign for its clinical use.

In conclusion, it was demonstrated that the hydroxyapatite coating was an effective method to improve the bone pin interface. A substantial improvement of the stability of the bone screw shaped implant interface, in many clinical situations, could be obtained.

REFERENCES

1. Pettine, K.A., Chao, E.Y.S. and Kelly, P.J. Analysis of the external fixator pin-bone interface. *Clin Orthop* 1993, 293,18-27, 1993.
2. Aro, H.T., Markel, D.M. and Chao, E.Y.S. The effect of fracture gap conditions on pin reaction. Transactions of the 37th Annual Meeting, Orthopaedic Research Society, Anaheim, CA, Vol.16, March 4-7, 1991, 447.
3. Cook, S.D., Thomas, K.A. and Kay, J.F. Experimental coating defects in hydroxylapatite-coated implants. *Clin Orthop* 1991, 265, 280-290, .
4. Geesink, R.G.T. Hydroxyapatite-coated total hip prostheses. Two-Year clinical and roentgenographic results of 100 cases. *Clin Orthop* 1990, 261, 39-58.
5. Lintner, F., Huber, M., Bohm, G. and Scholz, R. Histology of tissue adjacent to an HAp-coated femoral prosthesis. *J Bone Joint Surg* 1994, 76-B, 824-830.
6. Moroni, A., Caja, V.L., Egger, E.L., Trinchese, L. and Chao, E.Y.S. Histomorphometry of hydroxyapatite coated and uncoated porous titanium bone implants. *Biomaterials* 1984, 15, 926-930.
7. Moroni, A., Caja, V.L., Maltarello, C., Nicoli Aldini, N., Stea, S. and Visentin, M. Enhancement of the bone external fixation pin interface: a biomechanical and morphological in vivo experimental study. In: *Bioceramics* Vol. 7 Butterworth-Heinemann, Oxford 1994, 229-234.
8. Moroni, A., Caja, V.L., Stea, S., Visentin, M. and Nicoli Aldini, N. Improvement of the bone external fixation pin interface by hydroxyapatite coating. Transactions of the 41st Annual Meeting Orthopaedic Research Society. Orlando, Fl, February 13-16, Vol 20-1, 1995, 253-42.

ARTIFICIAL TRACHEA MADE OF POLYMERS COATED WITH HYDROXYAPATITE

Kazuya Suzuki, Yoshihiko Kageyama, Futoru Toyoda, Hiroshi Nogimura, Yukio Harada, and Tadashi Kokubo*
First Department of Surgery, Hamamatsu University School of Medicine,
3600 Handa-cho, Hamamatsu, 431-31, Japan
*Division of Material Chemistry, Faculty of Engineering, Kyoto University
Sakyo-ku, Kyoto, 606-01, Japan

ABSTRACT

Fibrous tissue culture, which was performed as a fundamental study for biocompatibility showed that fibrous tissue attached tightly to amorphous type HA, and proliferation of fibroblasts occurred. In an experimental study of artificial tracheas, amorphous type HA-coatings showed significantly better results than non-coatings. Thus, amorphous type HA seemed to be useful as a material for soft tissue prostheses.

INTRODUCTION

Studies of the response of soft tissue showed that hydroxyapatite (HA) coated on polymers did not induce inflammatory reactions, and facilitated proliferation of fibroblasts which might have a close relation to strong adherence [1]. Amorphous HA was more stable in handling than other types, and changed quickly to a highly crystalline HA in soft tissue [2]. Amorphous HA is thought to be suitable for soft tissue prosthesis at present, therefore, we grew fibrous tissue cultures on amorphous HA and studied an artificial trachea coated with amorphous type HA [3].

MATERIALS AND METHOD

HA coating was performed according to the biomimetic process reported by Kokubo [4,5]. In coating of amorphous, a biomimetic solution with higher concentrations of calcium and phosphate ions were employed. Temperature of solution was maintained lower than 35°C, and drying was done quickly [2] (Fig. 1).

1) Structural change of amorphous type HA in culture medium (RPMI 1640, 10% bovine serum) was analyzed by thin film X-ray diffraction (XRD), scanning electron microscope (SEM) and electron probe X-ray microanalyzer (EPMA).

2) Fibrous tissue (pleura) was cultured on culture bottles coated with amorphous type HA, and proliferation of fibroblasts and formation of collagen were observed by a phase difference microscope and SEM (Fig. 2).

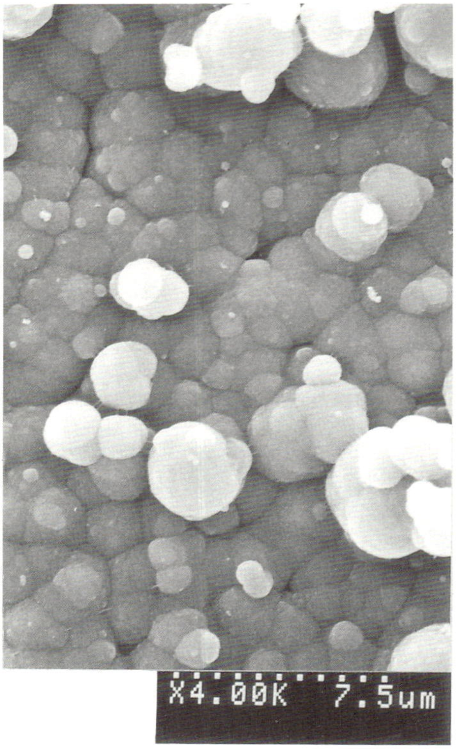

Figure 1. SEM photograph of amorphous HA.

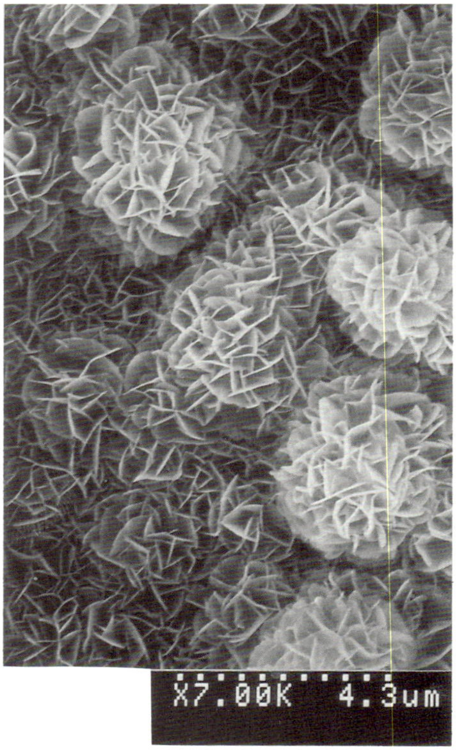

Figure 2. SEM photograph of crystallized HA. Amorphous HA coatings soaked in culture medium changed to highly crystalline type.

3) The shaft of a tracheal prosthesis was made of polyurethane. At both ends, nylon fibers were attached to prevent cutting in suturing. The internal diameters of the prosthesis were 12.5 mm, 15 mm and 16.5 mm, and the length of the prosthesis was 55 mm. In the coating group, all surfaces was coated with amorphous type HA. About 8-12 tracheal rings of cervical trachea of mongrel dogs were resected, and a prosthesis was interposed using a telescoped suturing technique. The clinical response and results of bronchofiberscopic examination and pathological findings were compared between the two groups amorphous HA-coating group (n=10) and non-coating group (n=10).

RESULTS

1) SEM and XRD showed that the rapid crystallization of amorphous HA in medium occurred, and the ratio of calcium to phosphorus in the coated HA increased (Fig. 3). The phenomena in culture medium were similar to the changes of amorphous HA implanted in soft tissue (Fig. 3).

2) Fibrous tissue, pleura, attached tightly to the coated HA layer. Proliferation of fibroblasts from cultured fibrous tissue and formation of collagen were observed in coated bottles with amorphous type HA (Figs. 4 and 5).

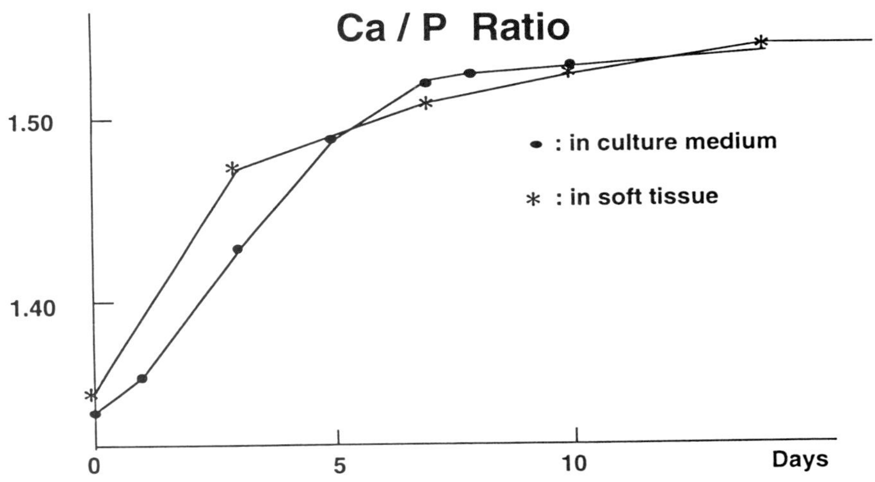

Figure 3. Ratio of calcium to phosphorus in coated HA increased rapidly.

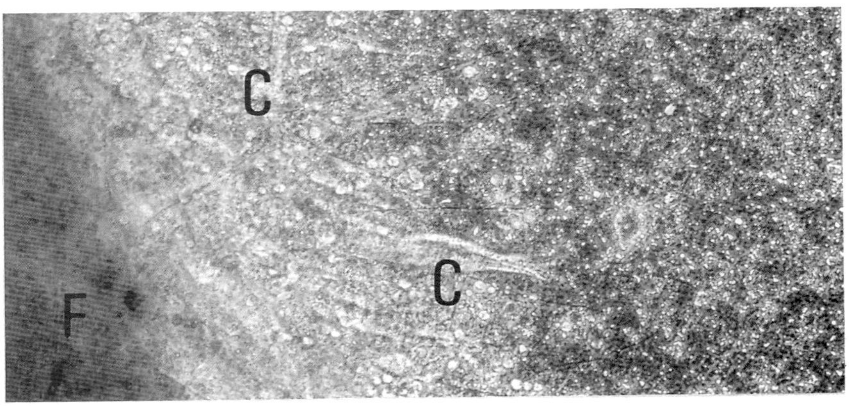

Figure 4. Photograph of a phase difference microscope (x 100). Proliferation of fibroblast from cultured fibrous tissue (F) and formation of collagen (C) were observed on amorphous HA layer.

3) Ten and twenty weeks survival rate were 90 % and 70% in coating group, 30% and 0% in non-coating group ($p<0.01$). Dehiscence of anastomosis, dislocation of artificial trachea, stenosis, and infection were more frequent in the non-coating group. Prostheses in long survivors were covered tightly by fibrous tissue. Coated HA protheses did not exfoliate 20 weeks after implantation (Figs. 6-8).

DISCUSSION

Previous studies revealed that any type of coated HA did not induce an inflammatory reaction and showed strong adherence in soft tissues [1-3]. These reactions had a close relation to proliferation of fibroblasts between the coated HA and native tissues [1]. Furthermore, amorphous type HA was more stable than other type in handling, and

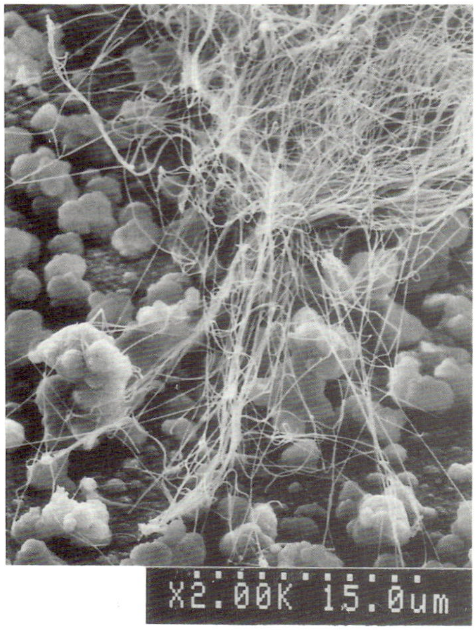

Figure 5a. SEM photograph. Collagen fibers produce by cultured fibroblasts grew as agglomerates around amorphous HA.

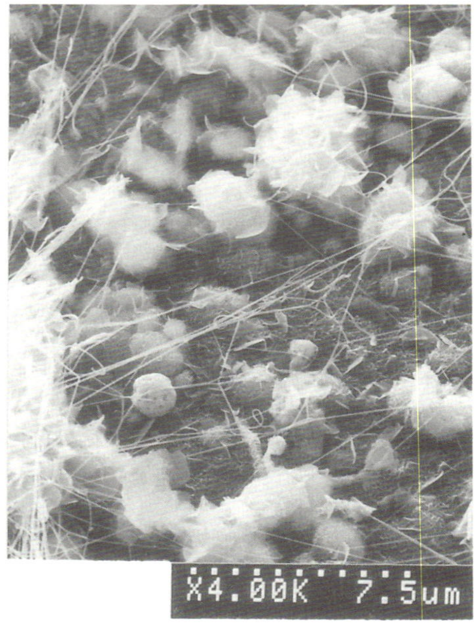

Figure 5b. SEM photograph. Collagen fibers grew around crystallized HA.

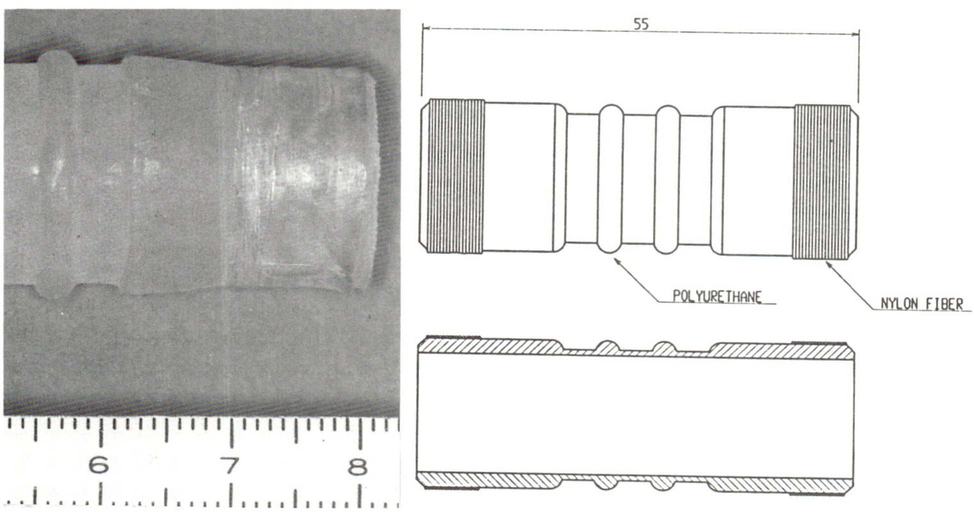

Figure 6. Photograph and schema of a artificial trachea.

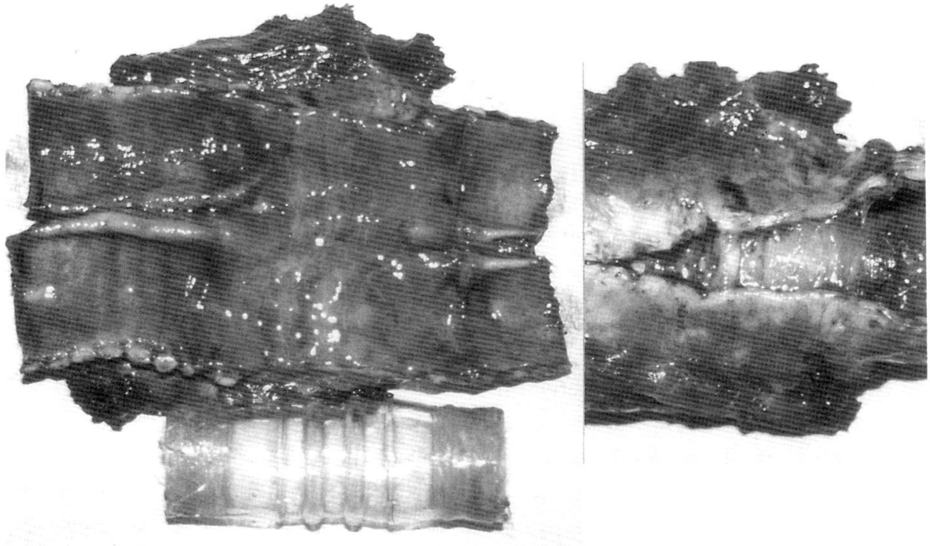

Figure 7. Photograph of a specimen resected 22 weeks after implantation. The HA coated prosthesis was covered tightly by fibrous tissue.

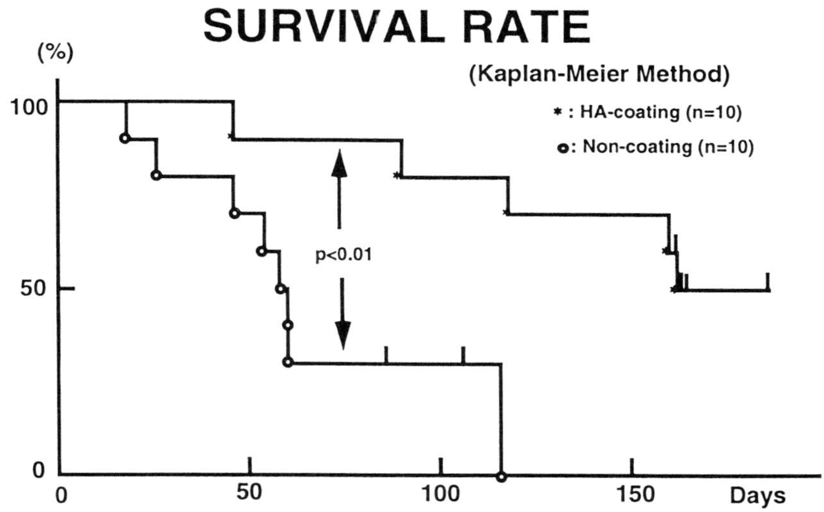

Figure 8. Survival rate after implantation of artificial trachea was significantly higher in the amorphous HA coating group.

changed to a highly crystalline type in soft tissue [2]. In this study, therefore, we investigated histocompatibility of amorphous HA using tissue culture technique in which reactions between coated HA and fibroblasts could be observed under the invariable conditions. Membranous and fibrous tissue, pleura, attached tightly to coated HA, then proliferation of fibroblasts and production of collagen occurred. Amorphous HA seemed to have histocompatibility as far as fibrous tissue was concerned, because these phenomena did not occur in the non-coating culture bottles. Amorphous HA is thought to be suitable for many applications at present, since amorphous HA did not exfoliate from materials when coated either on culture bottles and on soft tissue prosthesis. Tracheal reconstruction with amorphous HA-coated prosthesis yielded significantly better results than did non-coated prostheses, probably due to strong adherence and the good histocompatibility of amorphous HA [3]. In conclusion, amorphous HA can be useful for purposes which need tight attachment to soft tissue or cells.

REFERENCE

1. Kageyama, Y., Yokoyama Y., Suzuki, K., Harada, Y. and Kokubo, T. Jn: Bioceramics Volume 7, Butterworth-Heinemann, Oxford 1994, 165-170.
2. Suzuki, K., Kageyama, Y., Yokoyama Y., Harada, Y. and Kokubo, T. Jn: Bioceramics Volume 7, Butterworth-Heinemann, Oxford 1994, 113-117.
3. Suzuki, K., Kobayashi R., Yokoyama Y., Harada, Y. and Kokubo, T. Jn: Bioceramics Volume 6, Butterworth-Heinemann, Oxford 1993, 245-250 .
4. Kokubo, T., Hata, K., Nakamura, T. and Yamamoto T. Jn: Bioceramics Volume 4, Butterworth-Heinemann, Oxford 1991, 113-120 .
5. Kokubo, T. Jn: Biomaterials, 1992, 12,155.

COATING OF HYDROXYAPATITE ON BACTERIAL CELLULOSE

Y. Suwa*, H. Saito*, Y. Doi**, S. Yamanaka***, Y. Satoh****, and S. Niwa****

*:STK Ceramics Laboratory Corp., Tsukisan-cho, Minato-ku, Nagoya 465, Japan **:School of Dentistory, Asahi Univ., Hozumi-cho, Gifu 501-02, Japan***:AJI NO MOTO Co., LTD, Suzuki-cho, Kawasaki-ku, Kawasaki 210, Japan****:Dept. of Orthopaedic Surgery, Aichi Medical Univ., Nagakute, Aichi 480-11, Japan.

ABSTRACT

The present study investigated, coating of hydroxyapatite (HAp) on bacterial cellulose (BC) sheet for applying to adhesion blocking of the tendon from its surrounding tissues. HAp was deposited and grown by enzymatic hydrolysis of calcium ß-glycerophosphate (CaGP) on the sheet. Growth rate of HAp was found to be enhanced by grafting phosphoprotein to the BC, and the HAp deposited is considered to be chemically bonded with BC.

INTRODUCTION

The fibrils of BC produced by *Acetobacter aceti* are composed of pure cellulose which is devoid of lignin, hemicellulose or other substances, and is a biocompatible material [1,2]. Heat-pressed BC sheet has a high tensile strength and high Young's modulus, and is considered as a candidate biomaterial. In preliminary experiments, BC sheets were mechanically coated with HAp fine crystals on one side using an HAp sol [3]. This BC sheet was implanted surrounding the Achilles tendon of rabbit. After three weeks, the implant with tendon was removed and histologically examined. No impediment of the tendon repair was observed, and the HAp coated sheet was proposed as a tendon-adhesion blocking material [4,5]. However, coating of Hap homogeneously on local areas of the BC sheet, or on the inside or outside of BC tubes, was troublesome. Improvements in material and method are required.

Banks et al. [6] studied the growth of fibrous HAp by enzymatic hydrolysis of CaGP on reconstituted collagen which had been modified by the addition of a phosphoprotein, phosvitin (PVT), in the presence of a cross-linking agent, dimethylsuberimidate (DMSI) [6]. Doi et al. [7,8] developed this reaction process for formation of the composite of HAp and collagen.

The aim of this study is to examine whether or not HAp is deposited and grown by enzymatic hydrolysis of CaGP on BC sheet.

MATERIALS AND METHODS

A BC gelatinous mat was used as a substrate which is composed of microfibrils having about 20~50 nm width and over ten microns in length. Dry cellulose substance is about 1 % of the BC mat. The BC mat was soaked in a mixed solution of DMSI, PVT and alkaline phosphatase (ALP) at 37°C for 6 days. After rinsing with distilled water, the mat was again soaked in PVT and ALP solution at room temperature for 3 h and then transferred to a CaGP solution and incubated at 37°C for 20 h. Tris buffer solution (pH 8.5 adjusted with HCl) was used as the solvent for all solutions. The mat was alternately soaked in PVT and ALP solution and in CaGP solution. Each time, the mat was rinsed with distilled water. After several changes of the solution and a final washing, the calcified mat was dehydrated and heat-pressed to the sheet. For identification of deposited material, X-ray diffraction (XRD), Infrared (IR) spectrometry and scanning electron microscope (SEM) were used. Calcium and phosphate deposits were analyzed by inductive coupled plasma (ICP) spectrometry.

RESULTS AND DISCUSSION

XRD patterns and IR spectra of HAp coating BC sheet are shown in Figures 1 and 2, respectively, where HAp coating was performed by soaking alternately in PVT and ALP mixed solution for 3 h, and in CaGP solution for 20 h each three times, after soaking in DMSI, PVT and ALP mixed solution for 6 days (BCH-3d). These Figures show that the deposited material is typical carbonated HAp having a small crystallite size and/or defect structure similar to natural bone. Relative intensity of the XRD patterns indicates that there was no special oriented crystal growth of HAp on the coating. A piece of the HAp coating BC (BCH) sheet was dissolved in HCl, and Ca and P were analyzed by ICP. The Ca/P molar ratio of the deposits was 1.63~1.66 (approximately the same with Ca-deficient HAp). Thickness change of BCH sheet with cumulative soaking time is shown in Figure 3. Crystal growth rate of HAp increased by soaking in CaGP for 20 to 40 h, and saturated over 60 h.

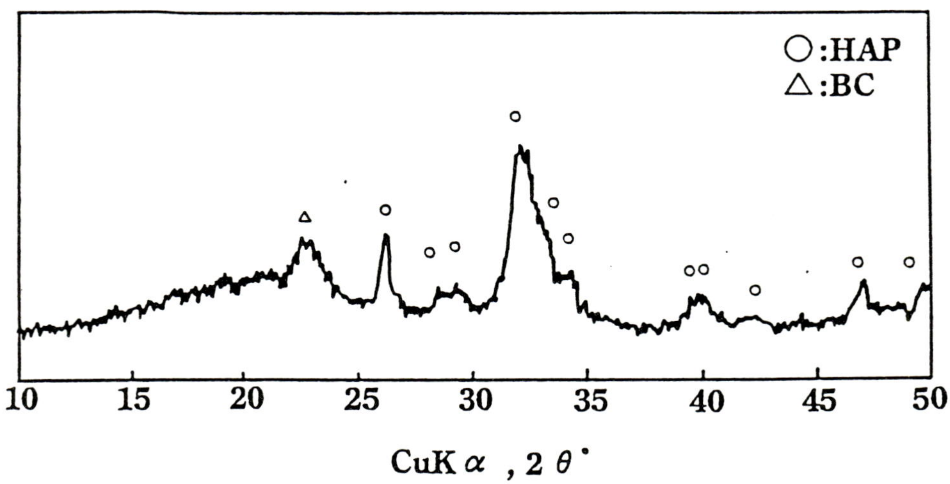

Figure 1. XRD patterns of HAp-coating BC sheet. Coating was performed by alternately soaking in PVT and ALP solution and in CaGP solution each three times, after soaking in DMSI, PVT, and ALP solution for 6 d.

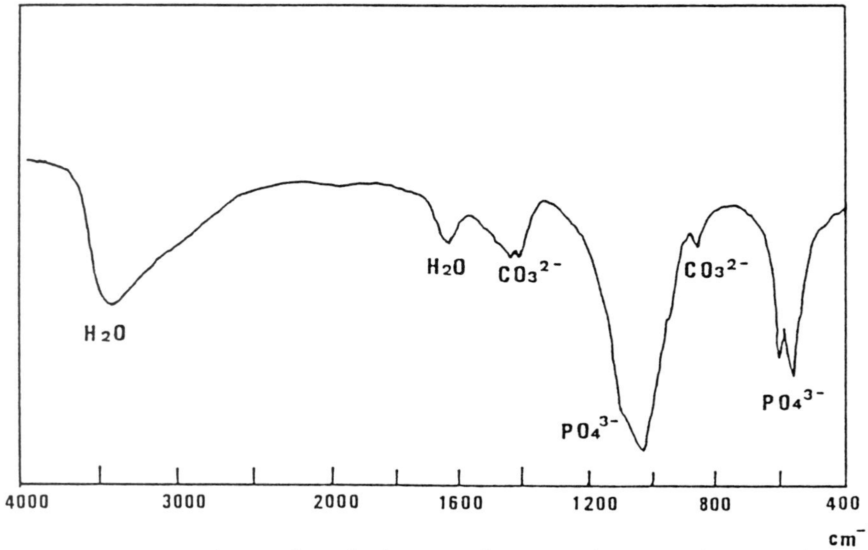

Figure 2. IR spectra of HAp deposited on BC sheet. Coating procedure was the same as described in Figure 1.

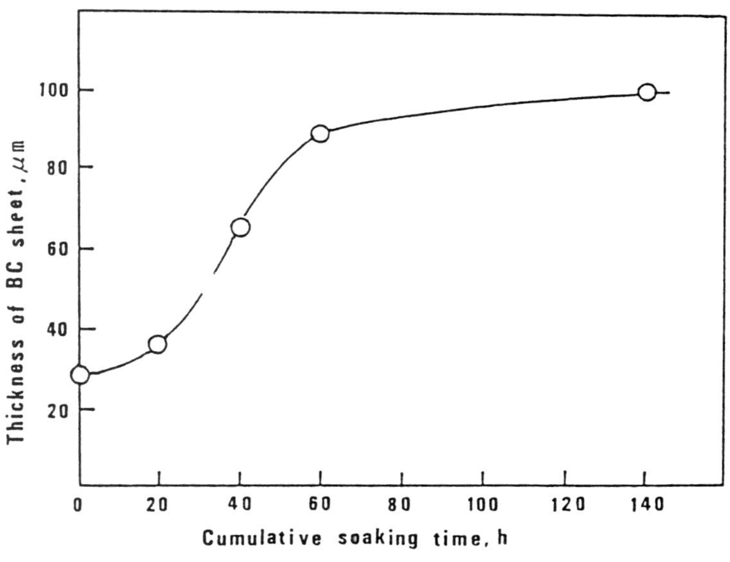

Figure 3. Change of thickness of HAp coating BC sheet with cumulative soaking time.

Banks et al. reported that the alternative soaking in enzyme, ALP and in CaGP affects the oriented crystal growth of HAp on a collagen layer, and also that the presence of a grafting agent, PVT, treated with cross-linking agent, DMSI, affects adhesion of HAp on collagen layer. In this study, the role of ALP on the oriented crystal growth of HAp on BC sheet is not clarified, but PVT seems to play a role on the chemical bonding of HAp on the BC sheet.

REFERENCES

1. Yamanaka, S., Watanabe, K., Kitamura, N., Iguchi, M., Mitsuhashi, S., Nishi,Y. and Uryuu, M., J.Mat.Sci., 1989, 24, 3141-3145.
2. Yamanaka,S. and Watanabe,K. in Cellulose Polymers, Blends and Composites, Gilbert,R.D. ed.,Carl Hanser Verlag 1994.
3. Japanese patent application No. 93-279625.
4. Satoh,Y., Niwa,S., Kawai, N., Suwa,Y. and Yamanaka,S., in 20th Ann. Meeting Soc.Biomaterials, Boston, 1994.
5. Satoh,Y., Niwa, S., Kawai, N., Suwa,Y., and Yamanaka, S., in 11th Ann. Meeting Symposium on Apatite, Japan, 1994.
6. Banks,E., Nakajima, S., Shapiro, L.C., Tilevitz, O., Alonzo, J.R., and Chianlli, R.R., Science, 1977, 1164-1166.
7. Horiguchi, K., Doi, Y., Kim, S.H., Wakamatsu, N., Adachi, M., Imura, S., Hayashi, K., and Gyotoku, T., J. Japanese Soc. Dental Materials and Devices, 1990, 9, 863-870.
8. Horiguchi, K., Doi, Y., Kim, S.H., Wakamatsu, N., Adachi, M., Imura, S., Hayashi, K., and Gyotoku, T., J. Japanese Soc. Dental Materials and Devices, 1991, 10, 814-819.

THE AMORPHOUS PHASE IN PLASMA SPRAYED HYDROXYAPATITE COATINGS

K.A. Gross and C.C. Berndt

The Thermal Spray Laboratory, Department of Materials Science and Engineering
Sate University of New York at Stony Brook, NY 11794-2275, USA.

ABSTRACT

Atmospheric plasma spraying of hydroxyapatite was carried out to investigate the influence of the plasma spraying parameters on the formation of the amorphous phase. The amorphous phase was investigated with X-ray diffraction and optical microscopy. The results infer that dehydroxylation of the molten particle and a high cooling rate produce a larger amount of the amorphous phase. Crystalline regions of the coating consist of partially molten particles and elongated recrystallized areas. The amorphous phase is commonly found at the substrate interface. It is shown that the amorphous regions vary throughout the coating which clinically could affect the process of bone deposition and successful implant fixation.

INTRODUCTION

Atmospheric plasma spraying is used for applying hydroxyapatite to dental implants and orthopedic prostheses. The feedstock in the form of a powder is fed to the plasma and accelerated to about 150 m/s before impacting the substrate [1]. These high impact velocities flatten the molten particles and cause rapid heat flow to the substrate. This results in a very fast cooling rate (> 10^5 °K/sec) which is sufficient to form an amorphous phase.

Crystallinity has been interpreted in different ways in the biomedical community. It was initially used as an indication of the crystal size or perfection of the crystal lattice in hydroxyapatite crystals [2]. Thermally sprayed materials typically have a small grain size and a high defect concentration due to the fast cooling rate, in addition to a residual stress. These variables give rise to a broadening of the X-ray diffraction peak, making it comparable to the spectra of the inorganic phase in bone, Fig. 1. A high crystallinity hydroxyapatite material is included as a reference.

The performance of a thermally sprayed hydroxyapatite coating depends upon the chemical phases and their distribution within the microstructure. A fine grain size has been shown to give a higher dissolution [3] and the residual stress further modifies the properties. The influence of these factors with respect to the clinical functionality of the implant has yet to be determined. The amorphous phase has been shown to dissolve more quickly than the crystalline phase [4,5], and could lead to coating degradation [6].

The purpose of this paper is to focus on the amorphous phase represented by the broad diffuse peak in the x-ray diffraction pattern of Fig. 1. The formation of such amorphous phases and their location within the coating is important knowledge with regard to designing a coating with the desired properties, such as a functionally graded coating.

MATERIALS AND METHODS

A Metco 3MB plasma spray torch, with a GH nozzle was used to prepare hydroxyapatite coatings. Powder with a Ca/P ratio of 1.67, and a particle size distribution of 5 to 40 μm was sprayed under different conditions. Initially, the powder was sprayed at different power levels to ascertain the changes taking place in the material upon entering the plasma. When this was determined, various plasma spraying parameters were altered to investigate the effect on amorphicity. The parameters that were changed include stand-off distance (5 to 20 cm), particle size distribution (the small particle sized powder was mixed with a larger particle size powder with a mean of 80 μm), substrate angle (0 to 60 degrees), gas flow rate (35 to 55 slpm), air cooling of the coating and hydroxylation state of the starting powder. A powder with a lower hydroxyl content was produced by heating at 1200°C for one hour followed by sieving. A substrate angle of 90° represents a substrate with the face positioned perpendicular to the stream of molten droplets.

The calcium and phosphorous concentrations were determined with X-ray fluorescence using a hydroxyapatite powder as a reference. Coating crystallinity was ascertained with a calibration curve produced by measuring the crystalline peaks and the broad amorphous peak of standard mixtures.

Coatings were sectioned on a diamond cut-off wheel, mounted in epoxy resin, ground and polished using 0.05 μm alumina as the last step. The crystalline regions were viewed in the optical microscope using the Nomarski interference method to increase the depth of field and contrast of the features.

Two coatings with 98 wt.% amorphous phase were heated to 660 °C for 5 minutes in either dry or moist helium gas. The crystallinity was then measured using x-ray diffraction to ascertain the influence of the water content on the crystallization.

RESULTS AND DISCUSSION

The coatings produced at various power levels showed that decomposition takes place at higher temperatures. At lower power levels tricalcium phosphate (TCP) will appear but more severe heating will also produce tetracalcium phosphate (TTCP) and calcium oxide. The former two phases are the equilibrium phases at high temperature and low partial water pressure. The Ca/P molar ratio also increases, signifying preferential removal of the phosphate group from the hydroxyapatite structure in more intense heating conditions, Table 1. This calcium rich molten particle solidifies to form calcium oxide along with the two calcium phosphate phases predicted by the equilibrium phase diagram.

As the spray angle deviates from perpendicular to the spray stream by more than 30°, an increase in the amorphous nature of the coating is noted, Fig. 2. Less unmolten particles participate in the buildup of the coating as they ricochet from the surface, but more importantly, the lamellae thickness decreases, as evidenced from studies on other materials [7]. This leads to a higher cooling rate and is associated with an increase in amorphousness of the coating. Heat flow through the substrate material will be higher than

Table 1. Influence of power level on the decomposition of hydroxyapatite.

Power Level (kW)	18	25	30	35
Ca/P molar ratio	1.67	1.69	1.75	2.03
Phases	HAp, TCP	HAp, TCP	HAp, TTCP, CaO	

to the surrounding air, however convectional cooling of the coating offers a secondary means to increase the cooling rate.

The composition of the hydroxyapatite also influences the formation of the amorphous phase. Use of a slightly dehydroxylated powder increases the amorphicity of the coating. A hydroxyl deficient molten particle will more likely form an amorphous phase compared to a droplet with a high hydroxylation level. The hydroxyl ion concentration of the molten particle before impact can be controlled by increasing the amount of heat transferred to the particles. For example, using a smaller particle size or a larger spraying distance facilitates this compositional change with a larger heat transfer to the particles. Also, a lower gas flow rate gives rise to slower particle velocities and a higher heat transfer. However, only part of the dehydroxylated droplet forms the amorphous phase, the remaining portion forming oxyapatite. This effect is most easily observed as the left shoulder on the 004 reflection in the X-ray diffraction pattern, inset of Fig. 3.

The penetration of X-rays is dependent upon the energy of the beam. X-rays will not penetrate through the entire thickness of the coating. Observation of the microstructure is important in determining the properties of the material and can be used to identify the size, shape and location of the crystalline regions within the coating. Figure 4 shows the microstructure of a 50 wt.% and 100 wt.% crystalline coating, as determined by X-ray diffraction. A noteworthy feature is the amorphous phase (darker grey in color) which very often forms at the titanium substrate. This is important in the performance of the coating. Other phases such as tricalcium phosphate are present in small quantities, however this cannot be distinguished from the hydroxyapatite.

The crystalline phase consists of unmolten or partially molten particles and recrystallized particles. The former is represented by the angular particles. The elongated crystalline particles (arrow on Fig. 4 and Fig. 6) are recrystallized regions, which can be explained by another short experiment. The heat treatment of the amorphous phase shows complete crystallization in a wet atmosphere but partial crystallization in a dry atmosphere, Fig. 5. Thus the molten droplet will consist of a hydroxyl rich core surrounded by hydroxyl deficient regions as it spreads out to form the lamellae. These two regions are inseparable and are both identified as the amorphous phase. The heat in the coating is dissipated slowly due to the low thermal diffusivity (~ 5×10^{-3} cm^2/s) and is elevated by additional heat given off in the structural relaxation of the amorphous phase. When the temperature is sufficiently high, recrystallization will first take place in the hydroxyl rich areas; hence the presence of elongated crystalline regions.

As consecutive layers are deposited, the heat in the coating may build up slowly and lead to crystallization in different places within the coating. The coating is more crystalline at the surface compared to the area adjacent to the substrate, Fig. 6, and

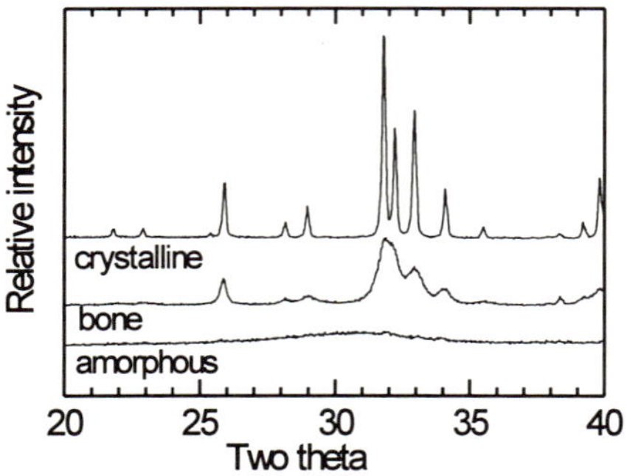

Figure 1. An X-ray diffraction pattern illustrates a) high crystallinity hydroxyapatite, b) inorganic bone and c) an amorphous phase found in hydroxyapatite coatings.

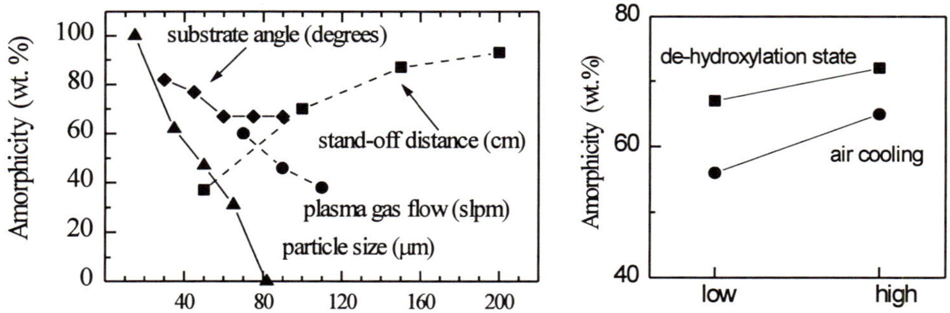

Figure 2. Influence of spray parameters on the amorphicity of the coating. (Abscissa is variable according to values or level of parameter).

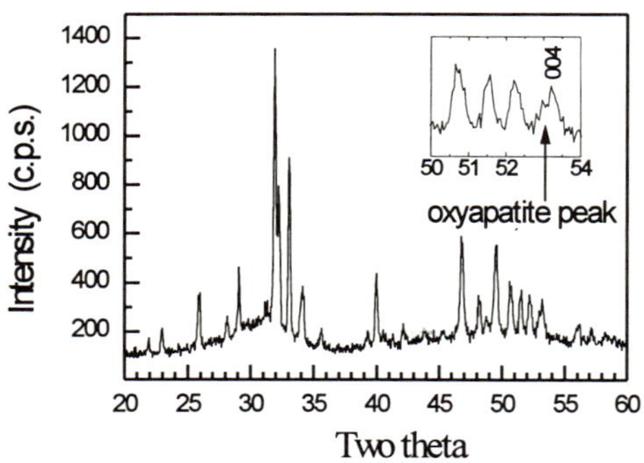

Figure 3. X-ray diffraction pattern showing the presence of the crystalline hydroxyapatite, oxyapatite and the amorphous phase.

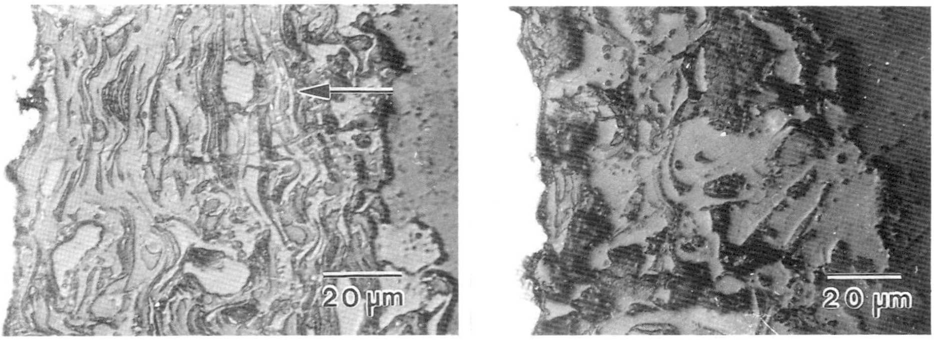

Figure 4. Microstructure showing the crystalline phase (indicated by higher plateaus of lighter color) in a 50 wt.% and 100 wt.% crystalline coating calculated from X-ray diffraction. (The titanium substrate is situated on the left hand side).

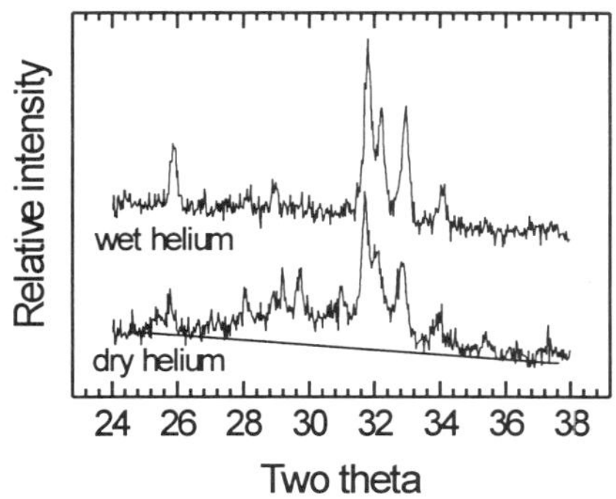

Figure 5. X-ray diffraction of the amorphous phase after heat treatment at 660 °C for 5 minutes in a dry and moist atmosphere.

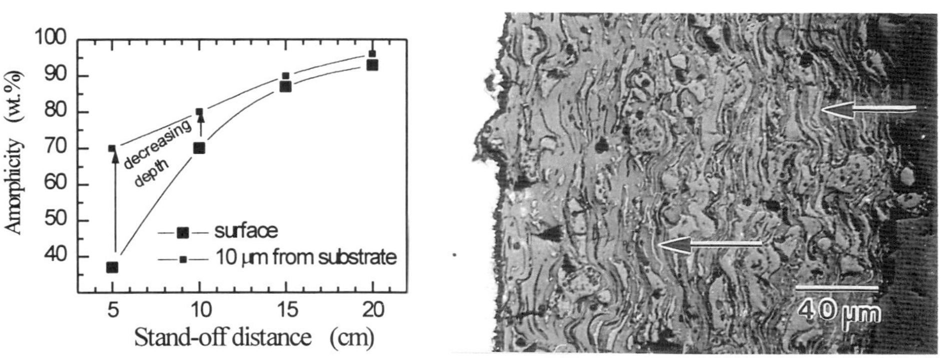

Figure 6. The variation of crystallinity close to the substrate and on the surface of the coating as identified by X-ray diffraction and shown in a micrograph.

becomes less noticeable with longer stand-off distances. The number of crystalline regions identified as recrystallized hydroxyapatite increases with thickness.

CONCLUSIONS

Plasma spray processing of hydroxyapatite is very sensitive to the spraying parameters. It has been shown that the crystalline phase consists of unmolten and recrystallized areas within the coating. The amorphous phase forms as a result of dehydroxlation taking place in the particle during spraying and the fast cooling rate at the substrate. Optical microscopy is suitable for discerning crystalline regions within the coating. The distribution of the crystalline phase is modified by a rise in temperature and form crystallinity-graded regions within the coating.

ACKNOWLEDGEMENT

The authors are grateful for the X-ray fluorescence conducted by Dr. H. Wang at Sherritt Gordon, Inc.

REFERENCES

1. Knight, R., Smith, R.W. and Xiao, Z., Proc. 7th Nat. Therm. Spray Conf., 1994, 331-337.
2. Le Geros, R., *Clinical Materials,* 1993, 14, 65-88.
3. Lelievre, F. and Bernache-Assolant, D., Proc. 4th World Biomaterials Congr., Berlin, 1992, 330.
4. Gross, K.A. and Berndt, C.C., *J. Mat. Sci.: Mat. in Med.* 1994, 5, 219-224.
5. Klein, C.P.A.T., Wolke, J.G.C., Blieck-Hogervorst, J.M.A., de Groot, K., *J. Biomed. Mater. Res.*, 1994, 28, 961-967.
6. Bauer, T.W., Geesink, R.G.T., Zimmerman, R. and McMahon, J.T., *J. Bone Joint Sur.*, 1990, 3A, 1439-1452.
7. Montavon, G., Sampath, S., Berndt, C.C., Herman, H. and Coddet, C., *J. Thermal Spray Technol.*, 1995, 4, 67-74.

NEW DIRECTIONS

MICROFRACTURE AND ACOUSTIC EMISSION IN PYROLYTIC CARBON HEART VALVE MATERIAL

J. Lankford[1], A. E. Nicholls[1], and J. Ely[2]

[1]Southwest Research Institute, San Antonio, TX 78238-5166
[2]Medical Carbon Research Institute, Austin, TX 78754

ABSTRACT

Improved techniques are needed to detect the possible presence of pre-existing flaws in mechanical heart valves. Accordingly, the acoustic emission (AE) associated with indentation-induced microfracture in pyrolytic carbon/graphite heart valve materials was investigated. It shows that AE is sensitive to the change in the types of microfracture patterns deriving from increasing indentation load. Moreover, additional loads applied to the same site appeared to produce no new cracks, but AE was nevertheless detectable, suggesting that the existing cracks may have extended, with associated stress wave generation.

INTRODUCTION

The concept of using AE to monitor damage initiation and/or growth is not new, and in fact has been used extensively for polycrystalline graphite [1,2]. However, it appears that similar experiments have never been performed using pyrolytic carbon (PyC). The microstructure of graphite consists predominantly of an isotropic, polycrystalline aggregate of fine, hexagonal symmetry grains [2]. Pyrolytic carbon, on the other hand, possesses a two-phase microstructure of p-SiC nanocrystals [3] (<20 nm) uniformly dispersed throughout carbon grains, which are about 0.5 1lm in diameter and are composed of turbostatic crystallites approximately 3.0 nm in size [4]. Samples for the indentation fracture tests described in this report were prepared by depositing such PyC onto machined graphite substrates in a fluidized bed process. This results in a composite structure consisting of an approximately 0.012-inch thick PyC coating wrapped around a 0.015-inch thick graphite core.

It should be noted that the as-grown outer surface of the composite is relatively flaw-free, while the pyrolytic carbon at the PyC-graphite interface is characterized by a significant flaw population. In particular, Schwartz and Haubold have shown [5] that collisions between neighboring graphite preforms early in the deposition process produce characteristic impact induced microcracks within the embryonic PyC coating. The cracks form a somewhat star shaped pattern, but their formation stops once the coating has built up sufficiently, and the earlier cracks are coated over.

Extensive sectioning experiments by Ely, et al. [6,7], have documented the fracture patterns induced in PyC-graphite slabs during indentation fracture experiments. He has shown that fracture first initiates at the PyC-graphite interface, followed at higher load levels by classical indentation microcracking.

EXPERIMENTAL PROCEDURES

Load-unload indentation fracture tests were run in an MTS serve-hydraulic test machine, with cross-head displacement controlled at a rate of 0.010 inches per minute. The loading history and displacement, the latter measured by placing an eddy current transducer (0.1 pm sensitivity) across the indenter/specimen couple, were recorded on a Nicolet digital transient recorder system. Both diamond pyramid and hardened steel ball indenters were used.

Indentation samples were prepared in the form of small beam-shaped slabs (1.12 inches long x 0.24 inches wide x 0.039 inches thick). The graphite core was softer and more compliant than the outer coating, so that indentation loading of the central sector of a simply supported slab essentially flexed the upper (loaded) portion of the PyC coating, placing the PyC-graphite interface in tension.

A piezo crystal, resonant at 160 KHz, was coupled to the specimen with silicone vacuum grease. The output of the crystal was fed into an acoustic emission device consisting of signal conditioner, 200 db gain filtered amplifiers with a 100 KHz to 1 MHz frequency range, a frequency-to-voltage converter, and a totalizing counter with a voltage output.

EXPERIMENTAL RESULTS

Typical diamond pyramid (DP) indentation load and acoustic emission versus displacement behavior for PyC is shown in Figure 1. In this case, indentations were performed to gradually increasing maximum load levels, each indentation site lying within a localized region of the slab, and each corresponding to a single load-unload cycle. The following observations can be made.

First, load-unload loops are nonlinear, i.e., convex upward. Although the unloading portion of each loop lies below the loading trace, all loops are observed to close (within the sensitivity of the displacement gage). Below a critical load level, approximately 23 N in this case (Figure 1), no acoustic emission is observed; above this level, one or more AE bursts are detected. At another characteristic load level, on the order of 85 N, the load-displacement trace experiences a change in slope that, if it were in terms of a stress-strain plot, would represent plastic yielding. Simultaneous with the "yield point" is an audible "click," and the nucleation of a set of optically visible microcracks emanating from the indentation corners, plus another set lying within and parallel to the four sides of the indent.

Multiple experiments of this sort yield results that are bimodal, with a transition at 70 N, above which the initial AE is in the form of the audible "click" associated with indentation microfracture; between 13 N and 70 N, inaudible AE is observed. Sectioning experiments were performed [8,9] to establish the origin of the latter emission, which was determined to derive from the initiation of subsurface tensile mode microcracks nucleated at the PyC graphite interface and lying within the PyC. Multiple pre -"click" AE appears to originate from an equivalent number of subsurface tensile microcracks

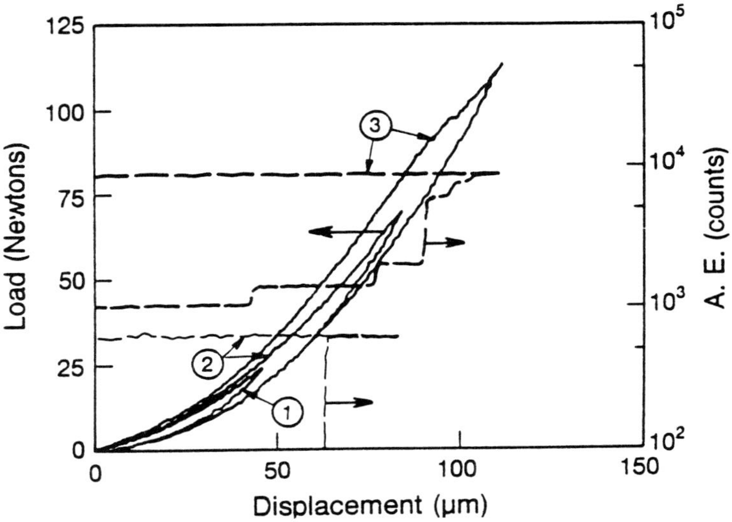

Figure 1. Load (P) and cumulative acoustic emission versus DP indenter displacement hysteresis loops; upper load-displacement traces are initial indentation, lower traces represent indenter withdrawal. "Yielding" due to indent microfracture occurs at $P \simeq 82$ N.

initiated at the PyC graphite interface. Above the "click" level, additional inaudible AE is detected, which may derive from crack extension. Similar observations hold for spherical indenters, which produce conical ring cracks (the origin of the "click") in addition to inaudible PyC-graphite interface tensile cracks (Figures 2 and 3).

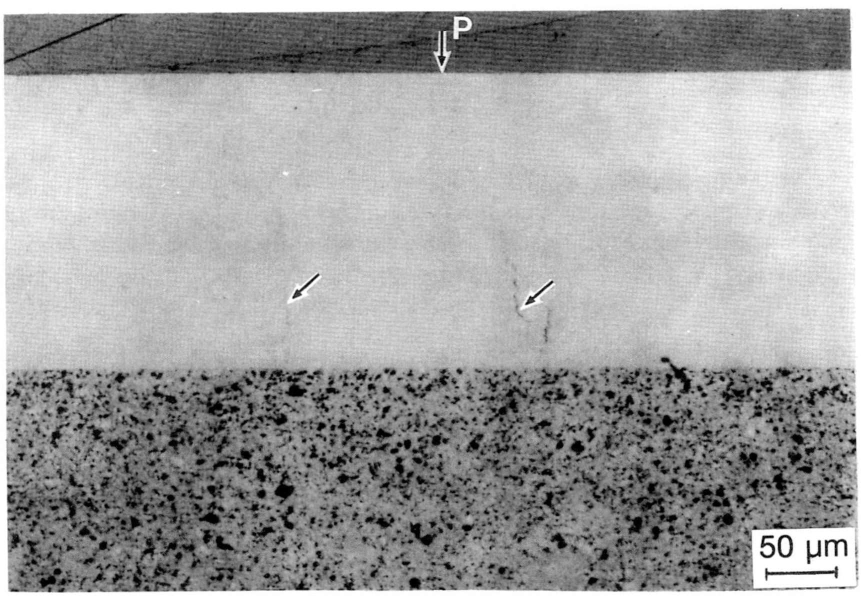

Figure 2. Flexural cracks (arrows) in PyC nucleated at PyC-graphite interface; load (P) applied via steel ball.

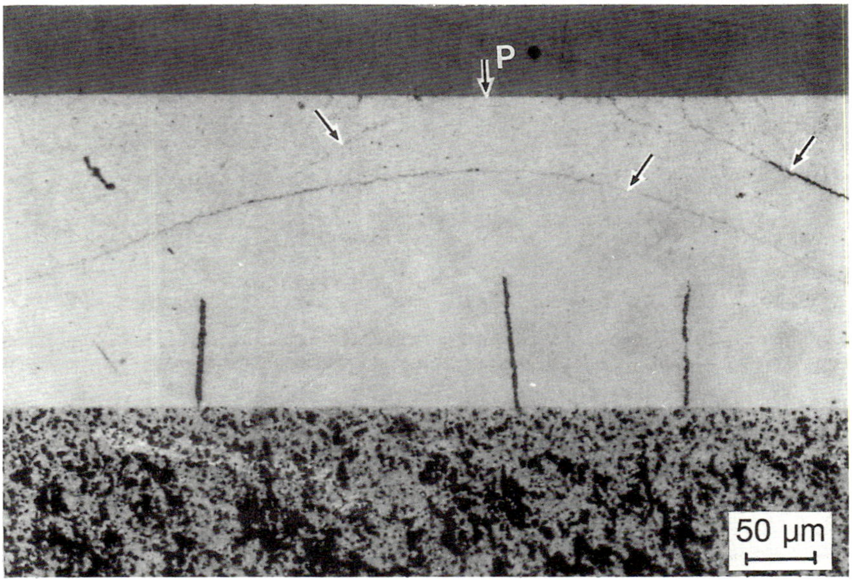

Figure 3. Flexural cracks at PyC-graphite interface and conical ring cracks (arrows) in PyC nucleated within audible AE regime; load (P) applied via steel ball.

Individual DP indentations in PyC-graphite were subjected to multiple loading. These cyclic load levels were chosen to range from no AE (Figure 4) to above the click level (Figure 5). It was observed that with repeated cycles, the number of AE counts decreases, the most marked drop usually occurring between the first and the second load cycle. As cycling continues, load-displacement loops gradually move toward an asymptotic value in permanent set (Figure 5), and the loops tighten (low load loops approach trace-retrace, Figure 4). Moreover, while the original AE usually occurs on a load cycle, later emission often is absent on loading, but is detected as the indenter is withdrawn.

DISCUSSION

The results suggest that the indentation load produces initial cracks by flexing the upper section of the composite beam, which is supported by the much more compliant graphite core, thus sampling the interface flaw population within the most highly stressed zone beneath the indenter. The wide range in stress required to generate the inaudible AE ($13 \text{ N} < P < 70 \text{ N}$ for the DP) associated with interface-nucleated flexural cracks suggests that the interface zone is characterized by a wide range of initial flaw severity, probably controlled by early, local impacts during fluidized load deposition.

It was observed that during indentation cycling, emission on cycles following the initial loading usually occurs as the indenter is withdrawn. This suggests, as per experience with regard to indentation fracture of ceramics [8], that previously nucleated cracks may be extending on the unload side of a loop, and that the AE system may be able to pick up relatively lower (compared to nucleation) stress wave emission associated with microcrack growth.

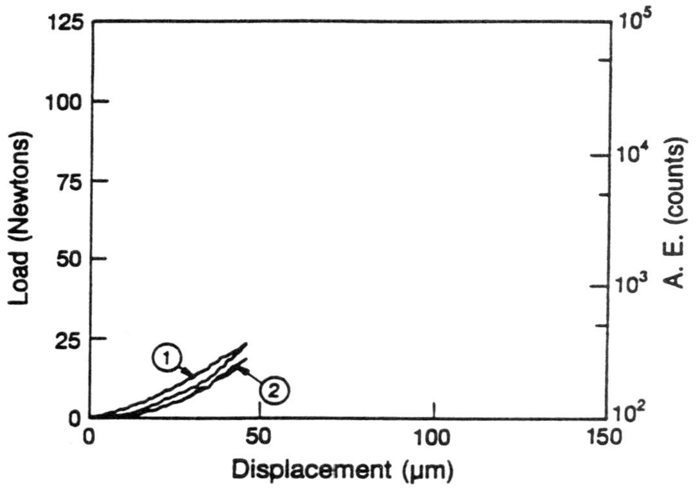

Figure 4. Load displacement hysteresis loops for cyclically-loaded DP indentation of PyC below thresholds for AE and indent microfracture: (1) N - 1; (2) N - 5.

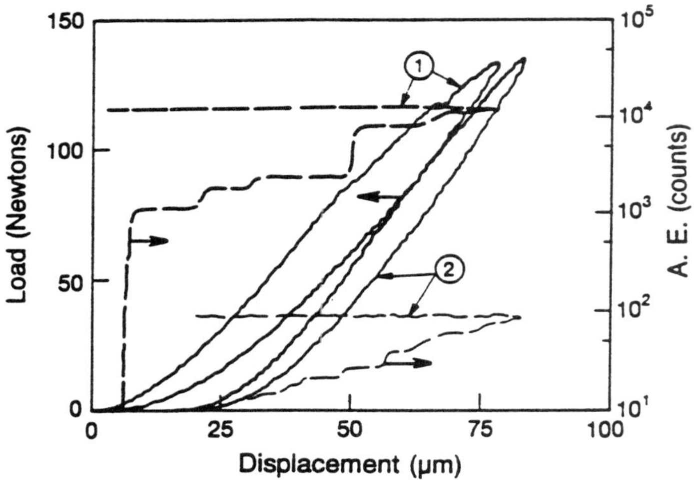

Figure 5. Load-displacement hysteresis loops and cumulative AE for cyclically-loaded DP indentation of PyC above the thresholds for AE and indent microfracture: (1) N - 1; (2) N 5. Acoustic emission count level decreases, and permanent impression is formed, with increasing N.

It should be noted that the load-displacement and associated microfracture behavior defined here for PyC is highly unusual. As shown in Figure 6, load-displacement loops for soda lime glass (and for metals and ceramics as well [8]) do not close upon unloading, evidence of a permanent remnant diamond pyramid impression. Above a fairly low threshold, AE occurs (Figure 6) that is the product of Palmqvist microfracture at inherent microscopic surface flaws near the corners of the indents. It is interesting that this is not the case for PyC-graphite, for which the first observed cracks originate at the PyC-graphite interface, with a much higher load required to initiate indent cone (ring) cracks.

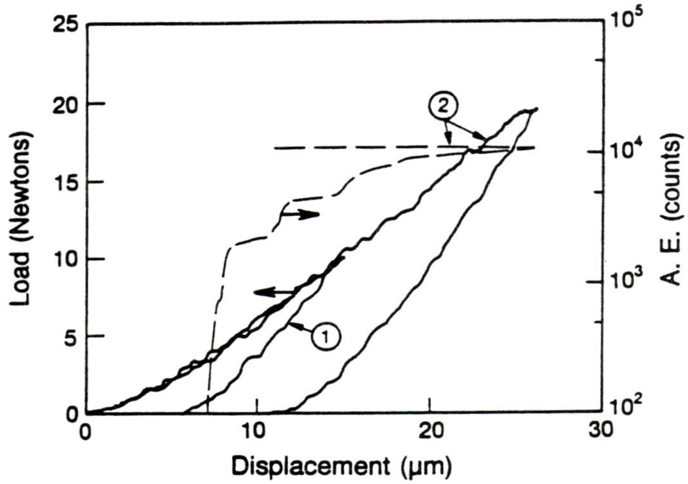

Figure 6. Load and cumulative AE versus displacement for DP indentation of soda lime glass loaded above (2) and below (1) AE threshold. Remnant displacement represents permanent indentation.

The difficulty of nucleating cracks in PyC is remarkable, in view of its low fracture toughness (~ 1.1 MPa√m) [9]. It seems likely that this must relate to the apparently large inelastic strains that can be accommodated by its open, nanoscale, turbostatic microstructure. The minimal permanent set associated with cyclic indentations, in fact, probably is not generated by continuum deformation, but rather by residual openings in the indent shear cracks. Preliminary SEM analysis suggests that the residual opening is caused by particulate (growth domain) debris that props the cracks open.

Finally, the exceedingly reversible indentation impressions, and indentation ring cracking instead of the median/radial indent fracture associated with classic ceramics, are virtually identical to the recent observations by Sakai [10] for glass-like carbon. In this case, the material was created by the reduction and hot isostatic pressing of phenolic resin powder. The resulting microstructure was "open", due to the presence of closed micropores (~8 nm diameter). This suggests that it is the moreopen, disordered constituent of the present turbostratic microstructure that is responsible for the observed purely elastic indentation behavior.

REFERENCES

1. Neighbour G. B., McEnaney, B., and Philips, M. *Carbon,* 1992, 30, 359-363.
2. Ioka, I., Yoda, S., and Konishi, *T. Carbon,* 1990, 28, 879-885.
3. Kaae, J. L., *Carbon,* 1975, 13, 51-53.
4. Kaae, J. L., *Carbon,* 1975, 13, 55-62.
5. Schwartz A. S., and Haubold, A. D., *Trans. Soc. Biomaterials, 1994,* 17, 219.
6. Ely, J. L., Haubold, A. D., and Stupka, J., *Trans. Soc. Biomaterials,* 1994, 17, 252.
7. Ely, J. L., Haubold, A. D., and Stupka, J., *Trans. Soc. Biomaterials,* 1994, 17, 252.
8. Cook, R. F., and Pharr, G. M., *J. Am. Ceram. Soc.,* 1990, 73, 787-817.
9. Gilpin, C. B., Haubold, A. D., Ely, J. L., and Ritz, J., *Proc. Cardiovascular Science and Technology Conference,* Dec. 12-14, Bethesda, MD (1992).
10. Saki, M., Hanyu, H., and Inagaki, M., *J. Am. Ceram. Soc.,* 1995, 78, 1006-1012.

PRESENT PROBLEMS, FUTURE SOLUTIONS

W. Bonfield

Interdisciplinary Research Centre (IRC) in Biomedical Materials, Queen Mary and Westfield College, University of London, Mile End Road, London, E1 4NS, (UK)

Biomaterials is now well established as a multidisciplinary subject which underpins the provision of implants and prostheses across a wide range of medical and dental applications. The report of The Institute of Materials Strategy Commission on Materials Technology Foresight in Biomaterials [1] starts with "Biomaterials save lives, relieves suffering and improves the quality of life for a large number of patients every year ---". In addition, the recent national exercise on technological forecasting performed by the UK Office of Science and Technology (OST) identified biomaterials as one of the eight priority areas within the sector of materials. The OST statement recommends "substantial increased resources in --- A new generation of biomaterials which encourage and enhance the restoration and repair of body tissue function"[2], which indicates that future funding prospects for biomaterials research remains bright. However, such statements should be put in the context of the overall mission statement of the relevant funding council (EPSRC in the UK), which seeks to "improve the competitiveness of industry and the quality of life". The implicit understanding in such a statement is that the fruits of biomaterials research will ultimately need to be transferred to the benefit of patients and, additionally, will add to the creation of industrial activity. It could well be argued that such deliverables in terms of patient care are likely to be essential if major research activities are going to receive continued funding into the next millennium. In most countries, there is an increase in the number of research topics meriting funding and, at the same time, at best, a maintenance of budget levels, or, at worst, a decline in the total funds available. Hence it is essential that the biomaterials community recognizes the need to influence both the population-at-large and the policy formers as to the merits of this particular research area. It could be suggested that much current biomaterials research is incremental rather than radical in scope, i.e., the aim is to contribute to a gradual optimisation of existing devices, rather than the introduction of new technologies which will produce a greatly enhanced patient benefit. Such a balance is perhaps inevitable given the need to form a truly multidisciplinary subject, which combines the trinity of materials sciences, biology and clinical medicine in an integrated and coherent form.

Within biomaterials, the topic of bioceramics has indeed been at the leading edge in terms of innovation. The pioneering work on Bioglass®, A/W glass-ceramic and hydroxyapatite has offered opportunities for bioactive implants, which have significantly altered the frame for clinical applications. However, it is equally recognised that monolithic ceramics often have restrictive mechanical properties and hence reduced applicability for major load bearing applications, while the design of appropriate bioceramic composites offers the opportunity for tailor making bioactive materials with special combinations of mechanical and biological performance. In this paper, a personal scientific stocktaking of the opportunities for bioceramics is presented, with the objective of focusing attention on the strategic opportunities for the coming decade.

MONOLITHIC BIOACTIVE CERAMICS AND GLASS CERAMICS

The conception of a bioactive glass by Hench and his colleagues[3] remains as the gold standard in the field. The particular insight was to design a range of glass compositions which could give either hard or soft tissue bonding or indeed a combination of the two. Following from this materials innovation, has been an extensive series of detailed studies in which the in vitro and in vivo behaviour of Bioglass® has been established and appropriate models for bone and soft tissue bonding developed. As a consequence, clinical applications have developed, in general stimulated by the rapid bonding achieved to the adjacent tissue by Bioglass®, which provides an important clinical benefit. The materials have found applications in both particulate and bulk form. The disadvantage of Bioglass® has remained its relative fragility and its invariant stiffness, which indeed is a feature of monolithic ceramics in general. The relatively low fracture toughness of Bioglass® restricts its general application to low load situations and requires careful handling by the surgeon to avoid failure during implantation. Hence the pioneering work of Yamamuro, Kobubo and associates[4] in developing a glass-ceramic (A/W glass-ceramic) with compositions design to improve mechanical strength has been another notable achievement. By combining bioactivity with enhanced mechanical performance, Yamamuro and associates have been able to introduce A/W glass-ceramic into more highly loaded clinical situations and indeed for larger artifacts. However, the general problem of designing with a brittle solid remains for A/W glass-ceramic as for Bioglass®. Such materials remain notch sensitive and hence use by other than highly skilled surgeons may introduce the possibility of a catastrophic failure due to imposed surface damage. Again, considerable contributions to bioceramic science have been made through understanding the biological mechanisms which produce bone bonding between A/W glass-ceramic and the surrounding bony tissue.

In parallel with the advances on bioactive glasses and glass-ceramics has been the development of hydroxyapatite as a biomaterial driven through the significant efforts of workers such as Jarcho[5], de Groot[6] and Aoki[7]. As a consequence, in twenty years the production of hydroxyapatite in powder or granule form has become a major activity and provides the basis for either subsequent sintering into hydroxyapatite artifacts or as the basis for plasma spraying orthopaedic implants. The latter technology was seen as a major means of promoting the concept of cementless implant fixation in orthopaedics, particularly for total hip replacement and hence as means for approaching the problems of limited prosthesis lifetime in the younger patient group (less than 45 years). It has been well demonstrated that hydroxyapatite coatings can have a beneficial effect in a suitably designed orthopaedic stem or cup in promoting bone bonding. In contrast, other adverse clinical results have been reported. At the moment there is no clear conclusion as to the efficacy of this particular approach. The clinical results are often obscured by a lack of characterisation of the starting hydroxyapatite and because of the variation between different commercial products. Again the biological mechanism has been well studied, and in particular, the role of the crystalline/amorphous ratio clarified. The mechanical constraints on hydroxyapatite are indeed similar to those for glass and glass-ceramics, but the delivery of "thin" coatings on orthopaedic stems has allowed the use of the material in one of the most highly loaded regions of the body. There is considerable potential in developing alternative "low temperature" production procedures to produce hydroxyapatite coatings on implants.

For a cementless implant, it is imperative to achieve bone bonding in the shortest possible time (ideally less than 1 day). Comparative in vitro and in vivo tests have often indicated that hydroxyapatite is slower in performance with respect to Bioglass® and A/W glass-ceramic. Such a result is not surprising given that bone mineral is indeed not hydroxyapatite, but a substituted apatite. Hence the initial period in vivo of a hydroxyapatite implant is surely to change the surface chemistry by an appropriate chemical and cellular mechanism, so as to become more biological in character. The early work by Le Geros and associates[8] indicated the possibility for a carbonate-substituted apatite. Recently this approach has been developed with some success by Barralet et al[9], such as to demonstrate the possibility of obtaining a relatively low temperature sintering route for apatite artifacts and production of a translucent material. Potentially the incorporation of enhanced bioactivity and, in particular, the speed of bone bonding as compared to available commercial hydroxyapatite, appears likely in suitably substituted apatites. It also appears possible to produce nanoscale substituted apatite precipitates, which with suitable post treatment, can be developed into artifacts with appropriate nanoscale structure.

MULTI-PHASE COMPOSITES

The original concept of a bioceramic reinforced polymer composite was introduced by Bonfield et al in 1981[10]. The approach was based on considering cortical bone as the template for a bone substitute material. As the major reinforcement in bone itself is a bone mineral resembling hydroxyapatite, then it seemed reasonable to form a composite utilising the same reinforcement. With the difficulties of handling collagen as a matrix material, at the onset it was decided to utilise polyethylene as a *ductile* polymer which allowed the incorporation of a brittle second phase, but still with a possibility of retaining some ductility. In addition the selection of a thermo plastic allowed the possibility of sophisticated polymer processing as a basis for producing a material with reasonable mechanical properties. It was demonstrated that such an approach did in fact yield a composite; i.e.' the Youngs modulus increased with the volume fraction of hydroxyapatite, while the strain to fracture correspondingly decreased. A ductile-brittle transition was demonstrated, but only after incorporation of a high volume percentage of reinforcement (40% by volume), representing in weight terms about 70% of hydroxyapatite. It could not be assumed that such a composite would demonstrate the bioactivity associated with 100% hydroxyapatite, but in vivo studies established that beyond a minimum volume percentage of about 20%, then indeed bone apposition and bone bonding was achieved in a loaded implant. The key advance obtained with this composite was the mechanical matching across the interface of the implant to the surrounding tissue. It should be emphasised that currently there is no other available bioceramic system which produces such mechanical matching into cortical bone. A particular advantage of this approach is that it is "surgeon friendly", in that the material can be readily shaped prior to implantation - a facility which is particularly appreciated when volume augmentation is required. As a consequence, the hydroxyapatite reinforced polymer composite found favour initially as a sub-orbital floor prostheses. With the establishment of the IRC, it proved possible to scale up the processing technology from laboratory scale to pilot scale. The material was licensed by the FDA in 1994 and has recently been commercialised as HAPEX®, as a cranial facial, maxilla facial and otologic implant. The projection is that in 1995/96, 60,000 patients will receive such a treatment. Beyond this application, it is planned that the material will find application for bone augmentation in a hip revision procedure.

An alternative approach to developing a hydroxyapatite composite is to induce precipitation of the hydroxyapatite in a suitable polymeric matrix, this has been the approach followed by the group in Leiden in developing Polyactivee®[11]. It has indeed been demonstrated that such mineralisation can be achieved with suitable levels of bioactivity. The disadvantage is that it is difficult to achieve both the homogeneity and volume fractions possible by a direct mixing procedure, but there is undoubted promise in this approach.

In some ways, the mineralisation of hydroxyapatite in a polymer matrix is equivalent to the approach of incorporating a bioactive element in a thermo setting polymer. Such methodology has value in terms of developing potentially bioactive bone cements. From a materials development standpoint, then again it would seem most appropriate to start with a ductile polymer. As current orthopaedic and dental bone cements are brittle then it is not immediately obvious that the incorporation of a brittle second phase will lead to suitable handling characteristics and indeed appropriate mechanical properties. For a bone cement, it is a prime requirement that a continuous layer should be developed at the interface. For this reason it has proved difficult to incorporate hydroxyapatite to a suitable level (i.e. greater than 20% by volume) in polymethylmethacrylate (PMMA) bone cement. However the selection of an alternative, mainly polyethylmethacrylate (PEMA), has yielded an interesting series of composites with some ductility[12]. The in vivo biological response of such a system is currently under evaluation.

Considerable progress has been made recently in this area in Japan with the incorporation of hydroxyapatite and A/W glass-ceramic into polymer matrices such as Bis GMA[13]. What has been remarkable about this work has been the high volume fractions achieved and the corresponding homogeneity of the composite material. Given the current emphasise on cemented systems as a route preferred by a number of surgeons, then it is likely that activity in this area will lead to some beneficial and significant clinical applications. In the limit, 100% calcium phosphate cement, setting at 37'C has been considered [14] but appears likely to be restricted to skeletal defect filling or, perhaps, as an injectable bone repair system.

The systematic development of hydroxyapatite reinforced polyethylene and associated modelling offers the prospects for other systems based on the same technology. A notable advance reported elsewhere in this volume is the incorporation of Bioglass® in particulate form into polyethylene. It has been demonstrated that a composite effect is achieved i.e. the Young's modulus increases with volume fraction of Bioglass®, while the strain to failure decreases. A ductile system can be delivered for volume percentages up to 40%. Of particular importance, has been the demonstration that the bioactivity associated with Bioglass® in bulk is retained in the particulate composite. While still at an early stage, there is every prospect that a Bioglass® reinforced polyethylene composite will extend the range of application of HAPEX®, by allowing a spectrum of bio-active implants, for applications ranging from cortical bone, through to cancellous bone, into soft tissue. It is apparent in many applications that rapid bonding between the implant and the tissue and the establishment of a secure interfacial bond is a necessary prerequisite for long term stability.

BONE SUBSTITUTE MATERIALS

In terms of skeletal implants the material most used and favoured by orthopaedic surgeons is bone itself. While there is considerable awareness of the prospects for synthetic materials in such applications, the major material source remains that of allographs and autographs. Both routes provide potential problems in the future. Clearly there is an advantage in using living bone (autographs), as the cellular activity can be delivered directly to the patient. However autographs require a second operation and consequently an extended operating time, when the trend is to contain the cost associated with each operation. In addition, there is the additional discomfort provided for the patient and the need to fill the defect created. With respect to allographs, there is considerable concern about the quality of some bone banks with the public awareness of the danger, however remote, of transmitted diseases; i.e., both of HIV virus and of Hepatitis B. Indeed it has been costed in the USA that a single procedure utilising allographs can cost as much as $1200, if a suitably stringent source of allograph is used. Hence, there is considerable potential for bone substitute materials, both of cortical and of cancellous bone. It should be emphasised that the mechanical properties of bone are critically dependent on the amount of porosity present. Hence cortical bone has very different values of stiffness than cancellous bone and, indeed, cancellous bone will demonstrate a range of Young's modulus values depending critically on porosity. For cortical bone, the approach based on hydroxyapatite reinforced polyethylene offers considerable prospects particularly as, with additional processing, it has proved possible recently to increase both the stiffness and strength to match the range of values associated with cortical bone. With respect to cancellous bone it is noteworthy that two materials currently on offer commercially as substitutes are biological derivatives, namely Endobon®, derived by calcining bovine cancellous bone, or Pro-Osteon®, derived from coral. Both materials require careful screening and have an intrinsic biological variability. The advantage of each derives from the particular architecture, which allows the interpenetration of newly formed bone. However it is envisaged that a completely synthetic porous template could be derived based on current technology which will be of enormous potential application for bone augmentation procedures.

CONCLUSION

Bioceramics have been at the forefront of radical research in biomaterials. Continued optimisation of the current monolithic bioceramics will extend the existing range of clinical applications. However, there is additionally the prospect of tailor made ceramic composites, utilising any or all of the monolithic bioceramics, so as to produce a comprehensive spectrum of bioactive materials, designed for particular clinical applications. This process is likely to be stimulated by current changes in the use of natural tissue in the coming years. Hence, the basis exists for a new golden age of bioceramics, which will ensure that biomaterials takes its place as the key science underpinning future medical provision.

ACKNOWLEDGEMENTS

The author acknowledges the contribution of colleagues in the IRC in Biomedical Materials and the continuing support of the Engineering and Physical Sciences Research Council.

REFERENCES

1. Materials Technology Foresight in Biomaterials, Institute of Materials, London, UK (1995).
2. Technology Foresight-Materials, Office of Science and Technology, HMSO (1995).
3. Hench, L.L. and Ethridge, E.C., *Adv. Biomed. Eng.,* 1975, 5, 35.
4. Kokubo, T., Ito, S., Sakka, S. and Yamamuro, T., J. *Mater. Sci.,* 1985,20, 200.
5. Jarcho, M. et al., J. *Mater. Sci.,* 1976, 11, 2027.
6. de Groot, K., *Bioceramics of calcium phosphate,* CRC Press, Boca Raton, FL (1983).
7. Aoki, H., *Science and medical applications of hydroxyapatite, JAAS* (1991).
8. Le Geros, R. Z et al., *Science* 1967, 155, 1409.
9. Barralet, J.E. et al., Bioceramics Volume 6, 1993, 179.
10. Bonfield, W. et al., Biomaterials 1981, 2, 185.
11. van Blitterswijk, C.A. et al., *Bone-bonding biomaterials,* Reed Healthcare Communications 1992, 13.
12. Khorasani, S.N. et al., Bioceramics Volume 5, 1992, 225.
13. Tamura, J. et al., Bioceramics Volume 7, 1994, 279.
14. Ginebra, M.P. et al., Bioceramics Volume 7, 1994, 273.

COMPOSITES

BIOGLASS®/HIGH DENSITY POLYETHYLENE COMPOSITE AS A NEW SOFT TISSUE BONDING MATERIAL

M. Wang*, W. Bonfield* and L.L. Hench**

*Interdisciplinary Research Centre in Biomedical Materials, Queen Mary and Westfield College, University of London, Mile End Road, London E1 4NS, U.K.
**Advanced Materials Research Center, University of Florida, One Progress Boulevard, Alachua, Florida 32615, U.S.A.

ABSTRACT

Particulate Bioglass® with an average size of 45.7μm was incorporated into a high density polyethylene (HDPE) for potential medical applications. Composites with Bioglass® volumes of 10%, 20% and 40% were produced by a manufacturing process consisting of blending, compounding, powderising, and compression moulding. The Bioglass® particles were well dispersed and an effective distribution in the polymer matrix was achieved after compounding, which was retained during subsequent composite processing. It was established that the Young's modulus of the composite increased with an increase in Bioglass® volume fraction, while the tensile strength and fracture strain decreased. Fourier-transform infra-red spectra obtained from Bioglass®/HDPE samples exposed for 20 hours at 37°C to a simulated body fluid (SBF-9) demonstrated that composites, of all the compositions examined, developed the surface biological apatite layer equivalent to that for bulk Bioglass®.

INTRODUCTION

Bioglass® is a family of bioactive glasses that elicit specific physiological responses, including the provision of surface-reactive silica, calcium and phosphate at interfaces with tissues [1]. A particular advantage of Bioglass® is the ability to bond to both hard and soft tissues, which has created a range of clinical opportunities. As for all monolithic bioactive glasses and ceramics, a disadvantage of Bioglass® is that it is a brittle solid and, as a consequence, its handling and mechanical properties may not be adequate for load bearing applications. In contrast, previous extensive experience on combining a bioactive ceramic, hydroxyapatite (HA) particles, with high density polyethylene (HDPE) [2] to form a composite has demonstrated an approach that allows appropriate mechanical properties, including ductility, to be developed, while retaining a bioactive response in vivo. The processing route developed for HA/HDPE has been used as a basis for producing a novel Bioglass®/HDPE composite, which offers a distinctive combination of mechanic/biological performance and hence some potential clinical applications [3].

EXPERIMENTAL

A particulate Bioglass® material (45S5 Bioglass®) supplied by U.S. Biomaterials Co. was incorporated into a high density polyethylene (Rigidex HM4560XP, BP Chemicals Ltd.). The manufacturing process for the Bioglass®/HDPE composite consisted of blending, compounding, centrifugal milling, and compression moulding, which has been established as the route to produce particulate ceramic/polymer composites as biomaterials. A Betol BTS40L co-rotating twin-screw extruder was used for composite compounding. Prior to composite processing, the Bioglass® particles were characterizedusing a Malvern Mastersizer X for particle size analysis. The particle morphology was examined using a JOEL 6300F field emission scanning electron microscope (SEM).

Composites with 10%, 20% and 40% by volume of Bioglass® particles and unfilled HDPE were produced. The dispersion and distribution of Bioglass® particles in the HDPE matrix was investigated for composites of the three particle volume fractions after compounding and compression moulding, using a JEOL 6300 scanning electron microscope on polished surfaces.

Tensile specimens were made from the 1.75 mm thick compression moulded composite plates according to the ISO standard 527. These specimens were subsequently heat treated at 80°C for 24 hours and were tensile tested 48 hours after the heat treatment. Normal tensile tests were conducted on an Instron 6025 testing machine at a crosshead speed of 0.5 mm/min. An Instron extensometer (maximum displacement: 1 mm) was mounted onto the test piece for the accurate measurement of specimen extension in order to determine Young's modulus. The extensometer was removed from the specimen when strain exceeded 1.0% and thereafter the strain was calculated from the crosshead displacement. The associated fracture surfaces of Bioglass®/ HDPE composites were subsequently examined using the SEM.

The bioactivity of composite having Bioglass® volumes of 10%, 20% and 40% was evaluated by subjecting the samples at 37°C to simulated body fluids (SBF-tris or SBF-9). The rate of formation of a biological apatite layer on the composite surface, which was measured using the Fourier-transform infra-red (FTIR) technique, was directly correlated with the level of bioactivity of the composite. Two simulated body fluids were used for the current investigation: SBF-tris which did not contain calcium or phosphate ions, and SBF-9 which did contain these ions.

RESULTS

The as-received particulate Bioglass® showed a monomodal particle size distribution with the average size being 45.7 μm, but the distribution peak located at approximately 69.7 μm. SEM examination of Bioglass® particles revealed their angular morphology.

It was found that Bioglass® particles were well dispersed and a reasonably homogeneous distribution of the particles in the polymer matrix was achieved after the compounding process (Fig. l). Subsequent composite processing by compression moulding preserved these characteristics.

During tensile testing, some specimens with 40% volume of Bioglass® particles failed at the extensometer contact points. However, composite specimens with lower Bioglass® volumes mostly broke within the gauge length. The values for Young's modulus, tensile strength and fracture strain of the Bioglass®/HDPE composite are shown in Table 1. The increase in the Bioglass® volume gives an increase in the Young's modulus, with corresponding reductions in both the tensile strength and the fracture strain. Necking was noted in composite samples with 10% volume of Bioglass® during the tensile testing, but

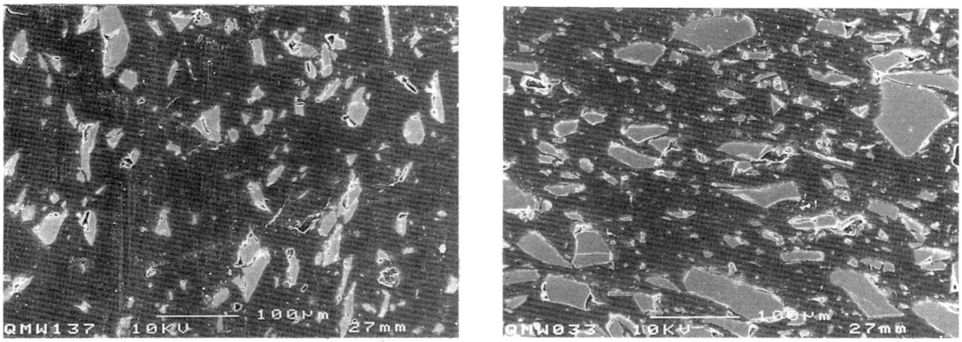

a. V = 20% b. V = 40%

Figure 1. Distribution of Bioglass® particles in high density polyethylene.

Table 1 Mechanical properties of the Bioglass@/HDPE composite.

Bioglass® Volume	Compression Moulded Material		
(%)	E(GPa)	σ(MPa)	ϵ(%)
0	0.65±0.02	17.89±0.29	>360
10	1.05±0.04	14.34±0.11	105.1±56.6
20	1.21±0.02	12.69±0.07	64.0±9.4
40	2.54±0.16	10.15±0.71	8.5±2.8

E: Young's modulus σ: tensile strength ϵ: fracture strain

was not observed for composite with higher Bioglass® volumes. Figure 2 compares the initial stress-strain curves of composite with different Bioglass® volumes (up to respective peak stress), showing different trends of Young's modulus and tensile strength with the incorporation of Bioglass® particles.

Fracture surfaces of composite with 40% of Bioglass® which are macroscopically flat exhibit long polymer fibrils microscopically, indicating large polymer deformation. Even at 40% volume of Bioglass®, the glass particles are separated and the surrounding polymer undergoes plastic deformation during tensile testing.

For SBF-tris treated composite samples, Figure 3a depicts three FTIR spectra obtained in the diffuse reflection mode for: (a) the Bioglass® particles in isolation, (b) the composite containing 40% Bioglass®, and (c) the composite containing 10% Bioglass® after reaction for 20 hours. The spectrum for composite with 20% of Bioglass® is not shown but is similar to spectrum (c). The 20-hour time period is clinically significant, and is used for quality-assurance testing of bioactive glasses intended to bond with soft connective tissue. The shaded regions correspond to the molecular vibrational modes characteristic of a microcrystalline biological apatite layer. The spectra indicate that only the composite with 40% of Bioglass® and a pure Bioglass® particle developed the

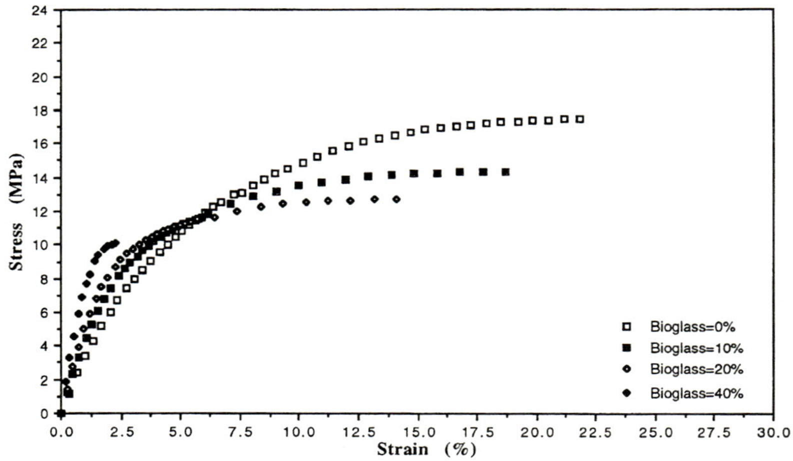

Figure 2. Initial stress-strain curves of the Bioglass®/HDPE composite with different Bioglass® volumes.

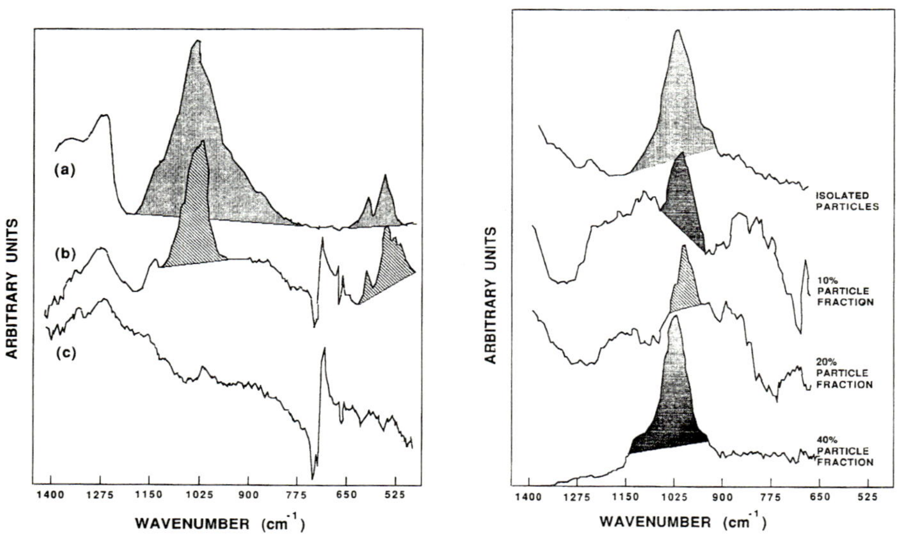

a. SBF-tris treated. b. SBF-9 treated.

Figure 3. FTIR spectra obtained from Bioglass® and Bioglass®/HDPE composite at 37°C for 20 hours for (a) SBF-tris, and (b) SBF-9.

biological apatite layer in SBF-tris within 20 hours. Because of the poor quality of diffuse reflection spectra from composite with low volume fractions of Bioglass®, infra-red microscopy (IRM) was subsequently used to determine the bioactivity of the composite. For SBF-9 treated composite samples, the resulting FTIR spectra are shown in Figure 3b. The strong P-O stretching vibration at 1020 cm^{-1} in all spectra demonstrates that all of the composite developed surface biological apatite layers equivalent to that for bulk Bioglass®.

DISCUSSION

The Betol BTS40L machine is a closely intermeshing, co-rotating twin-screw compounding extruder, developed for generating high shear forces to disperse hard particles in polymeric matrices. Enhanced "micromixing" is ensured when the material experiences a high level of shear as it flows through the passage of reduced area between screw channels inside the barrel. Therefore, a good dispersion and a homogeneous distribution of Bioglass® particles in the polyethylene matrix have been achieved after the compounding process for the Bioglass®/HDPE composite (Fig. 1). Such a distribution of the Bioglass® particles is important as, when a biological apatite layer develops between the Bioglass® and the surrounding tissue, these particles will provide uniformly distributed anchors for the prosthesis. It is also encouraging to note that the normal methods of mechanical abrasion, such as grinding and polishing, can expose Bioglass® particles on the composite surface, without experiencing the polymer smearing problem associated with some ceramic/polymer systems. Bearing in mind the envisaged biomedical applications, the homogeneous distribution of Bioglass® particles in the polymer matrix and the exposed Bioglass® particles on the composite surface together suggest considerable potential for the Bioglass®/HDPE composites as new, soft tissue bonding biomaterials.

It has been shown that the compression moulded Bioglass®/HDPE composite possesses considerable ductility when the Bioglass® volume is less than 30%. A higher filler loading reduces the ductility of composites drastically. As indicated in Table 1, composite with Bioglass® volumes of 30% or below exhibits levels of elastic compliance, tensile strength and fracture strain comparable to those of soft connective tissues. Composite with Bioglass® volumes in excess of 30% possesses mechanical properties comparable to cancellous bone. For the HDPE, the manufacturer quotes 0.68 GPa for the tensile modulus, and it has been determined that the Young's modulus of monolithic Bioglass® is 35 GPa. The incorporation of a particulate Bioglass® into the HDPE has resulted in a composite with a higher modulus than the unfilled HDPE. However, these modulus values are consistently lower than those of hydroxyapatite reinforced HDPE with corresponding hydroxyapatite volumes (Young's modulus of monolithic hydroxyapatite is approximately 80 GPa), although a similar ascending trend is observed with the increasing amount of Bioglass® in the composite.

Examination of polished surfaces and tensile fracture surfaces indicates that there is no chemical bond between the Bioglass® particles and the polymer matrix for the Bioglass® HDPE composite produced via the current manufacturing process. This effect may account for the decreasing composite strength with increasing Bioglass® content.

Bioglass® particles of irregular shapes can act as non-bonded, hard inclusions in the matrix, and the separation between the glass particle and the polymer matrix may begin at the sharp tips of the particle once mechanical load is applied. With increasing amounts of Bioglass® particles in the composite, there are more failure initiation sites, and the rapid coalescence of small cracks in test pieces during tensile testing leads to decreased strength of the composites. Nevertheless, the Bioglass®/HDPE composite has sufficient modulus and strength to find biomedical applications as soft-tissue prostheses.

It has been shown through FTIR analysis that the Bioglass®/HDPE composite develops a biological apatite layer after the treatment by a simulated body fluid, which confirms that the composite possesses bioactivity. The rate of apatite formation (i.e. the actual level of bioactivity), however, depends on the volume of the Bioglass® phase in the composite, which has been subjected to a systematic investigation employing various techniques [4].

Now that the processing route has been established and the composite microscopically and mechanically evaluated, further research on the Bioglass®/HDPE system will be directed towards the use of Bioglass® particles with smaller sizes and rounded shapes. The long term *in vivo* behavior of the Bioglass®/HDPE composite also remains to be investigated.

CONCLUSIONS

Bioglass®/HDPE composite containing up to 40% by volume of Bioglass® particles has been successfully manufactured. It has been established that the Young's modulus of the composite increases with an increase in Bioglass® volume, while the tensile strength and fracture strain decrease. A biological apatite layer develops on the composite surface when the composite is subjected to a simulated body fluid. By retaining the interfacial and chemical properties of bulk Bioglass®, the Bioglass®/HDPE composite offers unique advantages for applications as soft-tissue prostheses.

ACKNOWLEDGEMENTS

The authors acknowledge the contribution of Mrs. J. Huang in the examination of Bioglass® particle distribution in the composite. U.S. Biomaterials Co. supplied the Bioglass® powder for this project. Support from UK EPSRC is gratefully acknowledged.

REFERENCES

1. L.L. Hench and J. Wilson, eds., *Introduction to Bioceramics,* World Scientific Publishing Co., Singapore, 1993.
2. W. Bonfield, in *Annals of New York Academy of Science,* Vol. 523, New York 1988, 173-177.
3. W. Bonfield, M. Wang and L.L. Hench, US *Patent Application,* 1995.
4. J. Huang, M. Wang, I. Rehman, J. Knowles and W. Bonfield, in *Bioceramics,* Vol.8, Jacksonville, 1995.

ANALYSIS OF SURFACE STRUCTURES ON BIOGLASS®/POLYETHYLENE COMPOSITES *IN VITRO*

J. Huang, M. Wang, I. Rehman, J. Knowles and W. Bonfield

Interdisciplinary Research Centre in Biomedical Materials, Queen Mary and Westfield College, University of London, Mile End Road, London E1 4NS, UK.

ABSTRACT

The reaction of Bioglass® particles, in the Bioglass®/high density polyethylene (HDPE) composite, with simulated body fluid (SBF-K9) was investigated with Fourier transform infrared spectroscopy (FTIR), thin-film X-ray diffraction (TF-XRD), scanning electron microscopy (SEM) and energy-dispersive X-ray analysis (EDX). The existence of four main apatite peaks on the TF-XRD patterns confirmed apatite formation on the composite surface. FTIR spectra showed the appearance of C-O vibrations as well as P-O vibrations, which probably indicated the crystallization of hydroxyl carbonate apatite. It was also found that partial dissolution of Bioglass® particles provided the sites for apatite nucleation.

INTRODUCTION

Bioglass® is a bioactive implant material having an unique feature of bonding to soft tissue as well as to bone [1,2], although its brittle and fragile nature restricts wide clinical application. A new processing technology for ceramic-polymer composites provides a means for developing a Bioglass®/HDPE composite as a bioactive and relatively tough material [3]. Clinical applications of such a composite would benefit from the improved mechanical properties. Formation of an apatite layer on the Bioglass® surface *in vitro* is indicative of the bioactivity of the material *in vivo* [4]. The bioactivity of monolithic Bioglass® *in vitro* and *in vivo* has been considered [5], more recently, the bioactivity of individual Bioglass® particles has been investigated in relation to soft tissue augmentation [6]. For a Bioglass®/HDPE composite, it is essential to demonstrate a biological response and determine its surface structure both *in vitro* and *in vivo.* In this study, changes of the surface structure of the composites *in vitro* (SBF K9) are reported.

MATERIALS AND METHODS

Compression moulded Bioglass®/HDPE composite with 40% by volume of Bioglass® particles (with a mean diameter of 46 μm) was used in this investigation. All composite samples were finished by fine grinding with 4000# silicon carbide paper. Each sample (approximately 10 X 10 X 1.75 mm^3) was suspended in 20 ml SBF-K9 at 37°C for: 2 hrs, 4 hrs, 24 hrs, 4 days, 5 days, 6 days and 9 days. A Nicolet 800 system in conjunction with Nic-Plan Microscope was used to obtain FTIR spectra. The microscope was equipped with an ATR objective with which the surface properties can be analyzed.

Thin film analysis was performed on a Siemens D5000 diffractometer in the detector scan mode with a thin film analyzer. Samples were aligned at 1° to the incident beam. A step size of 0.02° (2θ) and a scan time of 12 seconds were used. A JEOL 6300 SEM with an EDX attachment was used for electron microscopy and elemental analysis.

RESULTS

TF-XRD analysis

Figure 1 shows the TF-XRD patterns of the composite before and after 6 days immersion in SBF. By comparison with standard pattern for hydroxyapatite (JCPDS 9-432), the existence of four main apatite peaks, with one at approximately 26° and the other three between 31~33° (2θ), confirmed apatite formation on the composite surface. The broad peaks indicated the low crystallinity of the apatite formed at this early stage.

FTIR analysis

Before immersion in SBF, the FTIR spectrum consisted of CH_2 vibrations of crystalline polyethylene and Si-O vibrations of Bioglass® for the composite, as shown in Figure 2a. After 2 hr immersion in SBF, a P-O stretching vibration peak at 1074 cm^{-1} together with a small peak associated with C-O stretching vibration at 872 cm^{-1} appeared (Fig. 2b), replacing the Si-O vibrations. The small and broad peak of the P-O vibration

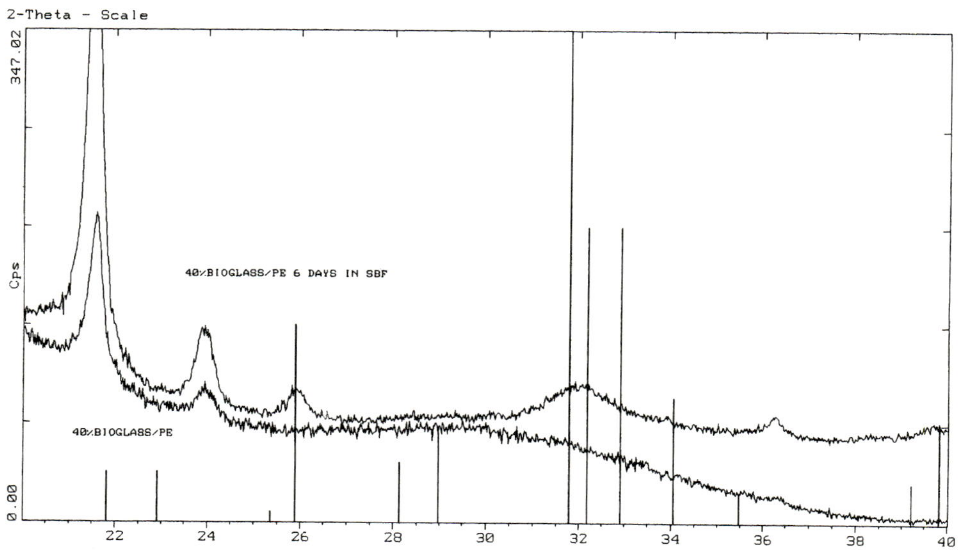

Figure 1. TF-XRD pattern of the surface of Bioglass®/HDPE composite before and after 6 days immersion in SBF.

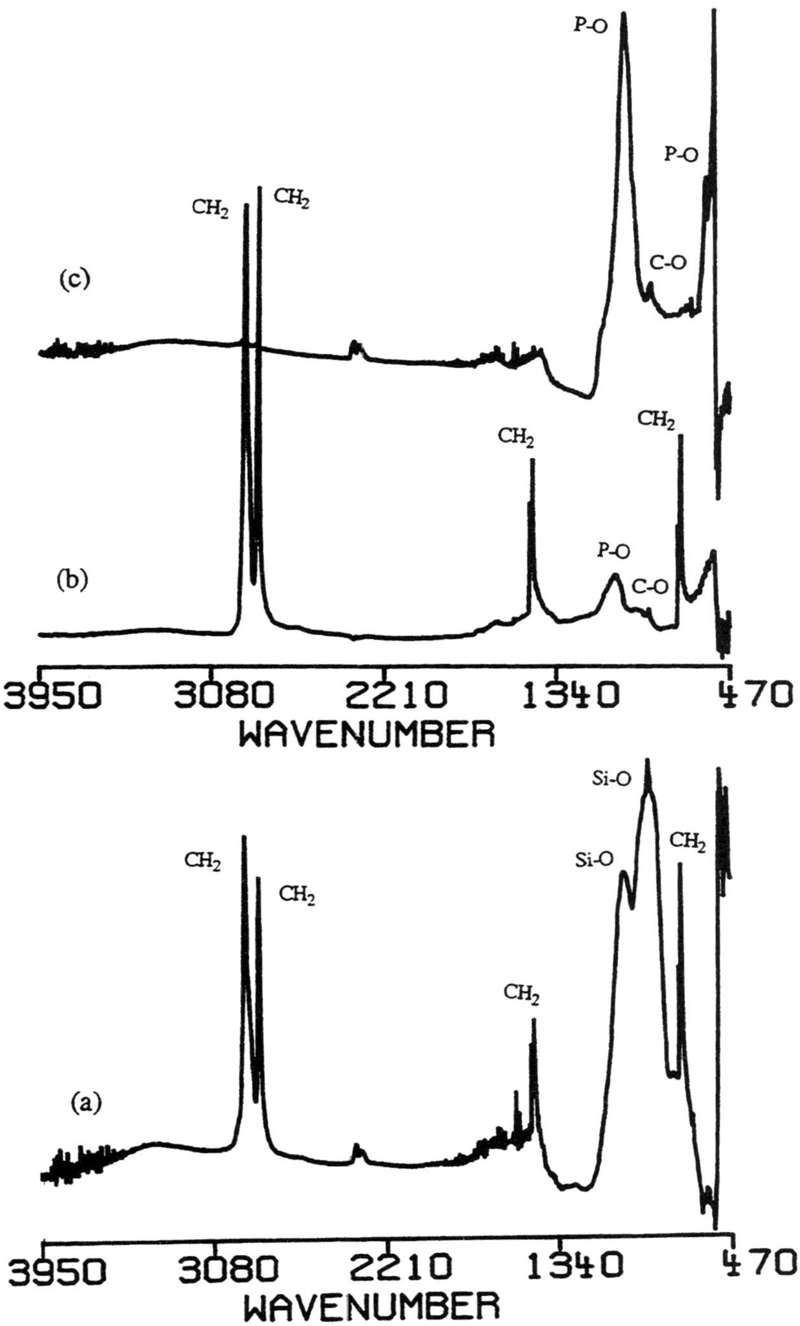

Figure 2. FTIR spectra of the surface of Bioglass®/HDPE composite after: (a) 0 hr, (b) 2 hrs, (c) 5 days immersion in SBF.

could be characteristic of an amorphous calcium phosphate phase. The increase in intensity and shift to 1013 cm^{-1} of the P-O vibration, and appearance of a P-O bending vibration at 615 cm^{-1} after 5 days in SBF (Fig. 2c) probably indicated the crystallization of hydroxyl carbonate apatite. Simultaneously, the intensity of CH_2 vibration peaks drastically decreased, which could have resulted from formation of an apatite layer on the polyethylene areas of the surface of the composite.

SEM observation

The surface of the composite before immersion in SBF is shown in Figure 3.1. Partial dissolution of Bioglass® particles was found after 2 hrs immersion in SBF (Fig. 3.2). Not only did the solution (or ions) attack the Bioglass®-HDPE interface, it also attacked the weak part of the particles, i.e. pores. This initial dissolution of silica provided the sites for apatite nucleation, where Ca and P first accumulated. A small amount of apatite crystals were formed on these sites after 4 hrs (Fig. 3.3) and covered these areas after 24 hrs (Fig. 3.4). The apatite continued growing and spread over the whole particles with further reaction time. Figure 4.1 shows the surface of the composite after 4 days immersion in SBF. Formation of apatite on the polyethylene matrix was also observed (Fig. 4.2). A thick and denser apatite layer at the Bioglass®-polyethylene interface (Fig. 4.3) is an indication of preferential nucleation and growth of apatite crystals at these sites. The morphology of the formed apatite crystals is shown in Fig. 4.4 at higher magnification.

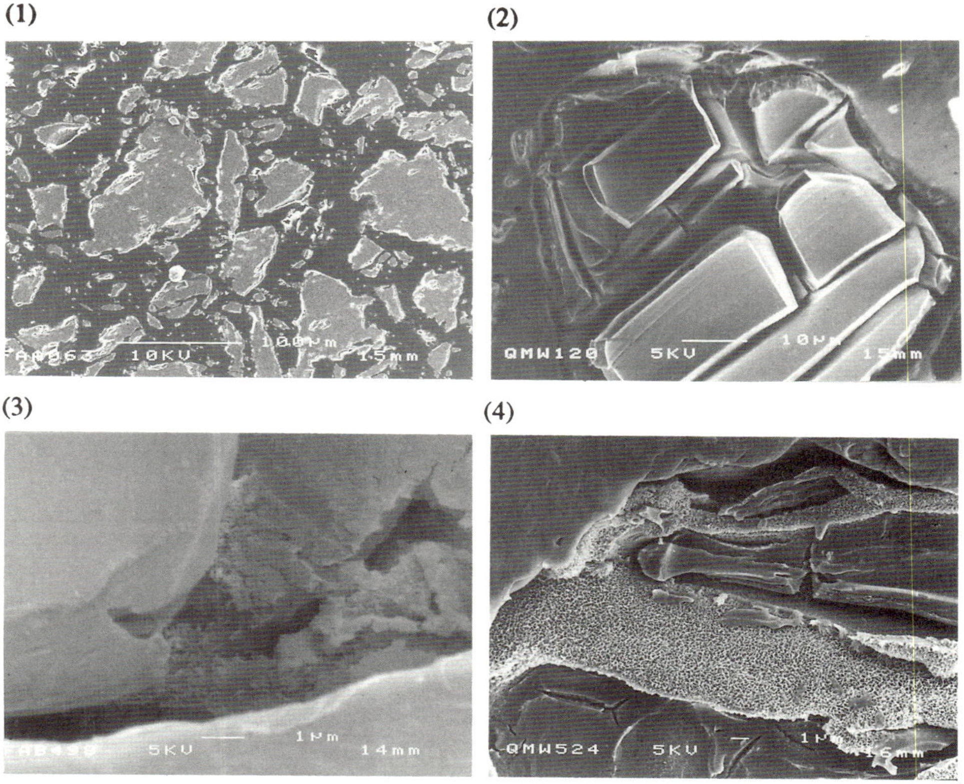

Figure 3. The surface Bioglass®/HDPE composite: (1) 0 hr, (2) 2 hrs, (3) 4 hrs, (4) 24 hrs immersion in SBF.

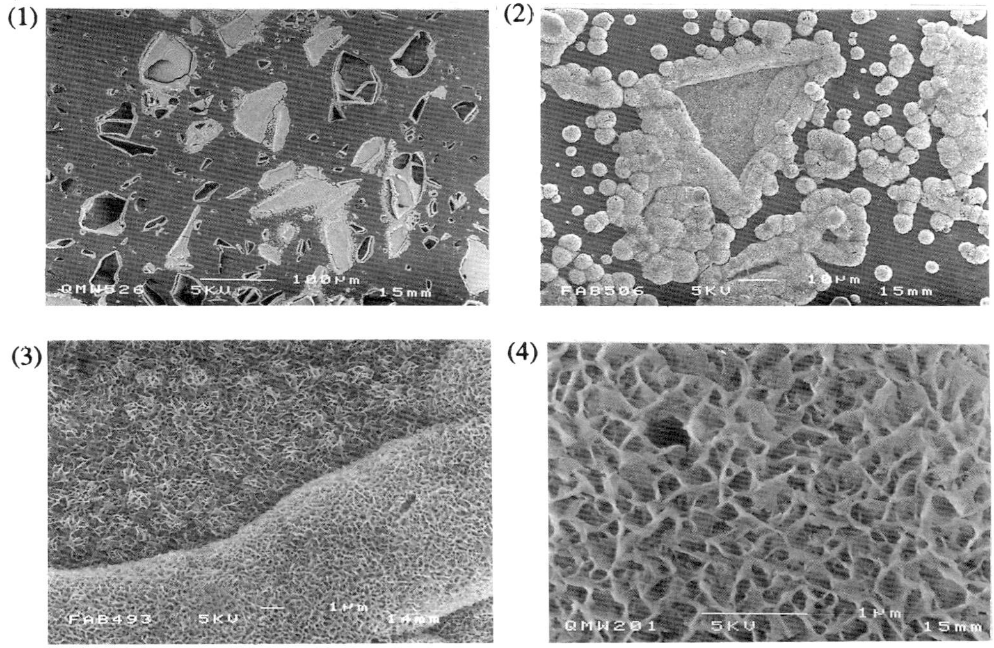

Figure 4. The formation of apatite crystals on the Bioglass®/HDPE composite surface after 4 days in SBF.

The spheroidal crystals (1-2 μm) were composed of small plate-like crystals (nm scale), which could provide a large surface area for bone apposition after implantation of the material.

The elemental spectra obtained by EDX from the composite surface are shown in Figure 5. The intensity of the major peaks in the spectra before immersion was Si > Ca > P = Na. The intensity of Si decreased during the reaction, while the spectrum gradually changed through Si > P > Ca, Ca > P > Si to finally only Ca > P for the apatite formation after 9 day immersion in SBF. Figure 5.4 indicates that the surface of the composite was covered by an apatite layer.

DISCUSSION

This study shows that the reaction of an individual Bioglass® particle (of micron size) in the composite with SBF is similar to that of bulk Bioglass® [7]. Exchange of Na^+ with H^+ from the solution occurred immediately on immersion in SBF. The Si-O-Si network broke down, leading to dissolution of particles, and subsequently Ca and P migrated into the silica gel. Initially, the C-O and P-O vibrations modes in FTIR spectra were characteristic of an amorphous calcium phosphate, which crystallized to carbonate apatite with further reaction. This was confirmed by the appearance of apatite peaks on the TF-XRD pattern.

The Bioglass® particles exist as isolated islands in the polyethylene matrix, and their size varies from less than 1 μm to 100 μm, which made their reaction with SBF complex. Dissolution did not occur evenly on the whole surface of Bioglass® particles.

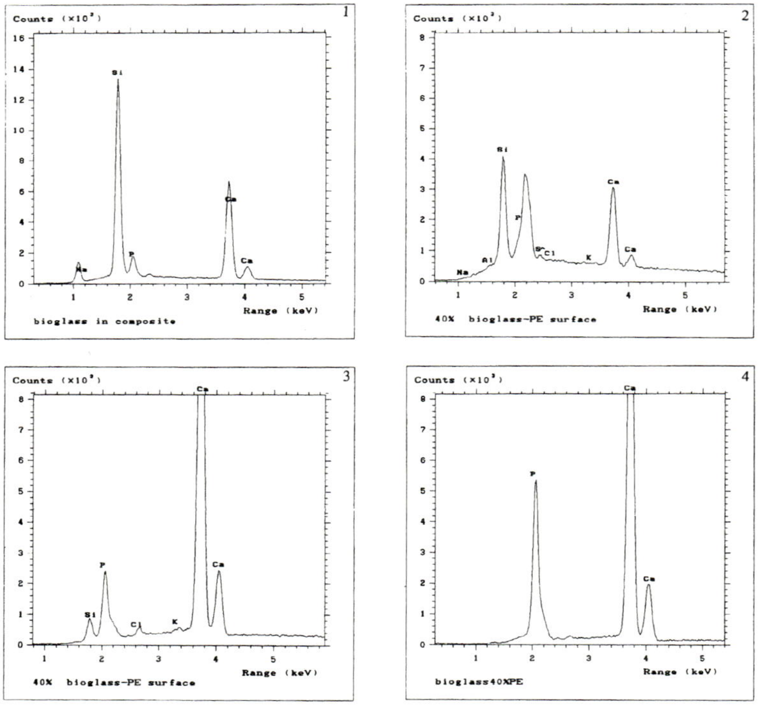

Figure 5. The elemental spectra of EDX for the Bioglass®/HDPE composite surface (1) O hr, (2) 24 hrs, (3) 2 days and (4) 9 days immersed in SBF.

Ions attacked the weak parts of the particles and the dissolution rate was higher on these sites. Dissolution dominated at the early stage of reaction. Accumulation of Ca and P on these sites was detected by EDX after 1 hr in SBF. The silanols resulting from initial dissolution of silica provided the sites for apatite nucleation, where apatite crystals grew quickly (Fig. 3.4). With reaction continuing, more nuclei provided for apatite formation on the surface. Apatite crystals not only covered whole Bioglass® particles, but also the polyethylene matrix. Apatite crystals on the polyethylene matrix in the vicinity of Bioglass® particles were found after 4 days immersion in SBF (Fig. 4.2), which is similar to the formation of an apatite layer on non-bioactive material surfaces [8]. Therefore, the tissue reaction to polyethylene in the Bioglass®/HDPE composite could not be totally 'inert'.

The growth rate of apatite on the particles in the composite surface varied (Fig. 4.1): a layer of apatite completely covered whole particles while a band of apatite crystals existed around particles. It seems that apatite crystals formed preferentially on relatively larger particles, while the dissolution dominated for small particles, which may need longer time for developing an apatite layer. The influence of Bioglass® particle size on the formation of the apatite layer on the composite surface is being investigated. The surface bioactive area on the composite increased with reaction with SBF, which could be an advantage of the Bioglass®/HDPE composite.

ACKNOWLEDGEMENTS

The financial support from U.S. Biomaterials Co. for this project is gratefully acknowledged.

REFERENCES

1. Wilson, J., *et al, J. Biomed. Mater. Res.,* 1981, 15, 805.
2. Hench, L.L., *et al,* in Biocompatibility of orthopaedic implants, 2, 1982
3. Wang, M., Bonfield, W. and Hench, L.L., in Bioceramic 8, Jacksonville, 1995
4. Filgueiras, M.R., LaTorre, G. and Hench, L.L., *J. Biomed. Mater. Res.,* 1993, 27, 445-453.
5. Hench, L.L., *J. Am. Ceram. Soc.,* 1991,74, 1487-1510.
6. Wilson, J., *et al, in* Bioceramic 4, London, 1991, 99-103.
7. Hench, L.L., Annals of New York Academy of Sciences, New York, 1988, 523, 54-71.
8. Abe, Y., Kokubo, T. and Yamamuro, T., *J. Mater. Sci. Mater. Med.,* 1990,1, 233238.

OSTEOGENIC POTENTIAL OF ALLOGENEIC RAT MARROW CELLS IN POROUS CALCIUM PHOSPHATE CERAMICS: A PRELIMINARY STUDY

T. Sempuku, H. Ohgushi*, M. Okumura* and S. Tamai*

Department of Orthopaedic Surgery, Saiseikai Chuwa Hospital, 323 Abe, Sakurai, Nara 633, Japan and *Department of Orthopaedic Surgery, Nara Medical University, Kashihara, Nara 634, Japan

ABSTRACT

Osteogenesis in hydroxyapatite combined with syngenic marrow cells was reported in our previous studies. The present experiment was conducted to determine osteogenic capacity of allogeneic marrow cells. Coralline hydroxyapatite discs were soaked in marrow cell suspensions harvested from each of seven-week-old male ACI, Lewis and Fischer 344 rats and were implanted in the subcutaneous space of Fischer 344 rats. Under immunosuppression with FK-506, the mismatched marrow cells formed bone in the ceramics, and allogeneic marrow could therefore be useful in repair of massive bone defects which need a large number of cells.

INTRODUCTION

Recently, hydroxyapatite ceramics are used extensively as a substitute for bone grafts in reconstructive surgery because of their biocompatibility and osteoconductivity [1-6]. Since the material is itself not osteoinductive [1,6-9], it has been attempted to implant the ceramic in combination with some osteogenic factor [10-14]. We previously showed that subcutaneous implantation of porous hydroxyapatite ceramics combined with murine bone marrow cells resulted in consistent bone formation in the ectopic sites [8,9]. Clinical application of this new concept of a bone substitute may be restricted to small regions of osseous defects because of limited amounts of autogenous bone marrow. If allogeneic bone marrow cells had osteogenic potency, larger regions could be repaired with the composite graft of the ceramic and the allogeneic marrow cells.

FK-506, a macrolide antibiotic isolated from the fermentation broth of a strain of Streptomycestsukubaensis has been proved to have stronger immunosuppressive properties than cyclosporine *in vitro* and *in vivo* [15,16]. We, in this study, investigated osteogenicity of the allogeneic bone marrow cells under immunosuppression with FK-506.

MATERIALS AND METHODS

Seven-week-old male ACI ($RT1^a$), Lewis ($RT1^l$) and Fischer 344 ($RT1^{lv}$) rats were used as donors. Each of five rats were sacrificed by ether inhalation and the femora and the tibiae were recovered. Both ends of the bone shaft were removed from the metaphysis and the cortex was cut with small bone cutting forceps. The marrow plugs were harvested and put into 1 mL heparinized phosphate buffered saline. The marrow was disaggregated by sequential passage through 18G and then 20G needles to obtain a single cell suspension. It was centrifuged (3,000 rpm, 5 min) and the sediment was mixed with 0.2 mL of the supernatant. Twelve coralline hydroxyapatite (Interpore 200, Interpore International, Irvine, California) discs, 5 mm in diameter and 2 mm thick, were soaked in the marrow cell suspension out of each strain of rats.

Twelve 7-week-old male Fischer 344 rats were used as recipients. Under sodium pentobarbital anesthesia (IP, 30 mg/kg body weight) given after light ether inhalation, three subcutaneous pockets were made in the back of the recipient rat. A ceramic combined with each of the three kinds of the marrow cells was implanted in the pocket.

Six of the recipient rats were given FK-506 (1 mg/kg/day) and the other six rats saline by intramuscular injection. The injection was done daily for two weeks starting at the day of the operation. All the rats were sacrificed by ether inhalation eight weeks after implantation. The removed implants were fixed in 10 % buffered formalin, decalcified in rapid bone decalcifier, K-CX solution (Falma Co., Tokyo), and sectioned in paraffin for staining with hematoxylin and eosin.

RESULTS

Without FK-506 administration, no bone or cartilage was formed in the pores of or outside any implants with ACI's or Lewis' marrow cells. In contrast, bone formation occurred in the pores of all of six implants with ACI's or Lewis' marrow cells with FK-506 administration (Table 1). The bone formation was in contact with the surface of the hydroxyapatite (Figure 1). These were the same findings as seen in the implants with the isogeneic marrow cells. Some pore areas, however, showed lymphocyte accumulation indicating an immunological response.

Table 1. Bone formation eight weeks after implantation

Donor	With FK-506	Without FK-506
ACI	6/6	0/6
Lewis	6/6	0/6
Fischer	6/6	0/6

Note. FK-506 was given for two weeks and the implants were harvested eight weeks after implantation. The number of implants with bone formation out of the total number of implants is shown.

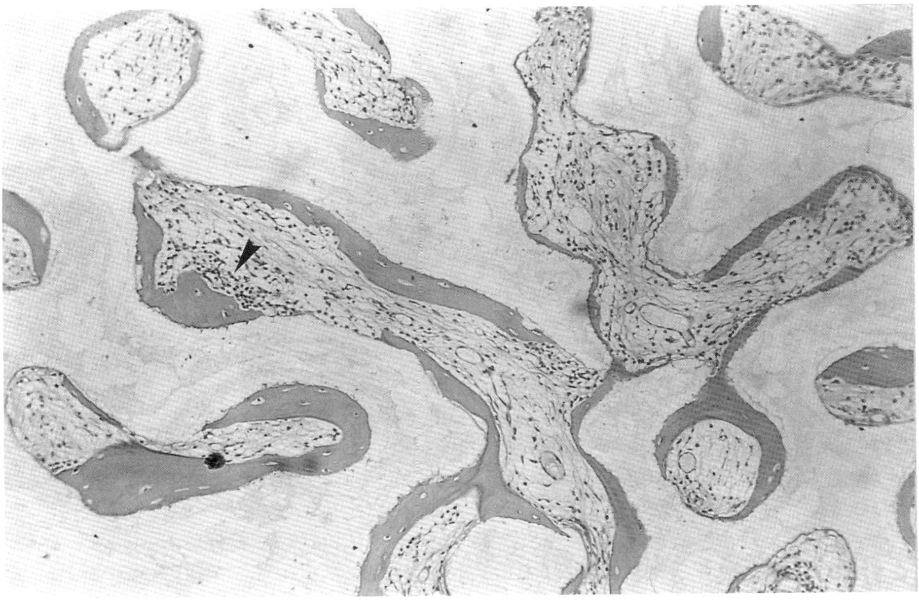

Figure 1. Photomicrograph of the implant with the marrow cells of ACI rats demonstrating lamellar bone (gray area) in contact with the surface of the hydroxyapatite (white area). Hematoxylin and eosin stain (x 125). The arrow indicates a cluster of lymphocytes.

DISCUSSION

Porous hydroxyapatite has been reported to facilitate osteogenesis when implanted into a bone and show no inflammatory reaction [1-6]. Although it is a useful material for a bone substitute in an orthotopic site, no bone formation occurs when it alone is implanted to an ectopic site [1,6-9]. We developed an experimental system such that consistent bone formation occurred in the coralline hydroxyapatite ceramic implanted to the murine subcutaneous space with syngenic bone marrow cells [8, 9]. The new bone was in direct contact with the ceramic and was formed centripetally towards the center of a pore. This ectopic and de novo bone formation can be useful not only as an experimental model, but also as a bone graft substitute for clinical use [17]. In most clinical cases, hydroxyapatite ceramics are, however, used alone and application of them is limited to small lesions surrounded with large bony tissue. The composite graft of hydroxyapatite and autogenous bone marrow cells could be applied to larger osseous defects or the regions in little contact with bone, because the graft is osteogenic by itself. However, it would be difficult to harvest such a large amount of bone marrow as to repair a massive defect. There are two alternative ways to procure a sufficient number of marrow cells: one is culture technology for autogenous marrow cells [18,19] and the other is transplantation of allogeneic marrow cells. We demonstrated the osteogenic ability of cultured human marrow cells in porous hydroxyapatite [18] and others reported the expansion of the osteogenic ability of cultured cells [19]. In the current study, we investigated osteogenesis of allogeneic marrow cells. They showed no bone formation without immunosuppression but did produce consistent bone formation with immunosuppression. This fact indicated that some of the grafted bone marrow cells survived, differentiated to osteoblastic cells, and contributed to bone formation. It supports our hypothesis that bone marrow contains the stromal cells that differentiate to osteoblasts and that the bone formation in the ceramic is attributed not to recipient's cells but to donor's marrow cells.

A new immunosuppressant, FK-506 (tacrolimus hydrate) was isolated from the fermentation broth of Streptomyces tsukubaensis in 1984 and this agent was reported to inhibit the production of T cell-derived soluble mediators such as interleukin 2, interleukin 3 and gamma-interferon as does cyclosporine and to inhibit the humoral and cellular immunity and alloantigen-driven proliferation across strong histocompatibility barriers [15, 16]. FK-506 has much higher potency *in vitro* and *in vivo* than cyclosporine and since about a hundred times lower concentration of FK-506 is needed for immunosuppression it is less toxic.

Many authors have demonstrated the osteogenic potential of autologous bone marrow cells [20-25]. Diduch et. al. [26] isolated two cloned cell lines from cultures of mouse bone marrow cells and showed that one of them exhibited osteogenic properties and synthesized type-I collagen. However, feasibility of osteogenesis supported by the allogeneic bone marrow cells has never been evaluated to date. The present study is the first evidence for the osteogenic effect of allogeneic marrow cells.

Coralline hydroxyapatite was thought to play, in the bone formation process, some important roles such as a vehicle for the osteogenic marrow, an adherent surface for osteoblasts or precursors of osteoblasts and a scaffold for apposition of new bone. Recently, we reported that the surface of hydroxyapatite supported osteoblastic cell differentiation [27]. The composite graft of hydroxyapatite combined with allogeneic marrow cells under proper immunosuppression could be a useful bone substitute especially for large bone defects. Although the composite grafts showed consistent bone formation in this study, some immunological response was seen in spite of administration of FK-506. Further studies are, therefore, desired to develop a more selective, more effective and safer immunological tolerance and practical method of selecting cells capable of differentiating into osteoblasts.

REFERENCES

1. Jarcho, M. *Clin. Orthop.* 1981, 157, 259-278.
2. Kato, K., Aoki, H., Tabata, T. and Ogiso, M. *Biomat. Med. Dev. Art. Org.* 1979, 7, 291-297.
3. Holmes, R.E. *Plast. Reconstr. Surg.* 1979, 63, 626-633.
4. Cameron, H.U., Macnab, I. and Philliar, R.M. J. *Biomed. Mater. Res.* 1977, 11, 179-186.
5. De Groot, K. *Biomaterials* 1980, 1, 47-50.
6. McDavid, P.T., Boone, M.E., Kafrawy, A.H., Mitchell, D.F. J. *Dent. Res.* 1979, 58, 1478-1483.
7. Nade, S., Armstrong, L., McCartney, E. and Baggaley, B. *Clin. Orthop.* 1983, 181, 255-263.
8. Ohgushi, H., Goldberg, V.M. and Caplan, A.I. J. *Orthop. Res.* 1989, 7, 568-578.
9. Okumura, M., Ohgushi, H. and Tamai, S. *Biomaterials* 1991, 12, 411-416.
10. Urist, M.R., Lietze, A. and Dawson, E. *Clin. Orthop.* 1984, 187, 277 280.
11. Miller, T.A., Ishida, K., Kobayashi, M., Wollman, J.S., Turk, A.E. and Holmes, R.E. *Plast. Reconstr. Surg.* 1991, 87, 87-95.

12. Grundel, R.E., Chapman, M.W., Yee, T. and Moore, D.C. *Clin. Orthop.* 1991, 266, 244-258.
13. Horisaka, Y., Okamoto, Y., Matsumoto, N., Yoshimura, Y., Kawada, J., Yamashita, K. and Takagi, T. *Clin. Orthop.* 1991, 268, 303-312.
14. Ripamonti, U., Ma, S.S. and Reddi, A.H. *Plast. Reconstr. Surg.* 1992, 89, 731-739.
15. Kino, T., Hatanaka, H., Hashimoto, M., Nishiyama, M., Goto, T., Okuhara, M., Kohsaka, M., Aoki, H. and Imanaka, H. J. *Antibiotics* 1987, 40, 1249-1255.
16. Kino, T., Hatanaka, H., Miyata, S., Inamura, N., Nishiyama, M., Yajima, T., Goto, T., Okuhara, M., Kohsaka, M., Aoki, H. and Ochiai, T. J. *Antibiotics* 1987, 40, 1256-1265.
17. Ohgushi, H., Okumura, M., Miyauchi, Y., Mii, Y. and Tamai, *S. Pioceramics* Volume 3, Rose-Hulman Institute of Technology, Terre Haute 1992, 279-286.
18. Ohgushi, H. and Okumura, M. *Acta Orthop. Scand.* 1990, 61, 431 434.
19. Goshima, J., Goldberg, V.M. and Caplan, A.I. *Clin. Orthop.* 1991, 262, 298-311.
20. Goujon, E. *Journal de l 'Anatcmie et de* la *Physiologiques Norma les et Pa thologiques de l 'Homm e et desAnimaux* 1869, 6, 399.
21. Pfeiffer, C.A.Anat. *Rec.* 1948, 102, 225-237.
22. Urist, M.R. and McLean, C.C. *J. Bone Joint Surg.* 1952, 34A, 443 476.
23. Burwell, R.G. *J. Bone Joint Surg.* 1964, 46B, 110-140.
24. Friedenstein, A.J., Petrakova, K.V., Kurolesova, A.I. and Frolova, G.D. *Transplantation* 1968, 6, 230-247.
25. Owen, M. *Arthritis Rheum.* 1980, 23, 1073-1088.
26. Diduch, D.R., Coe, M.R., Joyner, C., Owen, M.E. and Balian, G. *J. Bone* Joint *Surg.* 1993, 75-A, 92-105.
27. Ohgushi, H., Dohi, Y., Tamai, S. and Tabata, S. J. *Biomed. Mater. Res.* 1993, 27, 1401-1407.

BONE ASH BASED COMPOSITE BIOCERAMICS OF GOOD MECHANICAL PROPERTIES AND HIGH BIOACTIVITY

M. Dimitrova-Lukács [1], Zs. Suba [2], L. Miklós [3], J. Mink [4] and P. Lukács [1]

1. ALUTERV - FKI Ltd. HUNGALU Engineering and Development Center, P.O.B.308, H-1502 Budapest; 2. Semmelweis Medical University, Clinic of Maxillofacial Surgery, Maria u. 52, 1085 Budapest; 3. Holy Margit Hospital, Bécsi út 132, 1032 Budapest; 4. Institute of Isotopes of Hungarian Academy of Sciences, P.O.B.77, H-1525 Budapest

ABSTRACT

The results of *in vivo* experiments of infrared (IR) analyses and of mechanical testing are reported for two pressureless sintered composite bioceramics containing 60 vol.% apatite ("in situ" fluorinated bone ash) and 40 vol.% Al_2O_3 or yttria stabilized tetragonal ZrO_2 (YTZP). The bioactive phase proved to be fluorapatite (FAp) with traces of hydroxyapatite (HAp). Both composites exhibit more than twice higher strength and toughness than dense HAp and excellent biocompatibility with living bone; moreover they promote new bone formation. The *in vivo* behavior of implants made from these two composite biomaterials was compared with bioinert magnesia partly stabilized zirconia (Mg-PSZ).

INTRODUCTION AND OBJECTIVES

Hot isostatically pressed HAp - YTZP bioceramics are being intensively studied while biomaterials consisting of HAp and Al_2O_3 phases have not been reported yet. Dense composites of both systems with retained initial phases are difficult to obtain mainly because decomposition of HAp to β-$Ca_3(PO_4)_2$ and CaO during sintering is enhanced in the presence of Al_2O_3 or TZP (both can react with CaO to form either aluminates or cubic ZrO_2). Recently pressureless sintered Apatite-Al_2O_3 and Apatite-YTZP composites have been developed and studied in a wide range of compositions, varying the bioinert phase content from 20 to 60 vol.% [1-4]. The apatite phase is "in situ" fluorinated bone ash according to X-ray analyses [2], consists mainly of FAp. The developed composites are 2-4 times superior in strength and toughness to dense HAp ceramics [2,4].

The objectives of the present work were: 1. To determine the presence (if any) of HAp in the apatite phase of two selected composite bioceramic materials (one from each developed system), both containing equal amount of Al_2O_3 or YTZP; 2. To compare the response of living bone tissue to the implants made from these two composite biomaterials with bioinert; 3.To choose between the two selected composites the better biomaterial in respect to mechanical properties, biocompatibility and potential production.

CHARACTERIZATION OF BIOCERAMICS SELECTED FOR IMPLANTATION

Among the developed FAp - Al_2O_3 and FAp - YTZP bioceramics the following compositions: 60 vol.% FAp - 40 vol.% Al_2O_3 (coded as 60F40A) and 60 - 40 vol.% YTZP (coded as 60F40Z) were selected for implantation. The reason: they exhibit more than twice higher bending strength (σ_f) and fracture toughness (K_{IC}) and only about 30 - 55 % higher Young's modulus (E) compared to dense HAp (Table 1); in both the required phases (apatite, corundum and YTZP) were entirely retained in the bulk of the sintered samples [2,3]; owing to their high apatite content they are expected to possess good bioactivity. As FAp is more stable than HAp, the behavior of 60F40A and 60F40Z composites were compared in living bone to a 50H50Z composite prepared from 50 vol.% bone ash HAp and 50 vol.% YTZP containing 25 wt.% biodegradable β-$Ca_3(PO_4)_2$ and 10 wt.% bioactive HAp - both known to stimulate new bone formation. The composite 60 vol.% HAp - 40 vol.% YTZP was not selected because of its worse phase composition including α-$Ca_3(PO_4)_2$. For comparison the results of implantation of high density bioinert Mg-PSZ samples are mentioned briefly. All implants were prepared from *medical grade* Hungarian powders: very well crystallized bone ash HAp with Ca/P ratio 1.65 (as a source of apatite); DIAKOR® Al_2O_3 ; ZrO_2 stabilized with 3 mol.% Y_2O_3 or 9 mol.% MgO. DIAKOR® prostheses and granular bone ash have been widely used in human implantation; the ZrO_2 powder is certified as free from hazardous radioactive contamination. A sintering aid and CaF_2 were used in FAp-based composites to provide better densification and in situ FAp formation. The compacts of composites and reference HAp were sintered at 1300-1350°C. Comparing the mechanical properties of 60F40A and 60F40Z composite bioceramics both have similar values of σ_f and K_{IC} and higher values of E and HV (Vickers hardness) in the case of 60F40A (Table 1). The higher strength of *60F40A* is a result of its properly tailored fine microstructure with average grain size less than 1 μm. The composite 60F40A is similar in properties even to the hot isostatically pressed HAp - 26 wt.% 3YTZP ceramics with K_{IC}=2.3 MPa $m^{1/2}$ and σ_f=290 MPa [5]. The toughness and strength of 60F40Z are lower than expected presumably because the extremely fine zirconia grains could not provide efficient transformation toughening. The IR spectra were recorded by means of a Bio-Rad FTS-60A/896 type spectrometer in the 4000-400 cm^{-1} range at a resolution of 4 cm^{-1}. The powdered samples were mixed with 150 mg KBr and pelletized. The bands of the main components in 60F40A and 60F40Z composites are shown in the range below 1400 cm^{-1} (Fig. 1a). Both spectra give the characteristic bands of FAp at 1095, 1040, 960, 603 and 574 cm^{-1} [6]. In 60F40A the bands at 768, 670, 601, 488 and 465 cm^{-1} belong to α-Al_2O_3 .The broad band at around 500 cm^{-1} in 60F40Z can be attributed to ZrO_2. The

Table 1 Mechanical properties of 60F40A and 60F40Z composites and dense HAp

Composite	Relative density,%	σ_f , MPa	K_{IC} , Mpa· $m^{1/2}$	E, GPa	HV,GPa
Dense HAp	97.8	160	0.8-1.0	94	3.5
60F40A	97.6	360	2.3	147	6.9
60F40Z	98.8	340	2.4	120	5.7

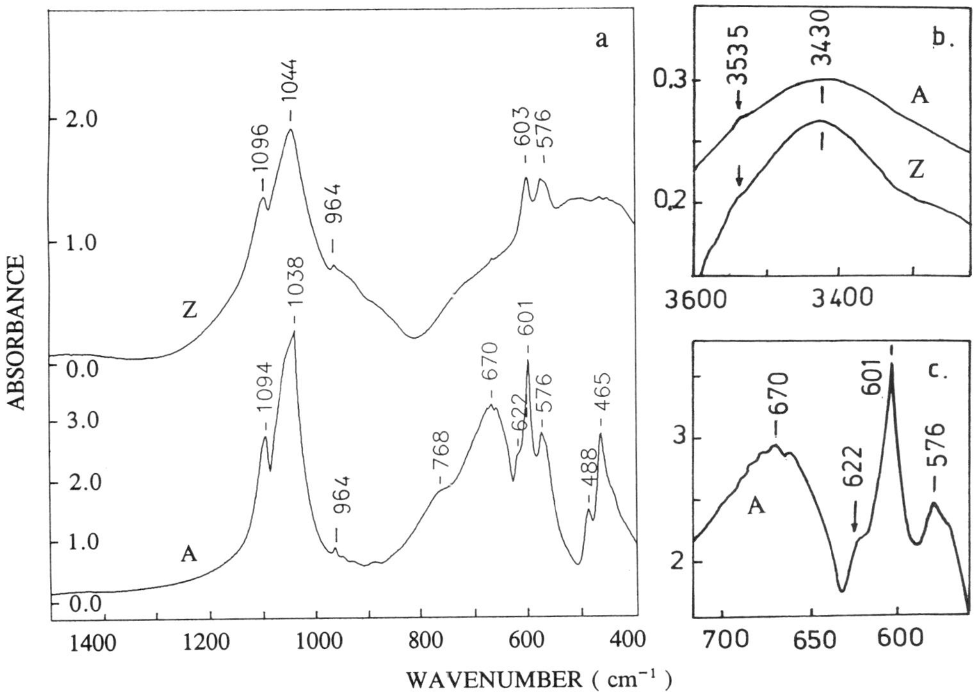

Figure 1. IR spectra of 60F40A and 60F40Z composites (curves A and Z respectively).

broad band of OH stretch at around 3430 cm^{-1} (Fig. 1b) belongs to the associated OH-groups of adsorbed water. The OH-stretch of HAp lies at 3573 cm^{-1} and the libration at 633 cm^{-1}. The interaction between OH and F in mixed HAp-FAp shifts the OH stretch to 3546 cm^{-1}. In heat treated samples (as ours) further shifting to higher energy gives an absorption at 3535 cm^{-1} [5]. In both composites the OH stretch appears as a weak shoulder just at 3535 cm^{-1} (Fig. 1c) and the OH libration is shifted to 622 cm^{-1}. Based on these results it can be concluded that only traces of OH were detected in both composites and their main apatite phase is FAp.

HISTOLOGICAL STUDY

Machined cylinder implants (5 mm long, 4 mm in diameter) were implanted into the parietal region of six pig skulls. Because of the restricted number of animals two different implants were placed in each scull: 60F40A - in pair with bioinert Mg-PSZ and 60F40Z paired with 50H50Z - for better comparison. The animals were sacrificed at three, six and nine months after the implantation. The implants with the surrounding bone tissue were excised and electrically decalcified; the implants - removed, the bone samples - embedded into paraffin. The histological evaluations were performed by light microscope on cut sections of 4-5 μm, stained with hematoxylin-eosin, azan and bone staining. Some characteristic sections are illustrated in Fig. 2 and Fig. 3. Necrotic bone was not observed in the tissue around all investigated implants. There was no connective tissue fibrous capsula in he vicinity of the bed of the bioactive-bioinert implants. Around them

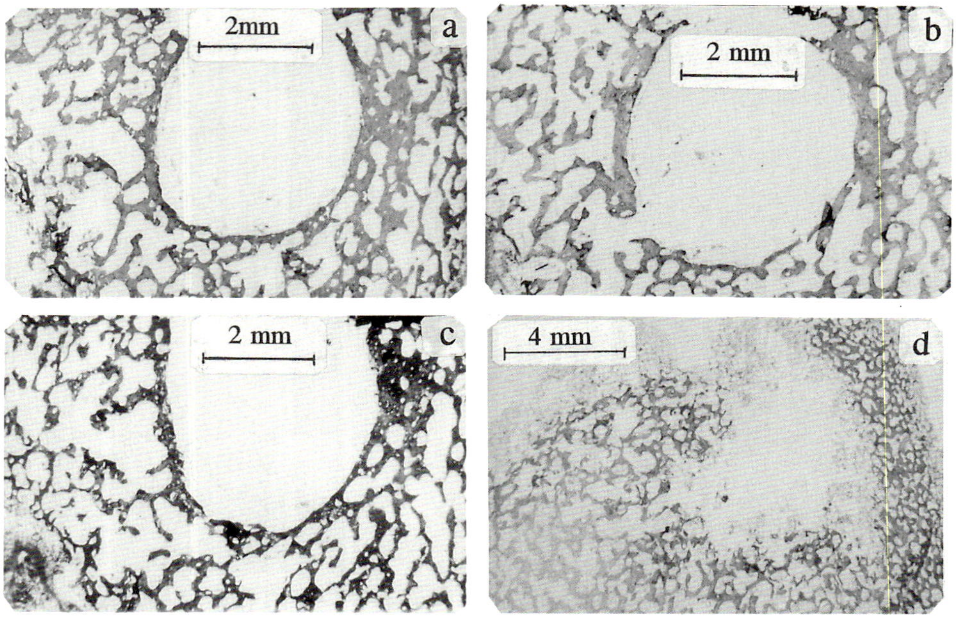

Figure 2. Micrographs of decalcified bone tissue around implants: 60F40A (a); 60F40Z (b); 50H50Z (c) and Mg-PSZ (d) three months after the implantation. Staining: hematoxylin-eosin (a,b,d) and azan (c)

new bone has formed even in three months after the implantation (Fig. 2 a-c). In contrast, thin connective tissue and decalcified bone matrix can be seen around the border of the bioinert Mg-PSZ implant (Fig. 2 d). Two types of newly formed bone tissue can be distinguished: continuous cortical bone along the border of the implants and spongeous bone around. The cortical-like bony layer has a lamellar structure and is about equally thick (150-200 μm) around all three composite implants (Fig. 2 a-c; Fig. 3 a,b). The added bone tissue exhibits advanced calcification: there is neither osteoblastic activity on the surface of the new bone trabeculae nor cellular activity in the marrow spaces (Fig. 3 a-d). Lamellar and non lamellar bony tissue can be observed around 60F40A and 60F40Z implants. Features of remodeling, mosaic structure and cementum lines, can be found both in the new bone adjacent to the implant and in the older bone trabeculae (Fig. 3c,d). Still the new bone tissue can be distinguished from the mature bone (often the first is differently stained, Fig.3 a). Six months after the implantation the new trabeculae are so well calcified that they do not differ from the original ones; around all composite implants homogeneous spongeous bone tissue can be observed (Fig.3 e,f). Nine months after the implantation similar results were obtained in the case of composite implants while around the bioinert Mg-PSZ implant the bone tissue was still not well calcified and connective tissue could be detected.

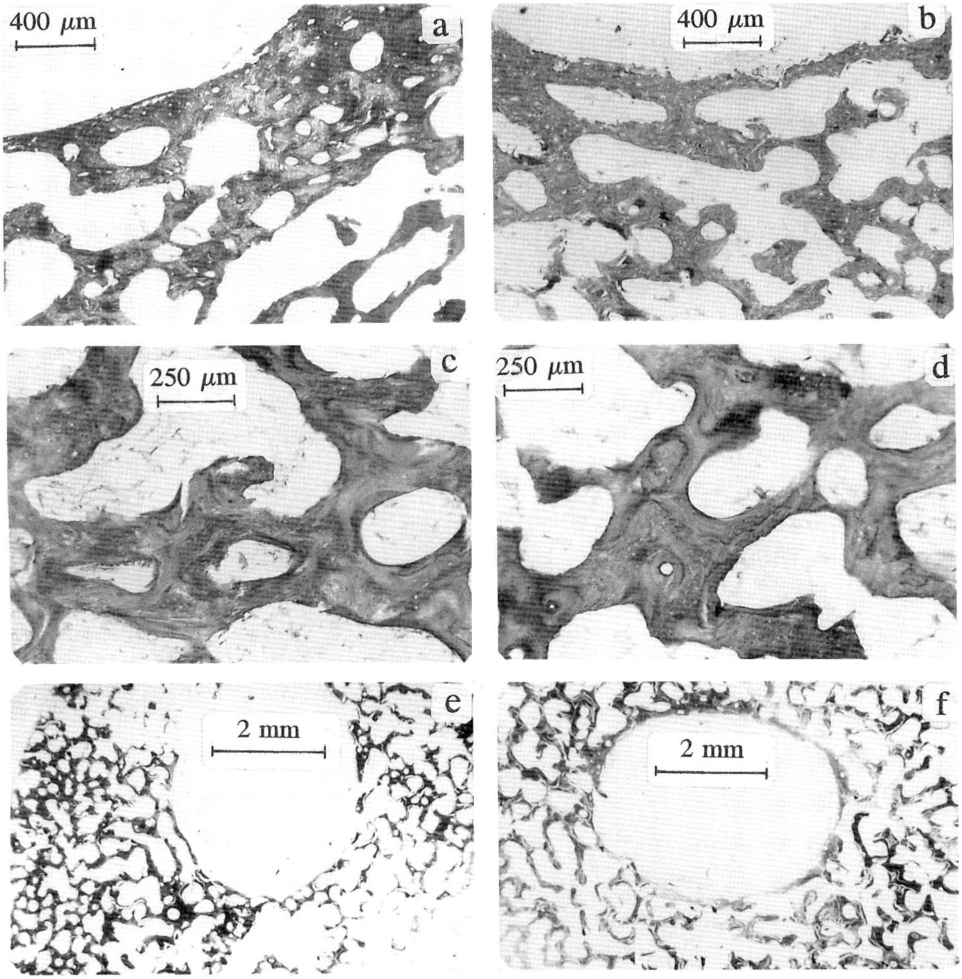

Figure 3. Micrographs of decalcified bone tissue around the implants 60F40A (a,c,e) and 60F40Z (b,d,f) removed three (a-c) and six (d,e) months after the implantation. Staining: azan (a,b); hematoxylin-eosin (c,d) and bone (e,f).

CONCLUSIONS

1. The results of IR analyses confirmed the presence of traces of HAp in the pressureless sintered FAp-based 60F40A and 60F40Z composite bioceramic materials.

2. During the *in vivo* experiments all ceramic implants including Mg-PSZ showed good compatibility with the living bone tissue. FAp in the composite bioceramic implants 60F40A and 60F40Z has promoted new bone formation to the same extent as the mixture of β-$Ca_3(PO_4)_2$ and HAp in the bone ash based 50H50Z composite implant. Around the bioinert Mg-PSZ implant thin connective tissue formed.

3. The composites 60F40A and 60F40Z exhibit similar mechanical properties, bioactivity and biocompatibility. Considering possible degradation of YTZP in a living

environment, concern about potential long term radioactivity of zirconia and the high price of ultra fine ZrO_2 powders, the composite 60F40A is recommended as the preferred biomaterial.

ACKNOWLEDGEMENT
This work was sponsored by the National Committee for Technological Development. The authors would like to thank Dr. J. Kristof for valuable scientific assistance

REFERENCES

1. Dimitrova-Lukács, M., Gillemot, L.in *Third Euro-Ceramics* Volume 3, Ed. Durán, P.- Fernández, J.F., Faenza Editrice Iberica 1993,179-184
2. Dimitrova-Lukács, M., Lukács, P., Sajó, I., to be published in the *8th CIMTEC Proceedings*, Ed. Vincenzini, P., Volume L, Faenza 1995
3. Dimitrova-Lukács, M., Lukács, P., Sajó, I., Migály, B. and Fodor, M. in *Ceramic - Ceramic Composites*, Extended Abstracts (3 pages), Mons 1994, 4.7
4. Dimitrova-Lukács, M., Juhász, A., Vörös, Gy.,and Arató, P. ibid, 2.12
5. Tagaki, M., Mochida, M., Uchida, N., Saito, K. and Umatsu, K. *J. Mater. Sci.: Mater. Medicine* 3, 1992, 199-203
6. *The Infrared Spectra of Minerals*, Ed. Farmer, V.C., Bartolomew Press, Dorking, Surrey, 1974, p. 391

PROCESSING AND CHARACTERIZATION OF BIOACTIVE POLYSULFONE-BIOGLASS® COMPOSITES

R. L. Oréfice, G. P. LaTorre, J. K. West and L. L. Hench

Advanced Materials Research Center, University of Florida, One Progress Blvd., #14, Alachua, FL 32615, USA.

ABSTRACT

The mismatch between mechanical properties of bioceramics and natural tissues has restricted a wider application of ceramics in medical and dental fields. In order to overcome this problem, polymer matrix composites can be designed to combine bioactive properties of some bioceramics with the excellent mechanical properties of some engineering plastics. In this work, Bioglass® powders were combined with a polysulfone (Udel®) matrix in different volumetric fractions. The composite was processed by a procedure including polymer dissolution and precipitation. The composite material was subsequently hot pressed and the samples were characterized by FTIR and SEM. Mechanical bending tests were also performed. SEM revealed a high degree of homogeneity of Bioglass® particles distributed within the polymer matrix. Fracture surfaces showed intimate contact between the phases with no pull-out of particles. An *in vitro* test demonstrated the bioactive behavior of the new material. Mechanical bending tests showed an increase of the elastic modulus of the composite and a decrease in mechanical strength and strain at failure with progressive addition of the Bioglass® phase. However, the mechanical properties of the composite are in the range of cortical bone, thus use of this new bioactive composite in some load-bearing applications is proposed.

INTRODUCTION

Even though the use of ceramics as an implant material has been widespread, the mismatch between the mechanical properties of ceramics in relation to the mechanical properties of natural tissues must be overcome in order to increase the number of load bearing applications. Ceramics have typically a higher elastic modulus and a lower fracture toughness than bone. The unique mechanical properties of bone are due to homogeneous distribution of a hydroxy-carbonate apatite phase in a collagen matrix. Therefore, the production of a molecularly tailored composite that can mimic the structure of bone is a potential path to solve the difference in mechanical properties between bioceramics and tissues [1]. The goal of this work is to investigate the processing, *in vitro* bioactivity and mechanical properties of a new bioactive composite. Polysulfone and a particulate Bioglass® were chosen to form the composite due to the high mechanical properties and stability in body environments of polysulfone [2] and the ability of Bioglass® to bind rapidly to bone and soft tissues.

COMPOSITE PROCESSING

The procedure used for processing the polysulfone composites involved two steps:

(1) Mixture of Bioglass® particles (125-106 μm) in a chloroform-polysulfone (Udel® - medical grade) solution (100 g of polysulfone/L of chloroform). A polysulfone non-solvent (ethanol) was then added to the mixture to precipitate the polymer. The obtained material is composed of well-distributed glass particles within a porous polymer matrix.
(2) Hot press the material prepared in the first step into a dense shape.

The process of polymer dissolution is well described in the literature involving the physical-chemistry of polymers and it can be atomistically viewed as a result of interactions between solvent molecules and polymer chains that reduce the effectiveness of secondary bonds to keep chains together. In terms of thermodynamics, the ability of a solvent to dissolve a polymer can be predicted by comparing solubility parameters of both solvent and solute. A good solvent should have a similar solubility parameter in relation to the polymer. Solubility parameters for polysulfone, chloroform and ethanol are respectively 20.6, 19 and 26 $MPa^{1/2}$.

Adding a non-solvent to a polysulfone solution in order to drive the system to phase separation is a procedure used to produce polysulfone membranes (commonly used in dialysis devices)[3,4]. The goal of using this technique was to enhance the mixing between polysulfone and Bioglass® particles. The effect of a non-solvent on the behavior of a solution can be described by a solvent-polymer-non-solvent ternary diagram. Systems involving polysulfone have been studied recently [3,4]. The addition of a non-solvent to a polymer solution leads initially to a region of one homogenous phase. The size of this region is a function of the type of system and was detected in this work for the polysulfone-chloroform-ethanol system to be less than 5% of ethanol. The boundary between one phase and two phase regions for polymer solutions is a function of molecular weight. Therefore, higher molecular weight chains come out of solution first and for the limit where infinite molecular weight is achieved the theta condition is defined. In this work, an excess of ethanol was added to the solution in order to avoid molecular weight fractionation. Very low molecular weight (MW) species, like lubricants, added during extrusion-based polymer processes, are eliminated during the solution quench process. Since the effect of low MW species in human body is always questionable, restricting the presence of these species in the composite is desirable for medical applications.

Bioglass® particles in the polysulfone solution act as nucleation sites for the precipitation of polysulfone. Consequently, the addition of ethanol leads to a preferential precipitation of the polymer on the glass particle surface and formation of uniformly coated particles. The precipitation process leads to an increase of the thickness of the polymer layer on the glass surface as in a growth process. Ultimately, the "growing" particles collide, forming a porous material with Bioglass® particles uniformly distributed within a polysulfone matrix. The porous material with Bioglass® particles was then fractionated and hot pressed in a mold. The temperature used in the hot press was only few degrees above the Tg of polysulfone (Tg polysulfone = 185°C) in order to provide flow of the polymer to fill voids.

Figure 1 shows a SEM photo of a fracture surface of a polysulfone composite with 40% volume fraction of Bioglass®. The homogeneity of particle distribution and the intimate contact between the phases are apparent.

IN VITRO BIOACTIVITY TEST OF THE COMPOSITES

Previous *in vivo* studies showed that the essential condition for a material to bond with bone is the formation of a hydroxy-carbonate-apatite layer in the body environment [5]. Reactions in simulated body fluids (*in vitro* tests) can predict the ability of a material to bond to bone [5]. The standard *in vitro* test [5] used on the composites includes: suspending a polished sample in a tris (hydroxymethyl) aminomethane buffered solution at 37°C for 20 hours (ratio between sample surface area and solution volume = 0.1 cm^{-1}) and FTIR reflection spectroscopy on the sample surface to identify the formation of an HCA layer. A polished sample was used to simulate the conditions of a machined shape, which may be the final processing step for this new composite.

Figure 2 shows the FTIR spectrum of polysulfone with 40% volume fraction of Bioglass®, obtained with a Nicolet 20SXB spectrometer. The spectrum in Fig. 2-a is for the unreacted composite and the frequencies of Bioglass® can be noted (between 1100-900 and 450-400 cm^{-1}) among others associated with the polymer. The result of a spectral subtraction between the spectrum in Fig. 2-a and a pure polysulfone spectrum is in Fig. 2-b, where the glass peaks are clearly identified. Figure 2-c is also a result of spectral subtraction between a reacted polysulfone with 40% volume fraction of Bioglass® and a pure polymer spectrum. The presence of a crystalline HCA layer on the composite surface is confirmed by the presence of its typical frequencies (between 600-550 cm^{-1}) [5], and the *in vitro* bioactivity of the composite is confirmed.

MECHANICAL PROPERTIES OF THE OBTAINED COMPOSITES

Figure 3 shows the effect of volume fraction of Bioglass® particles on the flexural elastic modulus and stress at failure of the composite (yield stress for pure polysulfone), obtained by four-point bend test (ASTM 790M-92). The elastic modulus is enhanced when Bioglass® particles are introduced into the pure polysulfone, since the applied stress is shared between the polymer and the higher-elastic modulus glass [6]. The reduction in strength as the amount of Bioglass® particles is increased can be associated to the fact that particles may be acting as source of flaws that would decrease the necessary stress to fracture the material [7]. Figure 4 shows the engineering stress-strain curve for two composites. Both Figures 3 and 4 reveal that the composite mechanical properties evaluated in this work (elastic modulus, strength and strain at failure) are between the range of cortical bone values [5].

The fracture surface of the composite, in Fig. 1, yields information related to the interfacial properties. The strength of the interface between components of a particulate composite can be divided into three types [8] by using fractograph analysis: (a) weak (where few particles are noted without matrix on them), in this case the crack propagates around the particles; (b) strong (a thin layer of polymer covers the particle surface), where the crack "climbs over" the particles; and (c) intermediary between weak and strong (few pull-out particles can be seen and the matrix can be observed on the surface of particles).

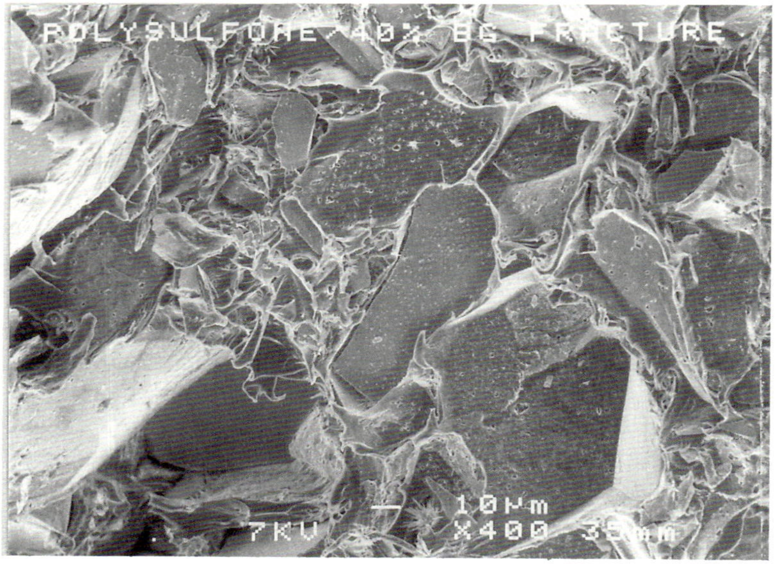

Figure 1. SEM of polysulfone with 40% volume fraction of Bioglass® fracture surface.

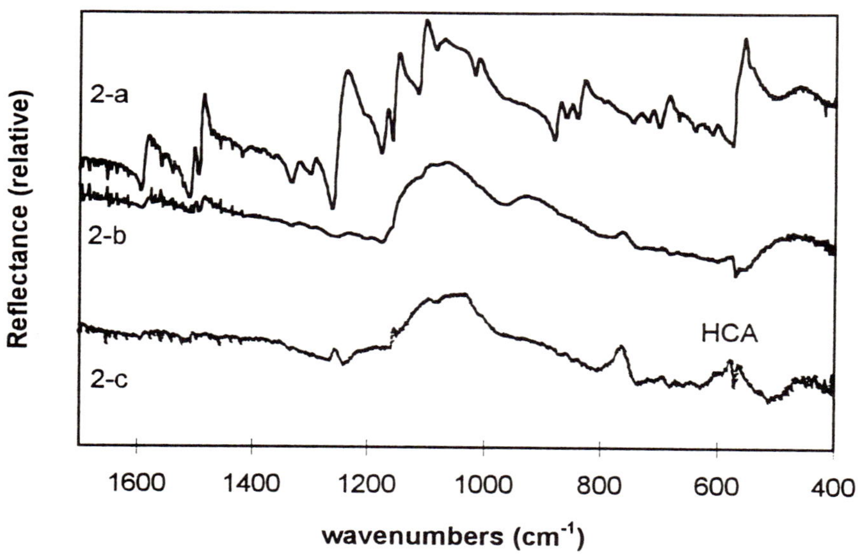

Figure 2. (a) FTIR spectrum of unreacted polysulfone 40% Bioglass® composite; (b) Bioglass® particles in the composite (subtracted spectrum); (c) reacted composite (subtracted spectrum) after 20 hs. in tris-buffer solution.

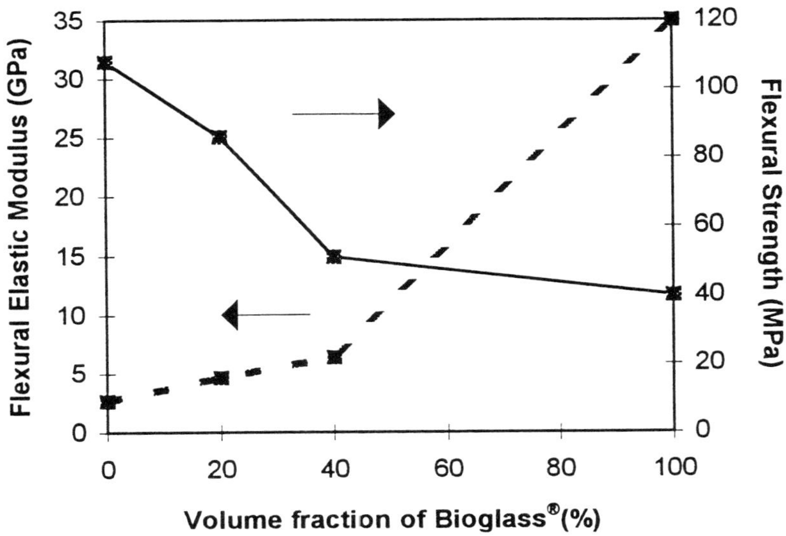

Figure 3. Flexural elastic modulus and stress at failure for polysulfone-Bioglass® composites.

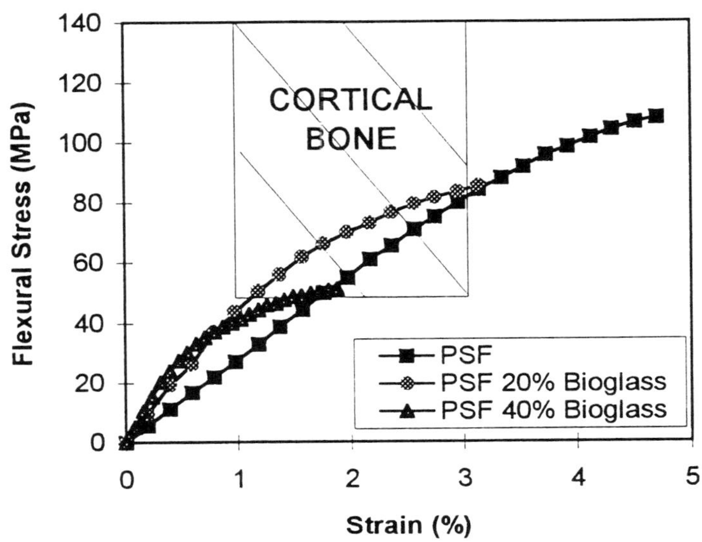

Figure 4. Engineering stress-strain curve for polysulfone-Bioglass® composites.

The micrograph shown in Fig. 1 shows no pull-out particles and some polymer on the Bioglass® particle's fracture surface. Therefore, the interface between polysulfone and Bioglass® can be described as having intermediate values of strength. Since no coupling agents were used, this information obtained by fractograph analysis suggests that the processing developed in this work leads to a high degree of interaction between the components of the composite.

CONCLUSIONS

Polysulfone-Bioglass® composites were fabricated by a method involving dissolution and precipitation of the polymer on the glass particle surface by addition of a non-solvent. This procedure enabled the preparation of composites with different amount of Bioglass® particles well-distributed within polysulfone matrix. An *in vitro* bioactivity test showed the presence of a HCA layer on the composite after 20 hs. in tris-buffer solution. The composite mechanical properties are within the range of cortical bone properties. Therefore, this new polysulfone-Bioglass® bioactive composite can be potentially used in load-bearing applications.

ACKNOWLEDGMENTS

The authors acknowledge the support of the Air Force Office of Scientific Research (AFOSR) grant F49620-92-0351. One of the authors (RLO) would also like to acknowledge the financial support from Conselho Nacional de Desenvolvimento Científico e Tecnológico (CNPq) of the Brazilian Government.

REFERENCES

1. Bonfield, W. In: *An Introduction to Bioceramics*, World Scientific, 1993, Chapter 16.
2. Spector, M. In: *Non-cemented total hip arthroplasty*, Raven Press, New York, 1988, Chapter 19, 227.
3. He, D. and Jiang, B. *J. Appl. Pol. Sci.* 1993, 49, 617.
4. Lau, W. W. Y.; Guiver, M. D. and Matsuura, T. *J. Membr. Sci.* 1991, 59, 219.
5. Hench, L. L. and Wilson, J. In: *An Introduction to Bioceramics*, World Scientific, 1993, Chapters 1 and 18.
6. Amdouri, N.; Sautereau, H. and Gerard J. F. *J. Appl. Pol. Sci.* 1992, 46, 1723.
7. Wang, D.; Li, K.; Sourirajan, S. and Teo, W. K. *J. Appl. Pol. Sci.* 1993, 50, 1693.
8. Sinien, L.; Xiaoguang, Z. and Zongneng, Q. *J. Mat. Sci.* 1992, 27, 4633.

PREPARATION OF NOVEL CALCIUM PHOSPHATE CERAMICS CONTAINING ß-$(PO_3)_2$ FIBERS FOR BIOMEDICAL USE

Toshihiro Kasuga,* Kenji Tsuji,* Yoshio Ota,* and Yoshihiro Abe,* Atsushi Niimi** and Minoru Ueda**

*Department of Materials Science and Engineering Nagoya Institute of Technology Nagoya 466, Japan; **Department of Oral Surgery Nagoya University School of Medicine Nagoya 466, Japan

ABSTRACT

High-strength calcium metaphosphate (ß-$Ca(PO_3)_2$) fibers for biomedical applications are extracted from crystallized products of calcium ultraphosphate glasses by aqueous leaching. The fibers have high aspect ratios ranging from 10 to 100 with diameters of 2 ~ 10 μm. In the present work, new types of bioceramics containing the crystalline fibers were prepared by the sintering of the fibers. A novel dense ceramic was obtained by hot-pressing. It shows high strength of ≈200 MPa in bending and relatively low Young's modulus of 30 ~ 50 GPa. These values are close to those of human natural bone. On the other hand, a porous material for bone-in-growth with a skeleton composed of ß-$Ca(PO_3)_2$ fibers was obtained by a pressureless-sintering method. This porous ceramic has large-size pores of 50 ~ 100 μm and a large porosity of > 60%.

INTRODUCTION

Calcium phosphate ceramics show good biocompatibility in living tissues, so that today, they are used clinically as biomaterials for bone repair. We have been studying glass-related materials based on the calcium phosphate system for biomedical applications [1-9]. When the CaO-P_2O_5 glasses are reheated under a temperature gradient around the glass transition temperature (Tg), unidirectionally crystallized glass-ceramics having a fiber-reinforced composite structure are successfully prepared [2-5]. These glass-ceramics composed of crystalline ß-$Ca(PO_3)_2$ fibers with ~ 1 μm diameter show high bending strength of 400 ~ 600 MPa, low Young's modulus of 60 ~ 130 GPa, and bending behavior similar to that of natural bone. Animal tests showed that the glass-ceramics have good biocompatibility [4,6,7]. These results imply that the crystalline ß-$Ca(PO_3)_2$ is a high-strength and flexible fiber with biocompatibility. We expect that this fiber will be used for new composite biomaterials. This paper presents preparations of the calcium metaphosphate fibers and of novel dense and porous materials containing the fibers.

PREPARATION OF ß-$Ca(PO_3)_2$ FIBERS

Long ß-$Ca(PO_3)_2$ fibers can be prepared by reheating $CaO\text{-}P_20_5$ glasses. Calcium phosphate glasses around the metaphosphate composition crystallize even at temperatures below the glass transition temperature (Tg). The crystal growth rate is extraordinarily high owing to "stress-induced crystallization" [10], while the nucleation rate is low around Tg. Glass-ceramics converted from the calcium ultraphosphate glasses, of which molar ratio of CaO/P_20_5 is slightly less than unity, consist of crystals such as ß-$Ca(PO_3)_2$, $Ca_2P_6O_{17}$ and an ultraphosphate glassy phase [3]. The ultraphosphate phases are much poorer in chemical durability than fibrous ß-$Ca(PO_3)_2$ crystals. Therefore, ß-$Ca(PO_3)_2$ fibers are able to be released preferentially from the matrix phase by aqueous leaching. The existence of the ultraphosphate matrix phases in ß-$Ca(PO_3)_2$-containing glass-ceramics is essential for this treatment [8,9].

A batch mixture with CaO/P_20_5 = 0.85 in molar ratio was prepared by using raw materials such as $Ca(H_2PO_4)_2 \cdot H_20$ and H_3PO_4. The mixture was melted in a platinum crucible at 1250°C for 2 h. The melt was poured onto a carbon plate and cooled to a room temperature. The resultant glass was reheated at 600°C for 48 h for the crystallization. The crystallized glass block was crushed into powder below 850, μm using an alumina mortar. An aqueous solution of 0.1 N NaOH was used as leaching solutions to extract ß-$Ca(PO_3)_2$ fibers. The 100 g of pulverized crystallized glass powder was put into a stainless-steel container filled with 3000 mL of the leaching solutions. They were stirred at 70° ~ 80 °C for 70 h. The resultant products were filtrated and dried at 150°C in air.

The fibrous products are successfully extracted from the matrix phases as shown in Figure 1. They are straight in shape. X-ray diffraction (XRD) analysis showed that the products consist of ß-$Ca(PO_3)_2$. The fibers are of 2 ~ 10 μm-diameter with high aspect ratios of 10 ~ 100. The dimension of the fibers varies with composition of the mother glass and with some treatment conditions [9].

Evaluation of the fibers by implantation in rats is in progress [11]. This result will be reported in the near future.

NEWLY DEVELOPED CALCIUM PHOSPHATE CERAMICS CONTAINING 1= $Ca(PO_3)_2$ FIBERS

A high-strength dense ceramic with a low Young's modulus

Calcium phosphate ceramics such as hydroxyapatite or tricalcium phosphate do not show as high a bending strength and a toughness as natural cortical bone. Some works for

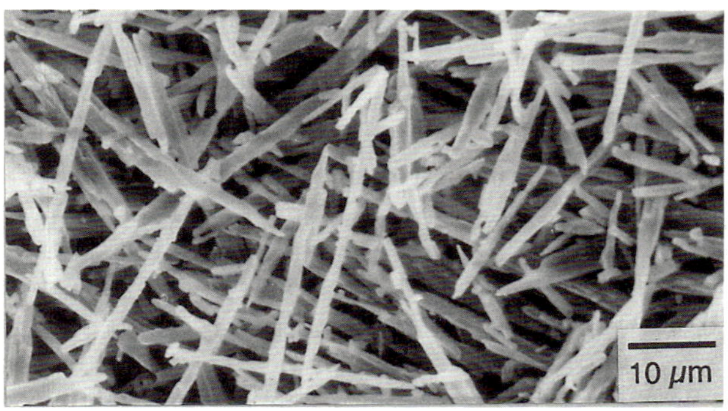

Figure 1. ß-$Ca(PO_3)_2$ fibers obtained.

microstructural improvement by introducing fibers or particles with high moduli of elasticity into the matrix phase have been done to improve the mechanical properties [12]. However, the disadvantage of this approach is that elastic moduli of the composites obtained are much higher compared to that of natural bone. Therefore, the problem of stress shielding is not solved. A great deal of attention is now being paid to high-strength and high toughness bioceramics with low moduli of elasticity.

In general, to obtain a ceramic with both a high toughness and a low modulus of elasticity, the fracture surface energy should be increased [10]. Abe et al. reported [4,13] that high-strength unidirectionally crystallized CaO-P_2O_5 glass-ceramics have critical strains of 4 ~ 7 x 10^{-3}, which are close to that (6 ~ 8 x 10^{-3}) of natural bone. They are composed of crystalline ß-$Ca(PO_3)_2$ fibers with ultraphosphate glass and crystals as the matrix phases. We believe that one of the most promising approaches for satisfying the biomechanical requirement of natural host tissues is to design microstructure of calcium phosphate glass-related materials containing the ß-$Ca(PO_3)_2$ crystalline fibers. Therefore, the objective in the present work is to prepare a new type of calcium phosphate bioceramic with high strength and low modulus of elasticity by using the ß-$Ca(PO_3)_2$ fibers extracted.

A crystallized product of a glass with composition of $Ca/P_2O_5 = 0.85$ was prepared by a method shown in a previous section. ß-$Ca(PO_3)_2$ fibers are obtained by leaching it with a dilute NaOH aqueous solution. To prepare a dense material, the matrix phases such as calcium phosphate glasses should be lain between the fibers. We prepared calcium phosphate fibrous products, in which a small amount of $Ca_2P_6O_{17}$ crystals remains, by using distilled water (DW) for the extracting treatment. $Ca_2P_6O_{17}$ crystal melts at 750°C ~ 770°C [14]. The melt is glassified on cooling. It is expected that the resultant glassy phase plays a role as a bonding agent to interlink the fibers.

The fibrous products were put into a carbon die of 40 mm-diameter and were hot pressed under a pressure of 40 MPa at 850°C. Figure 2 shows scanning electron micrographs (SEM photos) of fracture faces of a material obtained by the hot-pressing. No serious cracks, voids, or other defects are seen. A relative density of the material was estimated as ≈ 95%. ß-$Ca(PO_3)_2$ was identified as the only crystalline phase in the material by XRD analysis.

The material showed relatively high strength of 150 ~ 200 MPa in bending. The fracture toughness measured by using the single edge notched specimens was ≈4MPa·m^{05}. The value is as high as that of an alumina ceramic. Young's modulus of the material measured by a pulse echo overlap method showed 30 ~ 50 GPa. The modulus is one order of magnitude lower than that of conventional, high-strength ceramics such as a sintered alumina. The fracture surface energy of the material was estimated as 150 ~ 200 J·m^2 from the stress-strain curves in the bending test. This value is an order of magnitude higher than that of a hydroxyapatite ceramic or that of an alumina ceramic. Increase in the strength and the toughness is attributed to the extreme increase in the fracture surface energy. In Figure 2, a pull-out mechanism of the fiber is seen. It is found that the dense material obtained in this work has mechanical properties close to those of natural bone as shown in Figure 3.

A porous ceramic with ß-$Ca(PO_3)_2$ fiber skeleton

Porous bioceramics are very important materials in applications as artificial bones. The advantage is to anchor the ceramics mechanically by the high convoluted growth of natural bone into the pores. Some works reported that the open continuous pores with

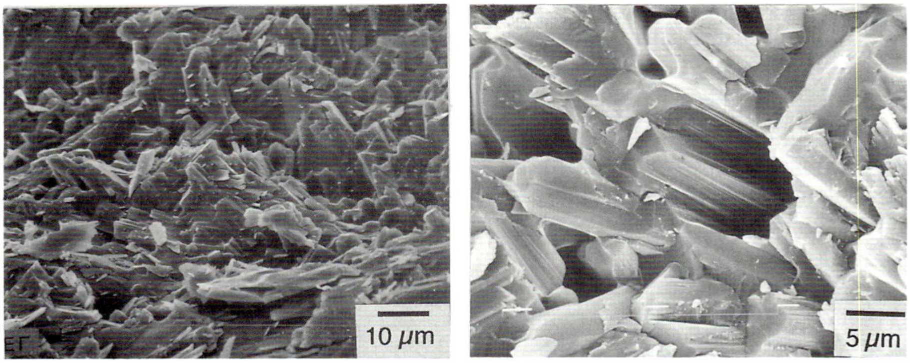

Figure 2. Fracture face of a dense material obtained in this work.

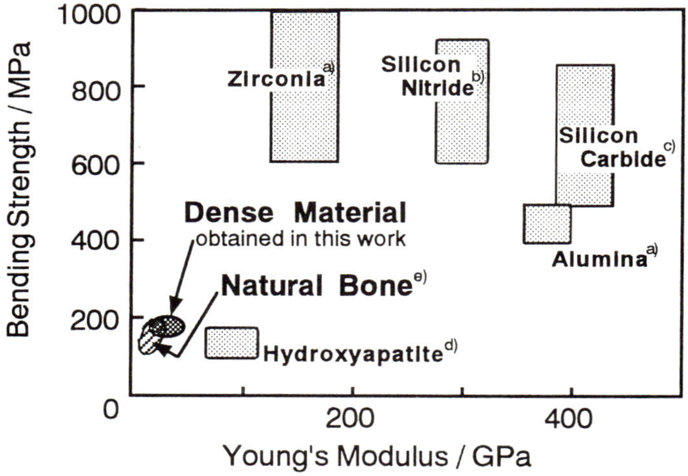

Figure 3. Bending strengths and Young's moduli of a dense material obtained, some dense ceramics, and human natural bone. a) Alumina, Zirconia (partially stabilized zirconia); Hulbert, S.F. in *An Introduction to Bioceramics,* World Scientific, Singapore 1993, 25-40. b) Silicon nitride (Si_3N_4); Komeya, K. in *Fine Ceramics,* Elsevier, NY 1988, 188-97. c)Silicon carbide (SiC); Iseki, T. and Hase, T. *ibid,* 188-97. d) Hydroxyapatite ($Ca_5(PO_4)_3OH$); Aoki, H. in *Medical Applications of Hydroxyapatite,* IshiyakuEuroAmerica, Tokyo 1994, 286-306. e)Cortical bone; Evans, F.G. and King, A. in *Biomedical Studies of the Musculoskeltal System,* Springfield, IL 1961, 49-53.; Bonfield, W. in *Natural and Living Biomaterials,* CRC Press, Boca Raton, FL 1984,43-60.

large pore-size in diameter (ex. 50 ~ 200 μm) and with large porosity (ex. > 60%) are required for development of new bone tissues in the ceramics [15-17]. Human bone comprises fractions of mineral tissues such as calcium phosphate and of organic tissues. The mineral framework in the bone is structured by long filaments which are connected to each other. It is expected that porous materials composed of a fibrous skeleton show high elasticity. We believe that the porous materials with a skeleton of long, high-strength calcium phosphate fibers have high potential in use as artificial bones. We tried to prepare new porous bioceramics composed of calcium metaphosphate fiber skeleton.

The fibrous products, which contain ß-$Ca(PO_3)_2$ with a small amount of $Ca_2P_6O_{17}$ crystals, as shown in section (a) were used for preparing the porous ceramic. Next, the fiber compact was prepared by pressing the fibers with ethanol of 20% in weight into a rod-shape of ≈ 10 mm-diameter X ≈ 20 mm-length under a hydrostatic pressure of ≈ 200 MPa. After drying, the compact was heated at 800°C for 5 h to prepare a porous ceramic.

Figure 4 shows scanning electron micrographs of the porous ceramic obtained. Shrinkage of the fiber-compact less than 10% in volume occurred during the heating. As seen in Figure 4, the ceramic has a network of filaments and contains numerous spaces with various sizes of 20 ~ 150 μm. The fibers are successfully interlinked to each other. ß-$Ca(PO_3)_2$ was identified as the crystalline phase in the material by XRD analysis. As mentioned in section (a), the calcium phosphate glassy phase interlinks the fibers. The porosity of the ceramic shown in Figure 4 was estimated as ≈ 65% from measurements of the densities. It was found that the pore size and porosity of the material are controlled by the preparation conditions of ß-$Ca(PO_3)_2$ fibers and their length.

Fracture of the porous ceramic with porosity of ≈ 60% began beyond the strain of 25% in the compressive test. The critical strain value is much larger compared to those (usually less than a few percent) of conventional porous ceramics. When compressive strain was smaller than the critical strain to failure, the shape of the ceramic was recovered to its original one after releasing the load.

SUMMARY

High-strength ß-$Ca(PO_3)_2$ fibers with low elastic modulus were successfully prepared. The crystalline fibers have high aspect ratios ranging from 10 to 100 with diameters of 2 to 10 μm. Two types of novel calcium phosphate ceramics were newly prepared by heating the fibrous products. A dense material was obtained by a hot-pressing method which has high bending strength and low Young's modulus. These values are close to those of human natural bone. Another material with large-size pores and a large porosity was obtained by a pressureless sintering method. The ceramic composed of ß-$Ca(PO_3)_2$ crystalline fiber skeleton exhibits high ductile behavior.

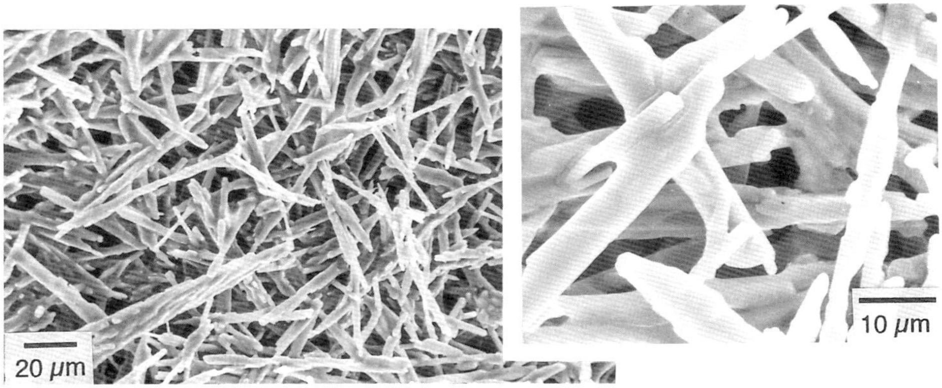

Figure 4. SEM photos of a porous ceramic with B-Ca(PO3)2 fibrous skeleton.

REFERENCES

1. Nagase, M., Abe, Y., Chigira, M. and Udagawa, E. *Biomaterials* 1992,13,172-75.
2. Abe, Y., Hosoe, M., Kasuga, T., Ishikawa, H., Shinkai, N., Suzuki, Y. and J. Nakayama, *J. Am. Ceram. Soc.* 1982, C5, C189-90.
3. Abe, Y., Kasuga, T., Hosono, H. and de Groot, K. *J. Am. Ceram. Soc.* 1984,67, C142-44.
4. Abe, Y., Hosono, H., Hosoe, M., Imura, S. and Tanaka, Y. In: *Handbook of Bioactive Ceramics* Vol. 1, CRC Press, Boca Raton 1990, 109-14.
5. Kasuga, T., Hosono, H. and Abe, Y. *Phos. Sulf. Silicon* 1993, 7C, 247-50.
6. Klein, C.P.A.T., Abe, Y., Hosono, H. and de Groot, K. *Biomaterials* 1984, 5, 362-64.
7. Idem *ibid* 1987, 8, 23436.
8. Kasuga, T., Ichino, A. and Abe, Y. *J. Ceram. Soc. Jpn.* 1992, 100, 1088-89.
9. Kasuga, T. and Abe, Y. *Phos. Res. Bull.* 1992, 2, 17-20.
10. Abe, Y., Arahori, T. and Naruse, A. *J. Am. Ceram. Soc.* 1976, 59, 487-90.
11. Niimi, A., et al. *unpublished.*
12. Davidge, R.W. In: *Mechanical Behavior of Ceramics,* Cambridge University Press, London 1979, 31-50.
13. Abe,Y. *to be submitted.*
14. Kasuga, T., Inoue, T., Tsuji, K., Ota, Y. and Abe, Y. *J. Am. Ceram. Soc.* 1995, 78 245-47.
15. de Groot, K., Klein, C.P.A.T., Wolke, J.G. and de Blieck-Hogervorst, J. In: *Bioactive Ceramics* Vol. 2, CRC Press, Boca Raton 1990, 3-16.
16. White, E.W., Webber, J.N., Roy, D.M., Owen, E.L. and Chiroff, R.T. and White, R.A. *J. Biomed. Mater. Res. Symp.* 1975, C, 23-27.
17. Hulbert, S.F. *J. Biomed. Mater. Res.* 1972, C, 347 74.

RAPID BONE FORMATION BY GRAFTING CULTURED BONE IN POROUS HYDROXYAPATITE

T. Yoshikawa, H. Ohgushi and S. Tamai

Department of Orthopedic Surgery, Nara Medical University, Kashihara City, Nara 634, Japan

ABSTRACT

Rat bone marrow cells obtained from femora were cultured in a standard medium. After ten days in the primary culture, the cells were released by trypsin treatment and combined with porous hydroxyapatite (HA) disks. The composites of HA disks and cultured cells were subcultured in a culture medium containing dexamethasone (Dex), which is known to induce osteoblastic differentiation of marrow stromal cells in culture conditions. After 17 days of subculture, the composites were subcutaneously implanted into syngeneic rats to examine *in vivo* osteogenic response of the composites. These implants were harvested 1, 2, 3, 4 and 20 weeks post implantation. The histological analysis showed active bone formation even at one week post implantation, followed by extensive bone formation, thereafter. The bone formation was evidenced by active osteoblasts lining and the appearance of tetracycline labeling which was injected 3 weeks after implantation. These results indicate that viability of the *in vitro* bone tissue generated by Dex-treated marrow cell culture in porous hydroxyapatite could be maintained and continue to produce *de novo* bone when grafting *in vivo*.

INTRODUCTION

The most ideal operative procedure in bone grafting is an autogenic bone graft. However, there are drawbacks: there is a limit to its mass and normal tissues have to undergo invasion. It would be ideal if we can employ *in vitro* cell culture techniques to generate bone tissue formation available for bone graft. However, active bone tissues seldom occur even if bone cells from bone are isolated and cultured in a regular medium. Maniatopoulos et al. succeeded in confirming differentiation of marrow cells into osteoblasts and osteocytes together with active formation of extracellular matrix by adding dexamethasone (Dex) into the medium of rat marrow cell culture [1]. The osteogenesis seen with this culture is morphologically and biochemically similar to the primary stage of *in* vivo osteogenesis [2-5]. Therefore, we speculate that this cultured bone can be clinically applied to bone reconstructive surgery. We have reported that ectopic membranous ossification is observed by combining freshly-isolated rat marrow cells with porous hydroxyapatite (HA) after subcutaneously grafting [6-10]. This means that the interior pores of HA localize the marrow cells in a particular area to help osteogenesis. If more osteogenesis can be achieved in an earlier stage through concomitant employment of some kind of culture technology, its clinical application will substantially expand. In this study, we demonstrate the osteogenic ability of the Dex-treated cultured marrow cells in porous HA.

MATERIALS AND METHODS

Materials: Coralline hydroxyapatite (HA) ceramic, Interpore 200, (Interpore International, Irvine, CA) was used. A hydrothermal chemical exchange reaction converts the original calcium carbonate exoskeleton into an inorganic replica of hydroxyapatite [11]. The average pore size of the ceramics is 200 μm in diameter and average void in volume is 60%. Disk-shaped ceramics with 5 mm in diameter and 2 mm thickness were used.

Marrow cells preparation and culture methods: Marrow cells were obtained from bone shaft of femora of 7 week old male Fisher 344 rats. Both ends of femora were cut away from the epiphysis, and the marrow was flushed out using 10 ml of culture medium [1]. The released cells were collected in two T-75 flasks containing 15 ml of the standard medium. The medium was changed after the first 24 hours to remove nonadherent cells. Subsequently, the medium was renewed three times a week. Cultures were maintained in a humidified atmosphere of 95% air with 5% CO_2 at 37°C. A standard medium consisted of Eagle-Minimal Essential Medium (MEM) containing 15% fetal bovine serum, and antibiotics (100 μg/ml Penicillin G, 50 μg/ml Gentamicine, and 0.3 μg/ml amphotericin B). After ten days in primary culture, marrow stromal cells were released from their culture substratum using 0.1% trypsin. The cells were concentrated by centrifuge at 900 rpm for 5 minutes at room temperature, resulting in 10^6 cells/ml. The HA disks were soaked in the cell suspension for 2 hours in a CO_2 incubator. After 2 hours of incubation, each HA disk was transferred into a 24 well-plate. One HA disk was subcultured in one well with 1 ml of the standard medium supplemented with 10 mM Na ß-glycerophosphate, 80 μg/ml vitamin C phosphate and 10^{-8}M dexamethasone. The medium was renewed three times a week and the cultures were maintained for 17 days. These subcultured marrow cells/HA composites were washed twice with 1 ml of Eagle-MEM and used for subcutaneous implantation into syngeneic 7 week old male rats.

Histological analysis: The subcutaneous implants were harvested 1, 2, 3, 4 and 20 weeks post implantation. The specimens were fixed in 10% buffered formalin, decalcified (K-CX solution, Falma Co., Tokyo) and stained with hematoxylin and eosin. These specimen were examined under light microscopy. To determine the bone dynamics in the composites, some rats were given one dose of tetracycline (50 mg/kg intramuscularly) 3 weeks after implantation. These specimens were harvested 4 weeks after implantation and used for undecalcified sections.

RESULTS

In the decalcified sectioned specimen of subcultured composites of marrow culture cells and porous HA disk, we could detect bone formation in some pores of HA in 8 of

12 implants one week after subcutaneous implantation (Table-l). In some pores, bone tissue together with active osteoblasts was observed in contact with the surface of the pores. The osteoblast layer in contact with bone was in close association with vasculature (Fig. l). At 2 weeks after implantation, mature bone areas could be detected. After 3 weeks and 4 weeks, consistent bone formation was observed in many pores (Fig. 2). At 20 weeks after implantation, almost all pores of the composite were filled with bone (Fig. 3). In this bone formation process, typical cartilage formation could not be found at any time, thus the process was so-called intramembranous bone formation. The bone formation was evidenced by active osteoblasts lining and the appearance of tetracycline labeling which was injected 3 weeks after implantation (Fig. 4).

Table l. Bone formation following subcutaneous implantation of subcultured composites. Ratio is number of implants with bone divided by number of total implants.

weeks post implantation	bone formation
1	8 / 12
2	9 / 12
3	10 / 12
4	8 / 8
20	8 / 8

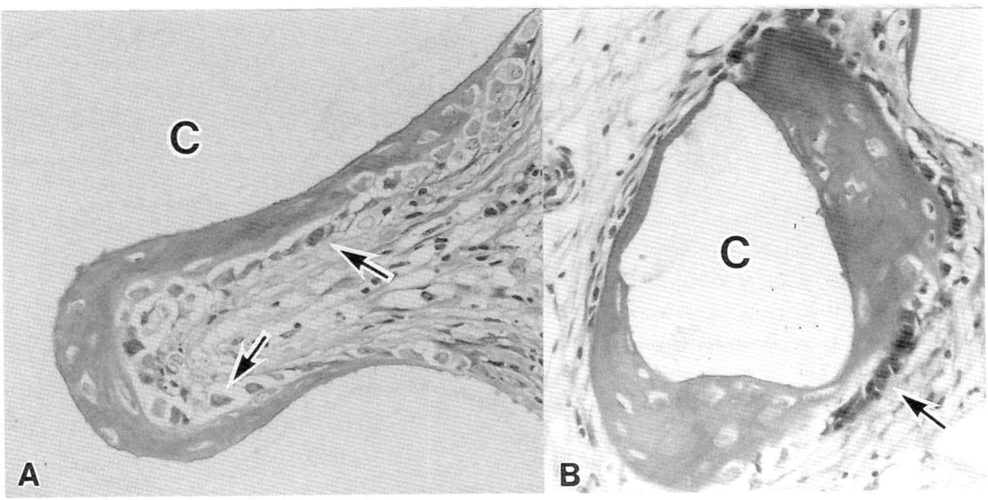

Figure l. (A, B) The subcultured marrow-cells/HA composite at 1 week after implantation White area shows the ghost of hydroxyapatite ceramic (C) produced by decalcification procedures. Black area indicates new bone appeared in porous area. (hematoxylin and eosin stain .x200). Arrows indicate active osteoblasts forming bone. Bone tissue together with active osteoblasts is seen in contact with the surface of the pores.

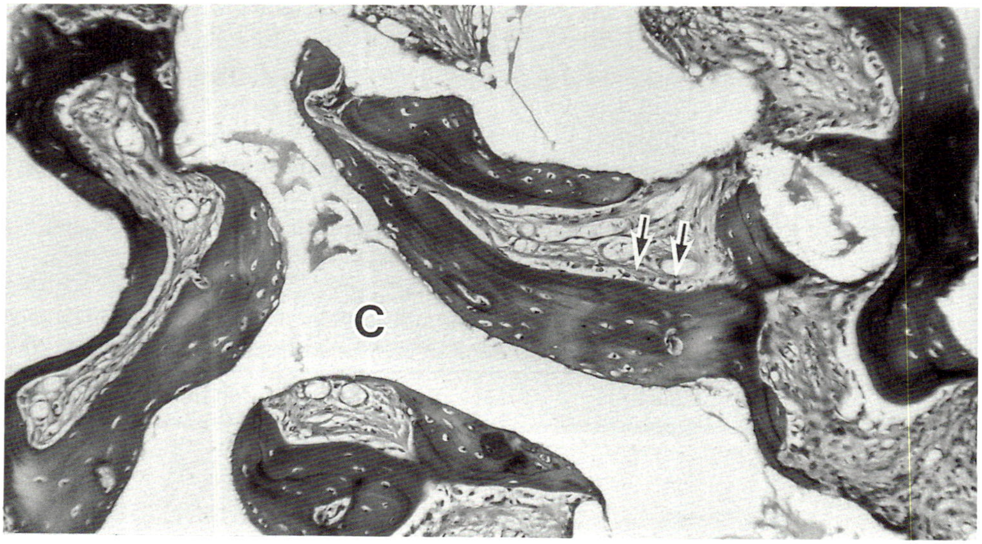

Figure 2. The subcultured marrow-cells/HA composite at 4 weeks after implantation White area shows the ghost of hydroxyapatite ceramic (C) produced by decalcification procedures. Black area indicates new bone appeared in porous area (hematoxylin and eosin stain x100). Arrows indicate active osteoblasts forming bone. Extensive bone formation are clearly seen in the pores.

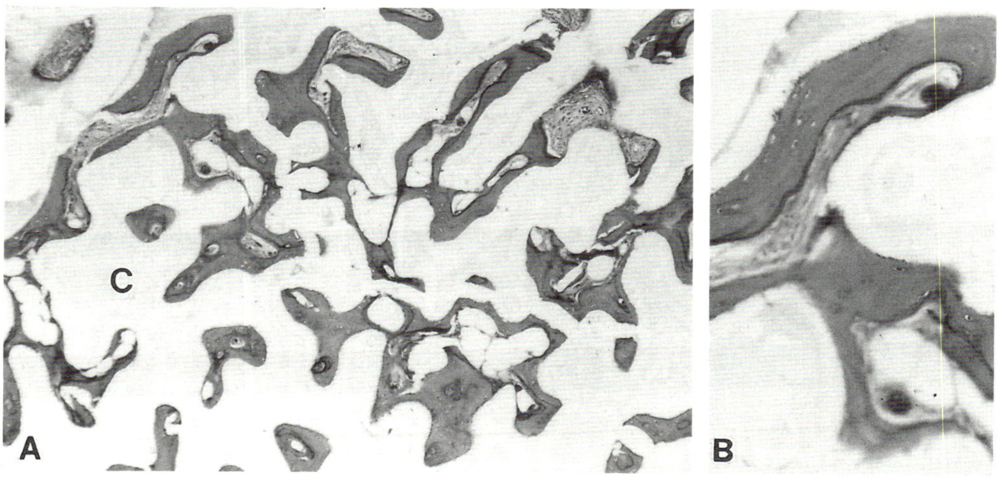

Figure 3. (A) The subcultured marrow-cells/HA composite at 20 weeks after implantation (hematoxylin and eosin stain x20). (B)Higher magnification (x50). Almost all pores of the composite are filled with bone.

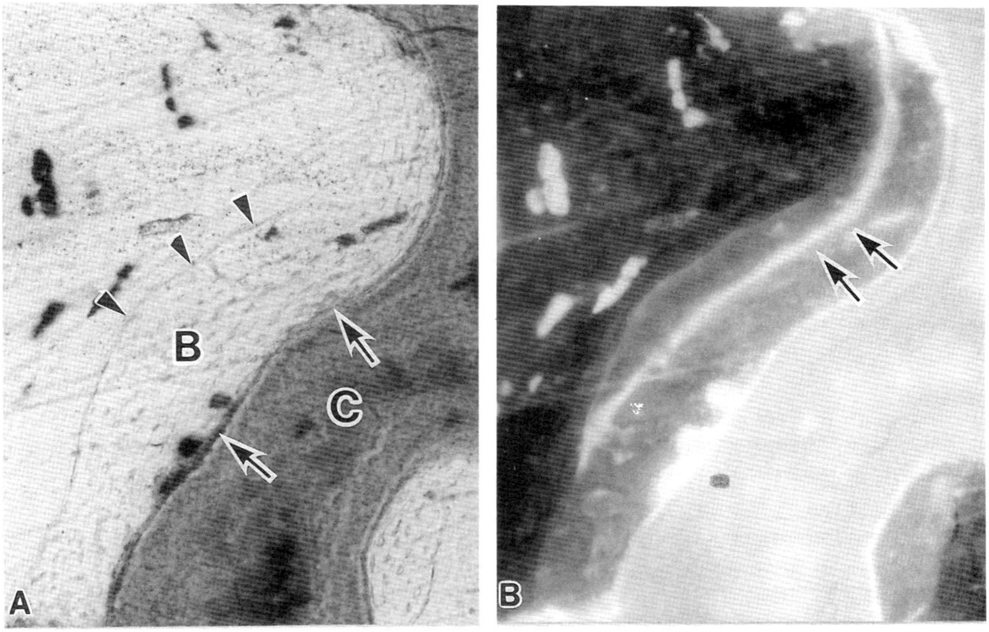

Figure 4. (A) Undecalcified section under microscopy at 4 weeks after implantation. Arrows indicate the interface between bone (B) and hydroxyapatite ceramic (C). Arrowheads indicate osteoid streams appearing as a black line (xl00).
(B) The same section under fluoroscopy. Arrows indicate tetracycline labeling, administrated 3 weeks after implantation. The fluorescent line is very sharp and not scattered.

DISCUSSION

In previous studies, it was reported that osteogenesis was observed inside the hydroxyapatite pores at 2 or 3 weeks post implantation when porous hydroxyapatite combined with freshly-isolated or cultured rat marrow cells was implanted at subcutaneous sites of syngeneic rats [6,8,12,13]. However, the composites did not show any bone formation at 1 week post implantation. In contrast, by using the culture technique presented here, osteogenesis could be detected even at 1 week after implantation. Also, more bone tissues were induced with less fresh marrow. Moreover, uptake of tetracycline was also observed and consistent osteogenesis was confirmed. This rapid *in vivo* bone forming capability of subcultured composites of HA and marrow cells was probably due to the pre existing *in vitro* bone tissue in the pore regions of the HA. In the subculture conditions, primary cultured marrow cells were needed on the porous structure of HA in the presence of Dex, which could induce osteoblastic differentiation of marrow stromal stem cells. Our preliminary experiments demonstrated the high alkaline phosphatase activity in the subcultured composite, indicating the osteoblastic differentiation. Based upon the fact that human cultured marrow cells possess osteogenic potential [14], the present method utilizing subcultured composite of HA and marrow cells can be applied for bone reconstructive surgery.

ACKNOWLEDGMENT

We thank Dr. Edwin C. Shor (Interpore International CA, USA) for supplying the ceramics.

REFERENCES

1. Maniatopoulos D., Sodek J. and Melcher A.H. *Cell Tissue Res.* 1988, 254, 317-330.
2. Davies J.E., Chernecky R., Lowenberg B. and Shiga A. *CellsMater.* 1991, 1, 3-15.
3. Davies J.E., Ottensmeyer P., Shen X., Hashimoto M., and Peel S.A.F., *The Bone Biomaterial Interface.* University of Toronto Press, 1991, 214-228.
4. Lowenberg B., Chernecky R., Shiga A. and Davies J.E., *Cells Mater.* 1991, 1, 177-187.
5. Yao K-L, Todescan R., JR. and Sodek J., *J. Bone and Minreral Res.,* 1994, 9, 231-240.
6. Ohgushi H., Goldberg V.M. and Caplan A.I. K. J. *Orthop. Res.* 1989, 7, 568-578.
7. Okumura M., Ohgushi H. and Tamai S., *Biomaterials,* 1991, 12, 411-416.
8. Yoshikawa T., Ohgushi H., Okumura M., Tamai S., Dohi Y. and Moriyama T. *Calcif. Tissue Int.,* 1992, 50, 184-188.
9. Yoshikawa T., Ohgushi H., Okumura M., Inoue K., Tamai S., Dohi Y. and Moriyama *T. Biomaterials-Tissue Interfaces,* Advances in Biomaterials, 1992, 10, 385-390.
10. Yoshikawa T., Ohgushi H., Okumura M., Tamai S., Dohi Y. and Moriyama T. *Bioceramoics* Volume 3, Rose-Human Institute of Technology, 1992, 157-162.
11. Holmes R.E., Buchololz R.W. and Mooney V. J. *Bone and Joint Surg* 1986, 68-A, 904-911.
12. Goshima J., Goldberg V.M. and Caplan A.I. K., *Clin. Orthop.* 1991, 262, 298-311.
13. Goshima J., Goldberg V.M. and Caplan A.I. K., *Biomaterials* 1991, 12, 253-258.
14. Ohgushi H. and Okumura M., *Acta. Orhtop. Scand.* 1990, 61, 431-434.

EFFECTS OF THE MIXING SOLUTION VOLUME ON ANTI-CANCER DRUG RELEASE FROM HOMOGENEOUS DRUG LOADED-SELF-SETTING CALCIUM PHOSPHATE CEMENT

M.Otsuka,[1] Y.Matsuda,[1] Y.Suwa,[2] J.L. Fox[3] and W.I. Higuchi[3]

Department of Pharmaceutical Technology,[1] Kobe Pharmaceutical University, Higashi-Nada, Kobe, Kyoritsu Ceramic Co. Ltd,[2] Minato, Nagoya and Department of Pharmaceutics and Pharmaceutical Chemistry,[3] University of Utah, Salt Lake City, Utah, U.S.A.

ABSTRACT

Effect of mixing solution volume (0.25-0.65 ml/g) on the *in vitro* drug release from a self-setting bioactive calcium phosphate cement containing the anti-cancer agent, 6-mercaptopurine (SMP) as a model compound was investigated. The drug release profiles from planar and whole surfaces of the cement systems containing 5% SMP were tested in simulated body fluid at pH 7.25, 37. °C. Drug release profiles from both the planar and whole surface of the cement matrix systems were analyzed using the Higuchi and Cobby equations, respectively, and the kinetic parameters were estimated using the nonlinear least-squares computer program. The relationships between the mixing solution volume and the drug release rate constants, or time required for 50% drug released, of the planar and whole surface cements showed a straight line.

INTRODUCTION

Polymethylmethacrylate cements have demonstrated clinical success as a combination bone filler and local drug delivery system for fixing non-bioactive prostheses to the surrounding bone [1]. However, this cement has several clinical problems for long-term application [2]. Hydroxyapatite (HAP) has an excellent bioaffinity with hard tissues [3] and would therefore be a viable candidate for long term use, which has led us to investigate drug delivery systems for various drugs [4-10] using a self-setting calcium phosphate cement [11,12] which is transformed from metastable calcium phosphate into HAP. In the present study, we tested the hypothesis that 6-mercaptopurine (SMP) release can be controlled by factors within the drug-containing cement, such as its porosity and geometrical structure.

EXPERIMENTAL

Materials

The cement powder system was an equimolar mixture of tetracalcium phosphate (TTCP, $Ca_4(PO_4)_2O$) and dicalcium phosphate dihydrate (DCPD, CaH $PO_4.2H_2O$) with added HAP seed crystals. (40%).

Procedures for cement formation

(A) Preparation of cement for release from a planar surface consisted of mixing calcium phosphate cement powder (0.5 g) with 0.125-0.325 ml of 20 mM H_3PO_4 for 1 min, then adding the drug powder (25 mg) to the paste. This mixture was then placed in a mold (8.5 mm in diameter, 3 mm in thickess) and stored at 37 C and 100% relative humidity for 24 h. The hardened cement pellet, with the mold, was mounted in a dissolution apparatus, so that only two faces of the pellet surface (1.13 cm^2) were exposed.

(B) The cement mixture was again placed in a mold (15 mm in diameter, 2mm in thickness) and stored at 37 C and 100% relative humidity for 24 h. The hardened cement pellet, without the mold, was mounted in a dissolution apparatus, so that the entire pellet surface (4.21 cm^2) was exposed.

Drug release test

Release profiles from all cement pellets containing the drug were measured as follows: A sample cement was placed in 25 ml of simulated body fluid (SBF)[14] (pH 7.25) in a 50 ml capped test tube at 37.0 ± 0.1°C. During the release test, the entire dissolution medium was replaced with fresh buffer at various intervals. The concentrations of 6-MP were measured spectrophotometrically (W 160A, Shimadzu Co., Kyoto, Japan) at 321 nm.

RESULTS AND DISCUSSION

Effect of Mixing Solution Volume on Drug Release from Planar- and Whole- Surface of Calcium Phosphate Cements.

The results of the effect of mixing solution volume on the drug release profiles from single planar surfaces and from the entire surfaces of the cement systems containing 5% SMP in pH 7.25 SBF at 37°C suggested that drug release rates from both cements increased with increasing mixing solution volume. This indicates that the volume affected the drug release rate, since the porosity of the cement matrix also depended on the volume. As reported previously [7-10], the drug release profiles from the planar surface of a homogeneous drug loaded calcium phosphate cement system followed the Higuchi equation [15]:

$$M_t = AM_0 \sqrt{C_s \frac{D_i \varepsilon}{\tau} (2C_d - \varepsilon C_s)t} = \mathrm{K}\, t^{1/2} \qquad \text{eq. 1}$$

where M_t is the amount of drug released from the cement at time t, K is Higuchi release rate constant, M_0 is the total amount of drug, A is the surface area of the tablet, D is the diffusion coefficient of the drug, C_s is the solubility, C_d is the concentration of drug, τ is the tortuosity and ε is the porosity. Therefore, the drug release was determined in part by the porosity and tortuosity of the cement pore.

For drug release from the entire surface, the area of the receding boundary implied in the Higuchi equation decreases with time. Cobby et al., [16] have developed a drug release equation (eq. 2) for various tablet shapes based upon Higuchi's equation (eq. 1) as follows;

$$f_1 = (q + 2)K_r\sqrt{t} - (2q + 1)(K_r\sqrt{t})^2 + q(K_r\sqrt{t})^3 \qquad \text{eq. 2}$$

where f_t is the fraction of the drug released at time t, K_r is the release rate constant and q is the ratio of the factors.

The drug release profiles from a planar surface and from the entire surface of the cement matrix systems were analyzed by using equations 1 and 2, and the kinetic parameters, K and K_r were estimated using the damping Gauss-Newton method and the nonlinear least-squares computer program MULTI[17].

Figure 1 shows the relationship between the mixing solution volume and the drug release rate constants for drug release from the planar surface and from the entire surface of the calcium phosphate cements. The drug release rate constants from both cements increase linearly with increasing mixing solution volume, indicating that it is possible to control the drug release by varying the mixing solution volume.

The T_{50} for drug release from the calcium phosphate cement exhibited a 50 fold difference between the minimum value from the planar surface cement and the maximum values obtained from the entire cement surface. For both systems, the values were proportional to the mixing solution volume, indicating that T_{50} could be controlled by a combination of the drug release style and variation of the mixing solution volume.

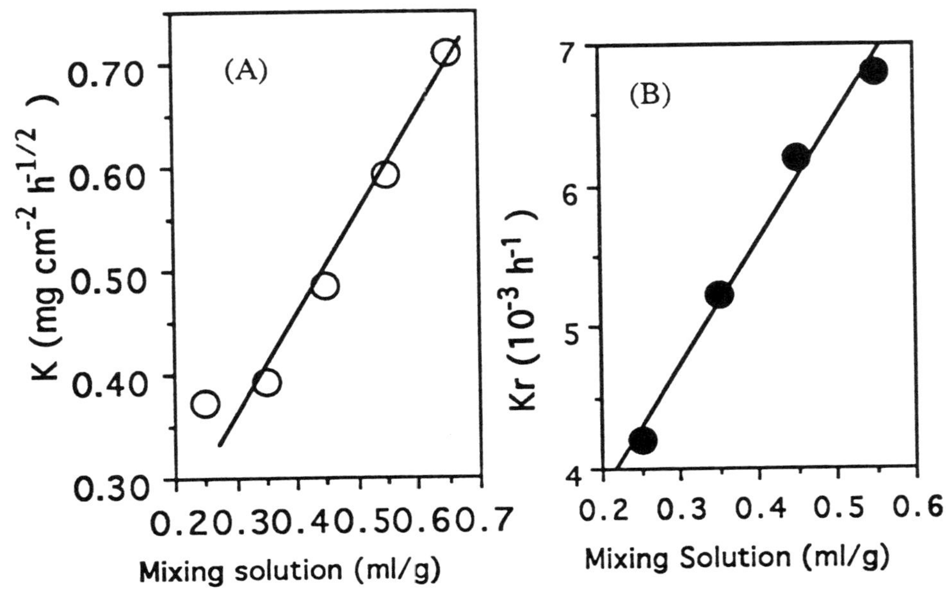

Figure 1. Relationship between mixing solution volume and drug release rate constants of 5% SMP-loaded calcium phosphate cements. (A) planar surface; (B) entire surface;

REFERENCES

1. Salvati, E. A. Callaghen, J. J. *et al., Clin. Orthop.,* 1986, 207, 83.
2. Petty, W. *J. Bone Jt. Surg.* 1978, 60 A, 752.
3. Aoki, H. "Science and Medical Applications of Hydroxyapatite", *Jpn. Ass. of Apatite Sci.*, Takayama Press. Sys. Cent. Co.,Tokyo; 1991 1-10.
4. Otsuka, M. Matsuda, Y. Yu, D. Wong, J. Fox, J. L. Higuchi, W. *I. Chem. Pharm. Bull.,* 1990, 38, 3500-3502.
5. Yu, D. Wong, J. Matsuda, Y. *et al., J.. Pharm. Sci.,* 81, 1992, 529-531.
6. Otsuka, M. Matsuda, Y. Suwa, Y. Fox, J. L. Higuchi, W. I. J. *Pharmn. Sci.,* 1994, 83, 259-263.
7. Otsuka, M. Matsuda, Y. *et al., Pharm. Phartnacol.* ***Lett.,*** 1994, 3, 173-175.
8. Otsuka, M. Matsuda, Y. et al. *Pharm. Pharmacol. Lett.,* 1994, 3, 183-185.
9. Otsuka, M. Matsuda, *et al., J. Pharm. Sci.,* 1994, 83, 611-615.
10. Otsuka, M. Matsuda, Y. et al. *J. Pharm. Sci.,* 1994, 83, 255-258 (1994).
11. Brown, W. E. Chow, C. L. U.S. Patent 4,612,053 (1986).
12. Takezawa, Y. Doi, Y. *et al., Jpn. J. of Oral Biology,* 1989, 31, 240-247.
13. Wong, J. Otsuka, M. Higuchi, W. I. Powell, G. L. Fox, J. L. *J. Pharm.* Sci., 1990, 79, 510-514.
14. Kokubo, T. Yoshiwara, S. Nishimura, N. and Yamamuro, T., *J. Am. Ceram.* Soc., 1991, 74, 1739-1741.
15. Higuchi, T. *J. Pharm. Sci., 1963,* 52, 1145 1149.
16. Cobby, J. Mayersohn, M. and Malker, G., *J. phartn. Sci.,* 1974, 63, 725 732.
17. Yamaoka, K. Tanigawara, Y. Nakagawa, T. Uno, T. *J. Pharmaco-Dyn.,* 1981, 4, 879-885.

OSTEOGENIC RESPONSE IN POROUS 50 VOL% ZIRCONIA DISPERSED HYDROXYAPATITE CERAMICS

M. Takagi, A. Suda, T. Sato, A. Ishikawa, T. Osanai, H. Kato and H. Orui

Department of Orthopaedic Surgery, Yamagata University School of Medicine, 2-2-2 Iida-Nishi, Yamagata 990-23, JAPAN

ABSTRACT

Osteogenic response to porous 50 vol% zirconia dispersed hydroxyapatite ceramics (ZH-C) was examined histologically and compared to that of porous hydroxyapatite ceramics (HAP-C). Excellent osteogenic response to porous ZH-C was observed in rabbit femur as well as to HAP-C. This suggest an excellent biocompatibility of porous ZH-C as bioactive ceramics in addition to its excellent mechanical properties, and possible clinical application of porous ZH-C.

INTRODUCTION

Hydroxyapatite ceramic is bioactive and has an excellent affinity to the osseous tissues [1,2]. However, strength and toughness of hydroxyapatite (HA) are sometimes inadequate in clinical weight-bearing applications and in joint replacement [2-4]. Although zirconia ceramics (Zr-C) have been proven to have sufficient strength and toughness in comparison with of HA, it is biologically inert [1,3]. We have developed a ceramic material, using a novel technique, in which 50 vol% zirconia was dispersed in an HA matrix [3]. The biocompatibility of ceramic materials consisting of HA and 50% Zr by volume under static or load-bearing conditions has been studied and excellent osteogenic conduction around ZH-C was observed [3-10]. In this study osteogenic response of ZH-C in porous form was examined and compared with that of porous HA.

MATERIALS AND METHODS

ZH-C was sintered at 1400°C for one hour. The average porosity was 50% and the pore-size ranged from 40 μm to 150 μm. HA-C was sintered at 1250°C for one hour. The average porosity was 47% and the pore-size ranged from 40 μm to 150 μm. Columnar ceramic blocks of ZH-C and HA-C, 10 mm in length and 5 mm in diameter, were prepared (Figure 1) and inserted into the right and left femurs of six adult rabbits under anesthesia. The hole was made by drilling from the lateral to medial side of the cortex in the distal metaphyseal region. Three months after implantation, the rabbits were killed under anesthesia, and radiographs of femurs containing the porous implants were taken. The isolated femurs were immediately fixed with 70 % methanol. The samples were

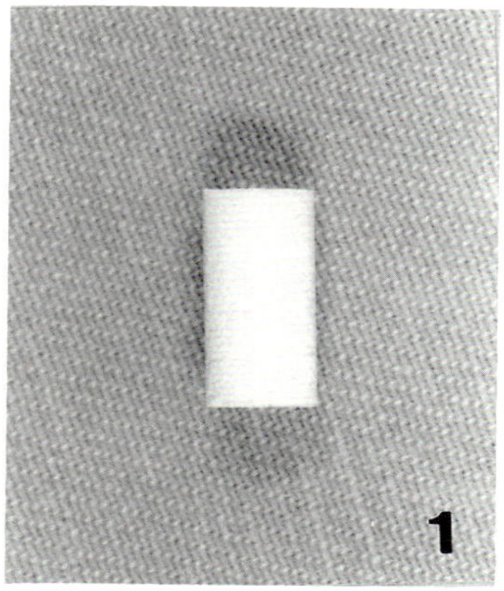

Figure 1. A columnar block of porous 50 vol% zircon is dispersed hydroxyapatite ceramics used in the study.

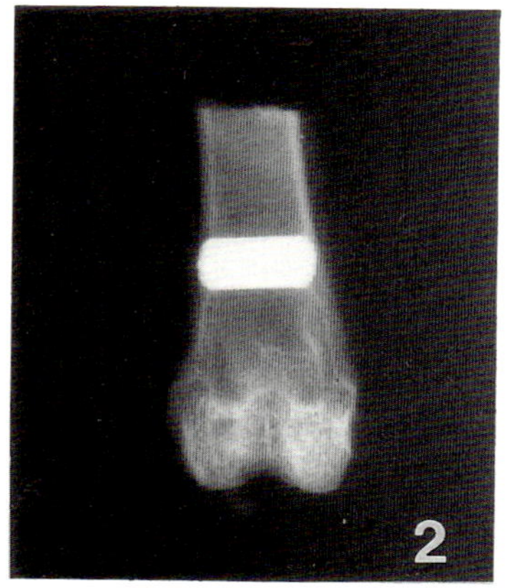

Figure 2. A radiograph of the distal femur of the rabbit with a porous 50 vol% zirconia dispersed hydroxyapatite ceramics after three months of implantation.

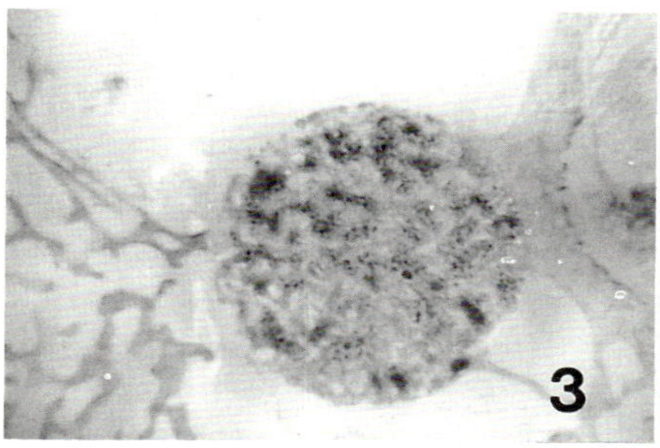

Figure 3. Osteogenic response in the pores of 50 vol% zirconia dispersed hydroxyapatite ceramic after three months of implantation.

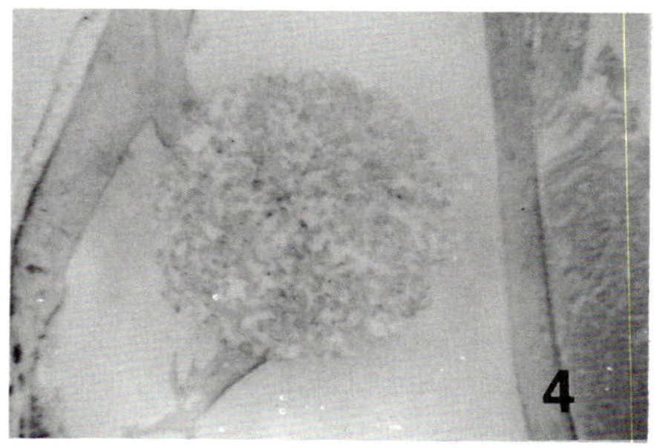

Figure 4. Osteogenic response in the pores of hydroxyapatite ceramic after three months of implantation.

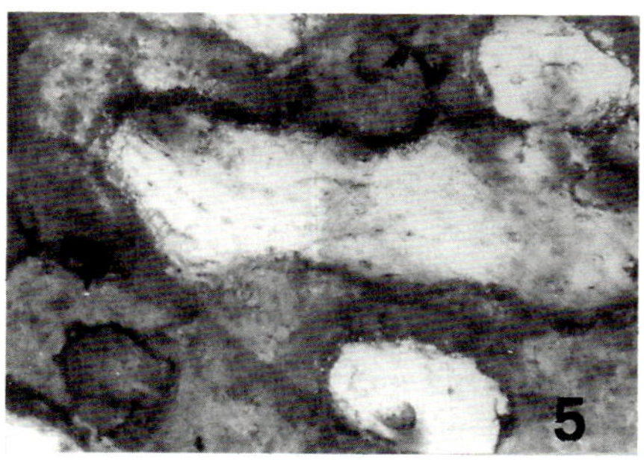

Figure 5. High power magnification of the osteogenic response observed in the pores of 50 vol% zirconia dispersed hydroxyapatite ceramic after three months of implantation.

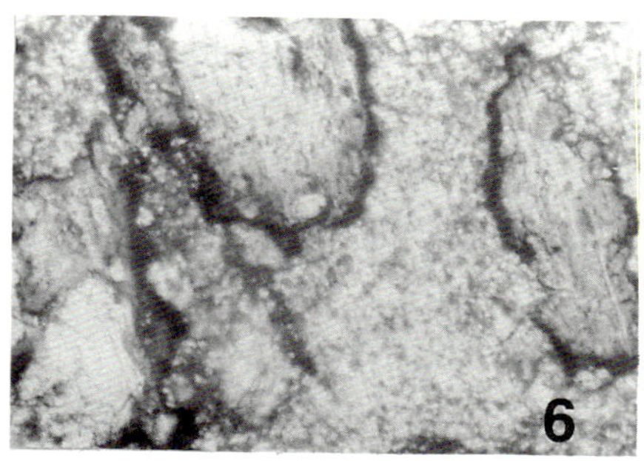

Figure 6. High power magnification of the osteogenic response observed in the pores of hydroxyapatite ceramic after three months of implantation.

sequentially dehydrated and embedded in methylmethacrylate resin, followed by the sectioning with a microtome (EXAKT Corp., Germany). The sections were stained with toluidine blue without decalcification and examined by an optical microscopy.

RESULTS

The radiographic observation showed osteointegration, and no evidence of loosening and bone atrophy around implant either type of after three months (Figure 2). In sagittal sections of the femurs, excellent osteogenic response in the pores was seen in porous ZH-C (Figure 3) as well as in porous HA-C (Figure 4). At high power magnification, osteogenic response was seen inside the pores, which was often filled by osseous tissue, where osteocyte arrangement and osteoblastic lining were observed, without intervening fibrous membrane between ceramic and host tissue in porous ZH-C (Figure 5) as well as in porous HA-C (Figure 6). No marked difference of osteoconduction into the pores was observed between ZH-C and HA-C.

DISCUSSION

Two main types of bioceramics, namely bioactive and bioinert ceramics have been reported. Bioactive ceramics, including HAP-C, have the property of direct chemical bonding to the host osseous tissues. However, this type of bioceramic is not mechanically strong enough, whereas, bioinert ceramics including Zr-C, are known to be stronger and tougher than other bioactive ceramics. We have developed a 50 vol% ZH-C material using a unique technique and have already reported the biocompatibility of 50 vol% ZH-C under static or load-bearing conditions [3-10]. In this study, the excellent osteogenic response of porous ZH-C and of porous HA-C. Niwa *et al.* [11] reported that porous HA-C with 90 μm pore size did not allow osteogenic conduction from surrounding bone into the center of the porous implants. In this study, we used a pore size ranging from 40 μm to 150 μm for the ceramics, which might encourage osteoconduction even into the whole area of the pores. In addition to the excellent osteogenetic response as good as that of HA-C, porous ZH-C may be less likely to produce microparticles under load-bearing conditions due to its mechanical properties. This would contribute to the prevention of unfavorable host responses, such as prosthetic loosening [12-14].

ACKNOWLEDGMENT

This work was partially supported by the Japan Society for the Promotion of Science, Grant-in-Aid for JPJS Fellows and Grant-in-Aid for Scientific Research, The Ministry of Education, Science and Culture, Japan, 1994-1995.

REFERENCES

1. Suda, A.: Orthopaedic Surgery, 42: 690-693, 1991.
2. Yamamuro, T.: Clinical Orthopaedic Surgery, 21: 1221-1224, 1986.
3. Suda, A., et al..: J. Jpn Orthop. Assoc., 64:250-259, 1990.
4. Suda, A., Osanai, T., Sato, T., et al. : Bioceramics, 5:191-196, 1992.
5. Suda, A., et al.: Orthopaedic Surgery and Traumatology, 33: 193-199, 1990
6. Suda, A., et al. : Orthopaedic Ceramic Implant, 7:165-168, 1987.
7. Suda, A., et al. : Orthopaedic Ceramic Implant, 8:135-138, 1988.
8. Iino, M., et al.: Orthopaedic Ceramic Implant, 10:171-175, 1990.
9. Iino, M., et al. : Orthopaedic Ceramic Implant, 9:153-159, 1991.

10. Fukuda, M., et al. : Orthopaedic Ceramic Implant, 11:23-27, 1991.
11. Niwa, S.: Clinical Orthopaedic Surgery, 21:1233-1240, 1986.
12. Jasty, M., et al.: Clin. Orthop. 308: 111-126, 1994.
13. Santavirta, S., et al.: J. Bone Joint Surg. (Br) 73(B): 38-42, 1992.
14. Takagi, M., et al.: J. Bone Joint Surg. (Am) 77-A: 16-25, 1995.

A HYDROXYAPATITE-POLYMER COMPOSITE PREPARED BY MIMICKING BONE MINERALIZATION

P.J. Li[1], D. Bakker[2] and C.A. van Blitterswijk[3]

Department of Bioengineering, University of Pennsylvania, Philadelphia, PA 19104[1]
HC Implants BV, Leiden, The Netherlands[2]
Biomaterials Research Groups, School of Medicine, Leiden University, The Netherlands[3]

ABSTRACT

We report here a method to produce hydroxyapatite-polymer composite at 37 °C by mimicking the mineralization of bone. The method involves the incubation of a synthetic polymer in a calcium phosphate solution. The polymer, which models the biological matrix, can swell and transform into a hydrogel in an aqueous environment. The calcium phosphate solution, which was used to imitate the physiological fluid, is supersaturated with respect to hydroxyapatite; but its supersaturation degree is not high enough for spontaneous precipitation to occur. The polymer powders were incubated in calcium phosphate solution at body temperature (37 °C), hydroxyapatite precipitation was then induced within the matrix of the polymer hydrogel. The formation of hydroxyapatite on a large scale in the entire polymer matrix produced a hydroxyapatite-polymer composite. The composite, which included a hydroxyapatite phase with concentration as high as 30% by weight, was fabricated in two weeks.

INTRODUCTION

Desirable biomaterials for implantation are those biologically and mechanically compatible with bone. Hydroxyapatite ceramics have proven to be bioactive. Resembling bone hydroxyapatite, they are capable of and chemical bonding to bone. So far, hydroxyapatite ceramics have been used successfully to manufacture prostheses which are required to bond to bone. However, these materials are not mechanically compatible with bone because of high Young's moduli. This can cause stress shielding in bone, leading to bone resorption when they are implanted to bear load. Polymeric materials have much lower Young's moduli than hydroxyapatite ceramics, but they are often unsuitable as implant materials because of a lack of bioactivity. A hydroxyapatite-polymer composite was proposed as an analogous material for bone replacement [1]. The a composite was expected to have the low Young's modulus of the polymer while retaining the bioactivity of hydroxyapatite. The retention of bioactivity requires a high content of hydroxyapatite in the composite which in turn deteriorates the mechanical properties of the material [2]. Therefore, the balance between mechanical properties and bioactivity has to be taken into account when such composite is made.

Bones are hydroxyapatite-polymer composites made by bone cells. Bone formation proceeds in a definite sequence [3]. Bone cells first secrete organic macromolecules which then assemble to form a polymeric matrix. Next, hydroxyapatite formation is initiated within the matrix from the physiological fluid that contains calcium and phosphate. Bone cells act as the manufacturer of the polymer matrix. The created polymer serves as a promoter of hydroxyapatite generation. The physiological solution functions as a source of calcium and phosphate for the formation of hydroxyapatite. Not surprisingly, the bone mineralization can be mimicked if (1) an appropriate polymer can be synthesized to imitate the polymeric matrix of bone; (2) a calcium phosphate containing solution can be prepared to model the physiological solution.

The objective of this study is to produce a hydroxyapatite-polymer composite by mimicking bone mineralization.

MATERIALS AND METHODS

A block co-polymer, composed of 80 wt% of hydrophilic soft segment poly(ethylene oxide) (PEO) and 20 wt% of hydrophobic hard segment poly(butylene terephthalate) (PBT), was selected to imitate the biological matrix, for it has been found to be biologically calcified [4]. The polymer powders ($< 300\ \mu m$) were then incubated in a calcium phosphate-containing solution, modeling the physiological solution. The calcium phosphate solution contains all the major inorganic compounds found in the body fluid and is buffered at pH 7.4 at 37°C with tris-(hydroxymethyl) aminomethane and hydrochloric acid [5]. This solution is metastable, it is supersaturated with respect to hydroxyapatite, but it does not precipitate spontaneously. Calcium phosphate precipitation took place from the solution only as the soaked polymer powders swelled and transformed into a hydrogel. This can be identified by a drop in the calcium concentration in the solution, which was measured by a calcium electrode. The mineralized polymer, or hydroxyapatite-polymer composite, was characterized by X-ray diffraction analysis (XRD), Infrared spectroscopy (IR), Scanning Electron Microscopy (SEM) and Transmission Electron Microscopy (TEM).

RESULTS AND DISCUSSION

The electrical potential of the calcium electrode which is proportional to the calcium concentration, decreased with the time of incubation (Figure 1). Since the calcium phosphate solution is buffered, there was no change in pH value during the precipitation. Analyses by XRD and IR identified the precipitate as carbonate containing hydroxyapatite (Figure 2). The hydroxyapatite deposited within the entire polymer matrix, left a hydroxyapatite-polymer composite behind (Figure 3).

The microstructure of such composite was studied by TEM. A TEM micrograph of the composite, containing up to about 30 wt% of hydroxyapatite, shows that the apatite was homogeneously dispersed in the matrix. The electron diffraction pattern confirms the formation of hydroxyapatite within the polymer. Since the polymer is Ca, P-free, the calcium and phosphate essential for the hydroxyapatite precipitation exclusively came exclusively from the calcium phosphate solution, which functions as the source of the calcium and phosphate for the formation of the hydroxyapatite mineral in the composite. As the calcium and phosphate transferred from the solution to the polymer,

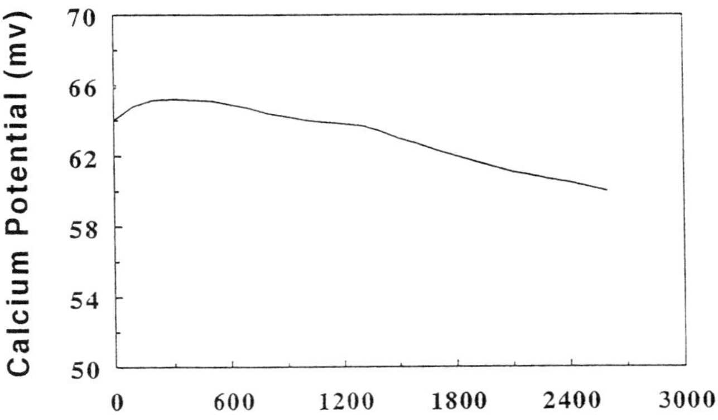

Figure 1 The Ca potential in the solution as a function of incubation time.

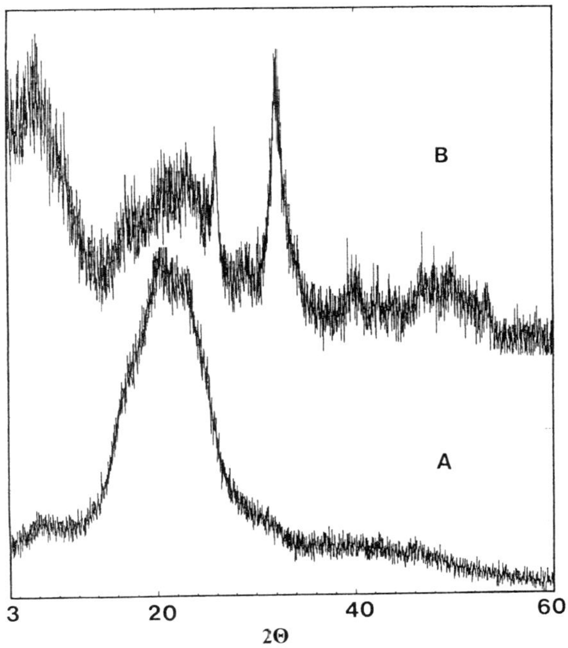

Figure 2. XRD pattern of the composite produced by *in situ* precipitation of hydroxyapatite within the polymer (B); the pattern of the polymer before incubation is given in (A).

their concentrations decreased in the solution. As a result, the hydroxyapatite deposition slowed and eventually came to stop, unless the solution was augmented with calcium and phosphate. This can be done on the principle of the constant composition method [6]. Hydroxyapatite phase density of mineralized polymer increased as the incubation time was prolonged. To date, we are able to produce the composite containing up to 30 wt% of hydroxyapatite in two weeks. Since biological composites usually have an extremely high fraction of inorganic minerals, for instance in cortical bone, hydroxyapatite accounts for 70% of its weight, a high content of hydroxyapatite seems to be needed to fabricate composite of comparable mechanical properties.

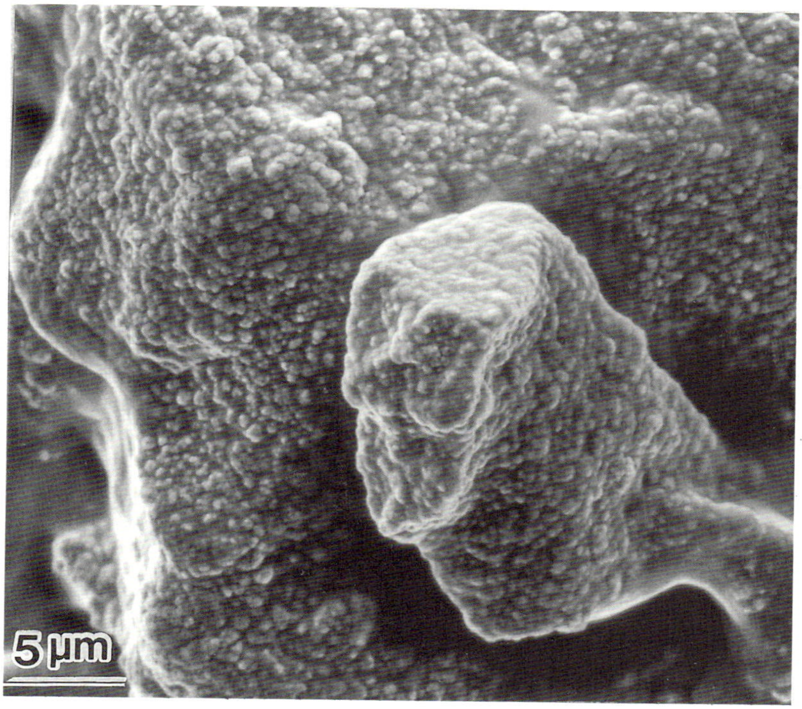

Figure 3. SEM picture for the hydroxyapatite-polymer composite in which nano-range hydroxyapatite needles were precipitated within the polymer matrix.

REFERENCE

1. W. Bonfield, M. D. Grynpas and A. E. Tully, Biomaterials 2(1981):185-186
2. W. Bonfield, in Bioceramics: materials characteristics versus in vivo behavior, P. Ducheyne and J. E. Lemons (eds), Annals of the New York Academy of Science Vol. 523 (1988) pp.173-177).
3. M. J. Glimcher, in The chemistry and biology of mineralized connective tissue, A. Veis (ed), Elsevier, Amsterdam (1981), pp.618-675.

4. C. A. van Blitterswijk, D. Bakker, H. Leenders, J. v.d. Brink, S. C. Hesseling, Y. P. Bovell, A. M. Radder, R. J. Sakkers, M. L. Gaillard, P. H. Heinze and G. J. Beumer,, in Bonebonding biomaterials, P. Ducheyne, T. Kokubo and C. A. van Blitterswijk (eds), Reed Healthcare Communications, The Netherlands (1992), pp.13-30.
5. T. Kokubo, H. Kushitani, S. Sakka, T. Kitsugi, T. Yamamuro, J. Biomed. Mater. Res. 24:721 734 (1990).
6. M. B. Tomson and G. H. Nancollas, Science 200:1059 (1978).

PREPARATION OF BIOACTIVE POLYMERS MODIFIED WITH SILANOL GROUPS

Akiyoshi Osaka, Chikara Ohtsuki and Kanji Tsuru

Biomaterials Lab., Faculty of Engineering, Okayama University Tsushima, Okayama-shi 700, Japan

ABSTRACT

Inorganic-organic composite polymers were prepared by polymerizing vinyl trimethoxysilane and incorporating Ca(II). Precipitation of apatite layer was confirmed within a day on the polymer surface after soaking in a simulated body fluid. Addition of calcium acetate was effective to provide bioactivity but not other salts like calcium chloride. Addition of silica sol derived from hydrolysis of tetraethoxysilane instantly solidified the polymers and the solids showed no bioactivity. This was attributed to condensation between the silanol groups of the polymer and the silica sol.

INTRODUCTION

Polyactive® [1], a block copolymer of poly(ethylene oxide) and poly(butylene terephthalate), is the only bone-bonding organic polymer known. Although some attempts were reported to provide polymers with bioactivity due to surface modification [2,3] various bioactive polymers are to be developed for enlarging the horizon of polymers for clinical application. Some ceramic materials, composed of CaO and SiO_2 as the major ingredients, are bioactive and form a bone-like hydroxyapatite layer through which they bond to living bones when they are embedded in the human body [3]. The Ca(II) ions dissolved from the material surface increase the degree of supersaturation concerning apatite, while the silica gel layer thus resulted serves nucleation and growth sites for apatite [3]. It is thus suggested that inorganic-organic composite polymers containing silanol groups and Ca(II) ions should be bioactive. Thus, we have synthesized silanol-modified polymers starting from vinyl trimethoxysilane (VTS-M). Calcium salts such as calcium chloride, nitrate and acetate are incorporated in the composite polymer and tetraethoxysilane (TEOS) is co-polymerized, and their effect on bioactivity is examined.

EXPERIMENTAL PROCEDURE

The synthesis route is illustrated in Figure 1. Vacuum-distilled VTS-M (9.8g or 0.66 mol in monomer unit) was placed in a 200 mL flask filled with dry nitrogen. Addition

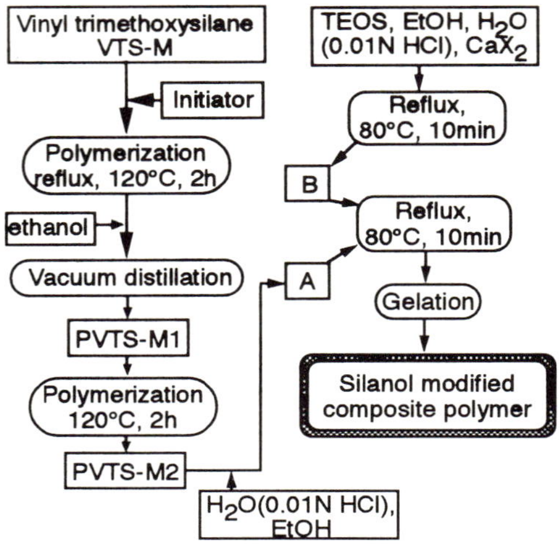

Figure l. Synthesis of bioactive silanol modified polymers.

of 0.49 g di-t-butyl peroxide (5 mol%) to the silane kept at 120°C initiated polymerization [4]. After 2 h reaction the resultant viscous liquid (PVTS M1) was dissolved into dry ethanol held in a 50 mL beaker and was kept further at 12°C for 2 h to remove lower molecular weight oligomers as well as the solvent and to deactivate the initiator. The obtained product (PVTS M2) was mixed with ethanol and H_2O where the molar ratio of PVTS M2: ethanol: H_20 was 1: 8: 3. In order to incorporate Ca(II) ions to the polymers CaX_2 (X=CH_3COO, Cl, and NO_3) was added to PVTS M2 so that the molar ratio Ca/VTS M =0.05/1 was attained, and was refluxed at 60°C for 80 min (solution A). Gel permeation chromatograms of the intermediates, PVTS M1 and PVTS M2, were taken on a Shodex System 11 with polystyrene as the standard. The resulted viscous liquid was cast into covered polystyrene boxes 3x3xl cm^3 in size and held at 40°C until gelation. The final mixing ratio VTS-M: ethanol: H_2O: Ca of the gel was 1: 8: 3: 0.05 (mol). Flexible gels resulted after drying at 40°C with removing the cover. Transmission FT-IR spectra of the dried gels were measured by the KBr method.

A simulated body fluid (SBF) was prepared by dissolving reagent grade NaCI, KCI, K_2HPO_4, $MgC1_2 \cdot 6H_2O$, $CaCl_2$ and Na_2SO_4 and adjusting pH to 7.25 as reported elsewhere [5]. The gel specimens 10x10xl mm^3 in size were soaked in 35 mL SBF kept at 36.5°C up to 14 days. Structural changes in the surfaces of the soaked specimen were examined by thin film X-ray diffraction (XRD), FT-IR reflection spectroscopy, scanning electron microscopy and energy dispersion X-ray analysis. SBF was analyzed for Ca(II), Si(IV) and P(V) using inductively coupled plasma photometry (ICP).

RESULTS

The gel permeation chromatographs of PVTS-M1 showed a broad and strong peak centered at 3000 in molecular weight (MW) and a shoulder at 55000 as well as a trace peak at 700. Thus PVTS-M1 consisted mostly of oligomers of 25 to 30 units since the vinyl trimethoxysilane monomer is 148 in MW. As PVTS-M1 was aged to be PVTS-M2, the 55000 MW peak grew at the expense of the 3000 MW peak indicating that polymerization still continued. FT-IR spectrum of the dried gel showed a peak at 3450 cm^{-1} assigned to H-O stretching whose intensity was lower than that of a silica gel prepared by an ordinary sol-gel reaction of H_2O and tetraethoxysilane under catalysis with hydrochloric acid. Moreover, a peak due to methyl C-H bonds in $Si(OCH_3)_3$ was observed at 2950 cm^{-1} with medium strength. It follows that a larger fraction of methoxy groups in the gels remained unhydrolysed despite the presence of H_2O in solution A.

Figure 2 shows FT-IR reflection spectra and thin-film XRD patterns of the surface of the gels soaked in SBF up to 7 days. The IR peak at 1080 cm^{-1} for the specimens was assigned to υ(Si-O) [6]. After 6h soaking a peak was observed at 600 cm^{-1}, assigned to δ(P-O) [6], above noisy backgrounds. Moreover, a peak appeared at 1130 cm^{-1}, assigned to υ(P-O), after 12h soaking. These two peaks suggested the precipitation of phosphate ions or compounds on the surfaces. Indeed, the thin-film XRD patterns for the specimen soaked in SBF for >6h showed two distinct peaks of (002) diffraction and an envelope of (211), (112) and (300) peaks of hydroxyapatite. The results indicated that the present gel was as bioactive as calcium metasilicate glass and Glass-Ceramic A-W® [7]. Scanning electron microphotographs of the gel surface after soaked in SBF for >3h exhibited a number of crystal chips that grew to agglomeration of petal-shaped crystallites covering the whole surface. Energy dispersion X-ray analysis of Ca, P and Si for the apatite-precipitated surface gave an almost constant atomic ratio Ca/P $\approx$ 2 while the fraction of Si decreased with the soaking period until it reached 3 atomic % for the 7 d-soaked specimen. This indicated continuous growth of the apatite layer.

DISCUSSION

In order to enhance bioactivity of the composite polymer, an attempt was made to hydrolyze the methoxy groups of PVTS-M2 by addition of 0.01N aqueous HCl solution instead of H_2O. However, it was solidified as soon as the addition of the HCl solution, probably due to condensation among silanol groups derived from the methoxy groups. Composition of solution B could control the properties of the composite polymer. Without the silica sol derived from TEOS the resulted polymers were very soft and flexible, while increasing the silica content in solution B not only hardened the polymer but reduced bioactivity. Mixture of solutions A and B having the 1 to 1 silica sol to PVTS-M2 ratio

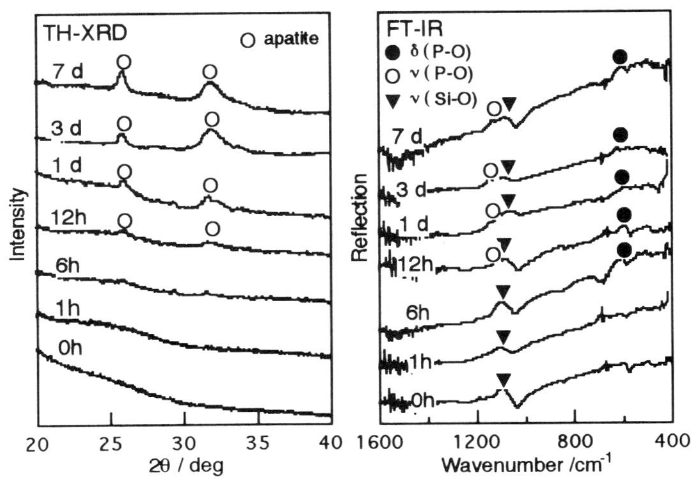

Figure 2. Thin film X-ray diffraction patterns and FT-IR reflection spectra of the composite polymers soaked in SBF up to 7 days.

gave brittle gels. This was attributed to consumption of silanol groups on PVTS-M2 in solution A due to condensation with the silica sol in solution B. Bioactivity of the composite polymer also depended on the calcium salts. Calcium acetate was only one that yielded a bioactive polymer. The other salts, nitrate and chloride, resulted in a brittle composite polymer with slight bioactivity. This was explained by a reduced number of active silanol groups in the polymer. Those salts may have acidified the mixture of solutions A and B and hence enhanced hydrolysis of the methoxy groups of PVTS-M2 to give many silanols to be condensed, as in the case of HCl addition. However, calcium acetate could keep solution B neutral to alkaline and thus a greater fraction of the methoxy group remained until they were hydrolyzed in SBF at soaking.

Mechanism of apatite formation

Figure 3 shows concentration of Ca(II), P(V) and Si(IV) ions in SBF as a function of soaking time. The specimen had a composition VTS-M: ethanol: H_2O: $Ca(CH_3COO)_2$ = 1: 8: 3: 0.05. The decrease in P(V) within 6 h indicated adsorption of phosphate species on the surface that started immediately after immersion in SBF. The increase in Ca(II) within 3 h represented release of Ca(II) from the specimen while the local minimum around 6 h corresponded to the rapid crystallization of apatite consistent with the decrease in P(V). Continuous crystallization of apatite gradually decreased the concentration of Ca(II) and P(V) after 1 day soaking.

ACKNOWLEDGMENTS

The authors gratefully acknowledge Professor T. Kokubo at Kyoto University for ICP analysis and thin film X-ray diffraction measurements.

REFERENCES

1. Bakker, D., van Blitterswijk, C.A., Hesseling, S.C., Daems, W.Th. and Grote, J.J. *J. Biomed. Mat. Res.* 1990, 24, 2M.
2. Tsuru, K., Nishiyama, C., Ohtsuki, C. and Osaka, A. *Memoirs Fac. Eng. Okayama Univ.* 1995, 29,77-81.
3. T. Kokubo, *J. Ceram. Soc. Japan* 1990, 99, 965-73.

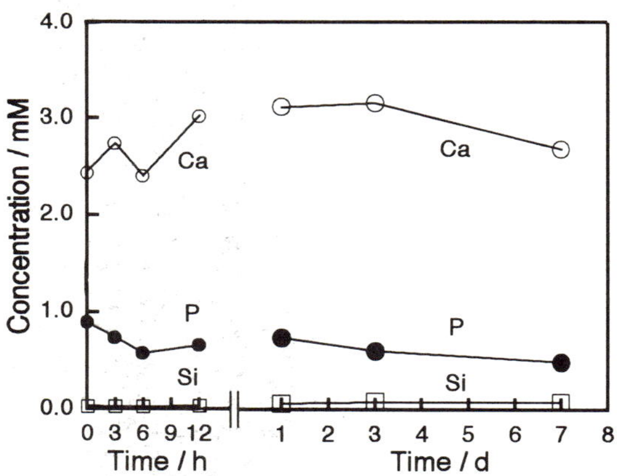

Figure 3. Concentration of Ca(II), P(V) and Si(IV) in SBF after soaking the composite polymer up to 7 days. Analysed with ICP.

4. Namiki, T., Nagao, Y., Abe, Y. in *"Extended abstracts for 9th Symposium on Inorganic Polymers,"* Polymer Society of Japan, November, 1990, Tokyo.
5. Ohtsuki, C., Kushitani, H., Kokubo, T., Kotani, S. and Yamamuro, T. J. Biomed. Mat.
6. *Res.* 1991, 25, 1363-1370. Hench, L.L. *J. Am. Ceram. Soc. 1991,* 74, 1487-1510.
7. Ebisawa, Y., Kokubo, T., Ohura, K and Yamamuro, T. *J. Mat. Sci.: Materials Med.,* 1990, 1,239-244.

CERAMIC PROCESSING OF TITANIA FOR BIOMEDICAL APPLICATIONS

K.-L. Eckert, S.-W. Ha, M. Mathey and E. Wintermantel

Chair of Biocompatible Science and Engineering (Prof. Dr. E. Wintermantel)
ETH Zurich, Wagistrasse 6, CH-8952 Schlieren

ABSTRACT

A ceramic powder for preparation of biocompatible porous titanium dioxide ceramics was developed, which has an average grain diameter of 7 µm and a narrow grain size distribution. The raw powder was a commercially available titanium dioxide powder. It was calcined in order to effect a defined crystal growth, then deagglomerated by milling. The milled powder was subjected to a sedimentation sizing procedure. A ceramic material which exhibited open porosity was prepared from the thus obtained powder. The powder is therefore appropriate for manufacturing porous cell carriers.

INTRODUCTION

It is known from titanium load transmitting implants such as hip endoprostheses and osteosynthesis devices that their surfaces allow direct ongrowth of local tissue. When applied to bone these surfaces demonstrate preferential growth of bone cells and not of connective tissue. Titanium dioxide surface layers of hip prosthesis stems have proven to be extraordinarily biocompatible [1]. This makes titanium dioxide ceramics a promising material for implant applications, especially for non-load bearing, microporous implants like cell carriers [2]. In a preceding work, ceramic cell carriers were developed out of a special aluminum oxide raw material. Those cell carriers were highly porous and had a specific shape which could induce directional vascularization if implanted into an organism. They were produced by a shaping process which used steam pressure to build up a hollow-sphere-morphology. It was the aim of this work to develop a titanium dioxide powder with properties adapted to the requirements of the above mentioned shaping process. Experience from preceding work shows that powders with rather coarse mean grain sizes 5-15 µm and narrow distributions are needed. Due to their narrow size distributions such powders exhibit low packing densities after green shaping. The rather coarse grain sizes lead to low sintering rates which allow close control of densification. Thus the development of pores can be controlled. Commercial titanium dioxide raw materials are not suitable for the preparation of porous ceramic raw materials because of their small crystallite size, which is due to the main use of these powders as white

Table 1: Powder properties of titanium dioxide Kronos 1171.

Purity standards EC-Standard 67/653/EWG FDA Regulation 21 CFR 73.1575	
Chemical composition	>99% TiO_2
Crystal modification	Anatase
Density	3.8 g/cm

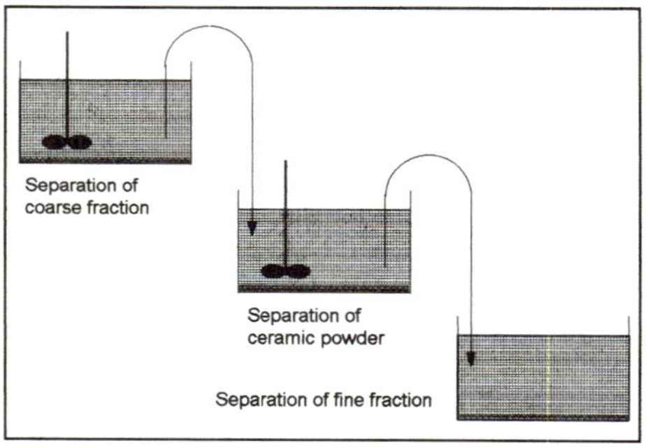

Figure 1. Experimental setup for the sedimentation procedure.

pigments. Furthermore the crystallites are agglomerated and thus not favourable for the shaping process used for angiopolar cell carriers. Monocrystalline grains can be produced by calcinating the powder at suitable temperatures, subsequent deagglomeration and sizing. Such a sizing process can remove large agglomerates as well as fine debris which would otherwise impair the shaping process or make sintering and pore formation less controllable.

MATERIALS AND METHODS

A titanium dioxide powder (1171, Kronos Titan, D-51373-Leverkusen) which is admitted for use in foods and drugs was used as a starting material. Powder properties are listed in Table 1. The powder was granulated by addition of binder solution (PVA 22000, Fluka, CH-Buchs) and mechanical stirring. The granulates were hardened at 180°C, crushed in a mortar and sieved to a granulate size of 140 µm (DIN 4188). The granulates obtained were calcined at temperatures between 950 and 1350°C (heating rate 3 K/min, soaking time 15 min). Deagglomeration of the calcined granulates was performed by dry milling in a ball mill with alumina balls. The powders obtained were analyzed by SEM and laser diffraction particle size measurement (Malvern). For obtaining sized fractions of the milled material a sedimentation process was applied (Figure 1). Sedimentation started with dispersing 3% of solid material in deionized water. After intensive stirring the coarse fraction of the material was allowed to settle for five minutes. The fraction remaining in suspension was carefully decanted and allowed to settle for another ten minutes. This powder fraction was investigated by SEM (Figure 2) and laser diffraction size measurements. It was then used for preparing ceramic samples. The sintering behaviour was assessed by a heating microscope (Leica). The material is pressed into a cube of 2 mm size and heated from room temperature to 1400°C while the cube dimensions are observed by a CCD video camera. Shrinkage is calculated by the decrease in cross-section area. Ceramic samples were prepared by dry pressing. 3.0 g of powder was mixed with 0.2 g of methylcellulose powder (Methocel 60 HG, Fluka, CH-9470 Buchs) and 0.2 g water. After drying, the granulates obtained were crushed, sieved 200 µm and pressed into cylinders 5 x 5 mm. For sintering, the samples were heated at a rate of 3 K/min to 1280°C with 15 min soaking time. Open porosity was measured as water uptake after boiling 10 min in deionized water.

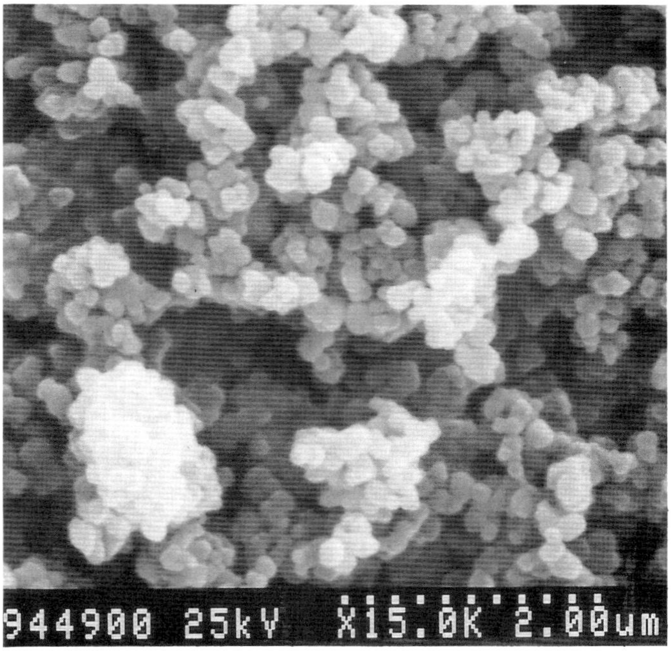

Figure 2. Titanium dioxide powder in pigment quality. The grain size is in the nm-range, mean agglomerate size is 1.7 µm.

RESULTS

Grain growth during calcination

The grain diameter rose continuously with increasing calcination temperature (Figure 4). The applied dry milling process was able to separate the grains of the granulates without producing large amounts of debris (Figure 3).

Effect of Sedimentation Sizing

Large agglomerates as well as fine debris were removed as shown in Figure 3. Removal of the finest and coarsest fraction resulted in narrower grain size distributions than the original grain size after calcinating and milling. After application the sedimentation process the grain size of the investigated calcination steps was nearly independent of the original size (Figure 5).

Preparation of ceramic material

Heating microscopy revealed that sintering of the powder only occurs at temperatures >1000°C (Figure 6). A continuous densification was found between 1000 and 1400°C. Sintering and pore formation can be controlled with the aid of the obtained densification curve. The ceramic material obtained exhibited 34.6% open microporosity. Figure 7 shows that the homogeneous grain size which was achieved in the sedimentation process lead to a loosely packed arrangement of grains with intergranular porosity.

CONCLUSIONS

Processing of titania pigment powders into a ceramic powder specially adapted to the requirements of a shaping process for porous cell carriers is possible by combined thermal

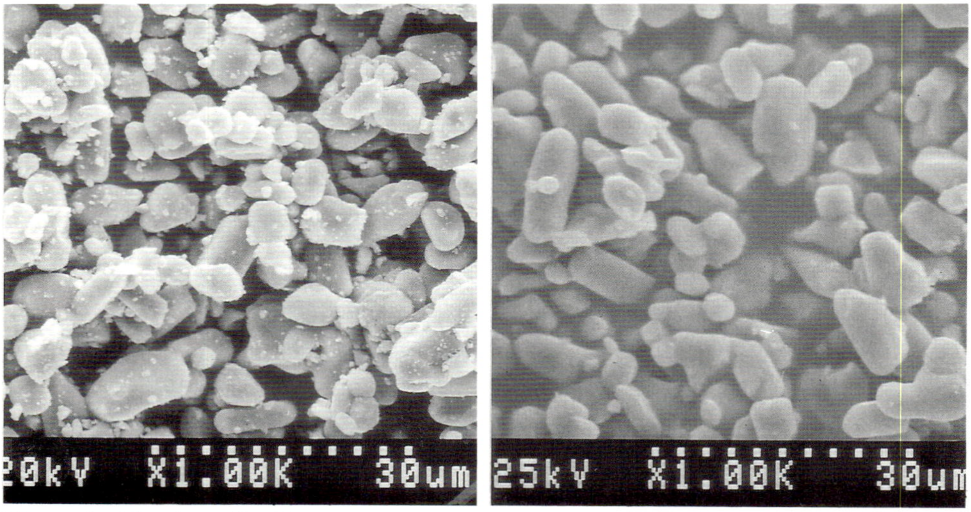

Figure 3. Titanium dioxide grains, calcined at 1300°C and milled, before (left) and after sedimentation process (right). The milled powder contains agglomerates and debris which are not present in the sedimented powder.

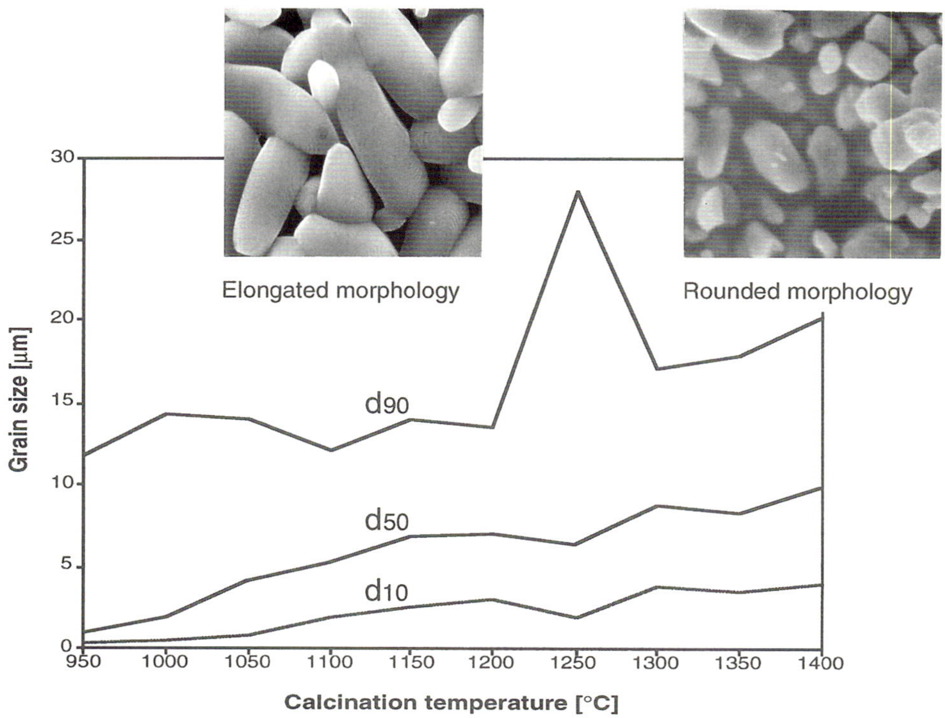

Figure 4. Grain size distribution after milling as a function of calcination temperature. The high value of d90 in the 1250°C-step is due to the elongated grain morphology which is the predominant at this calcination temperature. At 1300°C and higher temperatures a rounded grain morphology develops.

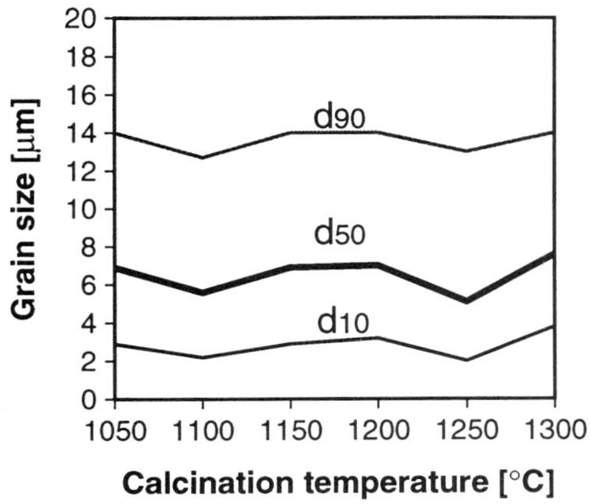

Figure 5. Grain size distribution after sedimentation sizing as a function of calcination temperature. The grain size is nearly independent from the original grain size distribution which is displayed in Figure 4.

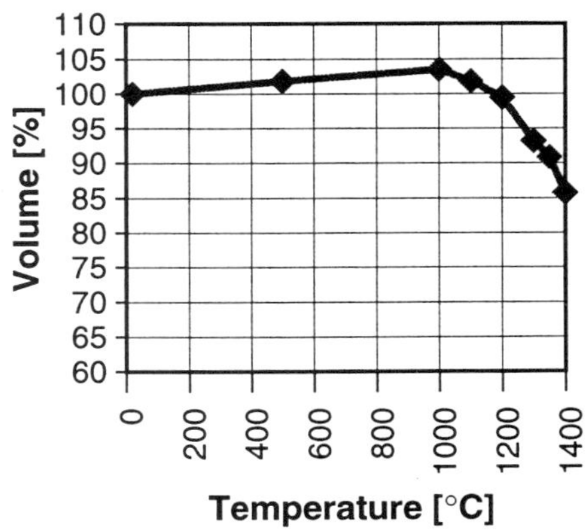

Figure 6. Thermal densification of ceramic powder. Between room temperature and 1000°C only thermal expansion can be detected. Densification starts at 1000°C.

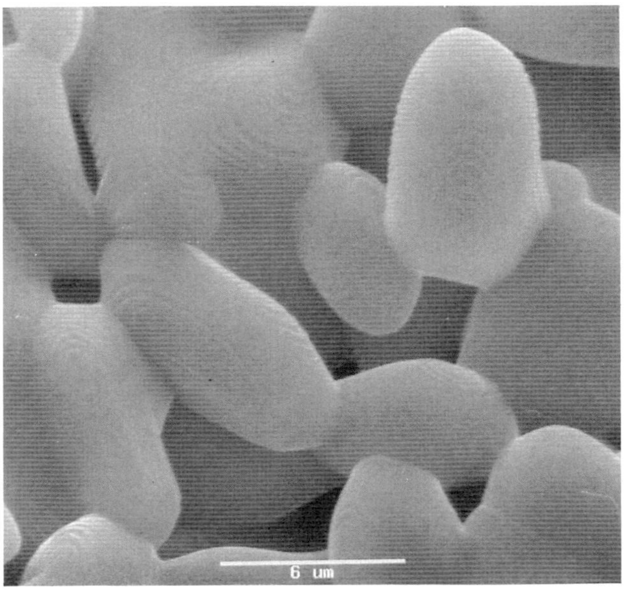

Figure 7. Microporous structure of the sintered ceramic material. Homogeneous size distribution and large grain size give an open-porous material with 34.6% open porosity

and mechanical processing. The applied sedimentation process is capable of supplying a narrow grain size distribution, which, transformed into a sintered ceramic material, leads to the formation of open micropores. In future work, a further optimization will have to be done in order to increase the efficiency of the process as well as working out parameters which enable the production of a range of grain sizes.

REFERENCES

1. Bauer, G., Dannheim, H., Oel, H.J., cfi/Ber.DKG 70 1993 233-237
2. Wintermantel, E., Cima, L., Schloo, B. and Langer, R. In *Angiogenesis, Key Principles: Science, Technology, Medicine* Steiner, R., Weiss, P. and Langer, R. (eds.) Birkhäuser Publishers Basel and Boston 1992
3. K.-L. Eckert, M. Mathey, U. Rösler, J. Mayer, E. Wintermantel, H. Hofmann, In *Bioceramics* Volume 6, Ducheyne, P. and Christiansen, D. (eds.) Butterworth-Heinemann, Oxford 1993, 251-255

RAPIDLY RESORBABLE MATERIALS BASED ON A NEW PHASE: $CA_2KNA(PO_4)_2$

G. Berger, R. Gildenhaar and U. Ploska

Federal Institute for Materials Research and Testing, Unter den Eichen 87, D-12200 Berlin, Germany

ABSTRACT

The basic composition field in the system of $Ca_3(PO_4)_2$-$CaNaPO_4$-$CaKPO_4$ is given, where glassy-crystalline materials that are developed for resorbable bone substitution are available, containing $Ca_2KNa(PO_4)_2$ as main crystalline phase. These glassy-crystalline materials crystallize spontaneously from the melt. A test method was developed to determine the solubility of the glassy-crystalline materials in comparison with those of hydroxyapatite (HA) and tricalcium phosphate (TCP) ceramics. The material eluates were analyzed for each component of the synthesis which indicates heterogenous solubility behavior. A few observations are made concerning biological tests.

INTRODUCTION

Bone substitution materials have to restore the functionality of the defective bone segment immediately and in these cases they remain in the organism permanently. But in examples of less mechanical load it is also possible that the bone itself restores functionality during a longer period of regeneration when a biocompatible and resorbable material occupies the place for bone growth. HA and TCP are well known to fulfil this task but only partially because biodegradation is not complete especially when the cysts are of a relative large volume as is the rule in the orthopaedics field. Thus, materials are sought which are of rapid resorbability but do not induce acute or chronic damage to the tissue when the material dissolves or degrades. The concentration of each dissolved component has to be within physiological variance. In this paper different materials in the system $Ca_3(PO_4)_2$-$CaNaPO_4$-$CaKPO_4$ were investigated relating to such requirements. The time dependence of solubility for all components were measured in a specially developed experimental arrangement for characterization of the biodegradability.

MATERIALS AND METHODS

TCP is a very well known resorbable bone substitution material. Also Rhenanite ($CaNaPO_4$) is composed of biocompatible ions whose degradation will not be expected to damage the surrounding tissue or organism. Therefore, the solution behavior of known and unknown materials in this basic system was investigated.

The new compounds result from combinations of $CaNaPO_4$ with potassium and/or magnesium orthophosphates to decrease the melting temperature below 1600°C. The compositions of the investigated materials are listed in Table 1. Their syntheses were realized from carbonates of the corresponding cations by adding phosphoric acid and subsequent sintering. The characterization of the glassy-crystalline materials was carried out with XRD, DTA, EMA and light microscopy. But the main investigations were focused on the solubility behavior.

A circulating reactor was developed for determining the solubility kinetics (see Figure 1). This reactor can operate both a quasi closed system and an open system, thus making possible a continuous approach to the conditions of the organism. The investigating material of 315 - 400 μm grain size is given into the sample vessel which has a volume of 7.5 ml and consists of two parts with sealed fritts in every section preventing sample movement in the whole circuit of 200 ml. The solvent is moved by a peristaltic pump 25 times per hour through the sample vessel (flow rate 5 l/h). The sampling is controlled by computer regulating the three-way valve and the fraction collector. The eluates were analyzed by AAS and photometry. The experimental arrangement is able to determine the solution kinetics very precise and reproducible (s_r = 0.056).

The total solubility and that of each ionic component are listed in Table 1. Furthermore, the influence of various solvents such as purified water (< 0.05 μS), 0.2 M TRIS-HCl buffer solution and 0.2 M TRIS-HCl buffer solution containing additional hydrogen carbonate ions. The buffer solutions were prepared by dissolving 48.6 g Tris (hydroxy-methylamino) methane in 500 ml purified water and adding 250 ml of 1 N HCl which is filled up to 2000 ml with purified water (20°C). Because the chloride concentration was kept constant the pH-value of the solution varies in the range of 7.4 ± 0.4.

Table 1. Compositions and solubilities of the investigated materials.

sample/ sample code	composition (ma%)					ions, eluted (μg/ml)					
	CaO	MgO	Na_2O	K_2O	P_2O_5	Ca^{2+}	Mg^{2+}	Na^+	K^+	PO_4^{3-}	Σ**)
HA*)	55.82	-	-	-	42.39	6.1	-	-	-	1.1	7.2
β-TCP	54.24	-	-	-	45.76	13	-	-	-	17	30
α-TCP	54.24	-	-	-	45.76	21	-	-	-	33	54
$Ca_5Na_2(PO_4)_4$	44.73	-	9.90	-	45.37	32	-	12	-	69	113
$CaNaPO_4$	35.48	-	19.61	-	44.91	32	-	23	-	73	128
$Ca_2KNa(PO_4)_2$	33.76	-	9.33	14.18	42.73	18	-	20	42	83	163
$MgKPO_4$	-	25.45	-	29.74	44.81	-	95	-	970	996	2061
GB 14	30.67	2.45	9.42	14.42	43.14	12	37	25	125	201	400
GB 15	27.53	4.95	9.51	14.45	43.56	14	145	20	252	613	1044
GB 16	24.32	7.49	9.60	14.60	43.99	9	179	17	357	849	1411
GB 18	17.72	12.75	9.79	14.88	44.86	8	257	25	444	1029	1763
GB 1 a	20.70	7.50	11.60	17.30	42.90	5	180	260	505	1278	2228

*) +1.79 ma% H_2O

**) 0 - 40 ± 5; >40 - 80 ± 10; >80 - 200 ± 20; >200 - 400 ± 40; >400 - 2000 ± 80; >2000 - 3500 ± 300

volume	200 ml
sample weight	2.0 g
flow rate	5.0 l/h
sampling	5, 10, 15, 20, 25, 30, 40, 50, 60 min; afterwards in steps of 30 min up to 6 h; 2.5 ml were analyzed
ratio of surface to volume	~ 2 cm^{-1}

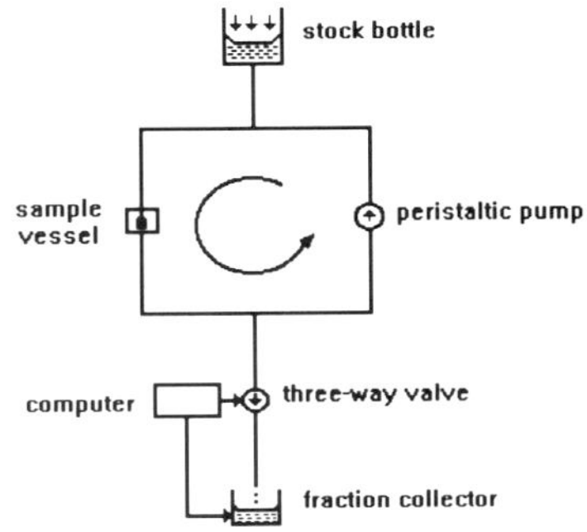

Figure 1. Scheme of circulating reactor

The hydrogen carbonate containing buffer solution was prepared by adding 0.027 M sodium hydrogen carbonate to the 0.2 M TRIS-HCl buffer solution. The solubility of the investigated materials was the lowest in purified water and the highest in 0.2 M TRIS-HCl buffer solution. If the carbonate concentration is similar to that of blood plasma the total solubility is only slightly diminished in relation to the 0.2 M TRIS-HCl buffer solution without changing the solution behavior.

RESULTS AND DISCUSSION

Ando and Matsuno [1] described that $CaNaPO_4$ reacting with $Ca_3(PO_4)_2$ forms the compound $Ca_5Na_2(PO_4)_4$ with a melting point widely above 1600°C just as $CaNaPO_4$ and $Ca_3(PO_4)_2$. As expected, the solubility of this compound in 0.2 M TRIS-HCl buffer solution determined with the circulating reactor is higher than ß-TCP but only slightly lower than ß-$CaNaPO_4$. But it is not absolutely correct to compare the measured solubilities directly because the preparation for getting materials with equal grain size (315-400 µm) in every case failed even if the ceramic method (solid reaction without total melting) was applied. During determination of the solubility, particles of the fine crystalline material are able to pass through the frit of the sample vessel thus leading to adulterated values. Such fine crystalline substances are not suitable for filling cysts. A strong washing out during the operation and perhaps even transport into the lymph nodes (producing macrophages) are possible. Materials for filling cysts also have to satisfy some mechanical stability.

$CaKPO_4$ and $CaNaPO_4$ react by forming $Ca_2KNa(PO_4)_2$ [2,3]. This compound also does not melt at temperatures below 1600°C but its sintering is much better than the material mentioned above. The solubility of $Ca_2KNa(PO_4)_2$ is not much higher compared with $CaNaPO_4$ but the ratio of single ion solubility differs. The partition of potassium ions of total solubility is much greater.

Partial substitution of calcium by magnesium, GB 14 - GB 18, leads to meltable and castable products at temperatures below 1600°C and are well granulated and fractionated and thus suitable for filling cysts. The XRD patterns of these compounds show line spectra shifting to greater angles as for $Ca_2KNa(PO_4)_2$ due to the partial exchange of calcium by magnesium. $Ca_2KNa(PO_4)_2$ already is described by the authors [3, 4]. Its lattice can evolve from α-$CaNaPO_4$ by triple the lattice parameters (superlattice structure). α-$CaNaPO_4$ itself is not obtainable at ambient temperatures. However, the superlattice structure is stable at ambient temperatures and changes into a high temperature form at

655°C. The cell parameters of this form lie between these of α-$CaNaPO_4$ and α-$CaKPO_4$ likewise not stable at ambient temperatures.

Besides the shifted line spectrum of the phase $Ca_2KNa(PO_4)_2$ the XRD patterns of samples GB 14 - GB 18 show more lines of the $MgKPO_4$ phase with increasing magnesium content. Further phases could not be identified but both DTA patterns and the extremely high solubility values give some indication of their existence. The DTA patterns show unidentified endotherm peaks between 1130 and 1160°C with increasing magnesium content. As for the samples GB 15 - GB 18 more magnesium ions are eluted than with $MgKPO_4$, as can be seen from Table 1 (determination of single ion solubility). The increased elution of sodium ions is also conspicuous, indicating the existence of further glassy and/or amorphous phase(s) in the sample set.

The substitution of calcium by magnesium leads to significant changes in morphology. A strong notable diminishing of the crystals is part of the increase of the solubility starting from $Ca_2KNa(PO_4)_2$. The controlled exchange of calcium by magnesium makes it possible to regulate the solubility of any material in the system. Because of the relatively simple preparation method and the solution characteristics these materials are qualified for filling bone defects. Implanted in soft and hard tissues there was no tissue damage even with materials of such a high solubility as GB 1 a [5]. Under the given conditions, the solution rate of GB 1 a, however, was shown to be higher than bone growth. A very positive assessment was given to the sample GB 14 in cell tests [6] as well as after implantation in soft and hard tissues.

ACKNOWLEDGMENTS

Financial support from the Federal Ministry of Research and Technology (BMFT) of the Federal Republic of Germany (project no.: 03 M 1501A) and the BIOVISION GmbH, Ilmenau, Germany, is gratefully acknowledged.

REFERENCES

1. Ando, J. and Matsuno, S. *Bull. Chem. Soc. Japan* 1968, 41, 342-347
2. Berger, G. et al., PCT, WO 91/07357, C03C 3/16. 30.05.91
3. Schneider, M., Gildenhaar, R. and Berger, G. *Cryst. Res. Techn.* 1994, 5, 671-675
4. Berger, G., Gildenhaar, R. and Ploska, U. *Biomaterials* (in press)
5. Hartwig, C, doctoral thesis, University Lipsia, 1992
6. Picker, H.-U. et al. *Z. Zahnärztl. Implantol.* 1993, 11, 111-116

PREPARATION OF CALCIUM PHOSPHATE BIOCERAMICS BY MOULDING AND SINTERING

E. Mejdoubi**, J.L. Lacout* and M. Hamad**

*Laboratoire des Materiaux-Physico-Chimie des Solides ENSCT URA CNRS 445 38, rue des Trente-Six Ponts 31400 Toulouse France. **Laboratoire de Chimie Physique, Department de Chimie, Faculte des Sciences, Universite Mohammed V, Rabat Maroc

ABSTRACT

We have developed a method for the preparation of an apatitic bioceramic which consists of the sintering of an apatitic cement. A mixture of ß-tricalcium phosphate (ß-TCP), of monocalcium phosphate (MCP) and tetracalcium phosphate (TTCP), added to water can be injected into moulds. After hardening the piece can be precisely tooled and then sintered. This method presents two advantages: first the possibility of easy moulding and then the possibility of working the piece accurately. In this paper we describe the different stages of preparation of such a ceramic and the physical and chemical modifications which occur during each of the stages.

INTRODUCTION

It is well known that the addition of water to a mixture of acidic and basic phosphates leads to materials which harden and slowly evolve to give apatitic phases. One of the important points is the control of the setting time which depends on the composition of the initial mixture, the liquid/solid ratio, the presence of additives, the addition of phosphoric acid. Here, we accurately studied, using a mathematical procedure, the conditions to obtain a cement with a definite setting time and hardness. So, it was possible to obtain a paste able to be moulded in a convenient form and which hardens. After hardening, the cement piece can be tooled; this stage is very important because it allows shapes to be machined which can not be obtained simply by moulding. The piece is then sintered.

SHAPING OF THE CERAMIC

Preparation of the cement

The cement is composed of a mixture of three calcium phosphates [1]: monocalcium phosphate monohydrate (MCPM: $Ca(H_2PO_4)_2{\cdot}H_20$), beta-tricalcium phosphate (ß-TCP:$Ca_3(P0_4)_2$ and tetracalcium phosphate (TTCP:$Ca_3(P0_4)_2$ and tetracalcium phosphate (TTCP:$Ca_4(PO_4)_2O$). When a determined quantity of water is added to the mixture of phosphates they react to form a hydroxyapatite $Ca_{10}PO_4)_6(OH)_2$, according to the following reaction:

$$a)\ Ca(H_2P0_4)_2,\ H_20) + b)\ Ca_3(PO_4)_2 + c)\ Ca_4(PO_4)_2O) \text{ ----> } Ca_{10}(PO_4)_6(OH)_2.$$

Previous work allowed us to define the conditions to obtain a paste with a setting time that is sufficiently slow to allow easy moulding and a homogeneous cement to be obtained. The initial solid mixture of phosphate powder with a Ca/P atomic ratio of 1.67, is previously treated with a mixture of water and ethanol (84/16), then dried and heated to 150°C for one hour. During this stage part of the solid evolves to a new phosphate: dicalcium phosphate $CaHPO_4{\cdot}2H_20$. At the temperature of 150°C, the condensation of $H_2PO_4^=$ ions into pyrophosphate ions ($P_20_7^{4-}$) begins. $P_20_7^{4-}$ ions are well known to inhibit or even to decrease the formation of phosphate compounds like apatite [2]. So the setting of the cement is slow and homogeneous.

MOULDING OF THE CERAMIC

A determined quantity of water is added to the previously treated and dried mixture; the quantity is calculated to allow the reactions of solubilization and precipitation of hydroxyapatite. In these conditions the paste has a convenient rheology to be injected into a mould. The setting and hardening of the cement then occur; evaporation of the water should be avoided, so the mould is maintained in a closed chamber with a water saturated atmosphere. To accelerate setting and hardening, this stage can be carried out at 40°C . The piece can be demoulded after 24 hours.

During this stage the main reactions of formation of the apatite take place. Figure 1 reports the X-ray diffraction patterns of the cement at various times.

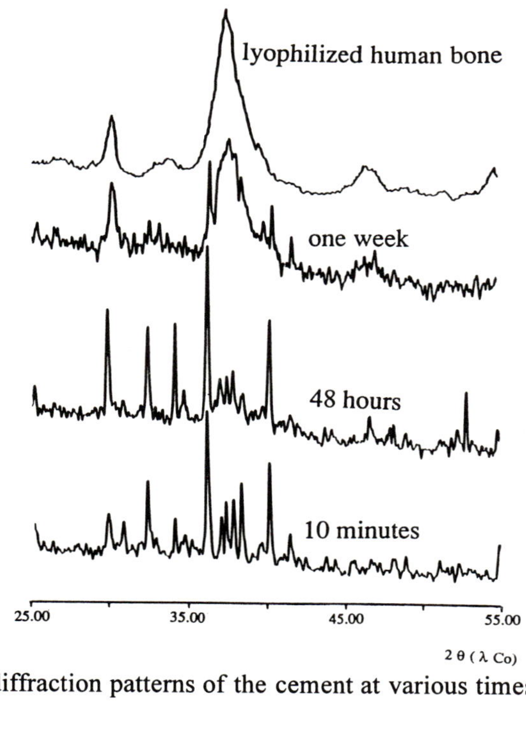

Figure 1. X-ray diffraction patterns of the cement at various times.

The initial phases disappear first, then the DCPD phase forms and finally weakly crystallized apatite appears.

SINTERING OF THE CERAMIC

The conditions of sintering are very important. The temperature cycle is reported in Fig. 2.

During the first stage, up to 900°C, the cement evolves to a well crystallized apatite. Hardening of the ceramic begins at 1150°C. Between 1150°C and 1250°C.sintering occurs without any modifications of the chemical structure, except the partial evolution of the hydroxyapatite into an oxyapatite according to the well known reaction:

$$Ca_{10}(PO_4)_6(OH)_2 \text{ ---------> } Ca_{10}(PO_4)_6\, O_x(OH)_{2-2x} + (l\text{-}x)\; H_2O$$

This reaction can be limited in a water saturated atmosphere.

Above 1250°C the apatitic structure collapses to form tetracalcium phosphate and α-tricalcium phosphate: annealing at 900°C allows the opposite reaction to form apatite. The Infra-red diagrams corresponding to the different stages of sintering are reported in Fig. 3.

Various sintering schedules were studied with the best reported in Fig. 2. In these conditions, the mechanical properties are similar to other apatitic ceramics.

During sintering the volume of the piece decreases. But the shrinkage is limited. This is due to the fact that the quantity of water added for cement setting and hardening corresponds exactly to the chemical reaction of apatite formation. Nevertheless, during sintering the initial porosity of the cement decreases and the final density of the ceramic is close to 99% of the theoretical maximum.

One special interest of the method is the possibility to prepare ceramics of various compositions. Easily and in a very homogeneous way addition of tricalcium phosphate improves the mechanical properties of the apatitic ceramics. The modification of the Ca/P atomic ratio of the initial mixture gives a cement and a ceramic containing tricalcium phosphate. In this case, the tricalcium phosphate is closely mixed with the apatitic phase in the cement.

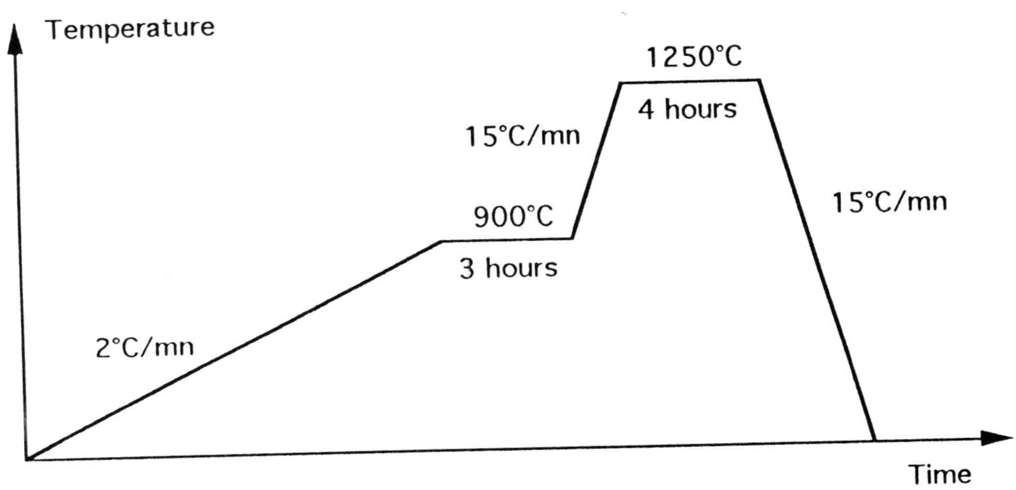

Figure 2. Temperature cycle.

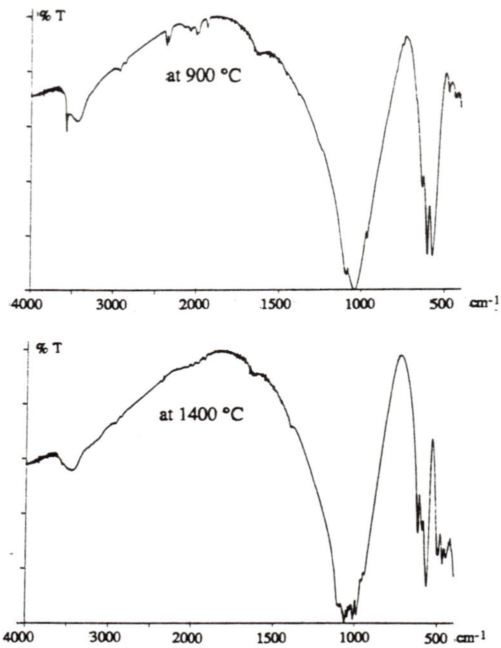

Figure 3. Infra-red diagrams corresponding to the different stages of sintering.

CONCLUSIONS

This method of preparation of dense bioceramics leads to materials with properties similar to those of other apatitic bioceramics. Moreover, some points seem to be of great interest. First, the intermediate stage of the cement, which permits the moulding of the piece. After hardening, the piece can be easily handed and tooled. This operation is particularly useful to obtain parts with very sharp angles or with axial holes. Secondly, the possibility to prepare homogeneous phosphate ceramics over a large range of compositions, containing various proportions of tricalcium phosphate as required.

REFERENCES

1. Lacout J.L., Mejdoubi E., Procede d'oblenlion d'hydroxyapatile phosphocalcique, application au comblement osseux ou au moulage de pieces et produits ulilises-Brevet Fr 92.090 1 9/PCT/FR.
2. Fleisch H., Russell R.G.G., Bisaz S., Termine J.D., Posner A.S., Influence of pyrophosphate on the transformation or amorphous to crystalline calcium phosphate. Calc. Tiss. Res., 2, 49-59, (1968).

ZrO_2/HAP GRADIENT CERAMIC BIOMATERIALS

Shaoxian Zeng, Wanpeng Cao, Guiju Liu,

Shanghai Institute of Ceramics, Chinese Academy of Sciences
1295 Ding-xi Road, Shanghai 200050,China
Bisheng Cheng, Changzhong Tao, Yuan Liu
Dept. Stomatology, Chang Zheng Hospital,
Second Military Medical University, Shanghai 200003

ABSTRACT

We have developed a new type of gradient ceramic biomaterial. ZrO_2 was selected as the substrate and Na_2O-SiO_2-B_2O_2-CaO system glass was chosen as a medium for bonding HAP and ZrO_2. On the surface of the substrate, several mixture layers were coated and sintered. The content of HAP in the coating increased gradually form the substrate to the surface. After three months implantation in dog's leg bone, the gradient bioactive implant bonded with the bone, the bonding strength between the gradient bioactive material implant and bone was much higher than that between a pure Ti implant and bone.

INTRODUCTION

In order to maintain function, many biomaterials are used to repair and reconstruct destroyed bone. In recent decades, more and more attention has been paid to bioceramics because of their good biocompatibility and chemical stability. In clinical applications, bioceramics with high strength and bioactivity are necessary [1], so gradient ceramic biomaterials have been developed to satisfy clinical needs. In this paper, a new type of bioceramic which combines the virtues of ZrO_2 and HAP was tested.

EXPERIMENTS AND RESULTS

Manufacture of ZrO_2 Substrate

The super-fine ZrO_2 powder (3%Y_2O_3) was shaped into cylinders of 3 mm diameter and 6mm height, sintered under 1600°C.

Selection of the Glass

According to the phase diagram, glasses of Na-Si-B-Ca system were chosen as a medium of bonding HAP and ZrO_2. The glass must have a thermo-expansion which matchs that of the ZrO_2 substrate and HAP coating and must wet ZrO_2 under the sintering temperature. The results showed that at temperatures up to 950°C, the wetting angle was smaller than 10°, indicating that the wetting property was good. The XRD and IR analysis demonstrated that the glass did not change the structure of the HAP during sintering.

Coating Technology

At an appropriate ratio, glass powder, organic binder and alcohol were mixed in a ball mill completely to get the mixture coating slurry, which was coated on the ZrO_2 substrate surface and sintered at 950°C for 10 minutes, then cooled to room temperature gradually, and then the second mixture slurry of HAP and glass, in a ratio of 1:1(wt%), was coated and sintered in the glass layer. With increasing HAP content of the slurry and coating several times, we could get a final coating in which the content of HAP increased gradually from the substrate to the surface.

SEM Observation of the Coatings

Figure 1,an SEM photograph of the gradient biomaterial implant, showed that the thickness of the coating was 40-50 μm. The element scanning photographs of Zr, Ca, P corresponding to the area of Fig. 1 are shown in Fig.2, Fig.3 and Fig.4, respectively. Comparing these photographs, it can be seen that Ca and P in the coating increased from the substrate to the surface, which indicates a gradient coating.

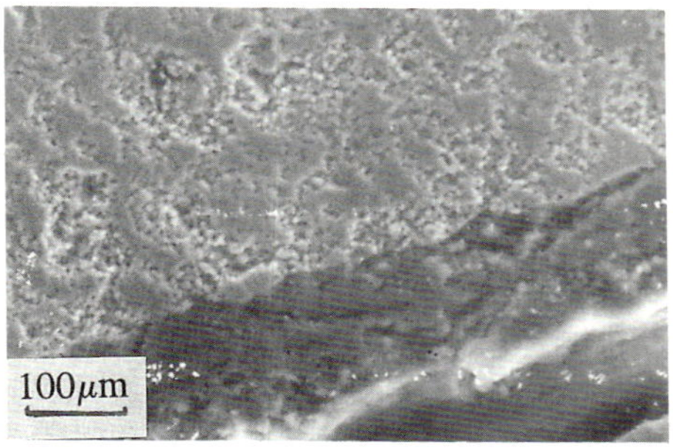

Fig.1 SEM photograph of implant

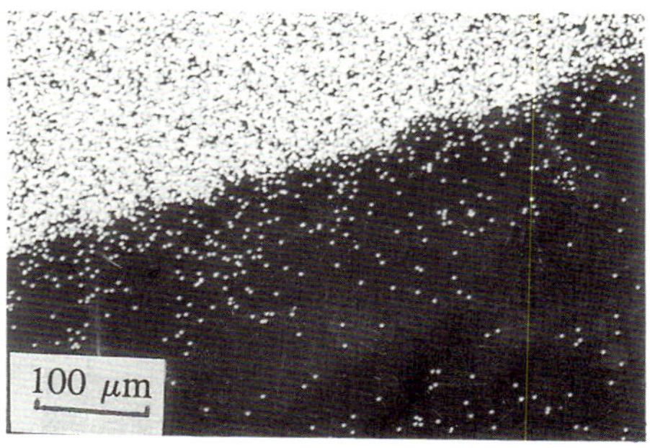

Fig.2 Zr scanning photograph

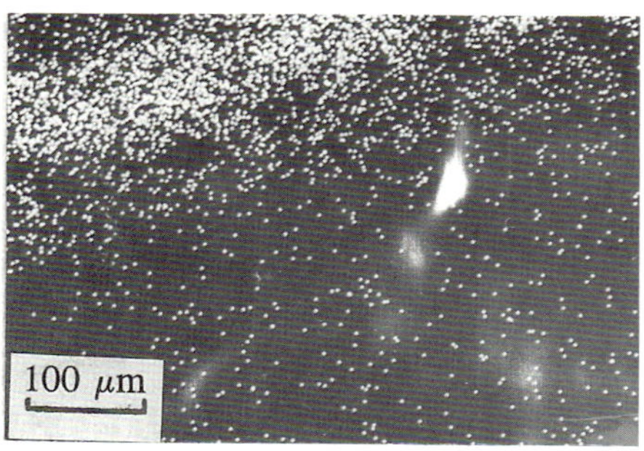

Fig.3 Ca scanning photograph

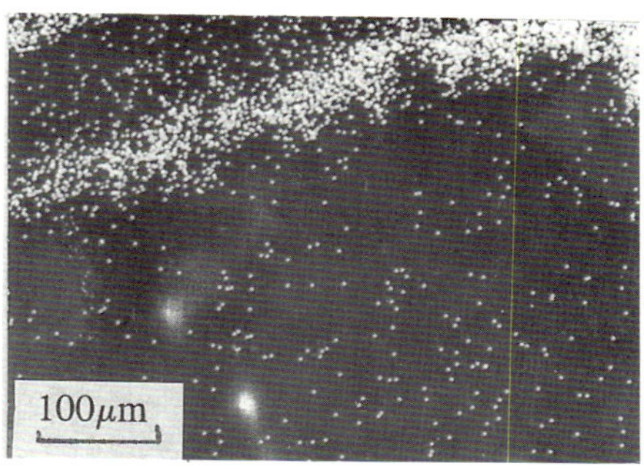

Fig.4 P scanning photograph

Animal Experiment

Two dogs were selected as the experimental animals. The implants were implanted in leg bone, and pure Ti implants were used as control implants. After 3 months implantation, the specimens were sectioned. The bonding strengths are listed in Table 1. In order to observe the bonding between implant and bone further, we prepared sections for optical microscopy. (Fig.5 and Fig.6)

Table 1 Results of bio-mechanical experiment

No.	L(mm)	D(mm)	F(N)	K(MPa)	$\overline{K}$(MPa)	Δ(MPa)
C_1	3.00	3.60	282	8.32		
C_2	3.50	4.00	366	8.33		
C_3	3.00	3.70	256	7.34		
C_4	2.40	3.80	286	9.00	8.14	1.08
C_5	2.70	3.50	156	5.26		
C_6	2.75	3.60	289	9.27		
C_7	3.33	3.64	347	9.12		
C_8	2.33	3.74	205	7.49		
T_1	3.45	4.00	122	2.82		
T_2	3.38	4.00	135	3.18	3.18	0.29
T_3	3.65	4.00	172	3.77		
T_4	2.88	4.00	107	2.97		

DISCUSSION

Because the coating and substrate are two different materials, their different thermo-expansion properties will cause stress concentration on the bonding interface sufficient to decrease the bonding strength. The stress concentration between coating and substrate can be expressed as following,

$$S=E(T-T_0)(a_g-a_s)(1-3J+J^2) \qquad \text{eq. 1.}$$

where E is the elastic modulus of the coating, T_0 is the room temperature, T is the treating temperature, a_g and a_s are the thermo-expansion coefficients of the coating and substrate, J is the thickness ratio of the coating and substrate, So the closer the thermo-expansion coefficients of the coating and the substrate are, the smaller the interface stress concentration will be. In this work, there are no cracks appearing on the glass layer on the surface of the ZrO_2 substrate when the thickness of the glass coating is up to 0.5 mm, which indicates that the glass and the substrate have thermo-expansion coefficients which match. In the coating, the content of HAP increases gradually from the substrate to surface, so the stress concentration in the coating is also greatly decreased.

Bio-mechanical testing of retrieved specimens showed that the implant-bone bonding was destroyed at both implant-bone interface and glass-substrate interface. The coating was also destroyed. The average gradient material implant-bone bonding strength was 8.14 MPa (maximum 9.99MPa), which was much higher than 3.18 MPa of Ti-bone (maximum 3.77MPa). The destruction pattern of the gradient biomaterial-bone bonding indicated that increasing the coating's strength and also the coating-substrate bonding strength was important to increase the biomaterial-bone bonding strength. The gradient ceramic biomaterial implant had greater bonding strength deviations than Ti implants mainly because the gradient material implant had more shape variation than Ti implants. On the other hand, because bone is a porous material, every implant has a different effective attaching area to bone, that can also cause the bonding strength deviation.

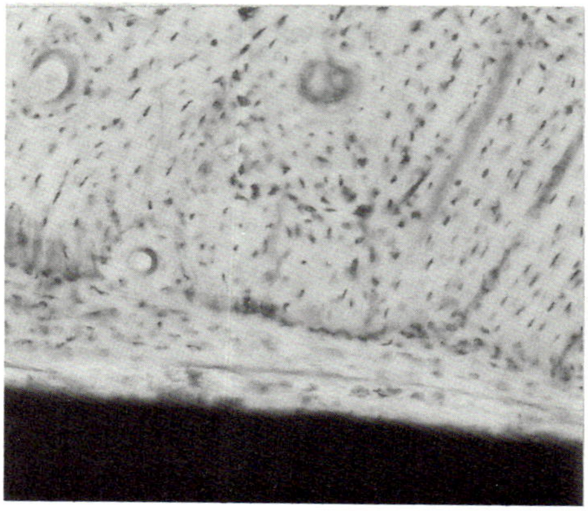

Figure 5. Interface of the implant and bone.

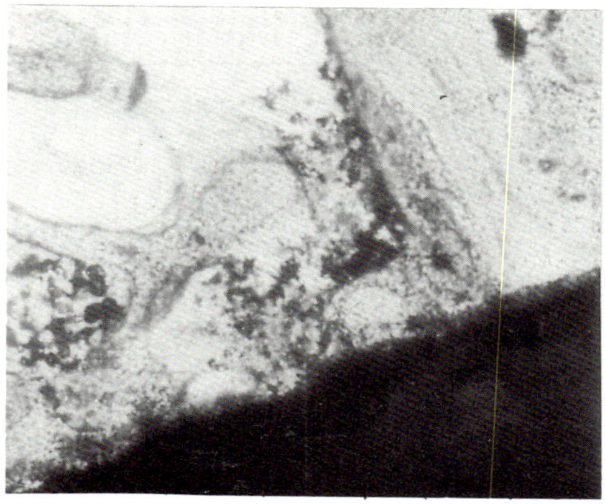

Figure 6 Interface of the implant and marrow space.

The histological observation and analysis showed that the gradient implant formed tight chemical bonding with bone without fibrous tissues at the interface. At the interface, there were interfacial blood vessels forming, showing that HAP had good biocompatibility (Fig. 5). Figure 6 showed that a new bone was formed on the implant in the marrow cavity indicating that HAP can facilitate new bone growth.

CONCLUSIONS

1. ZrO_2/HAP gradient material implants form a bond with bone. HAP has good biocompatibility and can facilitate new bone growth.
2. The bonding strength of ZrO_2/HAP gradient implant-bone is much higher than that of Ti implant-bone.
3. ZrO_2/HAP, a new type of gradient biomaterial possesses both the good mechanical properties of ZrO_2 and the bioactivity of HAP ceramics.

REFERENCES

1. L.L.Hench, Bioceramics: From Concept to Clinic, *J. Am. Ceram. Soc.*, 74(7)1487-510(1991)

BONE TISSUE REACTION ON 50 VOL% ZIRCONIA DISPERSED HYDROXYAPATITE CERAMICS IN OSTEOPOROSIS

A. Suda, T. Sato, A. Ishikawa, M. Takagi, T. Osanai, H. Kato and H. Orui

Department of Orthopaedic Surgery, Yamagata University School of Medicine, 2-2-2 Iida-Nishi, Yamagata 990-23, JAPAN

ABSTRACT

We have successfully developed 50 vol% zirconia dispersed hydroxyapatite ceramic (ZH-C) using a unique technique. Bending strength and fracture toughness of the new ceramic material were about 2 and 4.5 times greater than those of hydroxyapatite ceramics (HAP-C), respectively. In this study, we demonstrated that 50 vol% ZH-C had a perfect bond to the bony layer around the implants and showed significantly improved affinity to the bone when compared with that of Zirconia ceramic (Zr-C), in an experimentally induced osteoporotic rat model.

INTRODUCTION

Hydroxyapatite ceramic is bioactive and has an excellent affinity to the bone [1-3]. However, strength and toughness of hydroxyapatite (HA) may be inadequate [2,3]. Zr-C has been proven to be sufficiently stronger and tougher than alumina, alumina and Zr are both [1,3]. We have successfully developed a ceramic material, using a unique technique, in which 50 vol % zirconia was dispersed in an HA matrix [3]. We studied the biocompatibility of this material consisting of HA and 50% Zr by volume, under static or load-bearing conditions [3-9]. In this study, histomorphometrical analysis of 50 vol% ZH-C, HAP-C and Zr-C was performed to examine biocompatibility in an experimentally induced-osteoporotic rat model.

MATERIALS AND METHODS

The sintering temperatures and mechanical properties of the sintered products of each type of materials have been reported previously [1,3-8]. Bending strength and fracture toughness of 50 vol% ZH-C were about 2 and 4.5 times greater than those of HAP-C. After intraperitoneal anesthesia, ovariectomy and resection of the right sciatic nerve of adult rats (Wister strain, 27-28 months) were used to induce osteoporosis. Three months later a piece of columnar ceramic, 2 mm in diameter, and 6 mm long was inserted into a transverse hole in the proximal metaphyseal area of the right tibia under anesthesia. Five experimental groups were prepared. Three groups of 10 rate implanted with the three materials; 50% ZH-C, HAP-C and ZrC and two control groups of five rats each, with and

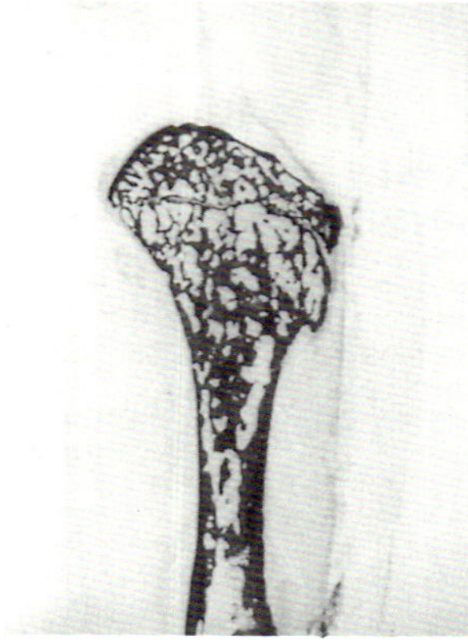

Figure 1. A tibia without ovariectomy and resection of a sciatic nerve with normal trabeculae.

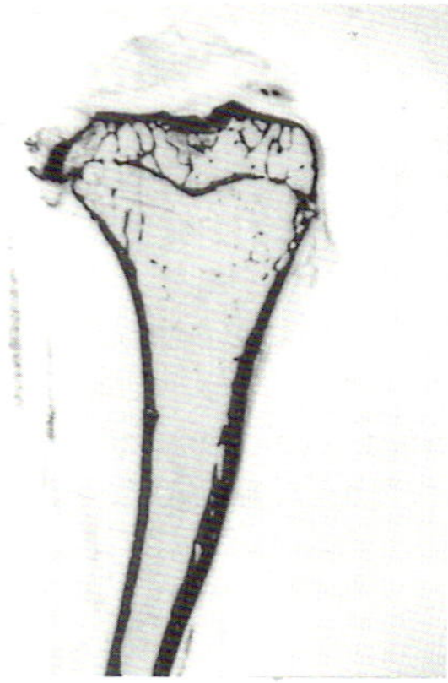

Figure 2. A tibia, 3 months after ovariectomy and resection of a sciatic nerve, with few trabeculae.

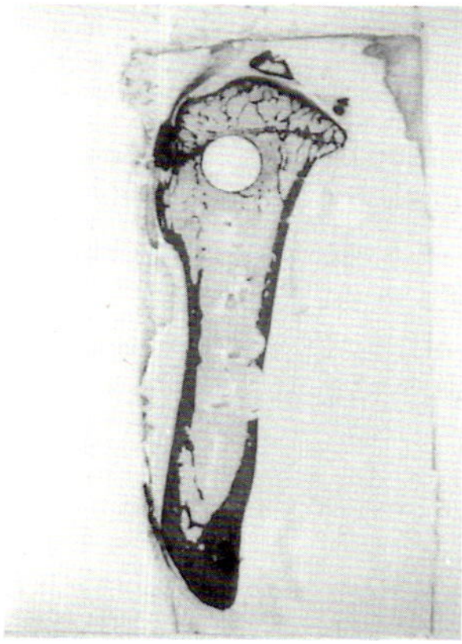

Figure 3. Three months after implantation, the 50 vol% ZH-C was surrounded with a thin osseous layer.

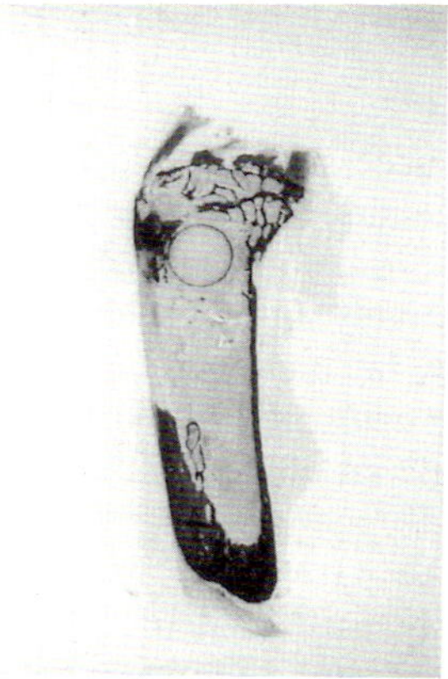

Figure 4. Six months after implantation, a thin layer of bone surrounded the 50 vol% ZH-C.

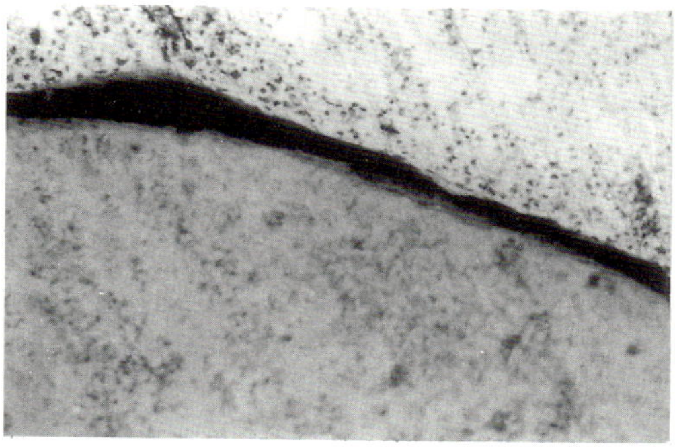

Figure 5. The section stained with toluidine blue without decalcification. Direct contact of bony trabeculae to the implant (X80).

without induced osteoporosis. The rats were killed with intraperitoneal anesthesia 3 and 6 months after implantation. The tibias were isolated and immediately immersed in 70% methanol. A radiograph of each tibia was taken and then the bone was dehydrated and embedded in methylmethacrylateresin, followed by sectioning with a microtome (EXAKT Corp., West Germany). The sections were stained with toluidine blue and examined by optical microscopy. They were also subjected to morphometry on COSMOZONE 98 image analyzer (Nippon Kogaku Co. Ltd.). The length of the bone-implant interface, which showed direct bonding of implant to the bone, was measured to calculate the affinity index (the length of the interface forming a direct bond to bone / the whole circumference of the implant (%)) observed in each section after 3 and 6 months of the treatments.

RESULTS

Rat tibias without ovariectomy and resection of a sciatic nerve had many osseous trabeculae, which indicated no evidence of osteoporosis (Fig. 1), whereas the tibias, 3 months after the treatments, had few trabeculae, confirming experimentally induced osteoporosis (Fig. 2). Three months and six months after implantation, the 50 vol% ZH-C implants were surrounded by thin layer of bone without interruption or by occasional contact of trabecular bone (Fig. 3, Fig. 4). The osseous layer was directly attached to the ceramic implants without any intervening membrane (Fig. 5). The bone affinity index was significantly greater in ZH-C as well as HAP-C than that of Zr-C after 3 and 6 months of implantation ($P< 0.05$, ANOVA Fisher's PLSD, Table 1 and 2).

Table 1

Affinity Index of Implant
(3 months after implantation)

Sample	n	Affinity Index (mean±SEM)
50vol% ZH-C	10	93.02 ± 0.97 *
HAP-C	10	94.62 ± 1.36 *
Zr-C	10	64.39 ± 2.95

* $P < 0.05$ versus Zr-C (ANOVA and Fisher's PLSD post hoc test)

Table 2

Affinity Index of Implant
(6 months after implantation)

Sample	n	Affinity Index (mean±SEM)
50vol% ZH-C	10	93.94 ± 1.09 *
HAP-C	10	95.01 ± 1.38 *
Zr-C	10	66.24 ± 2.63

* $P < 0.05$ versus Zr-C (ANOVA and Fisher's PLSD post hoc test)

DISCUSSION

There are two main types of bioceramics; bioactive ceramics and bioinert ceramics. Bioactive ceramics, including HAP-C, show a direct chemical bond to the bone. However, this type of bioceramic may not be mechanically strong enough. Bioinert ceramics, including Zr-C are sufficiently strong and tough as orthopaedic biomaterials, although they do not have the property of a chemical bond to bone. We have successfully developed 50 vol % ZH-C material using a unique technique and have already reported its biocompatibility of under static or load-bearing conditions [3-8]. In this study a perfect bond of 50 vol% ZH-C to the osseous layer around the implants, in an experimentally induced osteoporotic rat model, was demonstrated. In addition, bone affinity index of 50 vol% ZH-C, as well as that of HAP-C, was greater than that of Zr-C, which confirmed the bioactivity of 50 vol % ZH-C. This study suggested that the bioactivity of 50 vol% ZH-C, which was also strong and tough, was maintained in osteoporotic bone may be useful to patients with osteoporosis.

REFERENCES

1. Suda, A., Narisawa, I., and Suzuki, O. : J. Jpn Orthop. Assoc., 62:S120, 1988.
2. Yamamuro, T. : Clinical Orthopaedic Surgery, 21:1221-1224, 1986.
3. Suda, A., Sato, T., Takagi, M., Osanai, T. and Suzuki, O.: J. Jpn Orthop. Assoc., 64:250-259, 1990.
4. Suda, A., Sato, T., Takagi, M., Osanai, T. Narisawa, T. and Suzuki, O.: Orthopaedic Ceramic Implant, 7:165-168, 1987.
5. Suda, A., Osanai, T., Takagi, M., Narisawa, I., and Suzuki, O. : Orthopaedic Ceramic Implant, 8:135-138, 1988.
6. Iino, M., Fukuda, M., Suda, A., Osanai, T., Takagi, M., Ishikawa, A., Sato, T., Tanabe, H., Suzuki, O., Kakutani, K. and Harada, Y. : Orthopaedic Ceramic Implant, 10:171-175, 1990.
7. Iino, M., Suda, A., and Suzuki, O. : Orthopaedic Ceramic Implant, 9:153-159, 1991.
8. Fukuda, M., Iino, M., Suda, A., Osanai, T., Ishikawa, A., Sato, T., Tanabe, H., Suzuki, O., Kakutani, K. and Harada, Y. : Orthopaedic Ceramic Implant, 11:23-27, 1991.
9. Suda, A., Osanai, T., Sato, T., Ishikawa, A., and Takagi, M. : Bioceramics, 5:191-196, 1992.

BIOACTIVE GLASSES

PROTEIN ADSORPTION PROPERTIES OF BIOACTIVE GLASSES COMPARED TO THEIR BEHAVIOR IN RABBIT TIBIA

M. Brink, E. Söderling*, T. Turunen* and K. H. Karlsson

Department of Chemical Engineering, Åbo Akademi University, Biskopsgatan 8, FIN-20500 Åbo/Turku, Finland. *Institute of Dentistry, University of Turku, Lemminkäinengatan 2, FIN-20520 Åbo/Turku, Finland.

ABSTRACT

The adsorption of proteins to bioactive glasses has been investigated, and the results are compared to glass reactions *in vivo*. The results from the protein adsorption tests are also compared to those for Bioglass® 45S5, hydroxyapatite and an inert glass. The protein profiles were obtained using a plasma protein adsorption test, and the glass reactions *in vivo* by implantation into rabbit tibia. Albumin was the main protein adsorbed to all bioactive glasses. The differences in the protein profiles for the bioactive glasses were not associated with their behavior *in vivo*. However, the protein adsorption properties of the bioactive glasses differed considerably from those of hydroxyapatite and the inert glass.

INTRODUCTION

In the development of bioactive glasses, the need for fast testing methods of biocompatibility is obvious. Nowadays, tests are usually performed by soaking the material of interest in buffer solutions [1], and the dissolution of ions as well as resorption rate and weight loss of the material are investigated. The *in vitro* tests are often followed by implantation, and the reactions *in vivo* are investigated by e.g. scanning electron microscopy (SEM), transmission electron microscopy (TEM) and energy dispersive X-ray analysis (EDXA).

In the present study, the adsorption of plasma proteins, mainly albumin, immunoglobulin G and fibrinogen, to eleven glasses containing 39-55 wt-% SiO_2 was investigated using a fast plasma protein adsorption test. These results are compared to the *in vivo* behavior of the glasses. Bioglass® 45S5 [2], hydroxyapatite (HA) and an inert glass were used as reference materials in the protein adsorption test.

EXPERIMENTS

The investigated soda-lime-silica glasses contained 39-55 wt-% SiO_2. Those containing more than 52 wt-% SiO_2 have a so called large working range while the other tend to devitrify. The durability of the glasses as well as their surface reactions after soaking in a simulated body fluid have recently been investigated [3]. The composition of the glasses is given in Table 1.

Glass preparation

All glasses were prepared by melting the raw materials in a Pt/Au crucible at 1300 - 1360°C for three hours. The raw materials used, all of analytical grade, were Na_2CO_3, K_2CO_3, MgO, $CaCO_3$, H_3BO_3 and $CaHPO_4 \cdot 2H_2O$. Belgian sand was used as raw material for SiO_2. The melt was cast into a pre-heated graphite mould, and the glass annealed at 490-550°C.

The glass was partly used for making cones, partly for particles. Truncated glass cones with length 4-6 mm and cross-section 4-5 mm were prepared for the implantation test, and sterilized in hot air. The remaining glass was crushed and sieved, and particles of the fraction 315-500 µm were used for the plasma protein adsorption test.

Implantation in bone

The glasses were implanted into rabbit tibia for eight weeks. Adult New Zealand rabbits of both sexes and a weight of 3.5-4.5 kg were used. The glass cones, four of each glass, were placed into conical holes drilled in the proximal side of the tibia using a dental drill (Frialit 4-0, Friedrichsfeld GmbH, Mannheim, Germany) irrigated with sterile saline solution. The surgical operations were performed under standard aseptic conditions and general anesthesia at the Institute of Dentistry, University of Turku, Finland. National guidelines for the use and care of laboratory animals were followed.

The rabbits were killed after eight weeks, and resected bone specimens were fixed in 4 % buffered formaline. The fixation was followed by embedding into plastic (Technovit, Kulzer GmbH, Wehrheim, Germany), and the contact between glass and bone was examined by SEM and EDXA.

Protein adsorption tests

The protein adsorption tests were performed as described elsewhere [4]. Human plasma was prepared from blood collected in heparinized tubes. The plasma was separated by centrifuging at 4000 × *g* for 10 minutes, and stored at -20°C. Before use, the plasma was diluted 1:4 in TBS (10 mM Tris-HCl, 150 mM NaCl, pH = 7.4). HA, with a grain

Table 1. Composition of the investigated glasses (given in wt-%).

Glass	Na_2O	K_2O	MgO	CaO	B_2O_3	P_2O_5	SiO_2
5-92	20	10	5	10	0	0	55
11-92	25	5	2	20	0	6	42
12-92	20	10	5	10	3	0	52
14-92	20	10	5	20	0	3	42
15-92	15	15	2	20	3	6	39
20-92	15	15	2	15	3	0	50
9-93	12	15	5	11	1	2	54
13-93	6	12	5	20	0	4	53
14-93	18	6	2	17	2	2	53
17-93	18	9	0	14	1	4	54
19-93	15	12	2	11	3	4	53

size of approximately 200 µm, was obtained from BDH Chemicals Ltd, Poole, England, Bioglass® 45S5, a commercially available bioactive glass, from the University of Florida, USA, and the inert glass from Hackman-Iittala, Finland. The Bioglass® 45S5 and the inert glass were crushed and sieved (315-500 µm). These materials were used as references in the protein adsorption tests only.

Glass particles (100 mg) and HA (50 mg) were incubated with 1 mL of diluted plasma in Nunc CryoTubes (Nunc, Roskilde, Denmark) for 30 minutes by rotation end-over-end at room temperature. After this treatment, the particles were washed with 2 mL of TBS by rolling end-over-end for 1 minute. The adsorbed proteins were analyzed with sodium dodecyl sulphate polyacrylamide gel electroforesis (SDS-PAGE, PhastSystem®, Pharmacia, Sweden). The particles were heated at 100°C for 5 minutes in 120 µL distilled water and 30 µL denaturating buffer (0.2 M Na-phosphate, pH = 7.0, containing 15% SDS and 5% glycerol). The cleared solutions were subjected to SDS-PAGE, and stained with silver according to the manufacturer's instructions. The protein standard was obtained from BioRad (Richmond, CA, USA).

RESULTS

Glass reactions *in vivo*

Rabbit tibia seemed to bond to all glasses, and the glass surface was transformed into silica gel to which calcium and phosphorous (Ca,P) were bonded. The layer of Ca,P

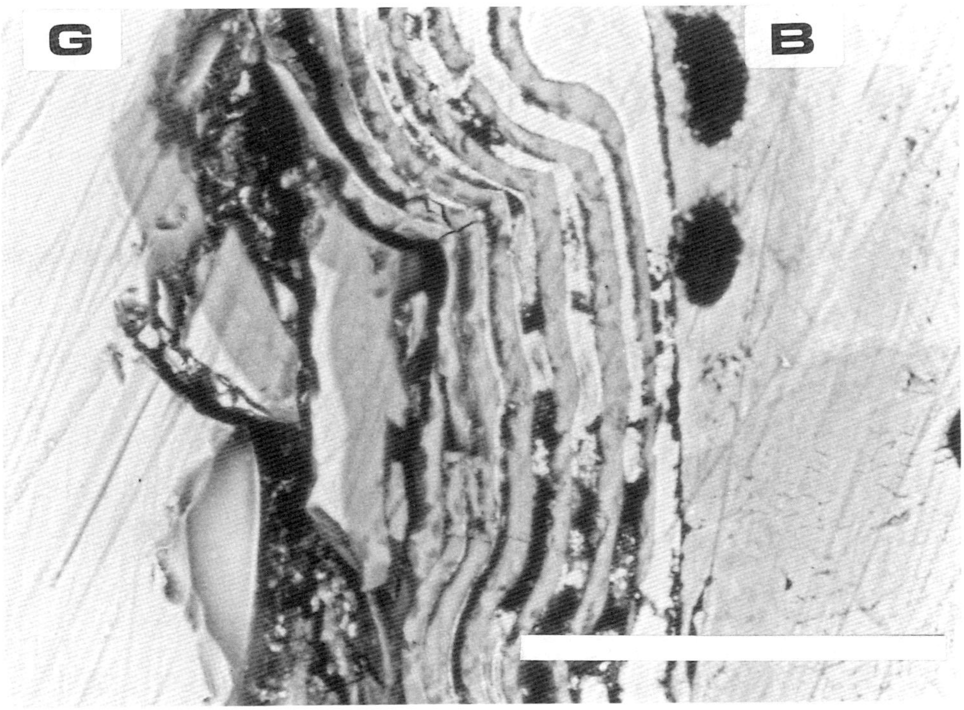

Figure 1. Glass 5-92 after eight weeks in rabbit tibia (bar = 65 µm). Altering layers of silica (dark stripes) and Ca,P (light stripes) are detected in the reaction zone between glass (G) and bone (B).

seemed to be in contact with the tibia. However, for the glasses 5-92, 12-92 and 20-92 altering layers of silica gel and Ca,P were found in the reaction zone between glass and bone. This may be due to the absence of phosphorous in these glasses. A glass showing this layered structure when implanted is presented in Fig. 1.

Protein adsorption

All bioactive glasses adsorbed mainly albumin from the plasma (Figs. 2 and 3). The inert glass (Fig. 2) showed a broad plasma protein adsorption profile. In addition to albumin, it adsorbed proteins from the molecular weight (M_W) range of immunoglobulins ($M_W \sim 150\ 000$) and fibrinogen ($M_W \sim 400\ 000$). HA showed also a broad plasma protein adsorption profile (Fig. 2).

Some differences in the protein adsorption properties were observed between the bioactive glasses. These differences occurred especially in the M_W-range of immunoglobulins and for proteins with a lower M_W than that of albumin ($M_W \sim 69\ 000$). No connection seemed to exist between the protein adsorption pattern, the behavior *in vivo* or the composition (e.g. the content of SiO_2) of the bioactive glasses.

DISCUSSION

Protein adsorption is a routine test to screen surface properties of various materials. A material adsorbing only albumin from the plasma is theoretically more biocompatible than a material that adsorbs several plasma proteins, including fibrinogen [5]. The bioactive glasses tested showed rather similar protein adsorption profiles with albumin as

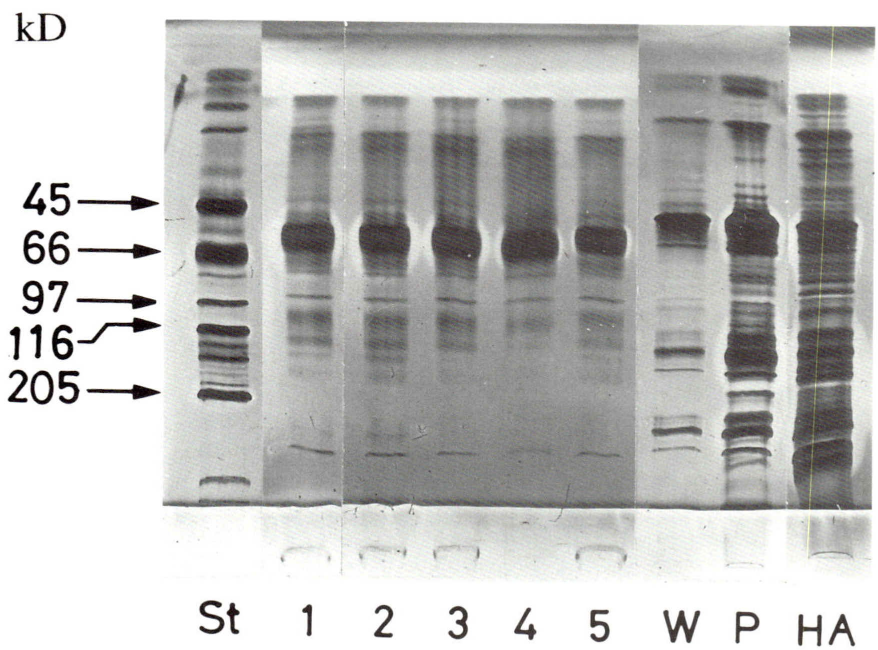

Figure 2. Adsorption of plasma proteins to various materials. St = molecular weight standard, 1 = glass 9-93, 2 = 13-93, 3 = 14-93, 4 = 17-93, 5 = 19-93, W = inert glass, P = plasma and HA = hydroxyapatite.

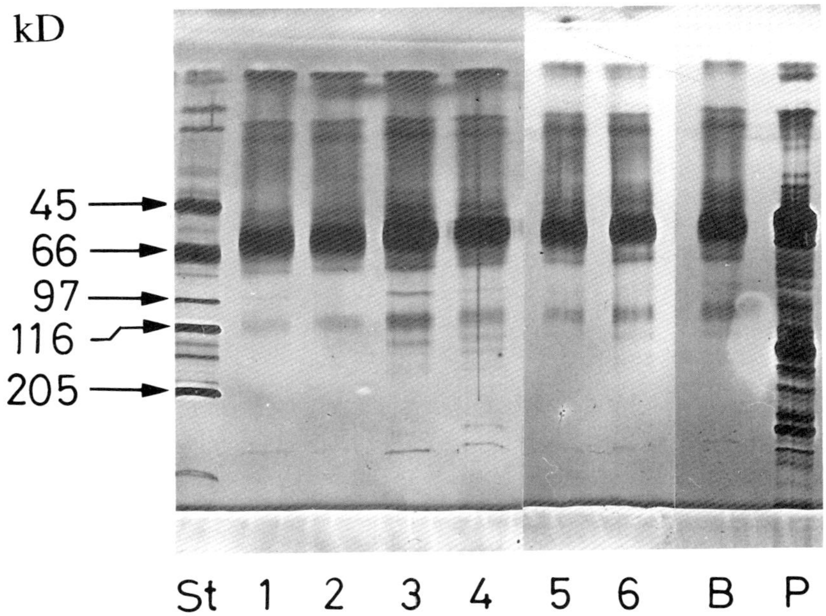

Figure 3. Adsorption of plasma proteins to various materials. St = molecular weight standard, 1 = glass 5-92, 2 = 11-92, 3 = 12-92, 4 = 20-92, 5 = 14-92, 6 = 15-92, B = Bioglass® 45S5 and P = plasma.

the main protein adsorbed. With regard to the plasma protein adsorption patterns, the glasses resembled the commercial reference, Bioglass® 45S5 and the bioactive glass S53P4 developed at Åbo Akademi University, Finland [4,6]. However, the protein adsorption to these glasses differed clearly from that of the inert glass and HA.

The differences in the protein adsorption to the materials may be due to differences in their surface potentials. In the experimental conditions used in the protein adsorption tests, both the proteins and the bioactive glasses are negatively charged. The glass surface is then supposed to attract calcium and sodium ions, and these may then attract the negatively charged proteins to the glass. Thus the protein adsorption tests may function as tests for large differences in surface potentials, e.g. due to corrosion, of bioactive glasses.

SUMMARY

The differences in the protein adsorption profiles of the bioactive glasses were not associated with their behavior *in vivo*. However, the protein profiles of the inert glass and HA differed clearly from those of the bioactive glasses. This indicates that large differences in surface potentials of glasses could be tested with the protein adsorption test used in this study. Such differences could be related to the bioactivity of the glasses.

REFERENCES

1. Kokubo, T., Kushitani, H., Sakka, S., Kitsugi, T. and Yamamuro, T. *J. Biomed. Mater. Res.* 1990, 24, 721-734.

2. Hench, L. L. and Paschall, H. A. *J. Biomed. Mater. Res. Symp.* 1973, 4, 25-42.
3. Brink, M., Brink, A. and Karlsson, K. H. Submitted to *J. Non-Cryst. Solids.*
4. Söderling, E., Herbst, K., Larmas, E. and Yli-Urpo, A. To be published.
5. Horbett, T. In: *Techniques of biocompatibility testing* Volume 2, CRC Press, USA 1986, 183-214.
6. Andersson, Ö., Liu, G., Karlsson, K. H., Niemi, L., Miettinen, J. and Juhanoja, J. *J. Mater. Sci. Mater. Med.* 1990, 1, 219-227.

THE EVALUATION OF SURFACE STRUCTURE OF BIOACTIVE GLASSES *IN-VITRO*

D. C. Greenspan[1], J. P. Zhong[1] and G. P. LaTorre[2]

[1]U.S. Biomaterials Corporation, One Progress Boulevard, #23, Alachua, FL 32615
[2]Advanced Materials Research Center, University of Florida, One Progress Boulevard, #14, Alachua, FL 32615

ABSTRACT

Evaluation of the surface structure of four compositions of bioactive glasses was conducted in this work. The formation of an hydroxyl carbonate apatite (HCA) surface layer on the bioactive glasses reacted in a tris buffer solution appeared to be related to the development of a high surface area. It was found that a surface area of at least 40 to 60 m^2/g was needed to induce the precipitation and crystallization of HCA. For the bioactive glass which can bond to either bone or soft tissue, the surface area ultimately attained was greater than 100 m^2/g. These *in-vitro* results could provide useful information for further investigations of bonding of biomaterials with living tissue.

INTRODUCTION

Bonding of bioactive glasses to living tissue is associated with formation of hydroxyl carbonate apatite (HCA) on their surface and is greatly influenced by the glass composition, especially the silica content [1]. Melt derived bioactive glasses with silica content from 45wt% to 52wt% can bond to either bone or soft tissue [2], glasses with silica content between 52wt% to 55wt% bond only to bone. For silica content greater than 55wt% [1], no bonding with tissue is observed and there is no formation of an HCA layer.

In previous studies, three characteristics: 1) surface charge [3], 2) surface pore size [4], and 3) surface silanol groups [5] were found to be key factors for the induction of HCA formation on the bioactive glasses and the resultant bonding of the glasses to tissue. However, all three factors are related to the surface structure of the silica gel layer which is formed from ion exchange, dissolution and polycondensation on the bioactive glasses.

In 1975, Walker and Hench found [6] that a high surface area resulting from the reactive gel layer formed on bioactive glasses was critical for bonding to bone. More recently, work on sol-gel bioactive glasses by Li [7] substantiated this finding. The current work was designed to evaluate the evolution of surface structure during *in-vitro* testing of four compositions of bioactive glass and to determine the relationship of the induction of HCA and their corresponding bonding behavior.

MATERIALS AND METHODS

The production of the four compositions of bioactive glasses used in this study are described in detail elsewhere [8,9]. Briefly, regent grade chemicals (SiO_2, $CaCO_3$, Na_2CO_3 and P_2O_5) were mixed, melted for 6 hours at 1350°C-1400°C and quenched in water. The resultant frit was then ball milled in alumina mill jars and sieved through -24mesh and +170mesh screen to produce a particle size range of 90μm to 710μm.

The properties of the four compositions of bioactive glasses have been also described in detail in an earlier work [8]. Their composition and bioactivity are listed in Table 1. The surface structure analysis was performed using N_2 adsorption/desorption isotherms (Autosorb-6, Quantachrome Corp., Boyton Beach, FL.). Based on a previous study [9] which established an *in-vitro* QA test model for 710μm -90μm powders, reactivity tests were conducted dynamically in tris buffer solution with SA/V of $0.4cm^{-1}$ at 37°C. After reaction at various time periods the samples were separated from solution by vacuum filtering and rinsed with acetone to dehydrate and halt the surface reaction. The samples were then subjected to FTIR and BET analysis.

RESULTS

Figure 1 shows the specific surface area and average pore radius of the four compositions of glass as a function of reaction time. There is a more higher surface area established for the low silica content glasses than the high silica glasses, with surface areas as high as 125 m^2/g for 45S5 after 20 hrs in tris buffer. As the silica content of the glass increased the resulting surface area decreased; pore size is relatively independent of silica content.

Figure 2 shows the FTIR reflection spectra of the four glasses. The appearance of the P-O vibrational modes for HCA with peaks around 602 cm^{-1} and 560 cm^{-1} indicates the development of crystalline HCA on the glass surface. The intensity of the Si-O bending vibration at 450 cm^{-1} is a measure of the thickness of the HCA layer. For 45S5 with the fastest change in surface area, HCA appeared after 6 hours reaction in tris buffer. As can be seen in FTIR spectrum, the Si-O vibrational mode at around 450 cm^{-1} disappeared after 20 hours which suggests that the HCA layer is well established and covered the entire surface of the glass. For 52S4, HCA appeared at 20 hrs and was well developed by 3 days. For 55S4, HCA appeared at 3 days and it took 7 days for the crystalline layer to cover the entire surface. For 60S3 with the slowest change in surface area, HCA never appeared even after reacted 20 days in tris buffer.

Table 1. Bioactive Glass Compositions and Their Bioactivity

Designation	Bioactivity Description	SiO_2 (Mol%)	Na_2O (Mol%)	CaO (Mol%)	P_2O_5 (Mol%)
45S5	Bond to Bone and Soft Tissue	46.1	24.4	26.9	2.6
52S4.6	Bond to Bone and Soft Tissue	52.1	21.5	23.8	2.6
55S4.3	Bond only to Bone	55.1	20.1	22.2	2.6
60S3.8	No Bonding	60.1	17.7	19.6	2.6

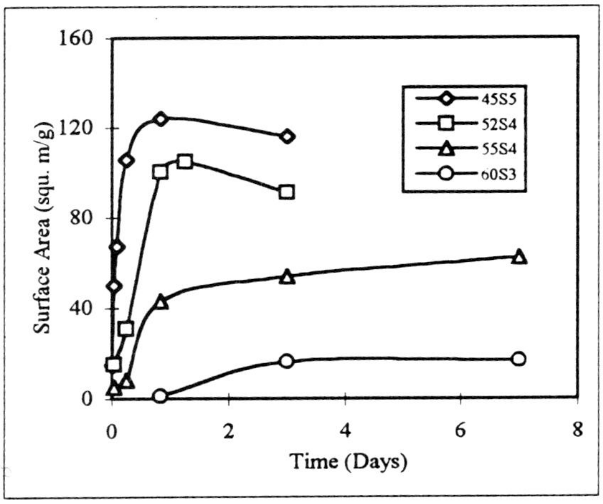

(a)

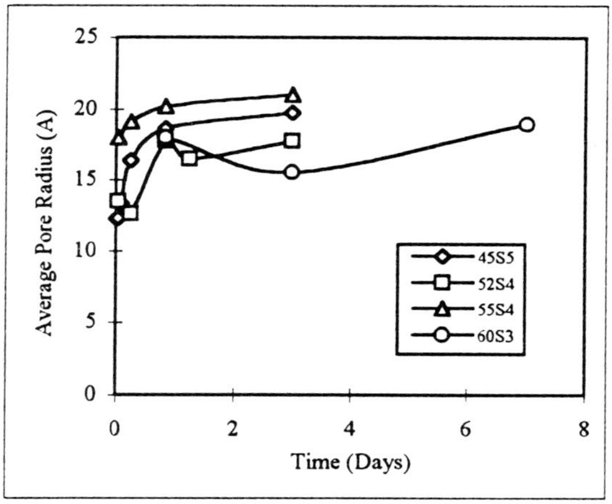

(b)

Figure 1. Specific surface area (a) and average pore radius (b) of four compositions of bioactive glasses as a function of reaction time.

DISCUSSION

Numerous authors have reported that a high surface area and a high concentration of silanol groups are required to grow crystalline HCA [4-7]. Bioactive gel glasses [7] and pure gel silica [5] with high surface areas and a high concentration of silanol groups were all found to induce the crystallization of HCA. When bioactive glass is immersed in physiological solution, ion exchange, dissolution and polycondensation takes place on the surface leading to formation of a silica gel layer which contributes high surface area and

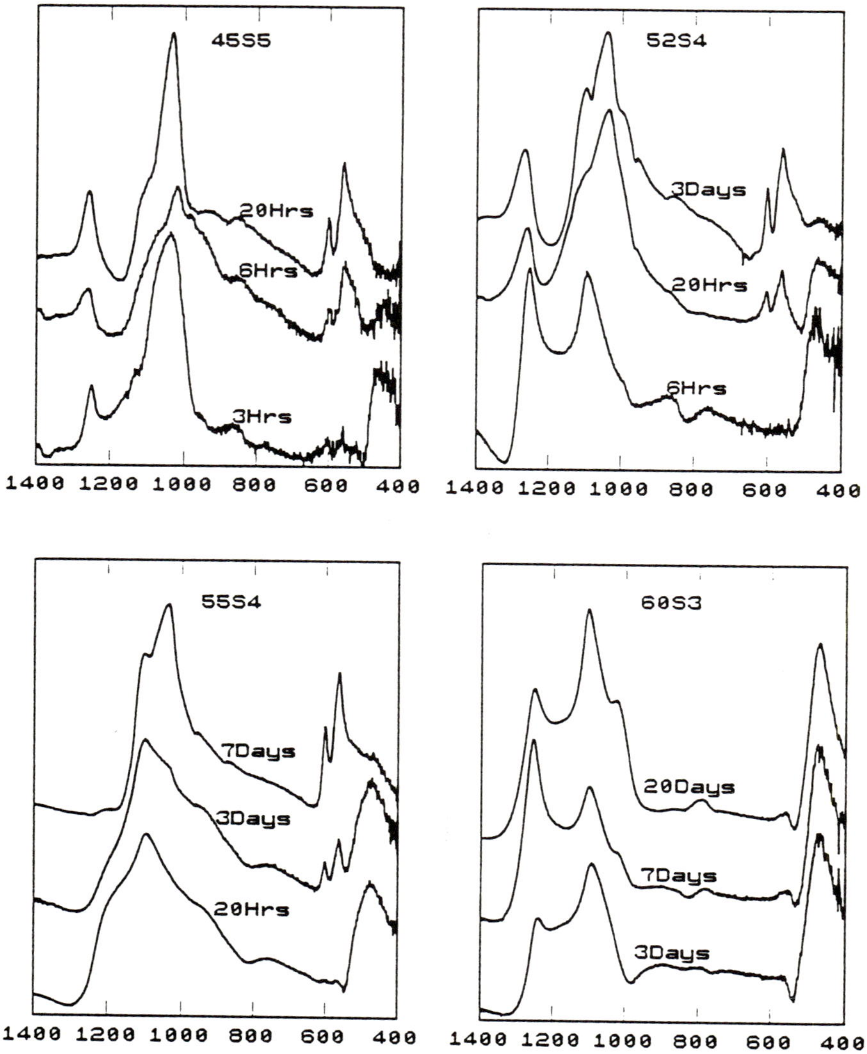

Figure 2. FTIR reflection spectra of the four compositions of bioactive glasses.

a high concentration of silanol groups. This silica gel layer with a high surface area is thought to be responsible for the formation of HCA [1].

As can be seen in Figs 1, and 2, HCA crystals appear for 45S5, 52S4 and 55S4 glasses when their specific surface area reaches a critical level of 40 m^2/g to 60 M^2/g. For 60S, no crystalline HCA layer can be observed and its specific surface area never reaches this level. It should be noted that only 45S5 and 52S4 reach a surface area of over 100 m^2/g. 55S4 only reaches a maximum of 60 m^2/g.

Hench has classified bioactive materials as either type A and type B [10], where, type A materials rapidly bond to bone <u>and</u> soft tissue and also function to enhance bone augmentation by releasing silicon into the local environment [11,12]. Since 45S5 and 52S4 are among type A biomaterials, the rapidly developed high surface area (> 100 m^2/g) could be another characteristic of type A biomaterials. In addition, the high surface area of 45S5 and 52S4 provides high concentration of silanol groups which could be sufficient for either inducing HCA formation as nucleation sites or binding tissue such as collagen and enable these glasses to bond to either bone or soft tissue.

Although 55S4, a type B biomaterial, can induce HCA formation, its surface area only reached a maximum of 60 m^2/g. It is likely that this surface area contributes to the bonding to bone, but is not sufficient to allow bonding to soft tissue. This could be related to the differences in silanol concentration and silicon release rates for high surface area (low silica content) versus low surface area (high silica content) glasses.

It was found that the average pore radius changed little as a function of glass composition. Previous work on sol-gel derived bioactive glasses by Pereira [4] has shown that large pore radii led to the early precipitation and crystallization of HCA. The data presented here indicates there is very little difference in average pore radius for 45S5 and 55S4 as a function of reaction time. If one assumes that the mechanisms responsible for the evolution of pore structure are similar (i.e., ion exchange and the dissolution and polycondensation of silica) then we would expect that the resultant pore radius for each of these compositions would be similar. Therefore, the most important factor influencing the formation of HCA with respect to surface evolution is the differences in surface area for low silica content versus high silica content glasses.

CONCLUSION

The surface area varied markedly for the four compositions of bioactive glasses which led to very different onset times and growth rates of crystalline HCA. For 45S5, 5254 and 55S4 glasses, crystalline HCA appeared when their specific surface area reached 40 m^2/g to 60 m^2/g, For 60S, no crystalline HCA can be observed and its specific surface area never reach this level. 45S5 and 52S4, type A bioactive materials, can reached over 100 m^2/g in specific surface area which could be responsible for their bonding to either bone or soft tissue.

REFERENCE

1. Hench, L.L., *J. Am. Ceram. Soc.*, 1991, <u>74</u>[7], 1487-1510
2. Wilson, J., and Nolletti, D., *Handbook of Bioactive Ceramics,* Vol. I, CRC Press, Boca Raton, Florida, 1990, 283-302
3. Zhong, J.P., LaTorre, G.P., and Hench, L.L., *Bioceramics 7,* O.H. Andersson and A. Yli-Urpo eds., Butterworth-Heinemann Ltd, 1994, 61-66
4 Pereira, M.M., Dissertation of Doctor of Philosophy, University of Florida, 1994
5. Li, P.J., Ohtsuki, C., Kokubo, T. *et al J. Am. Ceram. Soc.*, 1992, 75[8], 2094-97
6. Walker, M.M., Thesis for the Degree of Master of Science, University of Florida, 1977
7. Li, R., Clark, A.E., and Hench, L.L., *J. Appl. Biomater.,* 1991, 2 231-39
8. Ogino, M., Ohuchi, F., and Hench, L.L., *J. Biomed. Mater. Res.,* 1980, 14 55-64
9. Greenspan, D.C., Zhong, J.P., and LaTorre, G.P., *Bioceramics 7*, O.H. Andersson and A. Yli-Urpo eds., Butterworth-Heinemann Ltd, 1994, 55-60

10. Hench, L.L., *Bioceramics 7* , O.H. Andersson and A. Yli-Urpo eds., Butterworth-Heinemann Ltd, 1994, 3-14
11. Hott, M., Pollak, C. de, Modrowski, D., and Marie, P.J., *Calcif. Tissue Int.,* 1993, 53 174-79
12. Kubo, K., Kamada, T., Matsuyama, T. *et al. J. Biomed. Mat. Res.*, 1995, 29 503-09

SILICA RELEASE FROM BIOACTIVE GLASS

Örjan H. Andersson

Turku Centre for Biomaterials, Lemminkäisenkatu 2, FIN-20520 Turku/Åbo, Finland and Åbo Akademi University, Dept. Chem. Eng., Åbo/Turku, Finland

ABSTRACT

The Si-release in a tris-citric acid buffer was studied for glasses in the Na_2O-CaO-B_2O_3-Al_2O_3-SiO_2-P_2O_5 system. A polynom describing the relationship between Si-release and glass composition was developed. The model can be used to design glass compositions with controlled Si-release. This may be of interest since it recently has been suggested that soluble silicon might control intracellular mitogenic factors. The model is also useful when designing glasses of reduced solubility. It was found that the Si-release is mainly determined by the SiO_2 and Al_2O_3 contents of the glass. For Al_2O_3-free glasses the Si-release decreases linearly with increasing SiO_2. Without losing bioactivity, the solubility can be reduced more by increasing the SiO_2 content than by adding Al_2O_3.

INTRODUCTION

The first steps in the formation of a bond between a bioactive glass and bone are rapid ion exchange, loss of soluble silica to the solution and subsequent polycondensation of a Si-rich surface layer [1]. Reducing the rate of silica network dissolution by modifying the glass composition also reduces the rates of formation of the SiO_2-gel layer and of the hydroxylapatite surface layer required for bone bonding [2]. In addition to being essential for the bonding of a bioactive glass to bone, silica is also a constituent of many biological systems [3]. Carlisle showed that silica is essential for the development of bone [4]. Recent reports suggest metabolic function [5] and intracellular mitogenic effects [6] of soluble silicon. These aspects were recently discussed by Hench [7]. Thus, it may prove useful to be able to control the Si-release of bioactive glasses.

Control of the solubility is also important when developing e.g. glasses for long-term stable bioactive coatings. The chemical durability of silicate glass increases as the SiO_2 content is increased, or as Al_2O_3 is added. However, increasing the SiO_2 content decreases the rate of bone bonding (2,8) and Al_2O_3 has negative effects on bone formation (9-11). Thus, if the solubility is to be reduced, the addition with the smaller negative effect on the bioactivity should be chosen.

The dissolution of a glass involves several reactions. In addition to the ion exchange and network dissolution reactions, calcium phosphate forms at the surface of bioactive glasses. This reaction retards the dissolution [12]. If the chemical durability of the glass structure is to be tested, the calcium phosphate formation should be avoided. Since the rate of calcium phosphate formation depends on the glass composition, the choice of test time also greatly influence the results. By adding citrate to the solution, the calcium phosphate formation is prevented due to formation of soluble Ca-citrate [13]. Thus, the Si-release depends on the stability of the glass structure, not on calcium phosphate accumulation.

In the present work glasses within or near the bioactive composition region in the system Na_2O-CaO-B_2O_3-Al_2O_3-SiO_2-P_2O_5 were characterized with respect to their Si-release. The aims were to 1) compare the Si-release from bone bonding and non-bonding glasses, 2) develop a model which can be used when developing glass compositions with controlled Si-release and 3) determine whether the solubility expressed as Si-release is most efficiently decreased by Al_2O_3 additions or by increasing the SiO_2 content of the glass.

MATERIALS AND METHODS

The studied glass compositions (Table 1) were chosen by the Plackett and Burman method described by Montgomery [14]. Compositions 9, 10, 12, 14, and 15 are bioactive, whereas the others are not [8]. The raw materials used were SiO_2, Na_2CO_3, $CaCO_3$, $CaHPO_4 \cdot 2H_2O$, Al_2O_3 and H_3BO_3. The glasses were melted in a platinum crucible for 2-3 hours at 1340-1410°C, annealed, crushed and sieved to a grain size of 300-500 µm.

In order to remove glass dust, the grains were rapidly rinsed three times in demineralized water before they were immersed in the test solution. The test solution was tris-citric acid buffer (tris-c.a.), prepared by dissolving 50 mM tris(hydroxylmethyl-aminomethane) and 15 mM citric acid in demineralized water. The solution pH was 7.4, the temperature 37°C and the surface area to solution volume ratio 0.1 cm^{-1}. After 60 minutes the solutions were decanted and analysed photometrically for silicon by the molybdenum blue method.

RESULTS AND DISCUSSION

Si-release and the stabilizing effect of SiO_2 and Al_2O_3.

The mean Si-release during the 60 minute immersion period is shown in Figure 1. There is a trend toward a smaller release with higher SiO_2 content of the glass. It has been reported that the SiO_2-gel formation and calcium phosphate formation is more rapid for glass 10 than for glass 9 [15]. The present results show that the Si-release correspondingly is more rapid for the former glass. The bone bonding glasses 9, 10, 12, 14, and 15 released more silica than most of the non-bonding ones. However, for the non-bonding glasses 13 and 16, the Si-release was comparable to that of the bone bonding ones. Glasses 13 and 16 contain 3 and 2 wt-% Al_2O_3, respectively. Thus, for Al_2O_3 containing glasses a high Si-release cannot be taken as a sign of bioactivity. It has been reported that calcium phosphate accumulated at the surface of both glass 13 and 16 *in vivo* [8].

Table 1. Glass compositions by synthesis (weight-%)

Designation		Na_2O	CaO	B_2O_3	Al_2O_3	SiO_2	P_2O_5
#1	S63.5P6	15.0	14.0	0.5	1.0	63.5	6.0
#2	S57.5P5	16.0	18.0	3.0	0.5	57.5	5.0
#3	S63.5P1	17.0	13.0	1.0	2.5	65.5	1.0
#4	S52P3	18.0	24.0	0.0	3.0	52.0	3.0
#5	S56P6	19.0	16.0	1.5	1.5	56.0	6.0
#6	S51P7	20.0	17.0	3.0	2.0	51.0	7.0
#7	S51P2	21.0	21.0	2.0	3.0	51.0	2.0
#8	S64P0	22.0	10.0	2.5	1.5	64.0	0.0
#9	S53P4	23.0	20.0	0.0	0.0	53.0	4.0
#10	S45P7	24.0	22.0	2.0	0.0	45.0	7.0
#11	S52P8	25.0	12.0	0.5	2.5	52.0	8.0
#12	S46P0	26.0	25.0	2.0	1.0	46.0	0.0
#13	S38P8	27.0	23.0	1.0	3.0	38.0	8.0
#14	S48P2	28.0	19.0	1.5	1.5	48.0	2.0
#15	S55.5P4	29.0	11.0	0.0	0.5	55.5	4.0
#16	S45.5P5	30.0	15.0	2.5	2.0	45.5	5.0

The experimental data were analysed by linear regression. Each of the three parallel experiments for each glass was included. The Si-release could be fairly well described as a function of only the SiO_2 and the Al_2O_3 contents.

$$\text{Si (ppm)} = 43.677 - 0.705 \times SiO_2 - 2.257 \times Al_2O_3 \tag{1}$$

The regression coefficient (R^2) was 94.5 % and the residual standard deviation () 0.94 ppm. The most durable glasses in the series showed Si-release close to zero. The fit of the model to the experimental data (higher R^2) could probably be improved by extending the test time, so that clear differences would be seen also between these glasses.

The coefficients in the equation describe the internal relationship between the oxides with respect to their effect on solubility, whereas the intercept only serves to give the Si-release a numerical value. Thus, the stabilizing effect may be expressed as the absolute value of the sum of the SiO_2 and Al_2O_3 contents according to their weights given by equation 1 (Fig. 2). In terms of decreasing the Si-release, increasing the Al_2O_3 content by 1 wt-% unit has the same effect as increasing the SiO_2 content by 3.2 wt-% units.

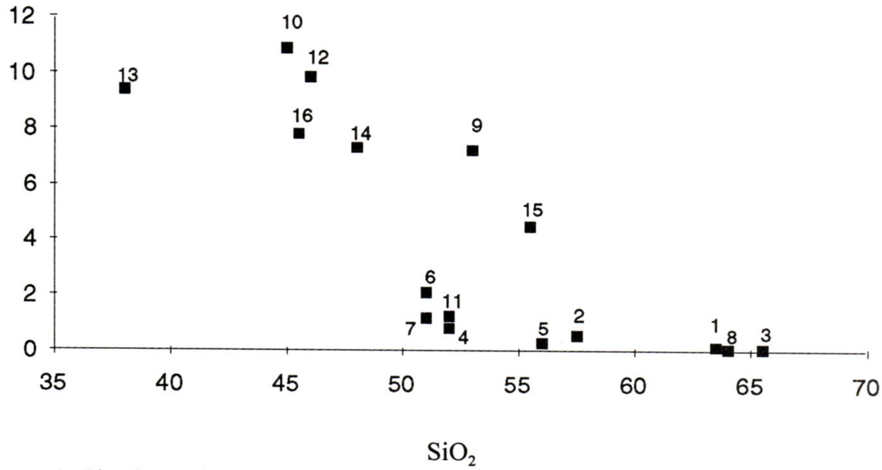

Figure 1. Si-release (ppm) during 60 minutes in tris-c.a, plotted versus the SiO_2 content of the glass. The designations of the points correspond to the compositions in Table 1.

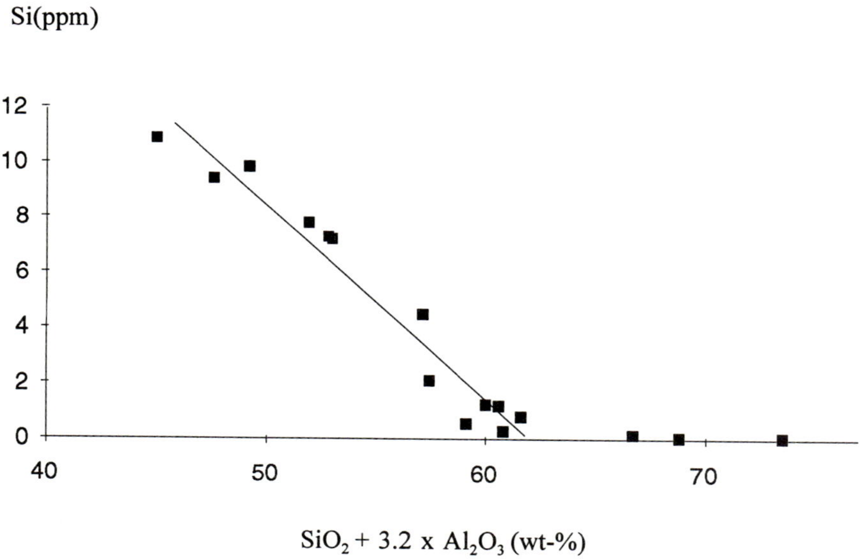

Figure 2. Same data as in Figure 1, plotted versus the sum of SiO_2 and Al_2O_3 contents according to their weights in equation 1.

Equation 1 shows that for Al_2O_3-free glasses, the Si-release decreases linearly with increasing SiO_2 content. Under the chosen experimental conditions, the Si-release Si(ppm) approaches zero as the SiO_2 content of the glass approaches 60-62 wt-% (Fig. 2). This suggests that compositions, in the studied system, with more than 60 weight-% SiO_2 are not bioactive, as also reported by Hench [2]. Thus, for Al_2O_3-free glasses there seems to be a correlation between Si-release and bioactivity.

It is well-known that Al_2O_3 increases the chemical durability of glass by altering the glass structure. It is also known that a strong retarding effect on the glass dissolution can result from the formation of an alumino-silicate surface film [16]. One could expect that the citrate in the test solution would interfere with the formation of such a film. However, according to Chappell and Birchall stable species of alumino-silicate can exist at pH 7.4 in the presence of citrate [17]. Whether an alumino-silicate film forms or not under the chosen experimental conditions, is a matter which requires further investigations.

Simulation of the effect of increased SiO_2 content or Al_2O_3 addition

The effects of increasing the SiO_2 content or adding Al_2O_3 to glass S53P4 [9] were simulated by combining equation 1 with a previously reported model for the biological behaviour [8]. In the latter model the biological behaviour of the glass is expressed as a reaction number, RN, where RN above 4.5 to 5 indicates bioactivity [8]. In the present simulation an RN value of 5 was taken as the criterion for bioactivity. The additions were made so that the other oxides decreased proportionally. Without losing bioactivity, the Si-release could be decreased by 47 % if the SiO_2 content of the glass was increased (Figure 3). If instead Al_2O_3 was added, the Si-release could be reduced by only 29 % before the bioactivity was lost (Figure 3). Thus, at the same degree of bioactivity the durability is more efficiently increased by SiO_2 than by Al_2O_3 additions. Therefore, if only the solubility of the glass is to be controlled it is preferred to increase the SiO_2 content. The addition of Al_2O_3 can be justified if other properties must be controlled. A greater number of oxides allows a greater number of properties to be controlled.

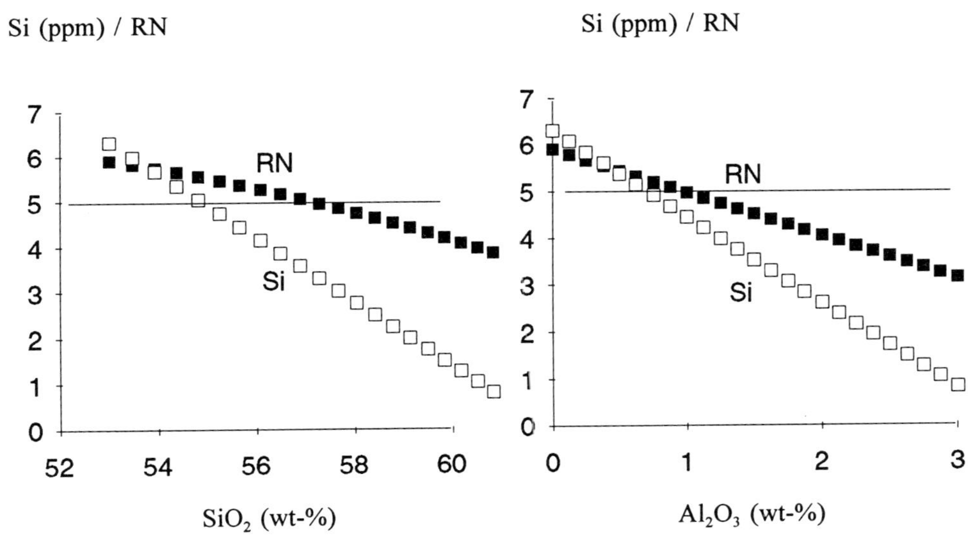

Figure 3. Simulation of the effect on Si-release () and biological behaviour, RN. (), of increasing the SiO_2 content or adding Al_2O_3 to glass S53P4 [9]. RN values above the horizontal line indicate glasses which are bioactive.

CONCLUSIONS

The Si-release from the bone bonding glasses was in general considerably higher than from the non-bonding ones. The results suggest that for Al_2O_3-free bioactive glasses there is a correlation between Si-release and bioactivity, whereas no such correlation was seen for Al_2O_3-containing glasses.

The Si-release was mainly determined by the SiO_2 and Al_2O_3 contents of the glass. The relationship between Si-release and composition could be described as a polynom. At the same degree of bioactivity, the durability is more efficiently increased by SiO_2 than by Al_2O_3 additions. Thus, if only the solubility of the glass is to be controlled, this should be done by increasing the SiO_2 content, not by adding Al_2O_3. For bioactive glasses in the Na_2O-CaO-(B_2O_3)-SiO_2-P_2O_5 system, the Si-release decreases linearly with increasing SiO_2 content under the chosen experimental conditions. The Si-release approaches zero as the SiO_2 content approaches 60-62 weight-%.

REFERENCES

1. Hench, L.L., *J. Am. Ceram. Soc.*, 1991, 74, 1487-1510.
2. Hench, L.L., *Ann. N.Y. Acad. Sci.*, 1988, 523, 54-71.
3. Iler, R.K. *The chemistry of silica*, John Wiley & Sons Inc, New York, NY., 1979.
4. Carlisle, E., In: *Biochemistry of Silicon,* Ciba Foundation Symposium 121. John Wiley & Sons, New York, NY. 1986
5. Keeting, P.E., Oursler, M.J., Wiegand, K.E., Bonde, S.K., Spelsberg, T.C., Riggs, B.L. *J. Bone and Mineral Res.* 1992, 7, 1281-1289.
6. Vrouwenwelder, W.C.A., Groot, C.G., de Groot, K., *J. Biomed. Mater. Res.* 1993, 27, 465-475.
7. Hench, L.L., in: *Bioceramics,* Vol. 7, Ö.H. Andersson, R.-P. Happonen, and A. Yli-Urpo (Eds.), Butterworth-Heinemann Ltd., Oxford, 1994, 3-14.
8. Andersson, Ö.H., Liu, G., Karlsson, K.H., Niemi, L., Miettinen, J., and Juhanoja, J., *J. Mater. Sci.: Materials in Medicine,* 1990, 1, 219-227.
9. Gross, U. and Strunz, V., *J. Biomed. Mater. Res.* 1985, 19, 251-271.
10. Gross, U. and Strunz, V., *J. Biomed. Mater. Res.* 1980, 14, 607-618.
11. Andersson, Ö.H., Karlsson, K.H., Kangasniemi, K., Yli-Urpo, A., *Glastech. Ber.* 1988, 61, 300-305.
12. Hench, L.L. and Clark, D.E., *J. Non-Cryst. Solids* 1978, 28, 83-105.
13. Andersson, Ö.H. and Karlsson, K.H. In: *Clinical Implant Materials*, G. Heimke, U. Soltesz and A.J.C. Lee (Eds.), Advances in Biomaterials, Volume 9, Elsevier Sciense Publishers B.V., Amsterdam, 1990, 259-264.
14. Montgomery, D.C., *Design and analysis of experiments,* 2nd ed. New York: Wiley 1984.
15. Hench, L.L. Andersson, Ö.H., LaTorre, G.P. In: *Bioceramics,* Vol. 4, W. Bonfield, G.W. Hastings and K.E. Tanner (Eds.), Butterworth-Heinemann Ltd. Guildford, UK, 1991, 155-162.
16. Dilmore, M.F., Clark, D.E., and Hench, L.L., *Cer. Bull.* 1978, 57, 1040-1044, 1048.
17. Chappell, J.S. and Birchall, J.D., *Inorganica Chimica Acta* 1988, 153, 1-4.

ALUMINUM INHIBITORY EFFECT ON THE FORMATION OF HYDROXYAPATITE

J. P. Zhong[1], G. P. LaTorre[2], D. C. Greenspan[1], L. L. Hench[2]

[1]U.S. Biomaterials Corporation, One Progress Boulevard, #23, Alachua, FL 32615.
[2]Advanced Materials Research Center, University of Florida, One Progress Boulevard, #14, Alachua, FL 32615

ABSTRACT
It was found in this work on porous silica gel that the addition of even a small amount ($2x10^{-4}$ M) of Al^{3+} in a SBF solution prevented the formation of HA on the gel's surface. Surface zeta potential data was obtained which indicated that the surface potential of silica changed from negative to positive when exposed to an aqueous solution with Al^{3+}. These results suggest that the surface binding of aluminum can establish a positive surface potential, which inhibits HA formation, bone mineralization and bonding of bone to bioactive implants.

INTRODUCTION
Clinically, osteomalacia, a bone disease, has been associated with aluminum present at the mineralization front in bone which inhibits mineralization[1]. In an *in-vitro* experiment, aluminum was shown to bind to hydroxyapatite (HA) and to amorphous calcium phosphate (ACP) and slow the HA crystal growth and transformation of ACP to HA [2]. 45S5 formula Bioglass® bonds rapidly to living tissue and the bonding appears to be related to the rapid development of a crystalline hydroxyl carbonate apatite (HCA) layer on its surface[3]. However, when as little as 3wt% Al_2O_3 is added to the 45S5 formula, HCA no longer forms on the glass surface and bone bonding is prevented [3]. Blumenthal [2] proposed that the binding of aluminum to HA interfered with the HA nucleation process by inhibiting the aggregation of calcium and phosphate ions required to form a critical nucleus. For bioactive glasses, Andersson suggested [4] that the favorable sites for calcium phosphate nucleation in the silica gel might be occupied by Al^{3+} ions and retarded HCA crystal growth by forming Al-containing crystals.

Recent work showed that a negative surface potential could be important in inducing HA formation [5,6]. We use a porous silica gel in this work to examine the effect of absorption of aluminum on a bioactive surface [7] and determine its effect on surface potential and formation of HCA.

MATERIALS AND METHODS

Type VI porous silica gel samples (from AMRC, University of Florida) were used for this study. The samples were TMOS derived with 4.5nm average pore radius and the preparation and characterization of this gel have been reported previously by Hench et al [8,9]. A simulated body fluid (SBF) was prepared for in-vitro test with ion concentrations nearly equal to those of human blood plasma [7] and pH buffered to 7.25 at 37°C. All in-vitro tests were conducted at 37°C by immersing the silica gel into the SBF solution in a polyethylene bottle with SA/V about $0.1cm^{-1}$ for 2 weeks (the surface area was calculated from the geometric shape). Another in-vitro test was conducted in parallel using a modified SBF solution with additional $2x10^{-4}$M Al^{3+}. The development of HA on the surface of all the samples was evaluated by FTIR reflection spectroscopy.

The zeta potential, ζ, of the electrical double layer in the gel surface was measured by means of a MATEC ESA 8000 System. For enough signals to be detected during the measurement, a suspension was made using 8 g of the gel powders (<38μm) in 200ml D.I. water. The pH was titrated for the suspension by 1N HCl or 1N KOH.

RESULTS AND DISCUSSION

In Fig.1, FTIR reflection spectra show the P-O vibrational modes of HA crystals at 560 cm^{-1} and 602 cm^{-1} for the silica gel exposed into SBF solution for 2 weeks. No HA crystal modes are found for the gel exposed in the modified SBF solution with $2x10^{-4}$M Al^{3+} for the same time period. The zeta potential of the gel vs. pH is shown in Fig. 2. It decreased from nearly 0mv at pH of 2.0, the IEP, to about -20mv at pH of 8.0 in the powder suspension without Al. However, the zeta potential versus pH was dramatically changed in the suspension with Al ions. The zeta potential at pH of 7.25 changes from negative to positive with Al^{3+} in solution.

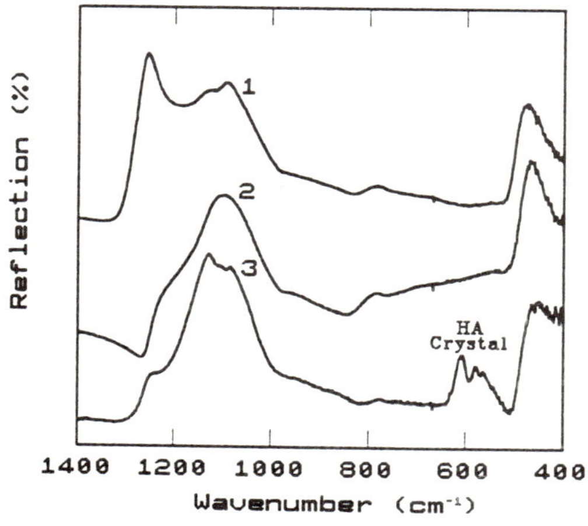

Figure 1. FTIR reflection spectra of silica-gel: 1) Unreacted; 2) 2 weeks in SBF with $2x10^{-4}$M Al; 3) 2 weeks in SBF.

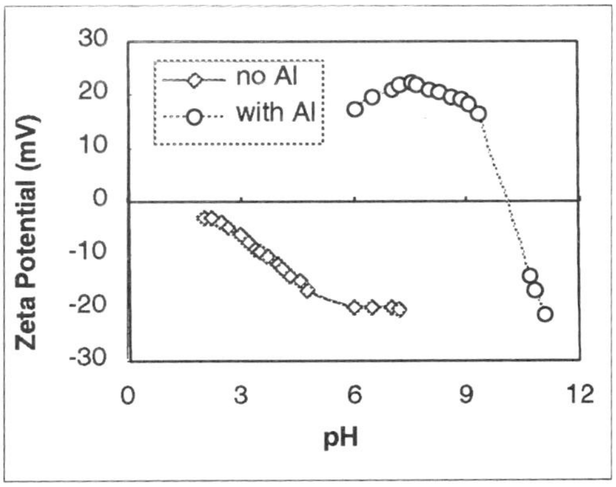

Figure 2. Zeta potential of silica in aqueous solutions vs. pH

Since indifferent counterions in the diffuse layer of an electrical double layer cannot contribute to a change in sign of ζ, the reversing change indicates a chemical adsorption of Al ions on the surface. In 1979, Dilmore *et al* [10], based on their studies of glass corrosion, reported that although Al^{3+} did not appreciably affect the ion exchange between glass and solution, the Al ions adsorbed onto and diffused into the silica-rich layer forming a protective film which minimized the corrosion by decreasing network dissolution. Iler reported [11] that the maximum amount of adsorbed alumna could reach about 3.1 aluminum atoms /nm^2 of silica surface. Since Al_2O_3 is a network former, the adsorbed Al on a gel surface could possibly substitute for Si and enter into a silicate network as shown in Fig.3. In this case, H^+ would tightly bound to the surface around Al which contributes to the positive surface potential.

For the zeta potential measurements, D.I. water was used instead of SBF buffer solution because the buffer solution needs a large amount of acid or base solution for titration which would result in an incorrect signal. However an assumption can be made that the zeta potential of the silica gel in modified SBF with 2×10^{-4}M Al^{3+} would be positive at pH of 7.25, the same as in D.I. water with the same amount of Al^{3+}.

In recent works, the surface negative potential of silica gel [7] and collagen fibrils [6] have been reported to accumulate calcium and phosphate ions leading to the formation of HA crystals. A positive surface potential can retard the accumulation of calcium and phosphate ions and therefore inhibit formation of HA.

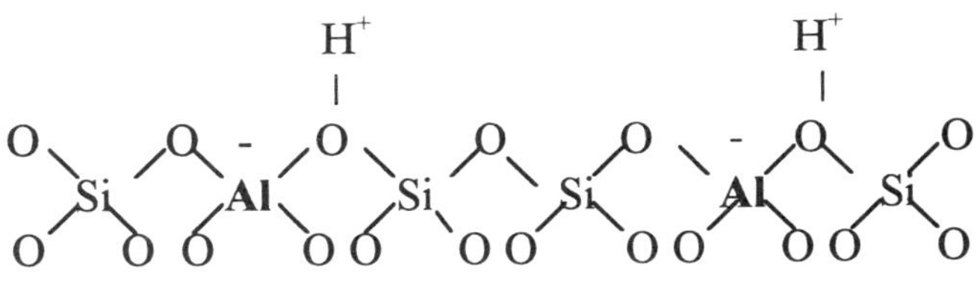

Figure 3. Surface structure of Al in silica.

The binding of aluminum ions to hydroxyapatite nuclei could also bring the surface to a high positive potential which could inhibit further precipitation and crystal growth. Aluminum could also bind to constituents of bone tissue such as collagen could build a positive potential on collagen fibrils and prevent the mineralization.

CONCLUSION

The binding of Al to the surface of silica gel converted the surface potential from negative to positive, which retarded the accumulation of calcium and phosphate ions and the formation of HA. Similarly, it could be assumed that the binding of Al on hydroxyapatite crystals and bone constituents, such as collagen, could also build a positive surface potential which is responsible for the inhibitation of HA crystal growth and bone mineralization.

REFERENCE

1. Hodsman, A.B., Sherrard, D.J., and Alfrey, A.C. et al, *J. Clin. Endocrinol. Metab.*,1982 54, 539-46.
2. Blumenthal, N.C., *The Chemistry and Biology of Mineralized Tissues*, W.T. Butler ed., Ebsco Media, Inc., Birmingham, AL, 1985, 385-88.
3. Hench, L.L., *J. Am. Ceram. Soc.,* 1991, 74 [7], 1487-1510.
4. Andersson, O.H., Rosenqvist, J., and Karlsson, K.H. *J. Biomed. Mat. Res.*, 1993, 27, 941-48.
5. Li, P.J., and Zhang, F.P. *J. Non-Cryst. Solids*, 1990, 119, 112-18.
6. Zhong, J.P., LaTorre, G.P., and Hench, L.L. *Bioceramics 7*, O.H. Andersson and A. Yli-Urpo eds., Butterworth-Heinemann Ltd, 1994, 61-66.
7. Li, P.J., Ohtsuki, C., Kokubo, T. et al *J. Am. Ceram. Soc.,* 1992, 75 [8], 2094-97.
8. Hench, L.L., LaTorre, G.P., and Donovan, S., et al, SPIE Sol-Gel Optics II Symposium, San Diego, CA, 7, 1992.
9. Hench, L.L., and Nogues, J.L., *Gel-Silica Optics,* L.C. Klein, ed., Kluwer Academic Publishers, Norwell, MA, 1994, 59-81.
10. Dilmore, M.F., Clark, D.E., and Hench, L.L., *Am. Ceram. Soc. Bull.,* 1979, 58 [11], 1111-14.
11. Iler, R.K., *J. Colloid and Interface Sci.,* 1973, 43 [2], 399-408.

APATITE FORMING ABILITY OF SILICATE ION DISSOLVED FROM VARIOUS SILICA GELS

S.B. Cho, F. Miyaji, T. Kokubo, K. Nakanishi, N. Soga and T. Nakamura,*

Division of Material Chemistry, Faculty of Engineering, Kyoto University, Sakyo-ku, Kyoto 606-01 Japan, *Department of Orthopaedic Surgery, Faculty of Medicine, Kyoto University, Sakyo-ku, Kyoto 606-01 Japan

ABSTRACT

A prerequisite for glasses and glass-ceramics to bond to living bone is the formation of biologically active bone-like apatite on their surfaces, and that a hydrated silica on their surfaces plays an important role in nucleating the apatite. In this study, the apatite forming ability of silicate ion dissolved from various silica gels was investigated. Poly-ether sulfone (PESF) substrate, pretreated with O_2 plasma was placed in parallel to a plate of the silica gels or silica glass with a distance of 0.5 mm between them in a simulated body fluid (SBF) with ion concentrations nearly equal to those of human blood plasma for 4 days, and then soaked in a solution with ion concentrations 1.5 times those of SBF for 6 day. The substrates faced with all the silica gels formed a bone-like apatite layer on them, but that faced with the silica glass did not form HA. The presence of silicon was detected on the surfaces of the former substrates after the first treatment by X-ray photoelectron spectroscopy. This indicates that a silicate ion dissolved from the silica gels induces the apatite nucleation on the surface of the substrate, irrespective of the kind of the silica gel.

INTRODUCTION

The prerequisite for glasses and glass-ceramics to bond to living bone is the formation of a layer of biologically active bone-like apatite on their surfaces in the body [1,2]. It has been proposed that hydrated silica which is formed on their surfaces in the body plays an important role in nucleating the apatite [3-5]. Actually, it was shown that even pure silica gel prepared by hydrolysis and polycondensation of tetraethoxysilane in aqueous solution containing polyethylene glycol forms the apatite on its surface in a simulated body fluid with ion concentrations nearly equal to those of human blood plasma [6]. The same gel, however, did not form the apatite when heat-treated above 900°C. Pure silica gels prepared by hydrolysis and polycondensation of the same tetraethoxysilane but in aqueous solution containing no polymer and polyacrylic acid also did not form the apatite [7]. These results indicate that only a limited type of the silanol group can induce the apatite nucleation. On the other hand, Abe et al. suggested that silicate ion dissolved from CaO-SiO_2 based glass into simulated body fluid can induce apatite nucleation on the surface of various substrates [8]. In the present study, the apatite forming ability of silicate ion dissolved from different kinds of silica gels into simulated body fluid was investigated.

EXPERIMENTAL PROCEDURE

Three kinds of pure silica gels, S-W, S-HPAA and S-PEG, were prepared by the hydrolysis and polycondensation of tetraethoxysilane (TEOS) as follow. First, 0.81 g concentrated nitric acid (62 wt%) was added with ion-exchanged distilled water in 8 g, or in aqueous solution containing polyacrylic acid (HPAA) having molecular weight of 30,000 or polyethylene glycol (PEG) having molecular weight of 10,000, respectively. Then 7 ml TEOS was added to the above solutions under vigorous stirring. After stirring for 5 min, the solution was transferred into a plastic petri dish with its top tightly sealed, and was kept at 40°C in air circulating oven for gelation. After it was aged for 18 h, the obtained wet gel was immersed in 1 mol/dm^3 nitric acid for 6 h to wash the gel and dried at 40°C for 6 days. The nitric acid was renewed every 2 h. After the obtained wet gel was dried, it was heated up to 600°C at a rate of 100°C/h for 2 h, then allowed to cool to room temperature.

Rectangular specimens of 10 x 15 x 2 mm^3 in size of the poly-ether sulfone (PESF) substrate was subjected to plasma treatment in O_2 gas for 5 min. The plasma treatment was carried out at a pressure of 30 Pa and 50 mW power, under an electric field of 13.56 MHz by using Plasma Polymerization System (BP-2, SAMCO Ltd., Kyoto, Japan).

The PESF substrate was placed in parallel to a plate of the silica gels described above or silica glass with a distance of 0.5 mm between them in 30 ml of a simulated body fluid (SBF) with ion concentration (Na^+ 142.0, K^+ 5.0, Mg^{2+} 1.5, Ca^{2+} 2.5, Cl^- 147.8, HCO_3^- 4.2, HPO_4^{2-} 1.0, SO_4^{2-} 0.5 mM) nearly equal to those of human blood plasma at 36.5°C and pH 7.4 for 4 days. Then the PESF substrate was successively soaked in 30 ml of a solution (1.5SBF) with an ion concentration 1.5 times those of SBF for 6 day. The 1.5SBF solution was renewed every 2 days.

After the first and second soaking, the PESF substrate was removed from the fluid and washed moderately with distilled water, and dried at room temperature. The surfaces were analyzed by thin-film X-ray diffraction (2651A, Rigaku Co., Tokyo, Japan), X-ray photoelectron spectroscopy (XPS) with an ESCA model MT5500 (ULVAC-PHI Co. Ltd., Chigasaki, Japan) and SEM observation.

RESULTS AND DISCUSSION

Figure 1 shows thin film X-ray diffraction patterns of the surfaces of PESF substrates faced to S-W, S-HPAA and S-PEG silica gels as well as to silica glass in SBF for 4 days. After the first soaking, no structural change was detected by X-ray diffraction on the surfaces of PESF substrates faced to all the kind of the silica materials.

Figure 2 shows XPS Si 2p spectra of the surface of PESF substrate before and after facing to S-PEG in SBF for 4 days. A new peak was observed around the binding energy of 102eV after the reaction. This peak is attributed to Si combined with oxygen atoms [9]. The same peak was also observed on the surfaces of the PESF substrates which were faced to S-W and S-HPAA silica gels, but not on that of PESF faced to the silica glass. This indicates that a silicate ion was dissolved from all the silica gels examined and adsorbed on PESF substrate in SBF. Inductive Coupled Plasma atomic emission spectroscopy showed that all the examined silica gels released about 30 ppm of silicate ion into SBF for 4 days, whereas silica glass released less than 1 ppm.

Figure 3 shows thin film X-ray diffraction patterns of the surfaces of PESF substrates faced to the different silica materials in SBF for 4 days and then successively soaked in 1.5SBF for 6 days. The PESF substrates faced to the silica gels formed a bone-like apatite layer on them irrespective of the kind of the silica gel, but those faced to the silica glass

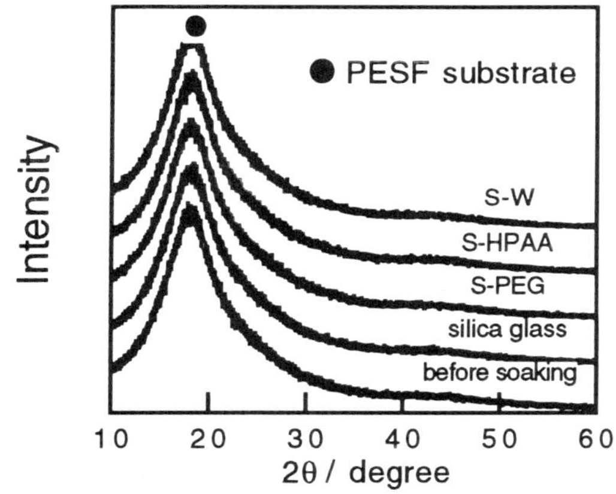

Figure 1. Thin film X-ray diffraction patterns of the surfaces of PESF substrates faced to different silica materials in SBF for 4 days.

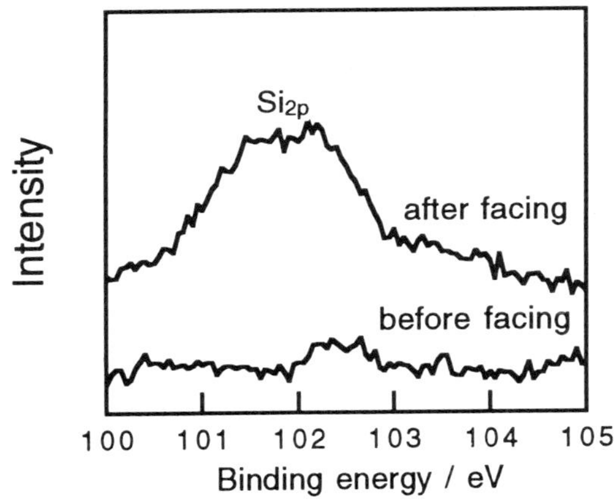

Figure 2. XPS Si_{2p} spectra of the surfaces of PESF substrates before and after facing to S-PEG in SBF for 4 days.

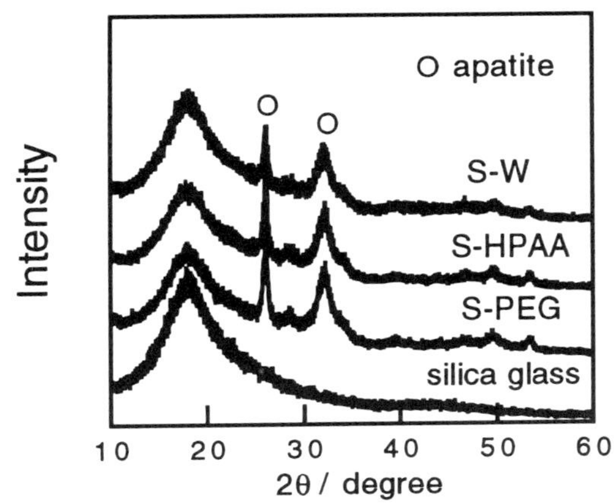

Figure 3. Thin film X-ray diffraction patterns of the surfaces of PESF substrates faced to different silica materials in SBF for 4 days and then successively soaked in 1.5SBF for 6 days.

did not form it. These results clearly show that a silicate ion dissolved from the silica gels can induce the apatite nucleation on the surface of the PESF substrate, irrespective of the kind of the silica gel.

ACKNOWLEDGMENT

This study was supported by a Grant-in Aid for Scientific Research of the Asahi Glass Foundation.

REFERENCES

1. T. Kokubo,Biomaterials, 1991, 12, 155-163.
2. L. L. Hench, J. Am. Ceram. *Soc.,* 1991, 74, 1487-1510.
3. L. L. Hench, In *Bioceramics: Material Characteristics Versus in vivo Behavior,* Annual of New York Academy of Science Vol. 523, New York, 1988, 54-71.
4. K. H. Karlsson, K. Froberg and T. Ringbom, *J. Non-Cryst. Solids,* 1989, 112, 69-72.
5. C. Ohtsuki, T. Kokubo and T. Yamamuro, *J. Non-Cryst. Solids,* 1992, 143,84-92.
6. P. Li, C. Ohtsuki, T. Kokubo, K. Nakanishi, N. Soga, T. Nakamura, T. Yamsmuro, J. Am. Ceram. *Soc.,* 1992, 75, 2094-2097.
7. T. Kokubo, S.B. Cho, K. Nakanishi N. Soga, C. Ohtsuki, T. Kitsugi T. Yamamuro and T. Nakamura, In *Bioceramics* Vol. 7, Butterworth-Heinemann, Finland, 1994, 49-54.
8. M Tanahashi, T. Yao, M. Minoda, T. Miyamoto, T. Nakamura and Yamamuro, J. *Appl. Biomater., 1991,* 74, 1487-1510.
9. C.D. Wagner, W.M. Riggs, L.E Davis, J.F. Moulder, *Handbook of X-ray photoelectron spectroscopy,* Perkin-Elmer Co., 1979, 12-28.

COMPLEXATION OF CALCIUM, MAGNESIUM AND ALUMINUM IONS ON SILICA GEL

Maria F.J. Zevenhoven-Onderwater, Jörgen Rosenqvist[‡], Kaj H. Karlsson

Åbo Akademi University, Laboratory of Inorganic Chemistry, Biskopsgatan 8, FIN 20500 Åbo/Turku, Finland
[‡]Currently at Umeå University, Department of Inorganic Chemistry, Umeå, Sweden

ABSTRACT

Silica gel can be used as a model substrate for bioactive glasses and glass-ceramics. Computer simulations with the Gibbs energy minimisation software SOLGASWATER® show that calcium, magnesium and aluminum ions can be adsorbed on silica gel. Simple adsorption experiments of calcium ions on silica gel confirm the calcium calculations. Adsorption of calcium ions reduces the negative charge of the surface, thus making it more attractive for bonding of anions, such as phosphates. The simulations show that small additions of aluminum and magnesium ions to a system containing calcium ions can inhibit the complexation of calcium to the silica gel by formation of magnesium or aluminum complexes with the surface.

INTRODUCTION

Several bioactive materials such as Bioglass®, Ceravital® and A-W glass ceramics have been developed over the last two decades. All these bioactive materials bond to bone in a similar way by formation of a Ca-P rich layer situated on top of or inside a Si-rich layer. Additions to the glasses such as Al_2O_3, MgO and B_2O_3 have or might have an influence on the bioactivity of the glasses by interaction with the silica rich layer. This paper describes an attempt to study the possible interactions of the ions present in the glass and surrounding body fluid with the Si-rich layer. To simplify the system silica gel is used as a model substrate. Since the complexation of calcium ions is of major importance in bone formation processes this ion is studied in more detail *i.e.* the complexation of Ca^{2+} is modelled by means of SOLGASWATER®, version 1992, and complexation experiments are carried out. Model calculations are also done for mixtures containing Ca^{2+}, Mg^{2+} and Al^{3+} to get an impression of their influence on the bonding of Ca^{2+} to an active surface.

SIMULATIONS WITH SOLGASWATER®

Model calculations of the adsorption of Ca^{2+}, Mg^{2+} and Al^{3+} ions are performed using the extended Gibbs energy minimisation software SOLGASWATER® [1].

Most of the equilibrium constants used were gained from literature [2-7]. They are recalculated for the appropriate ionic strength using the Davies equation [8]. Model calculations show that if a sufficient amount of surface active groups is present calcium complexes can be formed of the type $\equiv SiOCa^+$ or even $(\equiv SiO)_2Ca$, reducing the negative charge of the surface ($\equiv SiO^-$ groups present).

A simulation of the adsorption from a solution containing 1.5 mM Mg^{2+} and 2.5 mM Ca^{2+} as used in Simulated Body Fluid (SBF)[9] is shown in Figure 1. In this simulation a limiting amount of surface active groups, $\equiv SiOH$, is present, resulting in a competition between the formation of calcium and magnesium complexes. In the interesting pH range 6-8 for bone bonding $\equiv SiOCa^+$ and $\equiv SiOMg^+$ complexes are formed. Since magnesium forms stronger complexes than calcium complexes the formation of magnesium complexes will be favored. The formation of calcium complexes is found to shift to a higher pH- value. A simulation of the simultaneous complexation from a solution containing 2.5 mM Ca^{2+} and 0.025 mM Al^{3+} on a silica surface with a limiting amount of surface active groups is shown in Figure 2.

In the pH range 6-8 the formation of aluminum complexes of the type $\equiv SiOAl(OH)_2$ can inhibit the formation of calcium complexes, thus inhibiting the process of bone bonding.

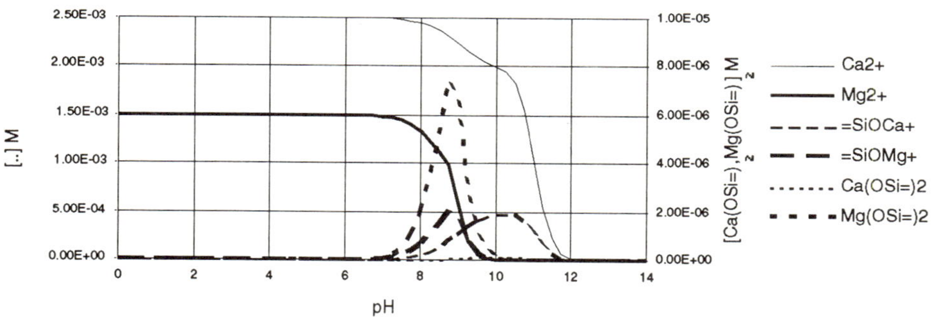

Figure 1. Simultaneous complexation of magnesium and calcium ions on a surface with a limiting amount of surface active groups

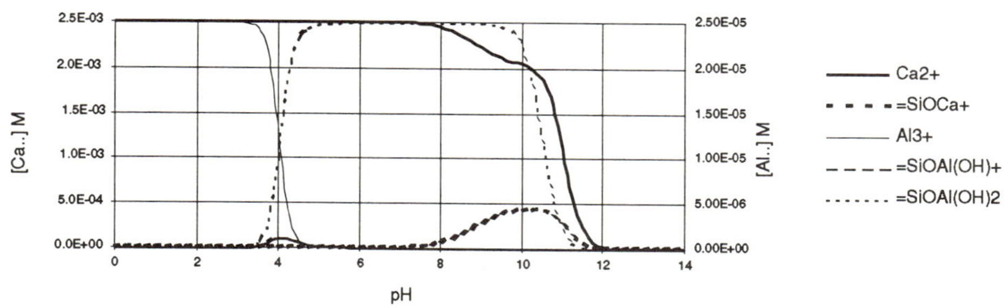

Figure 2. Simultaneous complexation of aluminum and calcium ions on a surface with a limiting amount of surface active groups.

ADSORPTION EXPERIMENTS

Adsorption measurements [10] of calcium ions on a silica gel with a BET surface area of 411 m^2/g are studied at 25 and 37°C in a concentration range of 0-35 mM and a pH range of 5-9. In this pH range the amount of $Ca(OH)_2$ present is negligible. The ion adsorption is established by stirring samples of silica gel in water at different pH values. After equilibrium between gel and solution is reached a çertain amount of $Ca(NO_3)_2$ is added. The change in pH is followed by means of an Orion pH-measurement device. The sorbed quantity of ions is obtained by determination of the ion concentration before and after the adsorption using Direct Current Plasma Emission Spectroscopy (DCP). The ratio between the liquid volume v and the amount of gel m was v/m=0.01 l/g. Data analysis was carried out with a linear regression method giving the ion concentration after the adsorption as a function of temperature, pH and ion concentration before the experiment. The experiments showed no temperature dependency. As the ions are added to the silica gel the pH decreases as a result of the ion exchange reaction:

$$n \equiv SiOH + Ca^{2+} \leftrightarrow (\equiv SiO_n\ Ca^{)2-n)+} + nH \qquad (1)$$

Analysis of the ion concentrations and release of H^+ ions before and after the experiments show that a part of the calcium ions become adsorbed in the above described way. For initial salt concentrations, $[Ca_{before}]$ below 7 mM, the concentration of Ca^{2+} after the experiments, $[Ca^{2+}{}_{after}]$ (mM), can be described mathematically as:

$$[Ca_{after}]=7.0+0.44\ x\ [Ca_{before}]-0.92\ x\ \overline{pH}\ \textit{the regression coefficient}\ R^2=0.87 \qquad (2)$$

Where pH is the negative logarithm calculated from the mean hydroxide concentrations before and after the experiment. For higher concentrations it is found that a mechanism other than described in (1) must be responsible for the adsorption of Ca^{2+} since no dependence on pH, and thus on the amount of surface active groups, could be found:

$$[Ca_{after}]=1.15\ x\ [Ca_{before}]-6.68\ \textit{the regression coefficient}\ R^2=0.92 \qquad (3)$$

Probably the ions are only physically bonded to the surface due to ion attraction. Rewriting the equation for the equilibrium constant for (1) and defining D as:

$$D = \frac{(\equiv SiO)_n\ Ca^{(2-n)+}}{[Ca^{2+}]} \qquad (4)$$

makes it possible to determine the number of active groups involved in the ion exchange reaction, n, from the slope of a log D vs. pH plot. In Figure 3, n is plotted as a function of the initial Ca^{2+} concentration. Figure 3 shows clearly that at a Ca^{2+} concentration of 2.5 mM, as used in SBF, only one surface active group is involved in the complexation reaction, thus leading to a complex of the type $\equiv SiOCa^+$. This is in accordance with the computer simulations as described above.

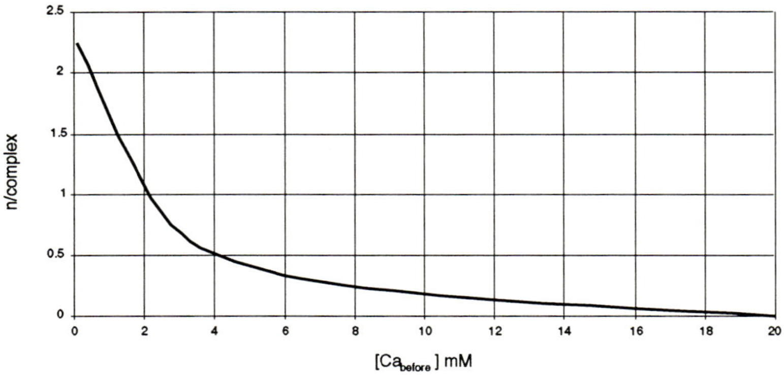

Figure 3. The calculated amount of surface active groups per complex involved in complexation of a calcium ion as a function of the initial calcium concentration.

CONCLUSIONS

This work shows that calcium ions become adsorbed to a silica gel surface. On the gel used in the experiments complexes of the type $\equiv SiOCa^{+}$ are formed when the initial calcium concentration corresponds to the concentration as in SBF. Calculations show that magnesium and aluminum ions can inhibit the formation of calcium complexes by formation of magnesium ($\equiv SiOMg^{+}$) and aluminum ($\equiv SiOAl(OH)_2$) complexes.

The amount of surface active groups present and the complexation strength are found to be the determining factors for the type of complexes to be formed.
The formation of calcium complexes can be seen as a first step in the bone bonding process, by reducing the negative charge of the silica gel, thus making the surface more attractive for complexation of anions such as phosphates.

ACKNOWLEDGEMENT

This work has been carried out with financial support of the Finnish Technology Development Centre, TEKES.

The authors are indebted to Prof. Paul Schindler, Bern University, Switzerland, for providing useful approximations of the equilibrium constants for the calcium and magnesium surface complexes as used in this work.

REFERENCES

1. Eriksson G., *Anal.Chim.Acta* 1979, 112, 375.
2. Sjöberg S., Nordin A., Ingri N., *Mar.Chem* 1981 10, 521.
3. Sjöberg S., Öhman L-O, Ingri N., *Acta Chem. Scand.* 1985, A39, 93.
4. Sjöberg S., Ingri N., Nenner A-M, Öhman L-O, *J.Inorg.Biochem.*1985, 24, 267.
5. Smith R., Martell A.,*Critical Stability Constants*, 4, Plenum Press, New York, 1979.
6. Charlet L., note to be submitted to *J.Coll.Interf. Sci.*.
7. Schindler P., University of Bern, private communication.
8. Davies C., *Ion Association*, Butterworths, London 1962.
9. Kokubo T., Kushitani H., Ohtsuki C., Sakka S., Yamamuro T., *J.Mat.Sci* 1992, 3, 79.
10. Ahrland S., Grenthe J., Noren B., *Acta Chem.Scand.* 1960, 14, 7.

GLASS FOR RADIOTHERAPY OF CANCER PREPARED BY PHOSPHORUS ION IMPLANTATION

M. Kawashita, F. Miyaji, T. Kokubo, G.H. Takaoka* and I. Yamada*

Division of Material Chemistry, Faculty of Engineering, Kyoto University, Sakyo-ku, Kyoto 606-01, Japan; *Ion Beam Engineering Experimental Laboratory, Faculty of Engineering, Kyoto University, Sakyo-ku, Kyoto 606-01, Japan

ABSTRACT

P^+ ions were implanted into a pure silica glass at 50 keV by various doses. The phosphorus was localized only in the regions deeper than 1.2 nm from the surface, giving a maximum concentration at 48.6 nm depth, in a form of phosphorus colloids for a dose of 5 x $10^{16}cm^{-2}$, whereas it was distributed up to the glass surface and a part of it near the surface was oxidized for doses larger than 1 x $10^{17}cm^{-2}$. The glass implanted at a dose of 5 x $10^{16}cm^{-2}$ released little phosphorus and silicon into water at 95°C for 7 d, although those implanted at doses larger than 1 x 10^{17} cm^{-2} released appreciable amounts of both elements. A chemically durable glass containing a large amount of phosphorus is believed to be useful for *in situ* irradiation of cancers, since it can be activated to be a ß-emitter with 14.3 d half-life by neutron bombardment.

INTRODUCTION

Radiotherapy is one of the effective treatments of cancers. External irradiation, however, often causes damage to healthy tissues. It has been reported that glass microspheres of 20 to 30 μm diameter of $40Y_2O_3$-$20Al_2O_3$-$40SiO_2$ (wt%) glass is useful for *in situ* irradiation of cancers [1]. Y-89 in the glass can be activated to a ß-emitter Y-90 with 64.1 h half-life by neutron bombardment. When injected to liver tumors through the hepatic artery, the glass microspheres can give large local irradiation of the short-ranged highly ionizing ß-ray to the tumors with little radiation dose of neighboring organs.

The Y-90, however, may result in substantial decay before the treatment owing to a short half-life of 64.1 h. P-31 with 100% natural abundance similar to Y-89 can be activated to a ß-emitter P-32 with 14.3 d half-life by neutron bombardment. Moreover, the biological effectiveness of P-32 is estimated to be about four times as large as that of Y-90. But highly phosphorus-containing glasses prepared by the conventional melting method are usually less chemically durable.

The authors previously proposed that P^+ ion implantation into a silica glass can be a useful technique for obtaining a chemically durable glass with high P content [2]. The glass implanted at 30 keV, however, released an appreciable amount of the phosphorus and silicon into hot water. In the present study, P^+ ion was implanted into a silica glass at 50 keV by various doses. The state and distribution of the phosphorus implanted, and structural change of the glass due to ion implantation were examined. Chemical durabilities of the glasses implanted with P^+ ion are discussed in terms of their structure.

EXPERIMENTAL

Highly pure silica glass (metallic impurities < 0.5 ppm, OH < 100 ppm) prepared by the vapor-phase axial deposition (SUMIQUARTZ SK-1300, Sumitomo Metal Industries Ltd., Tokyo, Japan) was cut into rectangular specimens 10 mm x 10 mm x 1 mm in size, and annealed at 1100°C for 1 h. The glass was implanted with P^+ ions at 50 keV by various doses 5 X 10^{16} to 1 x 10^{18} cm^{-2}. It is theoretically estimated that phosphorus takes a Gaussian distribution giving the maximum concentration at 48.6 nm in depth in the silica glass under this implantation energy [3]. After the ion implantation, every sample was preserved in a dry nitrogen atmosphere.

The content of the phosphorus implanted into the glasses were measured by Rutherford backscattering spectrometry (RBS) using 2 MeV $^4He^+$ ions with 170° incident angle. The state of phosphorus was investigated by measuring P_{2p} binding energies with an X-ray photoelectron spectroscope (XPS) (MT-5500, ULVAC-PHI Co. Ltd., Chigasaki, Japan), using MgKα X-ray as the source. Surface structures of the glasses were analyzed by a Fourier transform attenuated total reflection FT-IR ATR) spectrometer (System 200 FT-IR, Perkin-Elmer Ltd., Beaconsfield, England) with 45° incident angle.

The glasses implanted with the P^+ ion were soaked in 20 ml of distilled water at 95°C for 7 d in a polypropylene bottle, shaken at a rate of 120 strokes min^{-1} with a stroke length of 3 cm. The concentrations of the phosphorus and silicon released from the glasses were measured by an inductively coupled plasma atomic emission spectrometer (SPS-1500 VR, Seiko Instruments Inc., Tokyo, Japan).

RESULTS AND DISCUSSION

The area of the peak ascribed to the phosphorus on the RBS spectra of the glass implanted with P^+ ion increased with increasing dose of the P^+ ion implanted up to 5 X 10^{17} cm^{-2} and became almost constant for larger doses. This indicates that the amount of the phosphorus implanted into a silica glass is saturated at a dose of about 5 x 10^{17} cm^{-2} under 50 keV.

Figure 1 shows the P_{2p} XPS spectra of silica glasses implanted with P^+ ions by various doses. For a dose of 5 X 10^{16} cm^{-2} ((a)), no peak was observed at the surface, and only one peak ascribed to the elemental phosphorus (130 eV) was observed at regions deeper than 1.2 nm. This glass was colored brown which means that the phosphorus exists as colloids in this glass. For doses larger than 1 x 10^{17} cm^{-2} ((b)-(d)), two peaks, assigned to elemental phosphorus (130 eV) and oxidized phosphorus (134 eV), were observed at the surfaces. With increasing depth, the intensity of the peak ascribed to the elemental phosphorus increased while that ascribed to the oxidized phosphorus decreased. Thus, part of the phosphorus exists in an oxidized state near the surface although most of it exists as colloids in the glasses.

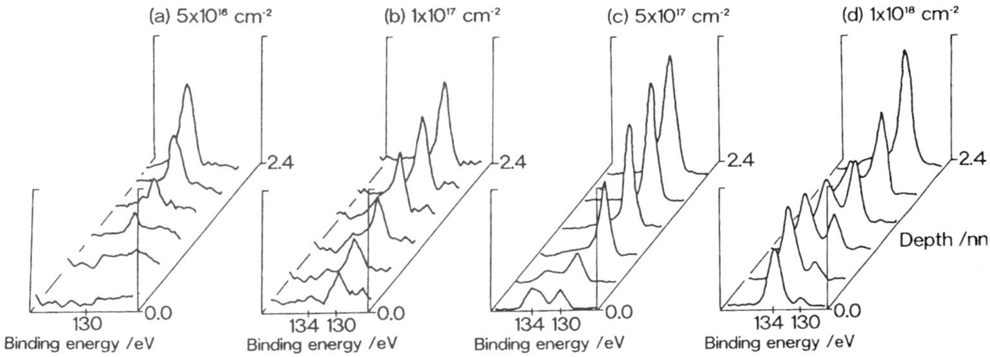

Figure 1. P_{2p} XPS spectra of silica glasses implanted with P^+ ions by various doses.

Figure 2 shows the FT-IR ATR spectra of the glasses implanted with P^+ ion by various doses. The 1150 cm^{-1}-band shifted to the lower wavenumber by the ion implantation. This means that a certain structural damage is produced at glass surfaces by the ion implantation.

Figure 3 shows the concentrations of the phosphorus and silicon released from the glasses implanted with P^+ ions by various doses into water at 95°C for 7 d. The glass as-implanted by a dose of 5 x 10^{16} cm^{-2} dissolved little phosphorus and silicon, whereas those implanted by doses larger than 1 X 10^{17} cm^{-2} released appreciable amounts of both elements. Figure 4 shows the RBS spectra of the silica glass implanted with P^+ ions by a dose of 5 x 10^{16} cm^{-2} before and after soaking in water at 95°C for 7 d. It is confirmed that most of the implanted phosphorus remained in the sample even after soaking.

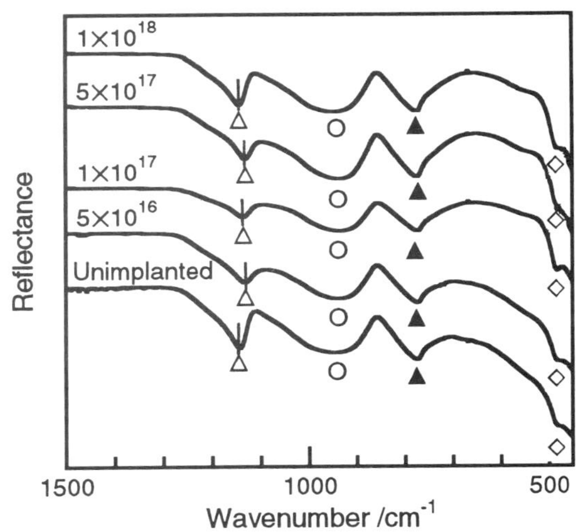

Figure 2. FT-IR ATR spectra of silica glasses implanted with P^+ ions by various doses. Δ: Si-O-Si asymmetric stretching (LO mode), O: Si-O-Si asymmetric stretching (TO mode), ▲: Si-O-Si symmetric stretching, ◇: O-Si-O bending.

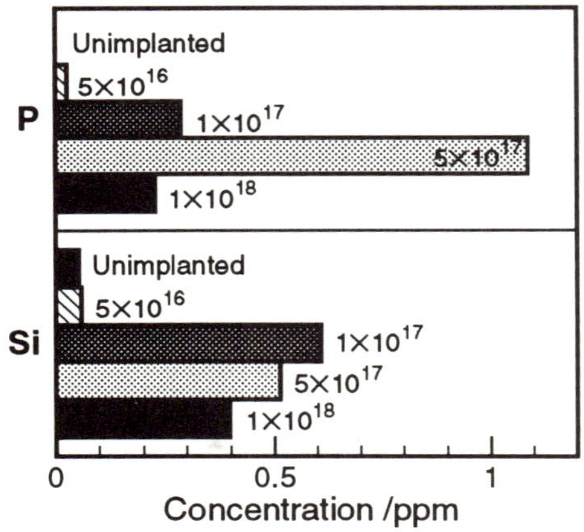

Figure 3. Concentrations of p and Si released from silica glasses implanted with P^+ ions by various doses into water at 95°C for 7 d.

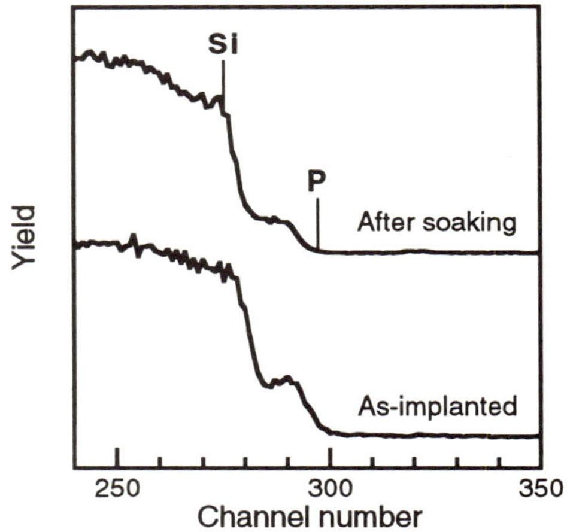

Figure 4. RBS spectrum of silica glass implanted with P^+ ions by 5 x $10^{16}cm^{-2}$ dose and soaked in water at 95°C for 7 d.

These results show that the low chemical durabilities of the glasses implanted by high doses are attributed to the presence of the phosphorus oxide near their surfaces, and that a highly chemically durable glass can be obtained if the phosphorus implanted is localized in its deep region even if the surface structure of the glass is damaged by ion implantation. This indicates that a highly chemically durable silica glass containing larger amounts of the phosphorus could be obtained if the P^+ ion implanted at higher energy. It is believed that the resultant glass might be useful for *in situ* radiotherapy of cancers.

ACKNOWLEDGMENT

We thank Radiation Laboratory of Nuclear Engineering, Kyoto University for RBS measurement.

This work was supported by a Grant-in-Aid for Scientific Research, The Ministry of Education, Science and Culture, Japan (No. 04559005).

REFERENCES

1. Ehrhardt, G.J. and Day, D.E. *Nucl. Med. BioL* 1987, 14, 233-242.
2. Kawashita, M. Yao, T. Miyaji, F. Kokubo, T. Takaoka, G.H. and Yamada, I. In: *Bioceramics* Volume 7, Butterworth-Heinemann, Oxford 1994, 35-40.
3. Wilson, R.G. and Brewer, G.R. In: *Ion Beams with Applications to Ion Implantation* A Wiley-Interscience Publication, New York 1973, 353-377.

STAINING CHARACTERISTICS OF BONE AND BIOACTIVE GLASS FOR MANUAL AND COMPUTERIZED HISTOMORPHOMETRY

JT Heikkila[1], N Beliaev[2], A Yli-Urpo[2], AJ Aho[1]

[1]Department of Surgery, University of Turku, Kiinannyllynkatu 4-8., [2]Turku University, Biomaterials Project, Lemminkäisenkatu 2., 20500 TURKU, FINLAND.

ABSTRACT
The aim of this study was to evaluate bone formation around bioactive glass cones using Toluidine blue, von Kossa and van Gieson staining methods with computerized automatic histomorphometry (CH) and semiautomatic histomorphometry (MH). Bioactive glass cones (BG, S56.5P4) were implanted in rabbit bone. The bone specimens were embedded in methacrylate and undecalcified sections were prepared. The histomorphometry was done using MicroScaleTC software with color detection in PC environment. Toluidine blue was found to be unsuitable for CH because of lack of contrast. Von Kossa stains mineralized tissue and gives good contrast, but stains reaction layer. Significant difference was observed between the measurements using CH and MH ($p. > 0.5$). Van Gieson does not stain the reaction layer of BG and produces a good contrast between bone and soft tissue together with good correlation between CH and MH ($p. > 0.5$). We suggest the use of van Gieson staining method for automatic color-based computerized histomorphometry.

INTRODUCTION
Bioactive glasses are osteoconductive having the capacity to produce bone at their surface. Evaluation of bone forming capacity is necessary when comparing the efficiency of bioactive materials with different compositions with each other. Systematic and unsystematic point classification, direct and semicircular line intersect systems and photographic or projection enlargement methods have been originally used for histomorphometry. All have their drawbacks and a manual digitizer using computer was developed. This was replaced by an automatic image analyser using gray levels. The modern and most reliable way to perform histomorphometry is computerized histomorphometry with color-based image analysing software. This technique is dependent on the staining method and especially the contrast of the tissue component to be measured. We compared three different staining methods and analyse bone formation adjacent to bioactive glass as well as automatic and semiautomatic computerized histomorphometry. For staining we chose a metachromatic glycogen stain (toluidine blue), a mineral stain (von Kossa) and a collagen stain (van Gieson).

MATERIALS AND METHODS

Bioactive glass cones were formed to fit the shape and size of Friolit 4 - O drill. They were manufactured in our laboratory and proven to be bioactive earlier [1,2]. The composition of the glass, in weight percentages, was: 56.5% SiO, 27.0% Na_2O, 12.0% CaO, 4.0% P_2O_5 and 0.5% Al_2O_3. Three cones were implanted with orthopaedic asepsis using a press fit technique in the distal femur subchondral weight bearing bone of adult New Zealand White Star rabbits [3]. The bone blocks were embedded in methacrylate and sectioned into two halves along the mid axis. Using a cutting-and-grinding technique described [4], 20 microns thick undecalcified sections were prepared. The sections were first stained with Toluidine blue, this was washed away and restaining performed with van Gieson method. The other sections were stained using von Kossa method [5] (Fig. 1.). The histomorphometric measurement was performed using MicroScaleTC (Digithurst Ltd., UK), a PC-based color image analysis system. The software operates in Windows™ (Microsoft, USA) environment. MicroScaleTC digitizes video signal under transputer control from light microscopy (Leitz Weitzlar, Germany) and stores a 24-bit data block in its video memory. Additionally 4 bits are used to hold graphic overlays. The resulting image, which consists of 28 bits per pixel is displayed on a separate image monitor (NEC

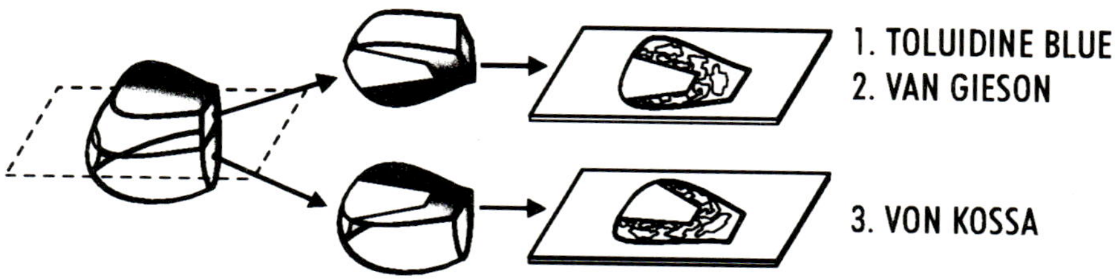

Figure 1. Schematic drawing of the sectioning of specimen.

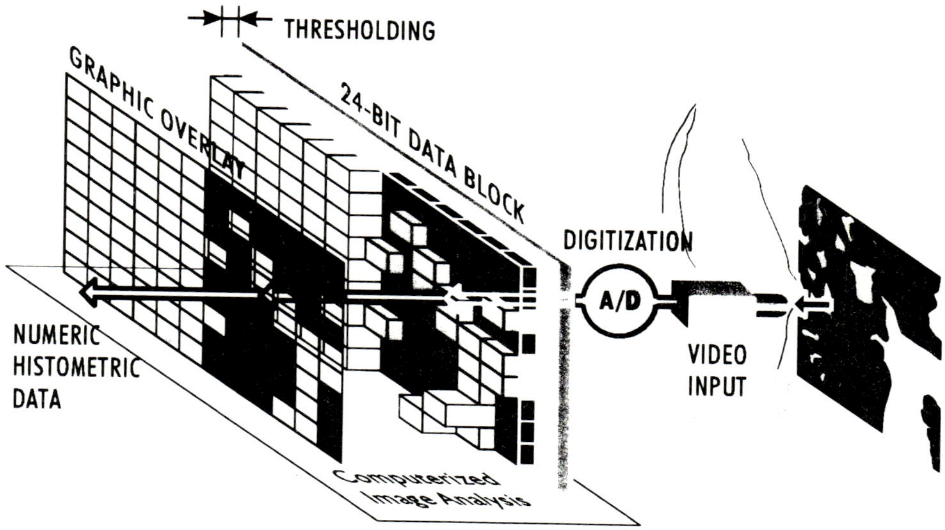

Figure 2. The image is digitized and thresholded into a graphic overlay and numeric histometric data.

Multisync 3D, Japan). It is necessary to adjust the threshold to make the graphic overlay match the original tissue component to be measured. This adjustment can be made by in putting numbers or by obtaining them directly as samples from the image monitor. The graphic overlay is transferred into quantitative data, which is saved in ASCII form. This data can be reorganised later using an Excel (Microsoft, USA) spreadsheet program (Fig. 2). Sta l istical analysis was made with analysis of variance and covariance with repeated measures using BMDP statistical software (BMDP Statistica l Software, Inc., USA) [5].

RESULTS

Toludine blue (Tb) stains acid polysaccharidesmetachromaticallyblue. Bone is stained light blue, but also the reaction layer is stained blue. Tb gives insufficient contrast between the different tissue components and bioactive glass. The graphic overlay achieved with color-based analysis is apparently not representative (Fig. 3A and B). In the Von Kossa method the Ca^{2+}-ions are replaced byAg^{2}-ions, which are turned black when exposed to light. Bone is stained black or dark brown, however reaction layer is stained black or dark brown. Contrast to soft tissue is good The reproducibility of MH results with CH is however not significant (p. >0.5). (Fig. 4A and B). Van Gieson method stains collagen types I and III red. The contrast between bone and soft tissues is good. However, collagen III in scar tissue disturbs the measurement of bone collagen I. The reproducibility of MH results with CH is good, significance p. <0.005. (Fig. 5A and B).

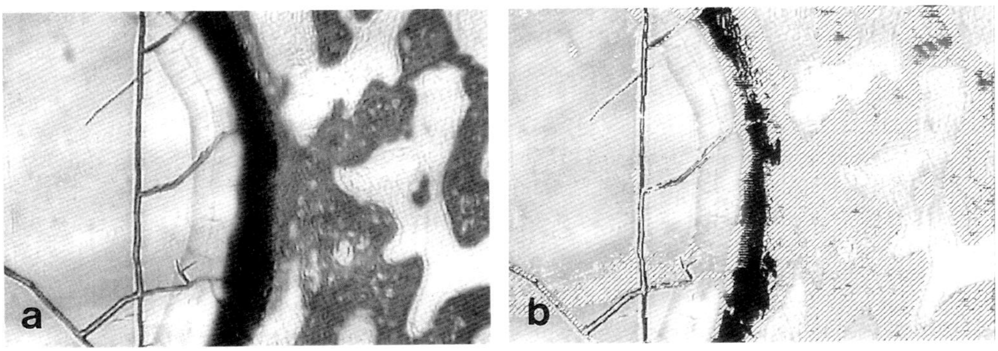

Figure 3A and B. Toluidine blue stain.

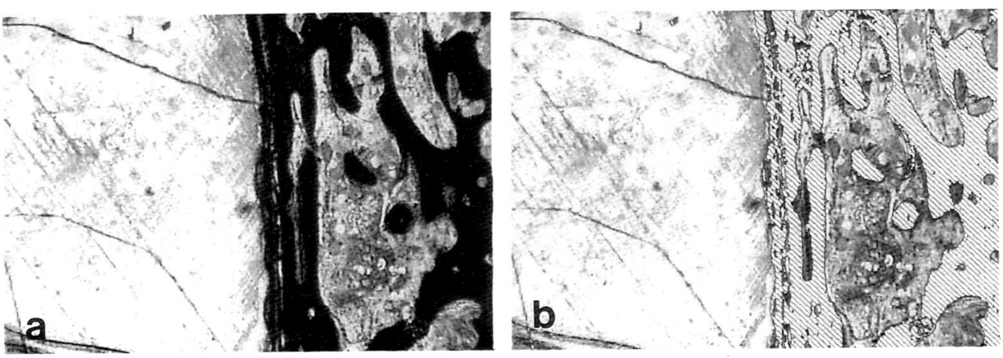

Figure 4A and B. Von Kossa stain.

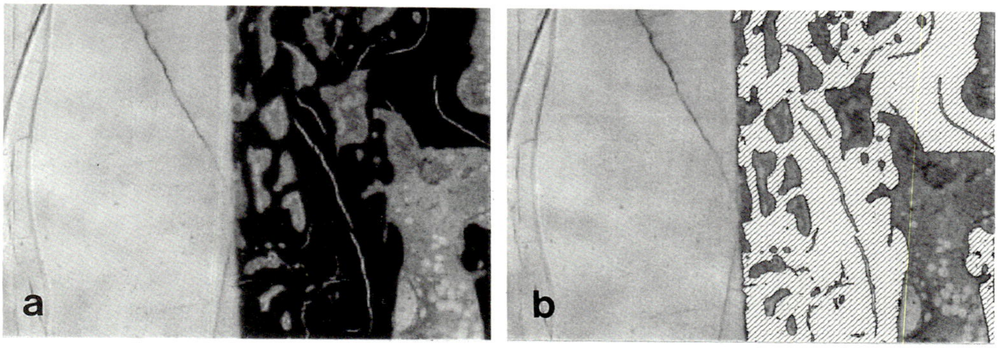

Figure 5A and B. Van Gieson stain.

Figures 3,4 and 5 display the original histologic image (A) and the resulting graphic overlay seen as hatched area. Bioactive glass on the left and new bone on the right side of each figure.

DISCUSSION

For reliable computerized automatic histomorphometry, it is necessary to use a staining method producing good contrast between the tissue to be measured and the other tissue components. The staining characteristics of the implant are also important in this respect.

Toluidine blue has previously been used for undecalcified sections embedded in methacrylate [6] and has also been used for manual histomorphometry [7,8]. It is a good staining method for histological evaluation of tissues and cells, but it produces insufficient contrast between the different tissue components, especially bone together with bioactive glass. It can well be used for manual histomorphometry, but it is a worthless staining method for CH. Von Kossa is an old staining method [9] widely used in bone histology and histomorphometry. With regard to bioactive glass it has the disadvantage of staining the part of reaction layer containing calcium phosphate. Because of this it is sometimes difficult to assess the real border of a CaP- layer and where newly formed bone starts to appear. This is the reason for the poor reproducability of MH with CH. The Van Gieson staining method was first described in 1906 [10]. As a collagen stain it stains only the biological component of the section, leaving the reaction layer unstained. It has the disadvantage to stain both collagen I and III, type I is typical for bone and type III for fibrous tissue. When measuring press fit implants, fibrous tissue formation is not a problem and does not intervene with the measurements. When analysing defects filled with bioactive glass granules this problem can be solved differently to what is presented here.

We suggest the use of van Gieson for automatic color-based computerized histomorphometry.

REFERENCES

1. Andersson ÖH, Karlsson KH. Int J Glass Sci and Techn 1988; 61, 300-5.
2. Andersson ÖH, Liu G, Karlsson KH, Niemi L, Miettinen J. Juhanoja J. J. Mater Sci, Mater Medicine 1990; 1:219-27.
3. Heikkilä JT, Aho AJ, Aho HJ, Yli-Urpo A, Happonen RP. Acta Orth Scand 1993;64:678-82.
4. Donath K, Breuner G., J Oral Pathol 1982;11:318-26.
5. Bancroft JD, Stevens A (Eds.): Theory and paractice of Histological Techniques. 2nd Edition. Churchill Livingstone, Edinburgh, London, Melbourne and New York, 1982.
6. BMDP statistical software manual. Los Angeles, USA, 1990, 489-492.
7. Aho AJ, Heikkilä JT, Aho HJ, Andersson ÖH, Yli-Urpo A., Ann Chir Gyn 1993;82:145-53.
8. Kossa von J. Beitr Path Anat 1904;29:163-202.
9. Gieson van I. New York Med J 1889; 50:57.

MULTILAYER COATING OF STAINLESS STEEL WITH INSOLUBLE AND BIOACTIVE GLASSES "*IN VITRO*" AND "*IN VIVO*" TESTS

J. Cavalheiro, R. Branco, A. Afonso and M. Vasconcelos

INEB - Instituto de Engenharia Biomedica, Pr.Coronel Pacheco 1 - 4050 Porto-Portugal

ABSTRACT

The use of bioactive coatings on metallic orthopaedic and dental prosthesis has proved to be useful for increasing osteointegration. The objective of this work was to produce a bioactive coating with good adhesion on AISI 316L stainless steel, avoiding open porosity and the possibility of contact between metal and body fluids. When the healing process is slow to cover the surface of implants, very active glasses are rapidly dissolved exposing the metal surface. To avoid this problem and adjust the difference of thermal expansion between the active glass and metal, a silica-aluminous intermediate layer of an insoluble glass was applied using a sintering technique. The active glass was sintered on this glass layer. The structure of the coating is free from open porosity. Oxidation of the substrate metal allows for chemical reaction and strong adhesion is promoted.

Solubility of P and Al in the intermediate layer of glass was evaluated through the cross section of the coating by SEM/EDS, and the interface between the silica-aluminous glass and bioactive glass was studied. Mechanical properties were determined using standard bend tests, the coatings began to crack at 460 MPa. Immersion tests showed that the intermediate layer was insoluble. The surface released Ca, Na and K.

"*In vivo*" tests were performed using pins implanted in the rabbit tibia, using uncoated samples as controls. Histological cuts of coated stainless steel pins were compared to uncoated control ones. An improved osteointegration was achieved with new bone growing in close contact with the bioactive surface of the implants. With this coating technique its possible to obtain a strong and active coating, and protect the metallic implant from interfacial attack.

MATERIALS AND METHODS

Using a sintering technique described elsewhere [1], a multilayer coating of stainless steel samples of AISI 316L was prepared. Two coatings were applied on the surface of the steel samples, based on the following glass system: SiO_2, Al_2O_3, Na_2O, CaO and K_2O.

A third layer of a bioactive glass whose composition was (% w/w) CaO 46.6, P_2O_5-14.2, MgO 4.7, Na_2O 3.3, CaF21.2 SiO_2(R) was applied on the surface of the previously coated materials.

Mechanical properties of this coating were evaluated in a three point flexural test (ASTM B 528), using rectangular 30 x 10 mm coated sheets.

Microanalyses by EDS was used to control the thickness of the diffusion layer of Al and P joining the metal and the first layer of glass.

Rectangular samples of 30 x 10 mm, one side coated, were used to perform degradation tests. Samples were immersed in 50 cc of DI water for 6, 12 and 24 hours at constant temperature - 37¼C - with continuous stirring. Atomic absorption was used to measure the concentration of Ca, Na and K in solution. Two groups of six Huila adult rabbits, with the same age were used for *in vivo* tests. Cylindrical pins, 2, 0 mm of diameter and 5 mm of length, were implanted in the tibiae of rabbits under sterile conditions. As control, an uncoated pin was implanted. X-ray observation was made to check the position of the implants. The animals were sacrificed after 1 and 3 months and the implants were excised with surrounding bone, fixed in alcohol and embedded in resin. Micro-slices with a thickness of about 50-90 μm were prepared using a diamond saw. The sections were stained with hematoxylin-eosin.

RESULTS AND DISCUSSION

In Figure 1a the surface of the coating is shown. An almost continuous layer of bioactive glass shows some roughness. This roughness can be modified by the duration and temperature of the coating procedure. In Figure 1b a perpendicular cut to the surface shows a completely closed porosity and good adherence between metal and glass. Electrical conductivity tests, carried out beforehand in samples with identical structure, show complete insulation between the metal and surface [2].

In Figure 2 is represented the change of composition of Al (from the binding layer), and P(from the bioactive glass), in a narrow layer of about 4 μm. Diffusion of the two glasses can be detected providing adhesion between the two materials.

As the thickness of the last layer, bioactive glass, is about 110 μm, almost all of the surface material keeps its original composition. This result agrees with those obtained from the surface composition: the chemical composition is the same as the bulk bioactive glass before coating.

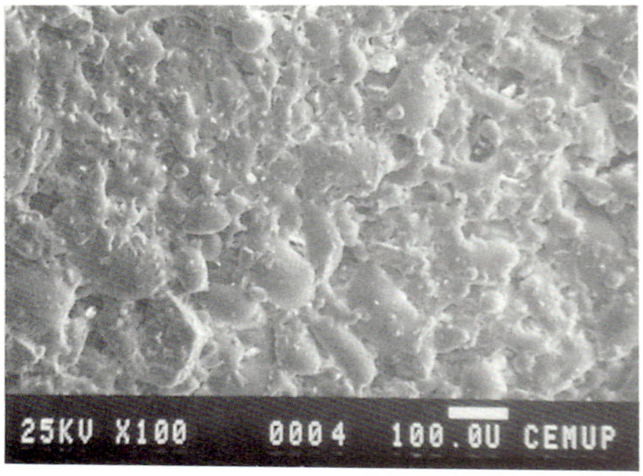

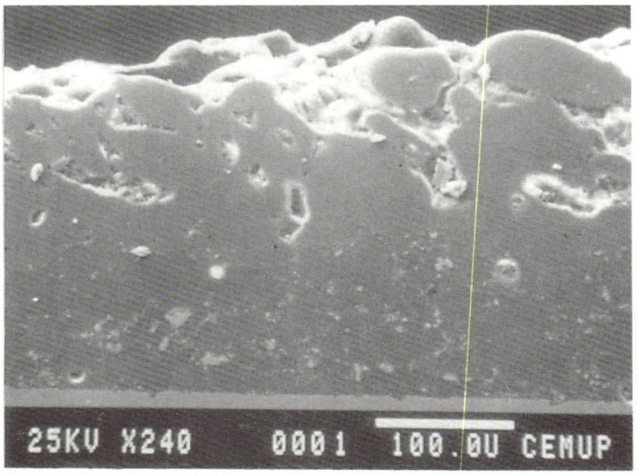

Figure 1a. Surface of bioactive glass coating. 1b. Cut of the coating B - Bioactive glass; G - Binding glass; M - Metal (316-S.S.)

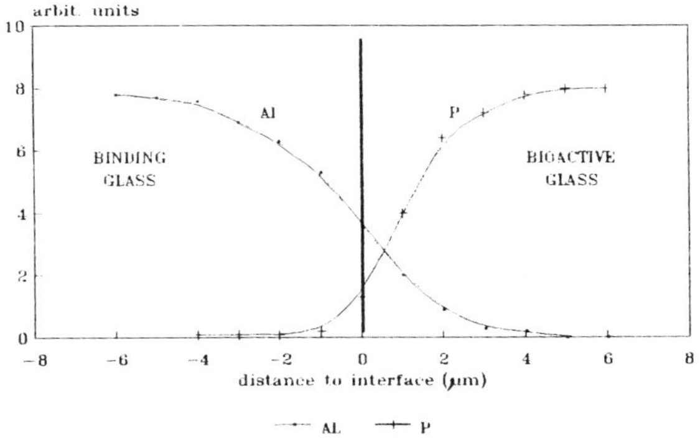

Figure 2. Interface glass/bioactive glass: diffusion of Al and P.

Mechanical tests showed that cracks on the surface of the material begins to appear with stresses of 460 MPa (average of 5 samples). Comparing these results to the interfacial stresses calculated for dental implants [3], the resistance achieved seems to be large enough for practical applications.

The ionic release of Na, Ca and K was measured (ppm in water) after samples immersion during 6, 12 and 24 hours. On this short term results (Table 1), the degradation rate is constant, and the concentration of Ca changes linearly with log, of time. Similar tests of the silica-aluminous layer not show detectable ionic release.

Observation with SEM back scattered electron image of samples immersed during 12 h in water shows an external layer of degradation, of about 4 μm, where the structure becomes porous and the chemical composition is different from the remaining material.

The graph of Figure 3 shows the effect of this ionic release on the surface of samples after 24 h of immersion, the concentration of P, Na, K and Ca decreased meaningfully. The surface concentration of SiO_2 and MgO, increase proportionally with time. Other degradation tests carried out from 24 h to 92 h proved that there was a change in the ionic release rate of Ca, Na and K after 24 h. Formation of thick layer of SiO_2 prevents release of other ions, and degradation proceeds with a decreasing rate.

The biological response to coated pins can be observed in Figure 4a compared to the uncoated stainless steel in Figure 4b. After 1 month of implantation in the rabbit tibia, the uncoated metallic surface (Fig. 4b) is covered with a thin layer of fibrous tissue (see arrows). The coated pin (Fig. 4a) is in close contact with the surface of the new bone. Three months later, this new bone will be well organized, growing directly on the implant surfaces.

Table 1. Ion concentration after degradation test.

	6h	12h	24h
Na	1.3	1.5	1.7
Ca	3.7	4.2	4.8
K	0.2	-	0.3

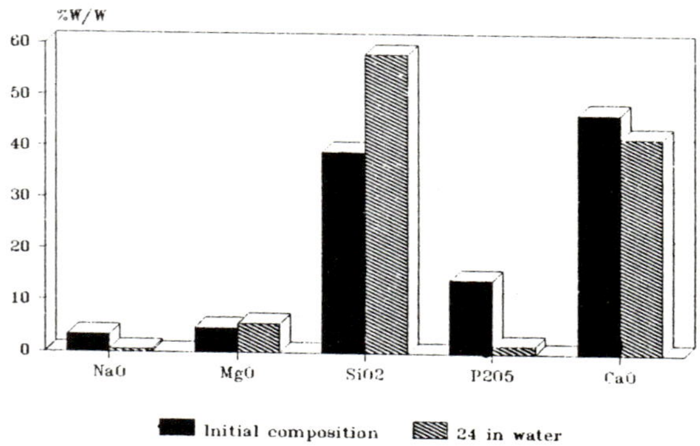

Figure 3. Bioactive glass degradation.

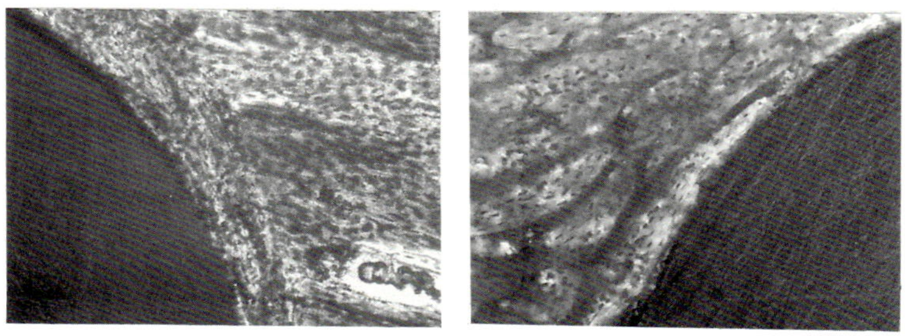

Figure 4a. Implanted coated pin one month after implantation. 4b-Uncoated, same time.

CONCLUSIONS

The coating technique and the materials used in this work produce an almost continuous layer of bioactive glass on the stainless steel. The intermediate layer of insoluble glass provides a barrier against the direct contact of fluids with metal, if for some reason the bioactive coating degrade before bone apposition. The coating process only changes the composition of the bioactive glass coating to a layer of about 4µm; the remaining bioactive glass did not change its original composition during processing. Flexural strength of 460 MPa seems to be enough for implant applications. Degradation tests show an important release of P, Ca, and K, mainly during the first hours. These results indicate that this process of coating can be considered promising for preparation of implants for orthopaedic or dental applications.

REFERENCES

1. Cavalheiro J., Branco R., Proc. of 1st Europ. Conf. on Biomedical Engin., Nice, France, 1991, 287-288.
2. Cavalheiro J., Ribeiro C., Branco R., Surf. and Coatings Technology 1991, 45, 209-213.
3. Ogino M., Fugino M., Oral Imp. and Biomat, Elsevier Science Publ., Amsterdam 1989, 139-144.

AUTHOR INDEX

Index of Authors

KEYWORD INDEX

Index of Keywords